Mental Illness and Substance Use Disorders

Mental Illness and Substance Use Disorders

Editor: Emma Russell

AMERICAN
MEDICAL PUBLISHERS
www.americanmedicalpublishers.com

AMERICAN
MEDICAL PUBLISHERS
www.americanmedicalpublishers.com

Cataloging-in-Publication Data

Mental illness and substance use disorders / edited by Emma Russell.
p. cm.
Includes bibliographical references and index.
ISBN 979-8-88740-261-1
1. Mental illness. 2. Substance abuse. 3. Mental illness--Diagnosis. 4. Mental illness--Treatment.
5. Substance abuse--Diagnosis. 6. Substance abuse--Treatment. 7. Psychology, Pathological. 8. Psychiatry.
I. Russell, Emma.
RC469 .M463 2023
616.890 75--dc23

American Medical Publishers,
41 Flatbush Avenue,
1st Floor, New York,
NY 11217, USA

ISBN 979-8-88740-261-1 (Hardback)

Contents

Preface ... IX

Chapter 1 **"...and How are the Kids?" Psychoeducation for Adult Patients with Depressive and/or Anxiety Disorders** ... 1
Marieke R. Potijk, Louisa M. Drost, Petra J. Havinga, Catharina A. Hartman and Robert A. Schoevers

Chapter 2 **Mental Health Literacy of Youth that have a Family Member with a Mental Illness: Outcomes from a New Program and Scale** ... 10
Joanne Riebschleger, Shane Costello, Daniel L. Cavanaugh and Christine Grové

Chapter 3 **Psychoeducational Intervention for Perinatal Depression** ... 20
Luca Steardo Jr., Vito Caivano, Gaia Sampogna, Arcangelo Di Cerbo, Giovanna Fico, Francesca Zinno, Valeria Del Vecchio, Vincenzo Giallonardo, Marco Torella, Mario Luciano and Andrea Fiorillo

Chapter 4 **Collective Impact on Prevention: Let's Talk about Children Service Model and Decrease in Referrals to Child Protection Services** ... 31
Mika Niemelä, Hannu Kallunki, Jaana Jokinen, Sami Räsänen, Birkitta Ala-Aho, Helinä Hakko, Tiina Ristikari and Tytti Solantaus

Chapter 5 **Improving Identification and Child-Focused Collaborative Care for Children of Parents with a Mental Illness** ... 36
Hanna Christiansen, Annette Bauer, Batool Fatima, Melinda Goodyear, Ingunn Olea Lund, Ingrid Zechmeister-Koss and Jean Lillian Paul

Chapter 6 **Developing an Intervention to Improve the Health Related Quality of Life in Children and Young People with Serious Parental Mental Illness** ... 49
Judith Gellatly, Penny Bee, Adekeye Kolade, Diane Hunter, Lina Gega, Craig Callender, Holly Hope and Kathryn M. Abel

Chapter 7 **Promotion of Wellbeing for Children of Parents with Mental Illness: A Model Protocol for Research and Intervention** ... 61
Charlotte Reedtz, Karin van Doesum, Giulia Signorini, Camilla Lauritzen, Therese van Amelsvoort, Floor van Santvoort, Allan H. Young, Philippe Conus, Richard Musil, Thomas Schulze, Michael Berk, Argyris Stringaris, Geneviève Piché and Giovanni de Girolamo

Chapter 8 **Adult Mental Health Outpatients Who have Minor Children: Prevalence of Parents, Referrals of their Children and Patient Characteristics** ... 71
Torleif Ruud, Darryl Maybery, Andrea Reupert, Bente Weimand, Kim Foster, Anne Grant, Bjørg Eva Skogøy and Solveig O. Ose

Chapter 9 **Children of Mentally Ill Parents at Risk Evaluation (COMPARE): Design and Methods of a Randomized Controlled Multicenter Study—Part I** ... 85
Hanna Christiansen, Corinna Reck, Anna-Lena Zietlow, Kathleen Otto, Ricarda Steinmayr, Linda Wirthwein, Sarah Weigelt, Rudolf Stark, David D. Ebert, Claudia Buntrock, Johannes Krisam, Christina Klose, Meinhard Kieser and Christina Schwenck

Chapter 10 **COMPARE Family (Children of Mentally Ill Parents at Risk Evaluation): A Study Protocol for a Preventive Intervention for Children of Mentally Ill Parents (Triple P, Evidence-Based Program that Enhances Parenting Skills, in Addition to Gold-Standard CBT with the Mentally Ill Parent) in a Multicenter RCT—Part II** ... 97
Markus Stracke, Kristin Gilbert, Meinhard Kieser, Christina Klose, Johannes Krisam, David D. Ebert, Claudia Buntrock and Hanna Christiansen

Chapter 11 **Protective Factors for Early Psychotic Phenomena among Children of Mothers with Psychosis** ... 111
Simon Riches, Louise Arseneault, Raha Bagher-Niakan, Manar Alsultan, Eloise Crush and Helen L. Fisher

Chapter 12 **Using Social Networking Sites in Research: An Emerging Approach to Engaging with Young People Who have a Parent with a Mental Illness and/or Substance Abuse Disorder** ... 121
Christine Grové

Chapter 13 **Identification of Children of Parents with Mental Illness: A Necessity to Provide Relevant Support** ... 129
Charlotte Reedtz, Camilla Lauritzen, Ylva V. Stover, Janita L. Freili and Kamilla Rognmo

Chapter 14 **Mothers with Postpartum Psychiatric Disorders: Proposal for an Adapted Method to Assess Maternal Sensitivity in Interaction with the Child** ... 143
Christine Heinisch, Mirijam-Griseldis Galeris, Sandra Gabler, Susanne Simen, Juliane Junge-Hoffmeister, Judith Fößel and Gottfried Spangler

Chapter 15 **Prenatal Alcohol Exposure and Child Psychosocial Behavior: A Sibling Fixed-Effects Analysis** ... 158
Kayoko Ichikawa, Takeo Fujiwara and Ichiro Kawachi

Chapter 16 **The Danish High Risk and Resilience Study—VIA 11: Study Protocol for the First Follow-Up of the VIA 7 Cohort −522 Children Born to Parents with Schizophrenia Spectrum Disorders or Bipolar Disorder and Controls being Re-Examined for the First Time at Age 11** ... 166
Anne A. E. Thorup, Nicoline Hemager, Anne Søndergaard, Maja Gregersen, Åsa Kremer Prøsch, Mette F. Krantz, Julie M. Brandt, Line Carmichael, Marianne Melau, Ditte V. Ellersgaard, Birgitte K. Burton, Aja N. Greve, Md Jamal Uddin, Jessica Ohland, Ayna B. Nejad, Line K. Johnsen, Anna Hester Ver Loren van Themaat, Anna K. Andreassen, Lotte Vedum, Christina B. Knudsen, Henriette Stadsgaard, Jens Richardt M. Jepsen, Hartwig Roman Siebner, Leif Østergaard, Vibeke F. Bliksted, Kerstin J. Plessen, Ole Mors and Merete Nordentoft

Chapter 17 **Prenatal Depression and its Associated Risk Factors Among Pregnant Women in Bangalore: A Hospital Based Prevalence Study....182**
B. Sheeba, Anita Nath, Chandra S. Metgud, Murali Krishna, Shubhashree Venkatesh, J. Vindhya and Gudlavalleti Venkata Satyanarayana Murthy

Chapter 18 **Key Informants Specify Core Elements of Peer Supports for Parents with Serious Mental Illness....191**
Joanne Nicholson and Anne Valentine

Chapter 19 **Identity in Personal Recovery for Mothers with a Mental Illness....200**
Rochelle Helena Hine, Darryl John Maybery and Melinda Jane Goodyear

Chapter 20 **Overcoming Clinician and Parent Ambivalence: General Practitioners' Support of Children of Parents with Physical or Mental Illness and/or Substance Abuse....212**
Marit Hafting, Frøydis Gullbrå, Norman Anderssen, Guri Rørtveit, Tone Smith-Sivertsen and Karin van Doesum

Permissions

List of Contributors

Index

Preface

Mental illness refers to a behavioral pattern which causes difficulty or impairment in personal functioning, which can occur as single, remitting or persistent episodes. There are various types of mental illnesses, which include mood disorder, psychotic disorder, personality disorder, eating disorder, sleep disorder, substance use disorder, developmental disorder and anxiety disorder. Substance use disorder (SUD) is a type of mental illness, characterized by continued use of drugs and alcohol despite significant harm and negative effects. They are associated with a variety of behavioral, mental, emotional and physical problems, including chronic guilt, physiological withdrawal symptoms and an inability to decrease or quit consuming the substances despite recurrent attempts. There are various categories of drugs with which a person can be involved, such as tobacco, opioids, phencyclidine, hypnotics, cannabis, inhalants, and stimulants. This book explores all the important aspects of mental illness and substance use disorders in the present day scenario. It presents researches and studies performed by experts across the globe. Those in search of information to further their knowledge will be greatly assisted by this book.

This book unites the global concepts and researches in an organized manner for a comprehensive understanding of the subject. It is a ripe text for all researchers, students, scientists or anyone else who is interested in acquiring a better knowledge of this dynamic field.

I extend my sincere thanks to the contributors for such eloquent research chapters. Finally, I thank my family for being a source of support and help.

Editor

1

"...and How are the Kids?" Psychoeducation for Adult Patients with Depressive and/or Anxiety Disorders

Marieke R. Potijk, Louisa M. Drost*, Petra J. Havinga, Catharina A. Hartman and Robert A. Schoevers

University Center for Psychiatry, University Medical Center Groningen, Groningen, Netherlands

***Correspondence:**
Louisa M. Drost
l.m.drost@umcg.nl

Depressive and anxiety disorders are highly prevalent and form a substantial burden for individuals and their family members. A recent study showed that approximately two-thirds of the children of patients with severe depressive and/or anxiety disorders develop one of these disorders themselves before 35 years of age. In the Netherlands, various preventive interventions are available for children of parents with mental illnesses. However, the actual reach of interventions is small (<1% of all children participate). A major barrier appeared to be parents' hesitancy to let children participate in preventive programs. In order to address this barrier, we designed a pilot study to implement a psychoeducation program on parenting and mental illnesses. The main aim of this study was to investigate how a preventive family-focused approach can be embedded in routine adult psychiatric care. The pilot started in April 2017 and has ended in September 2018. It was conducted in the University Center Psychiatry (UCP) in Groningen, The Netherlands. This article describes the implementation process so far. The main intervention was a monthly organized group-psychoeducation called "parenting and a mental illness," which could be attended by parents currently treated in the UCP. In 18 months, implementation activities were divided in four phases; (1) Creating awareness, (2) Adoption of the intervention, (3) Implementation and evaluation, and (4) Continuation phase. The program development process was evaluated using both qualitative and quantitative data. Based on the pilot study we were able to make recommendations for the further implementation of this approach so that more parents can be reached in future. Further study with follow-up activities is needed to measure the effects of the psychoeducation, for instance on parenting functioning and the quality of the parent-child interaction.

Keywords: anxiety, depression, implementation, parental support, child wellbeing, prevention

INTRODUCTION

Up to 45% of patients who receive adult psychiatric care are parents (1). Having a parent with a mental illness greatly affects children's wellbeing. Approximately two-thirds of the children of patients with severe depressive and/or anxiety disorders develop such a disorder themselves before their 35th year, and half of them even before their 20th year (2). These children form an important target group for prevention (3).

In the Netherlands, various interventions for prevention of mental health problems in offspring of depressive and anxious adults have been developed. Current interventions are aiming at the parents (psycho-education and parenting skills), the children (psycho-education, coping skills, mutual support), or the family as a whole (group sessions, online support) (4, 5).

However, the vast majority of children and parents does not receive the services they require (6). Regarding the Dutch preventive interventions aiming at the offspring of parents with a mental illness, no more than 1% of children take part (4, 7). The primary challenge, therefore, is to increase the reach of the preventive interventions for parents and children.

A first and crucial step in increasing the range of participants in preventive interventions is to get the offspring in the picture. A substantial group of these high-risk children can easily be detected; namely through the parent being treated. van Doesum et al. (8) found that mental health agencies are the most common source of referrals to preventive programs for offspring of parents with a mental illness. Moreover, screening on the presence of children in adult psychiatric care has already been improved in several countries. In Norway health legislation was altered in 2010, making it mandatory to assess whether or not psychiatric patients have children (9). In the Netherlands, it has been obliged to register the number of minor children of adult psychiatric patients, since 2017.

However, Skogøy et al. (10) underline that legal changes are helpful, but not sufficient to secure equal chances of protection and support for children of parents with mental illnesses. Research has indicated that both parents and professionals experience several barriers to be involved in prevention. Barriers of parents include: perceived lack of necessity for intervention, overburden, reluctance to bother their offspring, concern for shame and stigma, and practical problems such as lack of transport facilities (8, 11–13)

Professionals may perceive talking about parenthood with their patients as a sensitive topic (8, 14–16). Furthermore, between disciplines differences may exist in the ease with which professionals talk about parenting and wellbeing of the children. Findings of Maybery et al. (17) suggest that social workers feel more comfortable with talking about these family issues than nurses working in adult psychiatric care. Foster et al. (18) however, argue that nurses in mental health care are in prime positions to support parents who are patients. These authors proposed a framework for family-focused actions that psychiatric nurses can carry out at different phases of client care, such as providing age-appropriate information on mental illness to children and facilitating parental attachment with offspring. Furthermore, based on consultation with a group of senior clinical leaders in adult mental health services in Australia, Goodyear et al. (19) introduced essential and explicit practice standards for mental health nurses working with families. These efforts illustrate a growing knowledge base of what should be implemented into adult health care to serve patients who are parents and their children. However, papers on program development that investigate how knowledge can be successfully translated into clinical practice are scarce.

AIM OF THE CURRENT STUDY

The main aim of this pilot study was to investigate how a preventive family-focused approach can be embedded in routine adult psychiatric care. This aim resulted in the following research questions:

1) How can a preventive family-focused approach be made feasible and acceptable, for parents and professionals?
2) Which remedies can be identified in order to increase feasibility and acceptability?
3) Which recommendations can be given to further implement this approach?

METHODS

Design

We designed a pilot study to implement a preventive, family-focused approach for adult patients treated for depressive and/or anxiety disorders. We tried to build on existing routines so that changes were kept as small as possible. In the University Center Psychiatry (UCP) a psychoeducation program for parents already existed for a few years, but the program was not offered on a structured base, i.e., at maximum three to four times a year, at different times and dependent on the number of parents staying in the inpatient ward. A social worker of the inpatient ward coordinated these sessions and any other actions for patients regarding their children. Also, she led a special working group of professionals. Nurses were used to refer to this social worker, who invited parents to talk about the impact of parents' illness and to help explain the situation to children, on an age appropriate level.

In a four-phase implementation plan, we worked toward a situation in which all professionals mention patient's role as a parent at least once during routine treatment, and motivate parents to attend the group-psychoeducation "parenting and a mental illness" which was now offered monthly. Since it is known that parents may perceive different kinds of barriers to participate in preventive interventions, we listed common barriers and made a plan to address them in this pilot study (**Table 1**).

The medical ethical committee of the University Medical Center Groningen evaluated this study as not falling under the Medical Research Involving Human Subjects Act (WMO). Nevertheless, we followed the required procedures and obtained written informed consent for the qualitative components of the project. No written informed consent was requested for participation in a psychoeducation meeting because this option was offered as part of the treatment. Patients knew that their own therapist would be informed of their participation. Collection of participant information was kept to a minimum and reported at group level, such as the number of participants who joined the psychoeducation. In (online) registration the current privacy legislation was followed and only the necessary information was requested, such as an e-mail address confirming the registration, and the age category of the children to adjust the psycho-education on that particular evening.

TABLE 1 | Overview of the implementation process.

Barriers	Initial approach	Feasibility	Acceptability	Adjustment	Recommendations
Perceived lack of necessity to talk about parenthood and mental health	Creating awareness by providing information about the project e.g., flyers, newsletter, survey of professionals' attitudes	Overload of professionals	Professionals' view that talking about parenthood is important but does not belong to their core tasks Patients do not mention the subject spontaneously when the professional skips it	Involve management to make talking about parenthood part of the department policy Informative, normalizing online video (infographic) to increase awareness and acceptability Website with possibility for parents to sign up for a psycho-educative session themselves	Consideration of appointing an attention officer for patients' offspring Involvement of management needed to ensure that every patient who is a parent receives information about mental health and parenting Improvement of ICT facilities in electronic patient files, for e.g., a button "parenthood" and a treatment plan on parenting and child wellbeing
Reluctance to bother offspring; unfamiliarity with possibilities for prevention	Professionals should make the parent understand the importance of information for children.	Parents need support how to talk about their illness with their children	Parents' anxiety to loose custody	Relation building with parents, empathy for being reluctant while emphasizing the importance of information Peer exchange of parents' experiences; Information about further referral possibilities	Collaboration with other disciplines (public health, gp's) to continue and improve support for families
Feelings of shame and guilt ("being a bad parent")	Normalization of the attention for patients' children and their parenting roles	It appeared difficult for professionals to apply a family focused approach (which is broader than child safety procedures)	Different opinions among professionals regarding their task; who can best deal with family matters of patients and when?	Project leader attends the team meetings of all participating wards to discuss how this "child-aware" approach could best be implemented into work processes in their ward	Training of professionals how to introduce and talk about parenting with patients
Overload of the parent	Make professionals mention the topic at least once during therapy Refer to existing 2-h session of psycho-education	Acute phases of decompensation may ask for alternative ways and/or moments to raise the topic Group sessions can only take place with sufficient participation	Patients' feedback: timing is important when to talk about parenting	If there are reservations regarding the timing of mentioning parenthood, the timing will be discussed in the team meeting Psycho-education sessions are offered on a structural base to improve feasibility	Create guidelines how and when to talk about parenting and when to refer parents to the psychoeducation meeting Discussing parenthood should be adjusted to patient's condition (but will not be skipped) Automatic notifications in electronic patient file to reconsider action of practitioners at a later moment
It appeared difficult for professionals not to focus mainly on child safety procedures	Training for professionals	Due to an overcrowded training schedule, the training is postponed	Professionals differed in opinion about who could best deal with family matters of patients	Project leader attends the team meetings of all participating wards to discuss how this "child-aware" approach could best be implemented into the work processes in their ward	Postponed training will be scheduled Recommendation to document the working procedures for this point in each department

Participants

The target group consisted of adult patients who are parents of children in the age range of zero till 24 and who are currently being treated for depressive and/or anxiety disorders in an outpatient or inpatient ward. Patients will be informed by their own practitioner (psychologist, psychiatrist, psychology/psychiatry resident, or nurse practitioner), social workers, and/or nurses of the inpatient wards. The participating wards are one outpatient ward and two inpatient wards for patients with depressive disorders, 2 day-clinics for depressive disorders, one outpatient ward for bipolar disorders, an outpatient ward for anxiety disorders, and a day-clinic for anxiety disorders. Since the UCP is a tertiary care center, symptom severity of most patients is moderate to very severe.

In 1 year about 1,200 adult patients with depressive and/or anxiety disorders are treated in the UCP. It has been estimated that 30–50% of these patients have children. Systematically, information on the parent status of a patient is gathered when patients enter the UCP to receive care, via a general questionnaire. In this way practitioners know by forehand (a) whether the new patient is a parent, (b) how many children he or she has, and (c) what the age of the children is.

Primary Intervention: A Preventive, Family-Focused Approach

We performed this pilot to investigate the possibilities to permanently embed a preventive, family-focused approach in routine treatment protocols. In concrete terms, this meant that:

1. Practitioners and/or nurses mention patient's role as a parent at least once during routine treatment, and motivate parents to attend the group-psychoeducation "parenting and a mental illness."
2. Psychoeducation meetings for patient-parents are offered on a regular base.
3. We examined possibilities to permanently embed the preventive, family-focused approach in the organization and management structures.

Psychoeducation "Parenting and a Mental Illness"

We organized a monthly group-psychoeducation, on every first Thursday evening of the month, called "parenting and a mental illness." An experienced social worker of the inpatient ward for depressive disorders of the UCP and a child psychologist gave the psychoeducation, using a power point presentation. Project leader MP (resident psychiatry) coordinated applications for the evenings and was available to stand in when one of the group leaders was hindered to give the psychoeducation. Patients attended one meeting and were encouraged to bring their partners. The psychoeducation could only be attended by parents currently treated in the UCP. The content of the psychoeducation was theory-based and consisted of the following main items:

(a) Patients introduce themselves shortly (name, family situation, the current treatment status), followed by an introduction to the theme parenting and a mental illness. In particular, attention is paid to illness perception and the relation with the patient's role as a parent, before and during treatment. Group leaders pay attention to feelings of guilt or shame that may be present regarding shortcomings in the parenting role. Furthermore, the role of the other parent is a topic of conversation.
(b) How do parents tell their children about mental illness? This starts as an open conversation in which parents share their experiences. Later, group leaders give a summary and provide examples of how to talk with children about their mental illness, using age-appropriate information. Group leaders may notice barriers in talking with their children among parents, for example not wanting to bother their children and bring up these subjects.
(c) How do parents know when it is (not) going well with their children? Do they have worries about their children's wellbeing? For each age category, the group leaders provide information on signals of (ab)normal development. Sharing of experiences among parents is encouraged.

Additionally, at the end of the psychoeducation meeting further supportive options were offered to the parents, such as continued conversations about parenting with their current practitioner, or other professionals (e.g., the general practitioner, a social worker). If necessary, referral of the child for child psychiatric consultation was offered.

We estimated that 68 parents would have attended the group-psychoeducation after 1 year, based on data that about 1,200 patients with a depressive and/or anxiety disorder are treated in the UCP in a year. About 480 of the patients have children (40%) and we estimated that 336 parents could be motivated by practitioners to join the psychoeducation, with an eventual reach of 20% of the motivated parents.

Implementation Procedure

The pilot study started in April 2017 and was planned to end at the end of September 2018. In this time span of 18 months, implementation activities were divided in four phases; (1) Creating awareness, (2) Adoption of the intervention, (3) Implementation and evaluation (following an iterative process), and (4) Continuation phase. We described intended activities in these four phases in our implementation plan that we wrote prior to the start of the project. The implementation plan, including the four phases, was based on a workbook for guideline implementation in youth help and protection services (20).

Phase 1: Creating Awareness Among Parents and Professionals (April–October 2017)

During the first months of the project, we spread information about the project via various ways. In April we announced the project in the general newsletter of the UCP. During the next months, the project leader (MP) attended the regular team meetings of all participating wards, to discuss with colleagues how the family-focused approach could be embedded in their ward. In addition, these meetings served to spread flyers with practical information about the project and to present a flow chart of general procedures regarding children of patients and child safety. At the launch of the actual implementation (September 2017), more information on the project was given in a presentation for all professionals and researchers in the UCP. We stressed that the primary aim of the project was to pay more attention to patients' normal role as a parent, for example by asking how parents manage to perform this role now they are being treated for a mental illness. Existing child safety procedures were mentioned, but were not the main focus of the project.

Finally, we created awareness for the importance of implementing a preventive, family-focused approach. For both parents and professionals, we developed an infographic film of 3 min illustrating the impact on the family when one of the parents has a mental illness. This infographic was placed on the project website https://kopp.umcg.nl that we had developed in this first phase of the implementation. The launch of the project (including the infographic) was also spread as a local news item by the press agency of the UMCG, among others via Facebook. On the project website, more information was provided regarding the monthly group-psychoeducation on parenting and a mental illness. Recently, the infographic was translated to an English version which can be found via the following link https://www.youtube.com/watch?v=mZbsXjh2hYM.

Phase 2: Adoption of the Intervention (September–December 2017)

This phase predominantly focused on activities that promoted the adoption of the intervention, such as creating awareness and support of various groups, including the management.

First, via a survey among professionals of the department mood and anxiety disorders, we inventoried general practices regarding the attention for patients' role as a parent in routine treatment protocols. This raised awareness among participants and gave us an impression of the current state of preventive, family-focused care at the department. Second, in order to gain broad support for the project, we organized participation meetings with the client counsel, social workers, residents, the secretaries, and managers of the department. About once in 3 months, we wrote an update of the implementation process to publish in the UCP newsletter.

Phase 3: Implementation and Evaluation (September 2017–August 2018)

From September 2017 on it was possible to sign up for the group-psychoeducation sessions. Both parents themselves and practitioners were able to sign up, online via the project website, via an email or via a registration form on paper. The first psychoeducation session took place on the first Thursday in October 2017. After the start of the psychoeducation sessions, we constantly adjusted the original implementation plan to the actual situation in clinical practice, using an iterative approach. Feedback of parents and practitioners was essential during this phase. For example, after introducing the pilot project, the importance of the topic "parenting and a mental illness" was endorsed by many professionals. However, some of them indicated that they had not enough time to discuss parenting in the treatment sessions within the scheduled time. To solve this problem, we suggested that they could use the infographic film of 3 min to introduce the topic and refer parents to the group-psychoeducation. Another example of a change in the initial plan was prompted by the observed difference in working methods at the various wards. By attending team meetings of the wards, we explored together with the professionals how the family-focused approach could best fit the current working methods in their opinion. Furthermore, parents were asked to fill out a feedback form after attending a meeting (**Supplement 1**) and some of them were asked for a telephone interview. This information was used to help to define barriers and remedies (**Table 1**).

Parallel to the implementation of the family-focused approach, the experiences of nurses with talking about parenting were investigated by students of the School of Nursing (University of Applied sciences). They performed two qualitative research projects, in which nurses were interviewed both individually and in focus groups (which included other professionals). For the interviews, topic lists on the theme parenting were used. With respect to the aim of this study, we do not extensively report on the nursing projects in this article. However, these projects may have contributed to increased awareness of parenting and continued positive reinforcement. In general, nurses were highly motivated to participate in the interviews and brought up some interesting topics, such as task ambivalence. On the one hand they felt family-focused care as one of their core responsibilities, but on the other hand, many nurses found it unclear when and how specific tasks should be performed and by which professional.

Phase 4: Continuation (September–December 2018)

The main goals of this final phase of the implementation were (a) to create support and guidance for the intervention in the organization and management structures, (b) to realize professional guidance on the work floor and/or training, and (c) to make arrangements with management and stakeholders for continuation of the project. To date, we have taken the following steps. First, we have developed the parental questionnaire "parenting and a mental illness," involving questions on experiences of patients' role as a parent and wellbeing of the children (**Supplement 2**). The reason for developing this questionnaire was to ease conversations about parenting between parents and practitioners or nurses. It is now available for use as part of the routine outcome measurements (ROM) of the department. Patients who have started a treatment automatically receive an email with an invitation to fill out the parental questionnaire (online). When the questionnaire is completed, the practitioner of the patient can see the answers in the electronic patient file. In this way, we expect that practitioners will have a better view of the family situation, e.g., how patients perceive their parenting role, which may ease family-focused conversations with the patient. Evaluation of the use and effectiveness of the questionnaire will take place at a later stage. Second, to meet the wish of professionals who indicated they needed more practical support, we set up a targeted training. However, eventually, we decided not to schedule the training since it was not considered realistic in a year in which two new electronic patient registration systems were introduced.

Therefore, training programs have been designated as a future priority. Lastly, we asked the management and stakeholders to express the intention to continue the family-focused approach as part of routine treatment protocols. This has already resulted in initiatives such as including information on mental illness and parenthood in the training program of psychiatry residents.

Analysis

The implementation was evaluated using both quantitative and qualitative data. The quantitative part consisted of a survey among professionals of the department of mood and anxiety disorders and registration of the number of participants at the monthly group-psychoeducation meetings. The online survey (**Supplement 3**) was created using the program Survey Monkey and was accessible for the professionals via an email that was sent by the secretaries. We asked ten multiple choice questions which were determined through discussions in the project group (MP, LD, PH, CH, RS). MP analyzed the outcomes of the survey, which are documented in a word file (anonymous). Registration of the actual number of participants was done by social worker HH, who was present at all but one psychoeducation meetings, and further processed in an SPSS file by MP. All data were checked and verified by at least two researchers (mostly by MP and LD).

The qualitative part consisted of written evaluation forms of the psychoeducation meetings (filled out by parents) and semi-structured telephone interviews with some of the parents who participated in a psychoeducation meeting. Questions asked were for example: "What was the most positive of the evening and what are you least satisfied with?" and "Do you have any suggestions for us to improve this psycho-education?"

Lastly, we reflected on the barriers that we had listed, whether and how we addressed them and which remedies were found (**Table 1**).

RESULTS

Survey

In September 2017, at the launch of the implementation, we performed a survey among professionals of the department of mood and anxiety disorders. All professionals received an email with a link to the online survey which consisted of ten multiple choice questions about the general way of practice regarding family-focused care. Thirty-two professionals filled out the survey in a time span of 6 weeks. Most of them were nurses (13/32), followed by psychologists (7/32) and other professionals, such as creative therapists (5/21). Furthermore, three psychiatrists and four residents in psychiatry filled out the survey. Respondents were about equally spread among the different wards of the department of mood and anxiety disorders; professionals from the inpatient wards (12), the day-clinic wards (11), and the outpatient wards (13) were represented. Some professionals worked at more than one ward. Nineteen of the 32 respondents (59.4%) answered that they mostly or always mention parenthood when they talk to patients who have children in the age of 0–24 years. The other 13 respondents answered they do not mention the topic regularly. Regarding the timing for bringing up the topic, most respondents thought the beginning of treatment (until the third meeting with the parent) is most suitable. Although most professionals said to talk about parenting and/or child wellbeing, they indicate a need for further education or skills training in their current work. Eleven professionals want to have more general information on mental illness and parenthood; for example on the actual risk that children will develop problems if their parents have a mental illness. Furthermore, 19 professionals indicate that they miss practical information, such as to which organization they can refer parents and/or children if they signal any problems. Finally, skills training in conducting conversations about parenting and child wellbeing is wanted, as indicated by 11 professionals.

Psychoeducation "Parenting and a Mental Illness"

In **Table 2** we show the number of parents that participated in the psychoeducation meetings. The number of participants varied per meeting. In the meeting of June, the highest number of parents participated, i.e., 12 parents (**Table 2**). In July only one person applied, probably that was due to the summer holidays. Most patients came with their partner or, in exception, with another family member. Twelve patients came alone. After December 2017, when we had launched the online possibility for registration, the majority of the participants applied via this way. In total 64 parents participated in the psychoeducation meetings, which was lower than the estimated number of 68 at the start of the study. Regarding the age of the children that were reached via psychoeducation, we are only able to provide a rough estimate in age groups. Most parents that applied for a psychoeducation meeting had one or more children in the age ranges of 4–11 (at least 18 children) and 12–17 (at least 14 children). Fewer parents had one or more children in the age ranges of 0–3 (at least 9 children) and 18+ (at least 4 children). For 6 participants data were missing regarding the age of the children.

At the end of the psychoeducation meetings, we asked participants to fill out an evaluation form in which we asked whether parents regarded the meeting as useful and which needs they had regarding parenting and wellbeing of the children. Twenty-five participants filled out the evaluation form. All regarded the meeting as useful. Most of them further commented on this question, as shown in **Table 3**. Of the 25 participants, 12 regarded the information of the meeting as sufficient, 2 expressed the need for further information, 3 preferred to talk about parenting more frequently with a nurse of the ward, 6 would like to go to a social worker or therapist, and 2 had other preferences for further support. One patient who preferred to talk about parenting with a nurse said: "It keeps me bothering whether the situation at home is good, whether it is safe enough, comfortable, and also a bit "normal." A parent expressing other preferences wished for: "The possibility for our children to talk with someone."

In addition, we interviewed four participants by telephone after they had attended a group-psychoeducation session. The participants who were interviewed concerned one woman who had been treated for depression and her husband and two

TABLE 2 | Number of parents* participating in the psychoeducation meetings.

Date	Number of participants	Way of application			
	(Actual/ applied)	Via practitioner	Written form	Online form	e-mail or other
2017/10/05	8/10	2	2	NA	4
2017/11/17	4/4	.	.	NA	3
2017/12/17	4/6	0	0	4	2
2018/01/04	2/3#	0	0	3	0
2018/02/01	4/6	0	4	2	0
2018/03/01	8/8	.	.	5	1
2018/04/05	6/6	.	.	5	.
2018/05/03	4/4	0	0	4	0
2018/06/07	12/12	4	0	8	0
2018/07/05	1/1#	0	0	1	0
2018/08/02	9/9	4	1	4	0
2018/09/06	2/4	0	0	4	0
Total	**64/73**	**10**	**7**	**38**	**10**

**in most cases the other parent came along with the patient; in a few cases a grant parent or other family member was present.* #*individual appointment via social worker instead of the regular group psychoeducation.*

TABLE 3 | Reactions of parents who attended a psychoeducation meeting.

Question: what did you find useful of this meeting?
"It was nice to share our experiences with other parents"
"It was a relief to know that many things are going well in the way we approach the children regarding my illness"
"It gave me insights in the possible impact of my illness on the children, and that early signaling is important to prevent that they will have problems"
"The importance to keep in touch with our children"
"Some things I recognized, other things are not applicable to our family"
"It was confronting (we recognized the impact of my illness on our son), and we now have more knowledge than before this meeting"
"Now we know that we need to talk about it with the children"

women who were partners of patients in care. Beforehand they all consented to be interviewed about their experiences. All four were positive about the organization and contents of the evening. Exchange of experiences was mostly appreciated, although sometimes confrontational, for example when it appeared that other participants had received more familial support than the respondent. The timing (to offer this intervention during hospitalization) was seen as very important. Recommendations on which words to use to explain about the mental illness to their children were appreciated. One of the respondents suggested that this meeting should be mandatory for all patients with children.

Barriers and Remedies

Table 1 shows how the implementation process changed during the course of the project. The initial implementation plan was based on the barriers for parents to talk about their parenting we knew from the literature. With the help of the logbook, it was recorded which parts of the plan were feasible and acceptable and which were not (found barriers). Solutions were sought and found in consultation with those involved. Successful adjustments to the implementation procedure (remedies) were, for instance, the introduction of the online infographic, the discussions in the team meetings, involving the management, and the website with possibility for parents to sign in for a psycho-education session themselves. At the end of the project an overview could be made of the recommendations we deemed necessary for a successful continuation of the implementation, such as improvement of ICT facilities and the scheduling of the training that was postponed.

DISCUSSION

In this pilot study, we have described the development of a program to implement a preventive family-focused approach into routine care for adult patients who are parents and treated for moderate to severe depressive and/or anxiety disorders. The focus was on feasibility and acceptability. Most professionals expressed their sympathy to the project. Our survey showed that professionals consider it as important to inform patients who are parents about the possible impact of mental illness on parenting (nearly 60% of professionals already talked about parenthood and child wellbeing with their patients at the start of the implementation). The other 40% did not mention the topic frequently, and the need for additional training (education and/or skills) was indicated by a majority of professionals.

Team discussions revealed that opinions differed between disciplines whether talking about parenthood was part of their job. At wards where a social worker was part of the team, patients were preferably referred to the social worker for further consultation. However, the option of referral to a social worker is not present at all wards of the UCP. It gradually became clear that the family-focused approach fitted very well with the core business of nurses. First of all, the survey was filled out by nurses for 41% (13/32). This fits with literature on this topic, which shows that nurses are in a unique position to initiate conversations on parenthood and child wellbeing because of their direct, frequent, and sustained contact with patients and families (18). Nevertheless, family-focused care should not be reserved for specialized professionals. Small talk about normal life (events), including parenting, can, for example, be initiated by a secretary who can also hand over a leaflet with information about targeted psychoeducation. Furthermore, therapists of all kinds can stress that mental illness may have impact on parenting and that they, therefore, want to pay attention to it during therapy sessions. Management support and professional education in a positive organizational culture (13) are conditions to realize a therapeutic climate where support of patients who are parents becomes a normal part of treatment. This can benefit both parents and children (21).

As Foster and Isobel (14) have pointed out, talking about parenting involves special capacities. In our survey, 11 out of 32 professionals expressed their interest in training opportunities to address parenting and child wellbeing in conversations with patients. Other respondents mentioned (and perhaps rightly so) that they had enough conversation techniques to be capable to discuss parenthood. Interviews and case discussions during the team meetings provided more insight into the emerging dilemmas of professionals, such as the idea of having to choose between the good of the parent and that of the child (22). Reupert et al. (13) warn that professionals, including social workers and nurses, seem to avoid such dilemmas by arguing that talking about parenthood can harm the confidentiality of the relation between professional and patient. They also hold a plea to be creative in finding a solution when there is the conviction that these conversations are necessary.

The monthly organized psychoeducation meetings for parents were visited by 64 parents in 1 year. By far most of them (38) applied via the online registration form on the project website. Parents' reactions after the psychoeducational meetings were mainly positive, and they provided useful feedback to further improve the meetings. A good timing of the psychoeducation, for instance, was deemed indispensable. Parents' reactions were discussed in the team meetings by the project leader and once more colleagues were asked to draw their patients' attention (on time) to the educational evenings. This illustrates that the implementation of a preventive approach is not achieved after one or two actions, but requires continuous positive reinforcement (23).

The number of parents participating in the monthly psychoeducation meetings was variable. More professionals started to refer parents, but the most visible increase in registrations was in the number of parents who applied directly via the website. This may indicate that the psychoeducation meets the needs of, at least a subset of parents treated in the UCP, which also corresponds with the positive feedback of parents who had joined a psychoeducation meeting: all regarded the meeting as useful, and about half of the parents would like further support. Furthermore, feedback and interviews indicated that awareness among parents about the impact of the mental illness on child wellbeing has grown. We think that for e.g., better provision of information about the preventive offer may have facilitated parents to be more aware and to participate in the psychoeducation. Furthermore, the easy way of registration may also explain the higher number of online applications, or the fact that the involvement of a (busy) professional can be avoided.

A limitation of our research is that it was carried out in a specific setting under specific circumstances. It is unlikely that the same circumstances are present in any other organization for adult care, which could result in different outcomes. On the other hand, a strength of this pilot is that we were able to demonstrate how an iterative implementation method can be used to realize a translation from current knowledge to clinical practice. Further prospective studies with a control group are needed to assess whether preventive psychoeducation, as part of a family-focused approach, is effective. Findings of this pilot study provide useful information for setting up larger studies with a higher impact. Our aim is to continue the psychoeducation program in the UCP and to further develop it, using the outcomes of this pilot study. Regarding policy, we strive to offer more parents the possibility to attend the psychoeducation meeting on parenting and a mental illness at the UCP, for example by sharing our knowledge with other health care providers and governmental organizations.

In conclusion, our findings indicate that our preventive family-focused intervention met the needs of parents that participated in the psychoeducation meetings. Feedback of participants showed that they regarded the evening as useful, and more importantly, they seemed to be more aware of the potential impact of their illness on their children. However, a large number of parents were still not reached by our intervention and further study with follow-up activities are needed to measure the effects of psychoeducation on, for example, parenting, the quality of the parent-child interaction and child wellbeing. Lastly, we regard the structural embedment of interventions and continued positive reinforcement as essential elements for long-lasting attention for the prevention of mental health problems among children of parents that are treated for mental health disorders.

AUTHOR CONTRIBUTIONS

MP, LD, and PH set up the project, conducted the pilot study, and wrote the manuscript. CH supervised methodology, RS supervised it all.

ACKNOWLEDGMENTS

This project was financed by a grant of the Healthy Ageing Committee of the University Medical Center Groningen, The Netherlands. We would like to thank Henriëtte Hoving, social worker, and Dorien Rump, child psychologist, for their effort in giving the psychoeducation sessions and their expert comments on the study.

REFERENCES

1. Reupert A, Maybery D. The number of parents who are patients attending adult psychiatric services. *Curr Opin Psychiatry* (2018) 31:358–62. doi: 10.1097/YCO.0000000000000427
2. Havinga PJ, Boschloo L, Bloemen AJ, Nauta MH, de Vries SO, Penninx BW, et al. Doomed for disorder? High incidence of mood and anxiety disorders in offspring of depressed and anxious patients: a prospective cohort study. *J Clin Psychiatry* (2017) 78:e8–17. doi: 10.4088/JCP.15m09936
3. Hosman CMH, van Doesum KTM, van Santvoort F. Prevention of emotional problems and psychiatric risks in children of parents with a mental illness in the Netherlands: I. the scientific basis to a comprehensive approach. *Adv Mental Health* (2009) 8:250–63. doi: 10.5172/jamh.8.3.250

4. Dijkstra M. *Aard en Omvang GGZ-Preventie 2011 [Nature and Scope of Mental Health Prevention 2011]*, Utrecht: Trimbosinstituut (2012).
5. Goossens FX, Van der Zanden AP. *Factsheet KOPP/KVO [Prevention Factsheet: Children of Mentally Ill and Addicted Parents]*, Utrecht: Trimbosinstituut (2012).
6. Charles G, Reupert A, Maybery D. Families where a parent has a mental illness. *Child Youth Services* (2016) 37:95–7. doi: 10.1080/0145935X.2016.1104032
7. Romijn G, Graaf IM, de Jonge M. *Kwetsbare Kinderen: Literatuurstudie Over Verhoogde Risicogroepen Onder Kinderen van Ouders met Psychische of Verslavingsproblemen [Vulnerable Children: Review on High Risk Groups Among Children of Parents With Mental Illness or Addiction Problems]*. Utrecht: Trimbos-Instituut (2010).
8. Van Doesum KT, Riebschleger J, Carroll J, Grové C, Lauritzen C, Mordoch E, et al. Successful recruitment strategies for prevention programs targeting children of parents with mental health challenges: an international study. *Child Youth Serv.* (2016) 37:156–74. doi: 10.1080/0145935X.2016.1104075
9. Lauritzen C, Reedtz C, Van Doesum KT, Martinussen M. Implementing new routines in adult mental health care to identify and support children of mentally ill parents. *BMC Health Serv Res.* (2014) 14:58. doi: 10.1186/1472-6963-14-58
10. Skogøy BE, Sørgaard K, Maybery D, Ruud T, Stavnes K, Kufås E, et al. Hospitals implementing changes in law to protect children of ill parents: a cross-sectional study. *BMC Health Serv Res.* (2018) 18:609. doi: 10.1186/s12913-018-3393-2
11. Diaz-Caneja A, Johnson S. The views and experiences of severely mentally ill mothers. *Soc Psychiatry Psychiatr Epidemiol.* (2004) 39:472–82. doi: 10.1007/s00127-004-0772-2
12. Festen H, Schipper K, de Vries SO, Reichart CG, Abma TA, Nauta MH. Parents' perceptions on offspring risk and prevention of anxiety and depression: a qualitative study. *BMC Psychol.* (2014) 2:17. doi: 10.1186/2050-7283-2-17
13. Reupert A, Ward B, McCormick F, Ward C, Waller S, Kidd S. Developing a model of family focused practice with consumers, families, practitioners, and managers: a community based participatory research approach. *BMC Health Serv Res.* (2018) 18:66–75. doi: 10.1186/s12913-018-2844-0
14. Foster K, Isobel S. Towards relational recovery: Nurses' practices with consumers and families with dependent children in mental health inpatient units. *Int J Mental Health Nurs.* (2018) 27:727–36. doi: 10.1111/inm.12359
15. Grant A, Reupert A, Maybery D, Goodyear M. Predictors and enablers of mental health nurses' family-focused practice. *Int J Ment Health Nurs.* (2019) 28:140–51. doi: 10.1111/inm.12503
16. Houlihan D, Sharek D, Higgins A. Supporting children whose parent has a mental health problem: an assessment of the education, knowledge, confidence, and practices of registered psychiatric nurses in Ireland. *J Psychiatr Mental Health Nurs.* (2013) 20:287–95. doi: 10.1111/j.1365-2850.2012.01923.x
17. Maybery D, Goodyear M, O'Hanlon B, Cuff R, Reupert A. Profession differences in family focused practice in the adult mental health system. *Family Process* (2014) 53:608–17. doi: 10.1111/famp.12082
18. Foster K, O'Brien L, Korhonen T. Developing resilient children and families when parents have mental illness: a family-focused approach. *Int J Mental Health Nursing* (2012) 21:3–11. doi: 10.1111/j.1447-0349.2011.00754.x
19. Goodyear M, Hill T-L, Allchin B, McCormick F, Hine R, Cuff R, et al. Standards of practice for the adult mental health workforce: Meeting the needs of families where a parent has a mental illness. *Int J Mental Health Nurs.* (2015) 24:169–80. doi: 10.1111/inm.12120
20. Spoelstra J, Stals K, Foolen N. *Richtlijnen Jeugdhulp en Jeugdbescherming [Guidelines for Youth Aid and Youth Protection. Workbook Implementation for Creating an Organization-Specific Implementation Plan for the Guidelines Youth Aid and Youth Protection]* (2015). Available online at: richtlijnenjeugdhulp.nl/wp-content/uploads/2017/Implementatieplan.docx. (Accessed April 15th, 2017).
21. Reupert A, Price-Robertson R, Maybery D. Parenting as a focus of recovery: a systematic review of current practice. *Psychiatr Rehabil J.* (2017) 40:361–70. doi: 10.1037/prj0000240
22. Tchernegovski P, Hine R, Reupert AE, Maybery DJ. Adult mental health clinicians' perspectives of parents with a mental illness and their children: single and dual focus approaches. *BMC Health Serv Res.* (2018) 18:611. doi: 10.1186/s12913-018-3428-8
23. Grol R, Wensing M. What drives change? Barriers to and incentives for achieving evidence-based practice. *Med J Aust.* (2004) 180:S57–60.

2

Mental Health Literacy of Youth that have a Family Member with a Mental Illness: Outcomes from a New Program and Scale

Joanne Riebschleger[1], Shane Costello[2], Daniel L. Cavanaugh[1] and Christine Grové[2]*

[1] School of Social Work MSU, Michigan State University, East Lansing, MI, United States,

[2] Faculty of Education - Monash, Monash University, Melbourne, VIC, Australia

***Correspondence:**
Joanne Riebschleger
riebsch1@msu.edu

A program evaluation examined mental health literacy levels and coping outcomes for youth (ages 10–16), before and at the end of their participation in a manualized, school-based mental health literacy program called Youth Education and Support (YES). Most of the youth reportedly had a parent or other family member with a mental health disorder such as depression, anxiety, and/or substance abuse. The mental health literacy levels of program participants from pre to post were evaluated with the developing Knowledge of Mental Illness and Recovery (K-MIR) scale. This scale was validated using item-response theory, demonstrating good psychometric properties. Youth answered two coping questions about their use of positive coping during the program and coping skills compared from pre to post intervention. Findings revealed that youth levels of mental health literacy increased significantly from pre to post program participation. Over 90% of the youth reported an improved use of positive coping strategies from pre to post intervention. The program appeared to deliver enhanced levels of literacy and coping for this sample of youth. The scale appeared to be appropriate to measure youth mental health literacy. Recommendations for practice, policy, and research are offered.

Keywords: mental health, substance abuse, adolescents, children, families, psychoeducation

INTRODUCTION

Mental health disorders are one of the most common sources of disability in the world (1). The social, emotional, cultural, and economic costs of mental illnesses affect people across community, business, school, health care, family, and individual sectors (2, 3). Despite the magnitude of the impact, mental illness is an all-too-often a stigmatized topic all over the world. There is a need for mental health literacy programs that provide accurate, non-stigmatized information about mental health disorders and recovery (4). The programs provide practical application of how to seek help for mental health concerns and how to help others who may have mental health symptoms (5).

Children of a parent, or other family member, with a mental illness face particular risks for acquiring a mental health disorder such as depression, anxiety, schizophrenia, bipolar disorder, and/or substance (6). The children, including youth ages 10–16 included in this study, have for too long been "invisible" to services providers of mental health services (7, p. 86). Within individual medical model systems, mental health consumers are rarely if they are parenting minor children. In most of the world, there are little to no mental health literacy programs for youth with a parent or other family member with a mental health disorder (7).

This study is an evaluation of a new youth-focused mental health literacy program. Most of the youth have a parent or other family member with a mental health disorder. The current study includes the psychometrics for a developing scale to measure youth levels of mental health literacy.

BACKGROUND

Youth with a parent with a mental illness comprise a large population. One of five people have a mental illness and parenting rates are similar for adults with a mental illness, as compared to adults without a mental illness. England and Sim (8) explored government and private health care databases to find that over 22 million children in the U.S. have a parent with a diagnosis of major depression. Maybery et al. (9) used Australian national health care data to estimate that around 21–23% of young people have a parent with a mental illness.

Risk and Resiliency

Risk and resilience theorists have provided a theoretical framework to understand how to promote healthy psychological development in individuals that face increased levels of psychosocial adversity (10–15). Youth that have a parent with a mental illness are at a higher risk of developing a mental health illness when compared to their same age peers (16, 17). These youth can be at a higher risk of developing behavioral, developmental, and emotional difficulties (18). Young people of parents with a mental illness may experience school problems and difficulties with attention or self-regulation. For example, they experience higher dropout rates at school (19), an increased likelihood of being taken into foster care (20) and an increased risk of developing a substance abuse disorder (21). Self-harm and suicide rates are higher in young people who have a parent with mental illness (22). Some young people may need to be re-located if their parent is hospitalized and/or very unwell (23). The youth may face increased risk to acquire intergenerational mental illness (24).

Childhood development can be affected adversely when they take on caregiving for parents in a way that is long-term and disproportionate to the child's developmental level of emotional maturity and understanding (25). They can experience negative emotions including shame, fear of conflicts, loneliness feelings of abandonment, sadness, anger, or envy of peers (26). Sometimes, they may harbor resentment toward their parent (27). Often these youth do not receive developmentally appropriate information about mental health (28) and, similarly, do not have the opportunity to develop an adequate and accurate understanding of their parents' mental illness (29).

Not all children are affected adversely by parental mental illness, nor will all children in the same family be affected in the same ways (18). Young people also differ in their beliefs and understanding about the nature of mental illness, its causes and the ways to treat mental health difficulties (30). Darlington et al. (31) suggest that mental illness in a parent does not automatically result in negative outcomes in children. Many parents with mental illness can form healthy attachments and provide nurturing care to their children. Even some situations where children take care of their parents can lead to positive outcomes (25). Caregiving may help the youth build a sense of purpose, potentially supporting resiliency, and reinforcing the parent-child bond (32).

Despite the risks and outcomes that the young people of parents with mental illness may experience, many of these youth demonstrate resilience. Resilience appears when youth engage in positive adjustments to a situation that includes conditions of challenge, risk, and/or adversity (33–35). In general, the more that a young person are seen as resilient, the better their mental health (36). Youth can achieve resilience when there is a balance between adverse events and protective factors. The presence of protective factors can safeguard young people from the impacts of parental mental illness by potentially "buffering" the impact of the risk factors and reduce the vulnerability of a young person acquiring a mental illness. Protective factors include nurturing care by a parent, a close relationship with parents, the child's own problem-solving skills in response to stressors, psycho-education, and accessible social support from peers and other adults (such as teachers) or family members, such as aunts, uncles, grandparents, or siblings (37, 38).

Stress, Coping, and Adaptation

Another model for considering youth with a parent with a mental illness is stress and coping theory (39, 40). Youth that have a parent with a mental illness may share some of the secondary effects of living in a home where a parent has a mental illness such as underemployment, unemployment, poverty, and/or parental divorce and/or separation (41). Some youth report that it can be stressful living with a parent, sibling, grandparent, aunt/uncle, and other family member with a mental illness as family interactions may change as the family member's illness symptoms can increase or decrease from day to day (41, 42). Further, youth may worry the family may not be able to pay the bills if a parent or other breadwinner is unable to work due to mental illness symptom exacerbation; they may fear others will judge the family member harshly and make fun of the person and, sometimes, the family as a whole (41). They may worry they will inherit a relative's mental illness (43, 44). They may not know how to talk about the relative's mental illness (45).

Coping is part of health and wellbeing, that includes healthy environments, responsive parenting, sense of belonging, healthy activities, resilience, and if mental illness symptoms arise, treatment of the illness (46). Youth can learn to manage stress by engaging in healthy coping activities such as coping self-talk and positive self-talk (47, 48). For example, positive coping behaviors can include exercising, talking to friends, writing, making a craft, and/or listening to music. It can include seeking help for family mental health crises. Stallman (46) notes that youth can make a coping plan to recognize personal and family stress and then engage in stress-reducing coping behaviors. As youth increase their coping behaviors, they can learn to better manage stress and, over time, adapt to stressful situations. They can even move beyond mere adaptation as their crisis plan offers new buffers or protective factors toward youth developmental resiliency (49).

Mental Health Literacy Interventions and Measures

Mental health literacy interventions, sometimes called psychoeducation, aim to provide accurate, non-stigmatized information about mental illness and recovery to mental health consumers and/or family members. Jorm et al. (50) describe mental health literacy as consisting of several components such as the:

> ability to recognize specific disorders, knowledge of how to seek mental health information, knowledge of risk factors and causes, knowledge of self-treatments and of professional help available, and attitudes that promote recognition and appropriate help-seeking (p. 469).

Mental health literacy interventions can teach young people coping skill and strategies to help them reduce stress. They can also respond to specific requests of young people who often ask for more mental health information to help with their understanding about their parents' illness (28, 29). Many young people report that they do not receive enough information about their parent's mental health (28) and are left "guessing" or "figuring out" what is happening to their parent. Some youth may develop misconceptions about mental illness such as blaming themselves for their parent's illness, or believing the mental illness can be caught like a cold or be "passed" onto friends (51). A lack of understanding about parental mental illness hinders the recognition and promotion of appropriate help seeking and reduces the likelihood of young people pursuing help for their difficulties (52). Mental health literacy programs often offer social support; for example, youth may use the mental health information and supportive relationships acquired in mental health literacy programs to manage practical issues such as finding support when their parent is hospitalized and when they need a break from caring for their parent (23, 51).

Clearly, youth would like to be "kept in the loop" and informed about their parents' mental illness (53) and want to talk about their experience (29). However, they may be unsure of the implications of accessing support, such as discussing the impact of stigma for having a parent with mental illness (54). Each young person will process information about his or her parent's illness differently and so will have varying information needs. Young people's understanding of their parent's illness is constantly evolving and changing including the amount and type of information they acquire (55).

Gladstone et al. (29) suggest that psycho-education should attempt to include young people's views of their parent's illness and should recognize the youth's role within the family context. However, it is important to note that the kind of mental health knowledge, and how it is shared with youth, is mostly developed and implemented by adults who decide what youth need (56). Mental health information for youth should be examined from a child-centered approach; there is a need to investigate how mental health information is used by youth and whether this is helpful for the young person, if at all (29). The voices and experiences of young people and their families when developing mental health literacy programs also need to be heard (53, 57).

There are many emerging mental health literacy programs designed to promote resilience in children who are with parents or family members with mental illnesses (7, 18). For example, in Finland (58) and Sweden (59), there are national implementations of a family intervention program to encourage child and parent communication about the parent's mental health condition, recovery strategies, and social service coordination (58). However, in most areas of the world, only a small percentage of youth with a parent or other family members with a mental illness have access to mental health literacy programs. Even in Australia, where there are a number of family-, youth-, and parent- centered programs with mental health literacy content, there is limited access to the programs across many regions of the country. Many of the programs are emerging; they are not yet considered evidence-based (18). A lack of evidence-based programs that provide mental health information and support for youth, parents, and other family members could be a potential barrier to funding. Many private and government organizations prefer to fund evidence-based programs (60).

A lack of mental health literacy scales with sound psychometric properties are a barrier to building evidence-based practices, especially in evaluating interventions for young people with a parent with a mental illness. O'Connor et al. (61) conducted an extensive literature review of mental health literature scales. They found that of the measures they reviewed none covered all of the constructs of mental health literacy, such as disorder recognition, help seeking, risk factor identification, information seeking, causes of mental illness, self-treatment/coping, and risk factors. They also reported that most measures used had methodological gaps in psychometric validation and norming.

Since the publication of that article, new scales with increased rigor have been published (62, 63). The first measure was normed primarily on college students (62). The second measure was normed on a combination of health care practitioners and those in the general population ages 15 and up (63). Additionally, the second measure focused on three specific disorders (schizophrenia, anxiety, and depression). The most rigorous mental health literacy measures available appear to be normed only on adults (62). The work of Kutcher et al. (64) included a scale designed to measure mental health literacy as an indicator of increased mental health resiliency among high school students. However, the reading level appears to exceed that needed for middle school students.

Measures have been used to assess mental health literacy programs delivered to young people with a parent with a mental illness (5, 43, 65) or with young people without a parent with mental illness (66). However, these measures do not appear to capture all of the mental health literacy constructs. They also contain limited information about scale psychometric validation or norming. Therefore, building on these current works in the field comprehensive and robust mental health literacy scales are needed for youth of varying ages (4). Specifically, YES program services providers indicate that their evaluation of the program is need of a measure for youth aged 10–16 that have a parent or other family member with a mental illness. More evidence is needed for youth mental health literacy programs and scales to move the field forward toward building evidence-based practices.

METHODS

This study evaluated the outcomes of the YES mental health literacy program. The guiding research question asked, "What are the pre-post mental health literacy and coping outcomes reported by youth attending the Youth Education and Support program?" Given the lack of psychometrically validated measures of youth mental health literacy (4), the first phase of the evaluation study included development and analysis of an instrument to measure youth mental health literacy. The second part assessed youth participant self-reported levels of pre to post program mental health literacy and coping behaviors.

The Knowledge of Mental Illness and Recovery (KMIR) Scale

The KMIR scale items includes 36 questions. Eighteen are set in a true and false format. Eighteen use a four-item multiple choice response set. The primary aim of the scale is to assess the mental health literacy of children ages 10–16. The Flesch-Kincaid scale assigned the KMIR a 4.8 reading level. This means the scale is an appropriate reading level for youth 8 months into the fourth grade. In the US, most of these youth would be about 9 years old. Completion time is 11–14 min. The primary investigator used or modified questions found on mental health websites (67, 68), and as found within a nonfiction book written for teens with a parent with a mental illness (69). In addition, the scale author wrote 16 new questions, as the first version of the KMIR scale was pretested initially with six middle school children and who took the test and then offered suggestions for improvement. Their comments led to the second version of the scale administered to 39 YES program youth. Version two was then administered to 216 middle school students in three schools in the Midwest, which was used in the psychometric validation presented below. The validation sample included 55.10% female participants, with a mean age of 13.54 years (standard deviation 0.71 years, ranging from 11 to 16 years). The participants identified as Caucasian (80.10%), Black/African American (6.50%), Latino/Hispanic (6.00%), American Indian (2.30%), Asian American (0.50%), and other or did not answer (2.8%). Following the validation, the scale was administered to the 46 YES participants in the current study.

To determine the validity of the Knowledge of Mental Ill00ness and Recovery (KMIR) were evaluated for goodness of fit to a graded response model using Microsoft R Open version 3.4.2 (70) and R Studio version 1.1.383 (71). The M_2 limited information goodness of fit statistic (72) was calculated for each subtest, with significant results ($p < 0.01$) indicating less than adequate fit. However, when sample sizes are relatively small, a corresponding small Root Mean Square Error of Approximation value (RMSEA < 0.09) suggests that a lack of fit may be due to a limited amount of "model error" (73); common in strong parametric models (72). The Standardized Root Mean Square Residual (SRMR) is the square root of the difference between the residuals of the sample covariance matrix and the 0covariance model (74). Values range from 0 to 1.0, with well-fitting models obtaining values <0.06 (75). Marginal reliability coefficients (analogous to Cronbach's alpha coefficients) are calculated using Lord and Novak's true score model (76).

TABLE 1 | Rasch model fit statistics for KMIR scale.

	M_2	*df*	*p*	RMSEA	SRMR	Reliability
KMIR total score	1199.88	629	<0.001	0.06	0.11	0.87
Mental illness	83.79	65	0.06	0.04	0.08	0.69
Recovery	225.37	65	0.11	0.09	0.13	0.68
Stigma	147.34	65	<0.001	0.06	0.11	0.68

At the item level, fit was investigated further with $S\text{–}X^2$ item level diagnostics (77, 78); infit and outfit (79, 80); local dependency (81); and differential item functioning by gender (82). Non-significant $S - X^2$ item values are indicative of good item level fit, while infit and outfit scores between the range of 0.5 and 1.5 are considered productive for measurement. Local dependency indicates a relationship between items where the ability to answer one item is predicated on the ability to answer another item. For example, to demonstrate knowledge of bipolar disorders, one would likely need to be able to demonstrate knowledge of depressive disorders. Local dependency is identified using positive correlation coefficients of 0.20 or greater in a correlation matrix of residuals. Differential item functioning indicates a gender difference in likelihood of correctly endorsing an item for participants of the same underlying ability. One example of differential item functioning would be a question regarding the role of social support in recovery, which is generally answered correctly by females and not by males—reflecting differences in gendered experience and norms rather than knowledge.

The results of the Rasch analyses suggested that aside from a small number of locally dependent items (one item pair in *Mental Illness*; two pair in *Recovery*; and one item pair in *Stigma*), the subscales and total KMIR scales demonstrated reasonable model fit. There were no redundant items, no items demonstrated significant misfit, and no differential item functioning was observed. Infit and outfit statistics were all within the recommended range of 0.5–1.5. The fit statistics are presented in **Table 1**.

The Youth Education and Support (YES) Program

Forty-six youth participants were drawn from an urban, Midwest American middle school. Social workers employed by the school visited grade 5–8 classrooms to talk about students' opportunities to participate in the Youth Education and Support (YES) program to learn about mental health and recovery. If considering YES program participation, youth submitted a note of interest later to the mailbox of the social worker. This ensured that interested youth could not be identified as those turning in program inquiries at the time of the social workers visits to the classrooms. School social workers then met with inquiring youth and once their interests were confirmed, communicated with parents to explain the program, and if parents allowed, obtained signed informed consent for participation. The primary investigator trained the school social workers' in obtaining informed assent from youth and consent from parents in accordance with the overseeing university's Institutional Review Board. Parents also completed youth and family demographic information. Demographic information included parents' checking a general category of relative that they identified as having a mental health disorder. At no time were specific individuals identified by name.

Participation in the study did not require that youth have a parent or other family with a mental illness but it was a preferred criteria for inclusion in the program. Prior to the first group session of the YES program, school social workers obtained a pre-intervention youth completion of the Knowledge of Mental Illness and Recovery scale (KMIR) to assess youth beginning knowledge of mental health literacy information. The KMIR scale included knowledge about common mental illnesses, recovery, and stigma.

The Youth Education and Support (YES) program is a manualized, ten-session mental health literacy program for youth in grades 5–8. It was developed by the first author over a 12 year span of time with recommendations from children, youth, and adults that reportedly have a parent or other family member with a mental illness. Recommendations for the content were also drawn from mental health professionals, family members with a mental illness—especially parents, the professional literature, and reviews of existing mental health literacy program curricula from the United States, Australia, England, and Canada. The program continued to be modified over time in response to program evaluation data drawn from the comments of youth participants, their parents, other family members, middle school teachers, fidelity observers, and program facilitators.

Each session is about 50 min so there is around 8 h of total program time. Across the program, the content covers mental health literacy content including knowledge of mental illness in general, including risks/causes; specific mental health disorders, including major depression, types of anxiety, schizophrenia, bipolar disorder, and substance abuse, e.g., alcohol, marijuana, meth amphetamines, inhalants, and opioid addiction. It covers risks for mental illness such as stress and genetics, while emphasizing that it is difficult to know what causes any one individual to develop, or not develop, a mental illness. A holistic recovery model anchors the recovery-focused learning content. Youth discuss how to seek help for mental health concerns and how to help others with these concerns. Mental illness "truths" (facts) and "myths" (stigma) are included regularly within the program.

Words of the day guide session topics that include YES (introduction to the YES program), mental illness, coping, depression, recovery, substance abuse, co-occurring (mental illness and substance abuse), family (impacts of mental illness on family members), planning (for mental health crises and the future of the youth), and graduation (end of group celebration). Each session begins with attendance, word, of the day, and food and drink, i.e., cookies, fruit, cheese, and water. Every session includes a check-in on stress and coping, as well as discussion of ways to manage stress. Some kind of hands-on active learning activity takes place in each session. For example, youth construct a crisis mobile with drawings and names of behaviors that they believe will help them reduce stress and "stay in balance." They develop a customized individual coping plan with illustrations. They color pictures of a depressed vs. a non-depressed brain based on an MRI example. They engage in a hopscotch-like team competition to plan for ways to work toward their future goals. They watch a movie clip about a family with a parent with a mental illness and discuss what each family member may be feeling and/or thinking. They walk rapidly about the room in a circle demonstrating how substance abuse and depression can have a "circular" effect, sometime leading to increased levels of mental health symptoms.

All of these activities seemed to work well with all of youth, but those ages about 13–16 spent more time on discussion. For youth ages 10–12, facilitators talked at a slightly slower pace and used lower language levels. At each session end, each youth chooses a small item from a "prize box" to reward their participation. Each session ends with a take home educational document to share with parents. For example, some of the parent handouts are how to talk to a child/youth about mental illness and when and how to seek help should a parent have concerns about their son or daughter's mental health. These are general information handouts; no specific youth, parent, or family application is included.

The program was co-led by a school social worker and university faculty member with expertise in mental health practice and research. Sessions took place during the school day at varying days of the week and times of the day to reduce youth participants from missing too much of one class. Almost every session included a trained observer who completed a YES program fidelity scale that measures the extent the session met stated learning objectives. The observer sat in the rear of the classroom and did not participate in programming.

At the last session, facilitators asked youth participants to think about their coping at the beginning of the program. A pause followed for youth reflection. Then they were asked to think about their level of coping at the end of the program. The facilitator emphasized that honest responses were most helpful; youth were encouraged to choose the answer that seemed to fit their experience. Youth reported the extent they thought their pre to post coping met one of the following responses, i.e., a lot worse, a little bit worse, about the same, a little bit better, or a lot better. Facilitators also asked youth to report how frequently they were able to use positive coping behaviors during the time they were participating in the program. Positive coping behaviors are activities that youth choose to deal with their stress that are likely to make the situation better. For example, thinking positive thoughts or playing sports may help some youth reduce their stress. Negative coping behaviors such as hitting a window or yelling at someone are likely to make the situation worse. Youth circled a positive coping frequency estimate of not very often, sometimes or often.

These simple questions were included in the midst of developing the program. This was primarily because the

A-COPE, used in early YES program measurement, seemed to rely on youth implementing a wide array of coping measures to score higher in coping (83). Since the YES program focused on implementing one to three youth-selected coping behaviors regularly, combined with relatively short programming time and the fact that the A-COPE scale did not include computer and online coping behavior choices, this simplified coping measurement appeared to capture youth ideas about their coping.

RESULTS

Forty-six of fifty-two youth, ages 10–16, completed the YES program after development of the 2012, or third version, of the K-MIR scale. Reasons for non-completion were schedule conflict with team sports ($n = 1$), second parent withdrew consent ($n = 1$), not interested in continuing ($n = 2$), moved out of area ($n = 1$), and not known (n=1). **Table 2** notes the demographic composition of the YES participant youth. More than half of the sample were non-Caucasian. Most participants were in grades 6–8. About 59% of the sample reportedly had a relative with a mental illness, most frequently a parent with reported diagnoses of depression, bipolar disorder, or borderline personality disorder. Over 10 percent of the youth reported had a parent with a dual diagnosis of mental illness plus substance abuse (primarily alcohol abuse). Notably, parents reported that over 28% of the youth also had a mental health diagnosis, most commonly ADHD, anxiety, and depression.

TABLE 2 | Demographic and household details of the YES program sample ($N = 46$).

Demographic	% or mean
Female	63.00%
Male	32.60%
Age	13.07 years (SD 0.82)
RACE	
Black	21.30%
White	48.90%
Latino/Hispanic	12.80%
Mixed Race/Other	17.10 %
GRADE	
6th	19.60%
7th	8.70%
8th	69.60%
Missing	2.20%
REPORTED FAMILY MEMBER WITH DIAGNOSIS	
Parent	34.80%
Sibling	15.20%
Grand parent	4.30%
Aunt/Uncle	2.20%
Other family member	30.40%
None reported	30.40%
Missing	10.90%
Child reported to have a diagnosis	28.26%

Table 3 details the distributions of correct answers by item, subscale, and total scale; and statistical comparisons from pre to post intervention.

Youth reported how often they were able to use positive coping strategies across the program often (60.9%), sometimes (32.6%), and not very often (6.5%). Ninety three and a half percent of the youth said they were able to use positive coping strategies often or sometimes. Participant youth also rated their coping skills at the end of the program as compared to their skills at the beginning of the program; they said their coping skills were way better (51.1%), a little better (40.4%), and about the same (8.5%). Therefore, 91.5% of youth estimated their coping skills were way better or a little better from pre to post intervention.

The fidelity assessment revealed that fidelity objectives were met 94% of the time within the YES program delivery. For the 6% not met, it appeared that reduced session time available was a main barrier. Especially in the second semester and near holiday breaks, the schools sometimes shortened class hours to accommodate special activities such as pep rallies, standardized testing, and award ceremonies.

DISCUSSION

Data responded to the guiding research question: "What are the pre-post mental health literacy and coping outcomes reported by youth attending the Youth Education and Support program?" It appears that this sample of YES participant youth reported significantly increased levels of mental health literacy from pre to post program participation. Over 90% of the sample youth described the use of positive coping during the time they participated in the Youth Education and Support program. Over 90% of youth also reported improved coping skills from pre to post.

The YES mental health literacy outcomes align with the work of Kutcher et al. (64) who found participating in a mental health literacy program led to increased knowledge of mental health among Canadian high school students. The YES program youth participants showed less stigmatized assumptions from pre to post intervention. This result is similar to the work of Wahl et al. (66) in their implementation of a middle school mental health education curriculum. Since most mental health literacy programs are delivered to adults, this study may contribute to building knowledge about *youth outcomes* of mental health literacy programs. This is an important knowledge gap to address among mental health literacy program evaluations.

The Knowledge of Mental Illness and Recovery scale measuring levels of youth mental health literacy demonstrated promising psychometric properties including, reasonable model fit. Rasch analysis offers an approach to instrument development and validation that differs both conceptually and mathematically to the more commonly used classical test theory, where the aim is to measure across the range of the latent construct. Overall, the three subscales and the total scale score demonstrated adequate or good fit to the model. Reliability coefficients were generally fair for the subscales, and considered good for the total scale.

TABLE 3 | Repeated-measure *t*-test of KMIR by item, subscale, and total scale scores.

Items and scales	No. correct pre-program		No. correct post-program		*t*	*p*	Effect size	
	Mean	SD	Mean	SD			Cohen's *d*	95% CI
1. Mental illness is more common than...	0.63	0.49	0.78	0.42	1.86	0.07	0.27	0.16 to 0.66
2. The most common mental illness is...	0.22	0.42	0.61	0.49	4.32	<0.001	0.63	0.27 to 1.11
5. Mental illness most often begins when a person is...	0.72	0.47	0.84	0.4	1.30	0.20	0.21	−0.21 to 0.61
6. About one of _______ people develop a mental illness...	0.44	0.49	0.87	0.34	5.93	<0.001	0.80	0.26 to 1.11
10. What percentage of people with mental illness gets help?	0.26	0.43	0.54	0.5	3.49	<0.001	0.48	0.10 to 0.93
16. The mental illness of a person is likely caused by...	0.38	0.48	0.41	0.5	0.83	0.41	0.06	−0.35 to 0.47
20. In the U.S.A., more people go to the hospital because...	0.4	0.5	0.44	0.5	0.00	1.00	0.06	−0.35 to 0.47
21. People with mental illness often do fairly well in life...	0.46	0.51	0.85	0.36	4.12	<0.001	0.64	0.14 to 0.97
22. Parents can develop a mental illness when their kids...	0.34	0.47	0.52	0.51	2.14	0.04	0.29	−0.11 to 0.71
23. If someone in your family has a mental illness...	0.62	0.49	0.83	0.38	2.66	0.01	0.38	−0.07 to 0.76
30. Most people with mental illness are likely to get...	0.42	0.5	0.63	0.49	1.94	0.06	0.35	0.07 to 0.76
36. Epilepsy, or having seizures, is a mental illness...	0.5	0.51	0.67	0.48	1.64	0.11	0.27	−0.15 to 0.67
Mental Illness subscale	**5.35**	**1.9**	**7.96**	**2.04**	**7.4**	**<0.001**	**1.09**	**0.69 to 1.58**
3. One of the first steps to recovering from serious mental...	0.5	0.51	0.67	0.47	2.07	0.04	0.30	−0.12 to 0.70
7. Recovery from mental illness means...	0.35	0.48	0.39	0.49	0.47	0.64	0.06	−0.34 to 0.47
9. A lot of things can help a person recover from mental illness...	0.57	0.5	0.7	0.47	1.35	0.18	0.20	−0.22 to 0.60
13. One of the best combinations of things that can help people...	0.35	0.48	0.63	0.49	2.91	<0.01	0.43	0.02 to 0.85
15. Most people with mental illness...	0.44	0.5	0.44	0.5	0.00	1.00	0.00	−0.41 to 0.41
17. Family members can help a person with mental illness by...	0.28	0.46	0.59	0.5	3.18	<0.01	0.47	0.07 to 0.90
19. Getting help for mental illness works as well as getting help...	0.46	0.5	0.57	0.5	1.09	0.28	0.16	−0.24 to 0.57
28. If a person is trying to get attention by saying he or she will...	0.85	0.36	0.94	0.25	1.43	0.66	0.22	−0.22 to 0.60
31. Mental illness keeps a person from being able to develop...	0.53	0.5	0.8	0.4	2.60	0.01	0.40	−0.05 to 0.77
32. It is very important to know the cause of a person's mental...	0.2	0.4	0.24	0.43	0.63	0.53	0.09	−0.32 to 0.50
33. People with mental illness are usually able to make...	0.52	0.51	0.8	0.4	3.28	<0.01	0.48	0.02 to 0.84
35. Most people with a serious mental illness get well quickly...	0.85	0.36	0.89	0.31	0.63	0.53	0.09	−0.33 to 0.49
Recovery subscale	**5.89**	**2.06**	**7.65**	**1.84**	**5.87**	**<0.001**	**0.87**	**0.40 to 1.25**
4. The main reason people do not get help for their mental...	0.4	0.49	0.65	0.48	3.52	<0.001	0.46	0.04 to 0.87
8. People with mental illness...	0.52	0.51	0.74	0.44	3.16	<0.01	0.47	0.03 to 0.85
11. Some people think that people with mental illness are...	0.53	0.5	0.91	0.29	4.38	<0.001	0.67	0.13 to 0.96
12. Stigma toward people with mental illness happens when...	0.5	0.51	0.72	0.46	2.22	0.03	0.33	−0.10 to 0.72
14. People with mental illness...	0.35	0.48	0.59	0.5	2.69	0.01	0.40	−0.01 to 0.82
18. Most people with mental illness...	0.44	0.50	0.70	0.47	3.60	<0.001	0.53	0.10 to 0.93
24. Mental illness may be caused by being an emotionally...	0.33	0.47	0.61	0.49	2.93	<0.01	0.43	0.03 to 0.85
25. People with a mental illness are usually more dangerous...	0.67	0.47	0.89	0.32	2.66	0.01	0.40	−0.07 to 0.75
26. It is easy to tell if someone has a mental illness...	0.67	0.47	0.87	0.34	2.45	0.02	0.37	−0.09 to 0.74
27. People with a mental illness usually can't think well...	0.54	0.5	0.87	0.43	2.49	0.02	0.56	0.11 to 0.94
29. People with mental illness are more likely to be the victim...	0.48	0.51	0.37	0.49	−1.09	0.28	−0.16	−0.57 to 0.25
34. A person recovering from a mental illness is usually better...	0.7	0.47	0.87	0.34	2.43	0.02	0.35	−0.10 to 0.72
Stigma subscale	**6.12**	**2.23**	**8.67**	**2.1**	**7.14**	**<0.001**	**1.05**	**0.58 to 1.45**
Total KMIR scale	17.35	4.65	24.28	4.8	9.94	<0.001	1.47	1.03 to 1.95

Full items can be made available by the first author. For completeness, changes in score by item have been included, however interpretation is recommended at the subscale and total scale level. Cohen's d effect sizes calculated after correcting for the correlation between pre and post-program scores, as per (84).

Item redundancy were not found to be an issue for any item pair across all KMIR subscales. Given the relatively small number of items in each scale, this is somewhat expected, as the probability of redundant items increases with the number of items given that there are a finite number of ways in which a single construct can be represented in written language. However, even small numbers of items are not immune from the effects of redundancy, with items that are too similarly worded or of very similar difficulty likely to result in correlated residuals after accounting for the latent constructs. As noted earlier, differential item functioning was not explored given the sample size. Local independence was observed for several item pairs; however, given that there were no significant gains to be had from the removal of dependent items, all were retained.

There remain a number of areas for improvement, and it is important to note that the KMIR scale is still under development. Data collection is underway to measure test-retest and test convergence analysis of the KMIR compared to the Wahl et al. (66) knowledge scale. The development of scales with adequate psychometric properties is a key need for the development of evidence-based mental health literacy programs for youth.

The YES program does provide an early response to the requests for more mental health information echoed among youth that have a parent or other family member with a mental health disorder (57). The active learning format of the YES program and the readability of the KMIR scale seems aligns with the recommendation of parent mental health consumers for delivering mental health literacy programs that are fun and developmentally appropriate (85).

The YES evaluation includes youth-estimated coping skills is useful in beginning to collect behavioral change data. This is important since resiliency and coping theories include a need for knowledge and behavioral foci. The YES small group format may have provided an additional support network for the youth. Support networks are key components within resiliency and coping theories (11, 49).

However, it is not possible, even for this sample of youth, to know the extent that participation in a mental health literacy program may serve as a developmental factor in the prevention of mental health disorders or their reduction in symptoms severity. The YES program participant sample is relatively small and the KMIR scale is still undergoing psychometric testing. Family mental health disorders reported by parents were not subject to professional confirmation. Most critically, the study did not use a control group. It is likely that having the YES qualitative data analyzed by outside reviewers may have enhanced findings validity; an audit of the data using the trails of a codebook and raw data would also have contributed an external review of analyses (86). The findings cannot be generalized to all children of a parent or other family member with a mental illness.

There is a need for more funding, including long-term evaluation of mental health programs for youth. Specialized curricula may be needed for children that have a parent or other family member with a mental health disorder (4). The voices of youth, parents, and other family members should be included in the program development and evaluation. Intergenerational dialogue among family members may be helpful (87). Future research should include studies with matched comparison or control groups. The use of a randomized wait list controls may be an option. The inclusion of additional standardized scales to examine youth, parent, and family functioning would provide a stronger picture for assessing pre, post, and follow up intervention.

Mental health disorders one of the most common sources of disability in the world and mental health literacy may be able to build human developmental resiliency. Therefore, federal and state governments, as well as private funders of mental health research, should fund mental health literacy programs. Seeking this funding will require policy advocacy on the part of community members (30). It makes sense to build and test mental health literacy programs for youth, parents, and intergenerational family members (24, 88) to explore what works for whom, when, how, and for how long.

Despite many limitations, this study offers hope in findings that youth participating in a mental health literacy program reported increased levels of mental health literacy and coping skills. The target group was largely composed of youth that reportedly had a parent with a mental health disorder. The work is likely a small step of progress toward reducing the knowledge gaps for building evidenced-based mental health literacy programs for youth at risk of acquiring a mental health disorder. To do so, offers even more hope for a future world where mental illness is discussed respectfully, professional help is forthcoming, and accurate information about mental health is widely available.

ETHICS STATEMENT

The study was carried out in accordance with the recommendations of the human subject guidelines of the Michigan State University Institutional Review Board. The protocol was approved by the committee. All subjects gave assent (if minors) and their parents gave written consent.

AUTHOR CONTRIBUTIONS

JR lead the project and worked on all sections of the paper. SC author led the norming of the scale and wrote **Tables 1–3**. DC wrote the background section on scales and the information on resiliency and also coded all the data from which the paper was developed. CG wrote the background on children at risk and added to the discussion section. All authors helped with reviewing drafts.

FUNDING

This project was supported by the USDA National Institute of Food and Agriculture and Michigan AgBioResearch.

REFERENCES

1. World Health Organization. *Mental Disorders Affect One in Four People.* (2001). Available online at: http://www.who.int/whr/2001/media_centre/press_release/en/
2. Royal College of Psychiatrists. *No Health Without Public Mental Health: The Call for Action - RCP Position Statement* (2010). Available online at: https://www.rcpsych.ac.uk/docs/default-source/improving-care/better-mh-policy/position-statements/ps04_2010.pdf?sfvrsn=b7316b7_4
3. World Health Organization. *Social Determinents of Mental Health* (2014). Available online at: http://apps.who.int/iris/bitstream/handle/10665/112828/9789?sequence=1
4. Riebschleger J, Grové C, Cavanaugh D, Costello S. Mental health literacy content for children of parents with a mental illness: thematic analysis of a literature review. *Brain Sci.* (2017) 7:1–19. doi: 10.3390/brainsci7110141
5. Grové C, Reupert AE, Maybery DJ. Gaining knowledge about parental mental illness: how does it empower children? *Child Family Soc Work* (2015) 20:377–86. doi: 10.1111/cfs.12086

6. Serbin LA, Karp J. The intergenerational transfer of psychosocial risk: mediators of vulnerability and resilience. *Ann Rev Psychol.* (2004) 55:333–63. doi: 10.1146/annurev.psych.54.101601.145228
7. Riebschleger, J. A world tour of intervention programs for children of a parent with a psychiatric illness. In: Johnson DJ, Agbényiga DL, and Hitchcock RK, editors. *Vulnerable Children: Global Challenges in Education, Health, Well-Being, and Child Rights.* New York, NY: Springer (2013). p. 151–63. doi: 10.1007/978-1-4614-6780-9_11
8. England MJ, Sim LJ. *Depression in Parents, Parenting, and Children: Opportunities to Improve Identification, Treatment and Prevention. National Research Council (US) and the Institute of Medicine (US) Committee on Depression, Parenting, Practicing and the Healthy Development of Children.* Washington, DC: National Academies Press (2009).
9. Maybery J, Reupert A, Patrick K, Goodyear M, Crase L. Prevalence of parental mental illness in Australian families. *Psychiatr Bull.* (2009) 33:22–6. doi: 10.1192/pb.bp.107.018861
10. Greene R. Resilience. In: Mizrahi T, Davis LE, editors. *Encyclopedia of Social Work.* Washington, DC: National Association of Social Workers Press and Oxford University Press (2013).
11. Masten AS. *Ordinary Magic: Resilience in Development.* New York, NY: Guilford Press (2015).
12. Masten AS, Powell JL. A resilience framework for research, policy, and practice. In: Luthar SS editor. *Resilience and Vulnerability: Adaptation in the Context of Childhood Adversities.* Cambridge: Cambridge University Press (2003). p. 1–25. doi: 10.1017/CBO9780511615788.003
13. Rutter M. Psychosocial resilience and protective mechanisms. *Am. J. Orthopsychiatry* (1987) 57:316–31. doi: 10.1111/j.1939-0025.1987.tb03541.x
14. Rutter M. Resilience: some conceptual considerations. *J Adolescent Health* (1993) 14:626–31. doi: 10.1016/1054-139X(93)90196-V
15. Zimmerman MA. Resiliency theory: a strengths-based approach to research and practice for adolescent health. *Health Educ Behav.* (2013) 40:381–3. doi: 10.1177/1090198113493782
16. Edwards EP, Eiden RD, Leonard KE. Behaviour problems in 18- to 36-month-old children of alcoholic fathers: secure mother-infant attachment as a protective factor. *Dev Psychopathol.* (2006) 18:395–407. doi: 10.1017/S0954579406060214
17. Weissman MM, Wickramaratne P, Nomura Y. Offspring of depressed parents: 20 years later. *Am J Psychiatry* (2006) 163:1001–8. doi: 10.1176/ajp.2006.163.6.1001
18. Reupert A, Maybery D, Kowalenko N. Children whose parents have a mental illness: prevalence, need and treatment. *Med J Aust.* (2012) 16:7–9. doi: 10.5694/mjao11.11200
19. Farahati F, Marcotte DE, Wilcox-Gok V. The effects of parents' psychiatric disorders on children's high school dropout. *Econ Educ Rev.* (2003) 22:167–78.
20. Leschied AW, Chiodo D, Whitehead PC, Hurley D. The relationship between maternal depression and child outcomes in a child welfare sample: implications for treatment and policy. *Child Fam Soc Work* (2005) 10:281–91. doi: 10.1111/j.1365-2206.2005.00365.x
21. Mowbray CT, Oyserman D. Substance abuse in children with mental illness: risks, resiliency, and best prevention practices. *J Primary Prev.* (2003) 23:451–83. doi: 10.1023/A:1022224527466
22. Weitzman M, Rosenthal DG, Liu Y-H. Paternal mental health problems and depression and child emotional and behavioral problems in the USA. *Pediatrics* (2011) 128:1126–34. doi: 10.1542/peds.2010-3034
23. Maybery D, Ling L, Szakacs E, Reupert A. Children of a parent with a mental illness: perspectives on need. *Aust J Mental Health* (2005) 4:1–11. doi: 10.5172/jamh.4.2.78
24. Hancock KJ, Mitrou F, Shipley M, Lawrence D, Zubrick SR. A three generation study of the mental health relationships between grandparents, parents, and children. *BMC Psychiatry* (2013) 13:299–316. doi: 10.1186/1471-244X-13-299
25. Van Loon L, van de Ven MO, van Doesum K, Hosman CM, Witteman CL. Parentification, stress, and problem behavior of adolescents who have a parent with mental health problems. *Fam Proc* (2017) 56:141–53. doi: 10.1111/famp.12165
26. Bosch A, Riebschleger J, Van Loon L. Dutch youth of parents with a mental illness reflect upon their feelings of guilt and shame. *Int J Mental Health Prom.* (2017) 19:159–72. doi: 10.1080/14623730.2017.1315955
27. Foster K. 'You'd think this roller coaster was never going to stop": experiences of adult children of parents with serious mental illness. *J Clin Nurs* (2010) 19:3143–51. doi: 10.1111/j.1365-2702.2010.03293.x
28. Monds-Watson A, Manktelow R, McColgan M. Social work with children when parents have mental health difficulties: acknowledging vulnerability and maintaining the "Rights of the Child". *Child Care Prac.* (2010) 16:35–55. doi: 10.1080/13575270903369319
29. Gladstone BM, Boydell KM, Seeman MV, McKeever PD. Children's experiences of parental mental illness: a literature review. *Early Interv Psychiatry* (2011) 5:271–89. doi: 10.1111/j.1751-7893.2011.00287.x.
30. Jorm AF. Mental health literacy: empowering the community to take action for better mental health. *Am Psychol.* (2012) 67:231–43. doi: 10.1037/a0025957
31. Darlington YF, Fenney JA, Rixon K. Interagency collaboration between child protection and mental health services: practices, attitudes and barriers. *Child Abuse Neglect* (2005) 29:1085–98. doi: 10.1016/j.chiabu.2005.04.005
32. Williams C, Mfoafo-M'Carthy M. Care: Giving, receiving and meaning in the context of mental illness. *Psychiatry* (2006) 69:26–46. doi: 10.1521/psyc.2006.69.1.26
33. Campbell-Sills L, Cohan SL, Stein MB. Relationship of resilience to personality, coping, and psychiatric symptoms in young adults. *Behav Res Ther.* (2006) 44:585–99. doi: 10.1016/j.brat.2005.05.001
34. Luther S, Zelazo B. *Resilience and Vulnerability: An Integrative Review.* Cambridge: Cambridge University Press (2003). doi: 10.1017/CBO9780511615788
35. McGloin JM, Widom CS. Resilience among abused and neglected children grown up. *Dev Psychopathol.* (2002) 13:1021–38. doi: 10.1017/S095457940100414X
36. Ungar M. The importance of parents and other caregivers to the resilience of high-risk adolescents. *Fam Proc.* (2004) 4:23–41. doi: 10.1111/j.1545-5300.2004.04301004.x
37. Hosman C, van Doesum K, van Santvoort F. Prevention of emotional problems and psychiatric risks in children of parents with a mental illness in Netherlands. *Aust J Adv Mental Health* (2009) 8:250–63. doi: 10.5172/jamh.8.3.250
38. Pölkki P, Ervast SA, Huupponen M. Coping and resilience of children of a mentally ill parent. *Social Work Health Care* (2004) 39:151–63. doi: 10.1300/J010v39n01_10
39. Compas BE. Psychobiological processes of stress and coping. *Ann N Y Acad Sci.* (2007) 1094:226–34. doi: 10.1196/annals.1376.024
40. Compas BE, Connor-Smith JK, Saltzman H, Tomsen AH, Wadsworth ME. Coping with stress during childhood and adolescence: problems, progress and potential in theory and research. *Psychol Bull.* (2001) 127:87–127. doi: 10.1037/0033-2909.127.1.87
41. Riebschleger J. Good days and bad days: the experiences of children of a parent with a psychiatric disability. *Psych Rehab J.* (2004) 28:25–31. doi: 10.2975/28.2004.25.31
42. Mordoch E, Hall WA. Children's perceptions of living with a parent with a mental illness: finding the rhythm and maintaining the frame. *Qual Health Res.* (2008) 18:1127–44. doi: 10.1177/1049732308320775
43. Grové C, Melrose H, Reupert A, Maybery D, Morgan B. When your parent has a mental illness: children's experiences of a psycho-educational intervention. *Adv Mental Health* (2015) 13:127–38. doi: 10.1080/18387357.2015.1063637
44. Mordoch E. How children understand parental mental illness: "You don't get life insurance. What's life insurance?" *J Can Acad Child Adolesc Psychiatry* (2010) 19:19–25.
45. Sherman M. Reaching out to children of parents with mental illness. *Social Work Today* (2007) 7:26–30. Available online at: https://www.socialworktoday.com/archive/septoct2007p26.shtml
46. Stallman HM. Coping planning: a patient- and strengths-focused approach to suicide prevention training. *Aust Psychiatry* (2017) 26:141–4. doi: 10.1177/1039856217732471
47. Clarke AT. Coping with interpersonal stress and psychosocial health among children and adolescents: a meta-analysis. *J Youth Adolesc.* (2006) 35:10–23. doi: 10.1007/s10964-005-9001-x
48. Smith C, Carlson BE. Stress, coping, and resilience in children. *Soc Serv Rev.* (1997) 71:231–56. doi: 10.1086/604249
49. Van Breda AD. *Resilience Theory: A Literature Review.* Pretoria: South African Military Health Service (2001). Available online at: http://www.academia.edu/19596069/Van_Breda_A._D._2001_._Resilience_theory_A_literature_review._Pretoria_South_Africa_South_African_Military_Health_Service
50. Jorm AF, Korten AE, Rodgers B, Pollitt P, Jacomb PA, Christensen H, et al. Belief systems of the general public concerning the appropriate treatments for mental disorders. *Soc Psychiatry Psychiatr Epidemiol.* (1997) 32:468–73.

51. Fudge E, Mason P. Consulting with young people about service guidelines relating to parental mental illness. *Aust J Adv Mental Health* (2004) 3:50–4. doi: 10.5172/jamh.3.2.50
52. Rickwood DJ, Dean FP, Wilson CJ. When and how do young people seek professional help for mental health problems? *Med J Aust.* (2007) 187:S35–9. Available online at: https://www.mja.com.au/journal/2007/187/7/when-and-how-do-young-people-seek-professional-help-mental-health-problems
53. Grové C, Reupert A, Maybery D. The perspectives of young people of parents with a mental illness regarding preferred interventions and supports. *J Child Family Stud.* (2016) 25:3056–65. doi: 10.1007/s10826-016-0468-8
54. Pescosolido B, Martin J, Lang A, Olafsdottir S. Rethinking theoretical approaches to stigma: a framework integrating normative influences on stigma (FINIS). *Soc Sci Med.* (2008) 67:431–40. doi: 10.1016/j.socscimed.2008.03.018
55. Alasuutari M, Jarvi A. "My dad got depression, or something": how do children talk about parental mental disorder? *Qual Res Psychol.* (2012) 9:134–50. doi: 10.1080/14780880903414250
56. Gladstone BM, McKeever P, Seeman M, Boydell KM. Analysis of a support group for children of parents with a mental illness: managing stressful situations. *Qual Health Res.* (2014) 24:1171–82. doi: 10.1177/1049732314528068
57. Gladstone BM, Boydell KM, McKeever P. Recasting research into children's experiences of parental mental illness: Beyond risk and resilience. *Soc. Sci. Med.* (2006) 62:2540–50. doi: 10.1016/j.socscimed.2005.10.038
58. Solantaus T, Paavonen EJ, Toikka S, Punamäki RL. Preventive interventions in families with parental depression: children's psychosocial symptoms and prosocial behaviour. *Eur Child Adol Psychiatry* (2010) 19:883–92. doi: 10.1007/s00787-010-0135-3
59. Pihkala H, Sandlund M, Cederström A. Children in Beardslee's family intervention: relieved by understanding of parental mental illness. *Int J Soc Psychiatry* (2012) 58:623–8. doi: 10.1177/0020764011419055
60. Cooney SM, Huser M, Small S, O'Connor C. (2007). Evidence-based programs: an overview. In: *What Works, Wisconsin- Research to Practice Series.* Madison, WI: University of Wisconsin-Madison and University of Wisconsin-Extension. Available online at: https://wilenet.org/html/justice-programs/programs/juvenile-justice/library/what-works/what-works-practice-briefs-2007-10-evidence-based-programs.pdf
61. O'Connor M, Casey L, Clough B. Measuring mental health literacy – a review of scale-based measures. *J Mental Health* (2014) 23:197–204. doi: 10.3109/09638237.2014.910646
62. O'Connor M, Casey L. The Mental Health Literacy Scale (MHLS): a new scale-based measure of mental health literacy. *Psychiatry Res.* (2015) 229:511–6. doi: 10.1016/j.psychres.2015.05.064
63. Reavley NJ, Morgan AJ, Jorm AF. Development of scales to assess mental health literacy relating to recognition of and interventions for depression, anxiety disorders and schizophrenia/psychosis. *Aust N Z J Psychiatry* (2014) 48:61–9. doi: 10.1177/0004867413491157
64. Kutcher S, Bagnell A, Wei Y. Mental health literacy in secondary schools: a Canadian approach. *Child Adolesc Psychiatr Clin North Am.* (2015) 24:233–44. doi: 10.1016/j.chc.2014.11.007
65. Fraser E, Pakenham KI. Resilience in children of parents with mental illness: relations between mental health literacy, social connectedness and coping, and both adjustment and caregiving. *Psychology, Health, and Medicine* (2009) 14:573–84. doi: 10.1080/13548500903193820
66. Wahl OF, Susin J, Kaplan L, Lax A, Zatina D. Changing knowledge and attitudes with a middle school mental health education curriculum. *Stigma Res Action* (2011) 1:44. doi: 10.5463/sra.v1i1.17
67. Alaska Mental Health Board. *Test Your Knowledge of Mental Illness* (2004).
68. Center for Addiction and Mental Health. *Talking About Mental Illness: A Guide for Developing an Awareness Program for Youth.* Toronto, ON. (2001). p. 70. Available online at: www.camh.net
69. Sherman M, Sherman D. *I'm Not Alone: A Teen Guide to Living With A Parent Who Has a Mental Illness.* Edina, MN: Seeds of Hope (2006).
70. R Core Team. (2017). *R: A Language and Environment for Statistical Computing.* Vienna: R Foundation for Statistical Computing. Available online at: https://www.R-project.org/
71. R Studio Team. *RStudio: Integrated Development for R.* Boston, MA: RStudio, Inc. (2015). Available online at: http://www.rstudio.com/
72. Cai L, Maydeu-Olivares A, Coffman D, Thissen D. Limited-information goodness-of-fit testing of item response theory models for sparse 2P tables. *Br J Math Stat Psychol.* (2006) 59:173–94. doi: 10.1348/000711005X66419
73. Maydeu-Olivares A, Joe H. Limited and full-information estimation and goodness-of-fit testing in 2n contingency tables. *J Am Stat Assoc.* (2005) 100:1009–20. doi: 10.1198/016214504000002069
74. Hooper D, Coughlan J, Mullen MM. Structural equation modelling: guidelines for determining model fit. *Electr J Business Res Methods* (2008) 6:53–60. Available online at: http://www.ejbrm.com/issue/download.html?idArticle=183
75. Diamantopoulos A, Siguaw J. *Introducing LISREL a Guide for the Uninitiated.* Thousand Oaks, CA: Sage Publications (2000). doi: 10.4135/9781849209359
76. Lord FM, Novak MR. *Statistical Theories of Mental Test Scores.* Reading, MA: Addison-Wesley (1968).
77. Orlando M, Thissen D. Likelihood-based item-fit indices for dichotomous item response theory models. *Appl Psychol Measur* (2000) 24:50–64. doi: 10.1177/01466216000241003
78. Orlando M, Thissen D. Further investigation of the performance of S - X2: an item fit index for use with dichotomous item response theory models. *Appl Psychol Measur.* (2003) 27:289–98. doi: 10.1177/0146621603027004004
79. Bond TG, Fox CM. *Applying the Rasch Model: Fundamental Measurement in the Human Sciences* (3rd edn). London: Routledge (2015). doi: 10.4324/9781315814698
80. Linacre JM. What do infit and outfit, mean-square and standardized mean? *Rasch Measur Trans.* (2002) 16:878. Available online at: https://www.rasch.org/rmt/rmt162f.htm
81. Chen WH, Thissen D. Local dependence indexes for item pairs using item response theory. *J Educ Behav Stat.* (1997) 22:265–89. doi: 10.3102/10769986022003265
82. Cai L. SEM of another flavour: two new applications of the supplemented EM algorithm. *Br J Math Stat Psychol.* (2008) 61:309–29. doi: 10.1348/000711007X249603
83. McCubbin H. Adolescent Coping Orientation for Problem Experiences (A-COPE). Available online at: http://performwell.org
84. Morris SB, DeShon RP. Combining effect size estimates in meta-analysis with repeated measures and independent-groups designs. *Psychol Methods* (2002). 7:105–25. doi: 10.1037/1082-989X.7.1.105
85. Riebschleger J, Onaga E, Tableman B, Bybee D. Mental health consumer parents' recommendations for psychoeducation for their minor children. *Psychiatr Rehab J.* (2014) 37:183–5. doi: 10.1037/prj0000071
86. Marshall C, Rossman GB. *Designing Qualitative Research* (6th ed). Los Angeles, CA: Sage (2016).
87. Gladstone BM. Thinking about children of parents with mental illnesses as a form of intergenerational dialog and practice. In: Reupert A, Mayberry D, Nicholson J, Göphert M, Seeman MV, editors. *Parental Psychiatric Disorder: Distressed Parents and Their Families.* Cambridge: Cambridge University Press. (2015). p. 85–95.
88. Sin J, Jordan CD, Barley EA, Henderson C, and Norman I. Psychoeducation for siblings of people with severe mental illness. *Cochrane Database Syst Rev.* (2015). CD010540. doi: 10.1002/14651858.CD010540.pub2

3

Psychoeducational Intervention for Perinatal Depression

*Luca Steardo Jr.[1], Vito Caivano[1], Gaia Sampogna[1], Arcangelo Di Cerbo[1], Giovanna Fico[1], Francesca Zinno[1], Valeria Del Vecchio[1], Vincenzo Giallonardo[1], Marco Torella[2], Mario Luciano[1] and Andrea Fiorillo[1]**

[1] *Department of Psychiatry, University of Campania Luigi Vanvitelli, Naples, Italy,*

[2] *Department of Gynecology, University of Campania Luigi Vanvitelli, Naples, Italy*

***Correspondence:**
Andrea Fiorillo
andrea.fiorillo@unicampania.it

Perinatal depression (PD) is a severe and disabling condition impacting negatively on children in terms of adverse neonatal outcomes and on the well-being of women and their families. All pregnant women attending the unit of Gynecology and Obstetrics Service of the University of Campania "L. Vanvitelli" will be screened for PD using the Edinburgh Postpartum Depression Scale (EPDS). Women with a score $\geq$10 at the EPDS will be invited to receive a full psychiatric assessment. The required sample size is of 126 women with PD which will be randomly allocated to either an experimental group, receiving a uni-familiar psychoeducational intervention, or to a control group, receiving the Best Treatment Option (BTO). Patients will be evaluated through several assessment instruments: Hamilton Depression Rating Scale (HAM-D), Hamilton Anxiety Rating Scale (HAM-A), Global Assessment of Functioning (GAF), Clinical Global Impression (CGI), Manchester Short Assessment of Quality of Life (MANSA), Family Assessment Device (FAD), Family Coping Questionnaire (FCQ), and Pattern of Care Schedule (PCS). Patients will be evaluated at baseline, 3, 6, 9, and 12 months post-randomization. The severity of depressive symptoms at the HAM-D scale has been selected as primary outcome. Other outcome measures include improvement in the severity of anxiety symptoms, of global and personal functioning, an improvement in family members' coping strategies and in the level of quality of life. It has been highlighted the importance of developing screening and treating programs for PD, and our study will use rigorous study design to evaluate the efficacy of the adaption of a well-known family psychoeducational model to the treatment of PD. The aims of present trial are to: (1) develop an informative package for pregnant women with PD; (2) promote a screening programme for PD; (3) identify those (socio-demographic and pregnancy-related environmental) factors associated with a higher risk to develop a perinatal or postnatal depression; (4) evaluate the efficacy of a new experimental psychoeducational intervention in reducing the depressive symptoms during pregnancy compared to the BTO.

Keywords: perinatal depression, women mental health, severe mental disorders, family burden, coping strategies

INTRODUCTION

Depressive disorders represent the major cause of disability worldwide (1, 2). These disorders are prevalent in the perinatal period and about 12% of women are affected (3). However, prevalence rates of perinatal depression (PD) should be cautiously considered since this disorder is frequently underdiagnosed, mainly because patients experience delays and difficulties in help-seeking due to feelings of guilty and fear of stigmatization (4, 5). PD poses a significant burden on affected women, their families and on society at large; moreover, it carries serious long-term consequences on the mental health of the new born (6, 7). In particular, PD can have several detrimental effects including low birth weight, preterm birth, small development for gestational age, early childhood developmental delays, poor maternal fetal attachment, impairments in cognitive functioning, behavioral disturbances, and development of depressive disorders in the childhood or adolescence (8–16).

Different risk factors have been identified for PD, including low socioeconomic status (17–19), being a single mother (17, 20), poor social support (21), general life stress (17), and unplanned pregnancies (22). Indeed, PD is associated with a dysregulation and hyperactivity of the hypothalamic-pituitary-adrenal axis activity (HPA) (23), with an increased exposition to the corticotrophin-releasing hormone (CRH) during intrauterine development.

Several interventions have been developed for reducing the impact of risk factors and for preventing the development of PD (24), including professionally-based home visits, postpartum peer-based telephone support, interpersonal psychotherapy (25), and cognitive behavioral therapy (26). Although several of these interventions have been made available in clinical practice, research is needed in order to confirm their efficacy (27).

Symptoms of perinatal depression often include anxiety, irritability, sleep disturbance, low mood, and excessive concern for the child's care (28), in fact, PD is a multi-faceted and complex condition which can have heterogeneous clinical presentations (15). In particular, a significant number of women with PD experience comorbid anxiety (29, 30), obsessive-compulsive symptoms and post-traumatic stress disorders (31).

One of the main debated issues regarding the optimal prevention and treatment of perinatal depression is related to the opportunity to early detect the disorder through screening procedures (32, 33). In particular, it has been argued that screening programmes can be effective in reducing burden and disability associated with the disorder (34), although there is the risk to create false-positives (35). Screening procedures aim to detect people at high risk to develop a full-blown disorder, and therefore the clinical utility of the screening process is greatly influenced by the ability to accurately identify those patients (33–35).

However, screening programmes are considered acceptable and even desirable by most pregnant women, both depressed and non-depressed (36). Therefore, available guidelines (37, 38) recommend that healthcare professionals (including midwives, obstetricians, health visitors, and general practitioners) ask questions about past or present mental illness, family history of perinatal mental illness and previous psychiatric treatments including inpatient care. Moreover, the American Academy of Pediatrics also recommend that pediatricians screen new mothers for depression during their visits in the 6 months following childbirth (39).

According to a recent review (40), treatment of PD depends on symptom severity and functional impairment (41, 42). Cognitive behavioral therapy (43), interpersonal psychotherapy, and psychoeducation (44, 45) are usually adopted in case of mild to moderate forms of PD; while antidepressants, more often selective serotonin reuptake inhibitors (SSRI), are used for severe cases (46–51).

When available, pregnant women with PD prefer psychotherapy (52) and the effectiveness of psychological and psychosocial treatments for PD has been explored (53).

Several initiatives have been proposed worldwide in order to assess the efficacy and feasibility of psychoeducational interventions for women with PD. A recent meta-analysis by Sockel (26) found only one study (54) evaluating the efficacy of a psychoeducational programme for women with PD in improving depressive symptoms. More recently, other programmes have been proposed also in low-middle income countries (55).

Psychoeducational interventions are effective in reducing affective symptoms and the levels of stress, with low costs for the mental health department (56).

Based on these premises, the Department of Psychiatry of the University of Campania "Luigi Vanvitelli" is carrying out a study to develop and test the efficacy of a psychoeducational family intervention in pregnant women with perinatal depression and their close relatives.

To our knowledge no randomized controlled trial has been carried out so far in Italy on the effectiveness of psychoeducational interventions for women affected by perinatal depression, although psychoeducational intervention has demonstrated its efficacy in a wide range of severe mental disorders, such as bipolar disorder (57), schizophrenia (58), major depression (59), obsessive compulsive disorder (60), and eating disorders (61).

AIMS

The present trial aims to evaluate the efficacy and feasibility of a new psychoeducational family intervention compared to the Best Treatment Option (BTO) in a sample of women affected by perinatal depression and their family members. The Best Treatment Option (BTO) is provided according to the NICE guidelines (62). In particular, mild to moderate forms of depression may be addressed with self-help or psychological counseling. For moderate or severe forms of PD, high-intensity psychological intervention, or pharmacological treatments are recommended.

The secondary aims are to: (1) improve mental health literacy on the topic of perinatal depression, with a specific focus on risk and protective factors as well as on available therapeutic strategies for the management of perinatal depression; (2)

identify clinical, socio-cultural, and pregnancy-related predictive factors for the development of perinatal depression; (3) improve coping strategies and family functioning of family members participating to the intervention; (4) evaluate the long-term effects of the intervention.

METHODS

Design

This is a randomized controlled trial with two parallel arms for evaluating the efficacy and effectiveness of psychoeducational family intervention in improving depressive symptoms in patients with perinatal depression. The new psychoeducational intervention has been developed by the research staff, based on the Falloon model of psychoeducation for patients with schizophrenia and their families (63).

PATIENTS' RECRUITMENT PROCEDURE

Recruitment for the RCT will be conducted adopting a multistep strategy, as reported in **Figure 1**:

- Step 1. All pregnant women attending the outpatient unit of Gynecology and Obstetrics of the University of Campania "Luigi Vanvitelli" will be invited to participate in the study through the use of informative leaflets on perinatal depression (i.e., characteristics of the disorder, risks, long-term consequences, available treatments). Those interested in having more information will be referred to a research team member presenting a brief overview of study procedures and time commitment in order to obtain their informed consent. Once informed consent is obtained, patients will be officially enrolled in the study and will undergo the screening procedure, compiling the Edinburgh Postnatal Depression Scale (EPDS) (64).
- Step 2. Women with a score $\geq$10 at the EPDS will be invited to receive a full psychiatric assessment.
- Step 3. Patients will receive a full mental state examination by an expert clinician working at the Department of Psychiatry of the University of Campania "Luigi Vanvitelli," in order to evaluate the presence of any mental disorder.
- Step 4. Once a diagnosis of perinatal depression is made, patient's code will be given to the statistician for randomization in one of the two groups. Patients will be allocated through a randomized procedure (with a 1:1 ratio) to the experimental or to the control group.

INCLUSION CRITERIA

Starting from January 2019, patients attending the outpatient unit of Gynecology and Obstetrics of the University of Campania "Luigi Vanvitelli" will be invited to participate to the study. The eligibility criteria will be: (1) gestation age > 3 months or within 3 days of childbirth; (2) age $\geq$ 18 years; (3) absence of any disabling physical condition; (4) living with a relative for at least 9 months in the last year and continuously in the last 3 months.

EXCLUSION CRITERIA

Exclusion criteria will be: (1) intellectual disability; (2) diagnosis of schizophrenia, schizoaffective disorder, delusional disorder, or other not specified psychosis-spectrum disorder; (3) having experienced depressive symptoms before pregnancy.

INTERVENTION

Theoretical Background of the Experimental Intervention

Experimental intervention includes techniques derived from classic psychoeducation (63), motivational intervention (65, 66) and cognitive behavioral therapy (67). The intervention has been developed following the guidelines on the management of perinatal depression released by NICE (62), the American College of Obstetricians and Gynecologists (68) and the United States' Preventive Service Task Force (69). The adopted methodology included the following phases: (1) analysis of the scientific literature; (2) evaluation of available handbooks and manuals of other psychosocial interventions targeting perinatal depression; (3) focus groups with expert researchers, clinicians, users and carers, in order to identify the most relevant information to be included in the intervention; (4) development of an *ad-hoc* manual with a detailed description of each session of the intervention, booklets, and other written materials are provided to patients and relatives, whenever relevant; (5) evaluation of the feasibility of the "pilot" intervention in a small-size study.

Features of the Experimental Intervention

The intervention consists in a uni-familiar psychoeducational intervention, scheduled every 7–10 days. It includes six modules on:

1) Individual and family assessment. This module is focused on the assessment of patients' personal and social functioning, and on the identification of personal goals. Moreover, the communication skills adopted by family members are evaluated as well as the characteristics of family functioning.
2) Information on the clinical characteristics of the disorder and its treatment. In this module, information on the main clinical and epidemiological features of PD, including incidence, prevalence, long-term outcome, risk for the children, and negative impact on mother's mental health are presented. Moreover, available pharmacological and non-pharmacological treatment options are discussed, with a specific focus on the risk/benefit ratio for each approach and the importance to be compliant with the therapy. Moreover, during these sessions, the patient is invited to actively participate as the "expert," describing her own personal experience. At the end of the session, an informative booklet will be provided to patients and their family members, summarizing the main aspects discussed during the session.
3) Early warning signs. The third session is focused on the early warning signs of perinatal depression (e.g., changes in the number of sleeping hours; presence of irritability; anxiety;

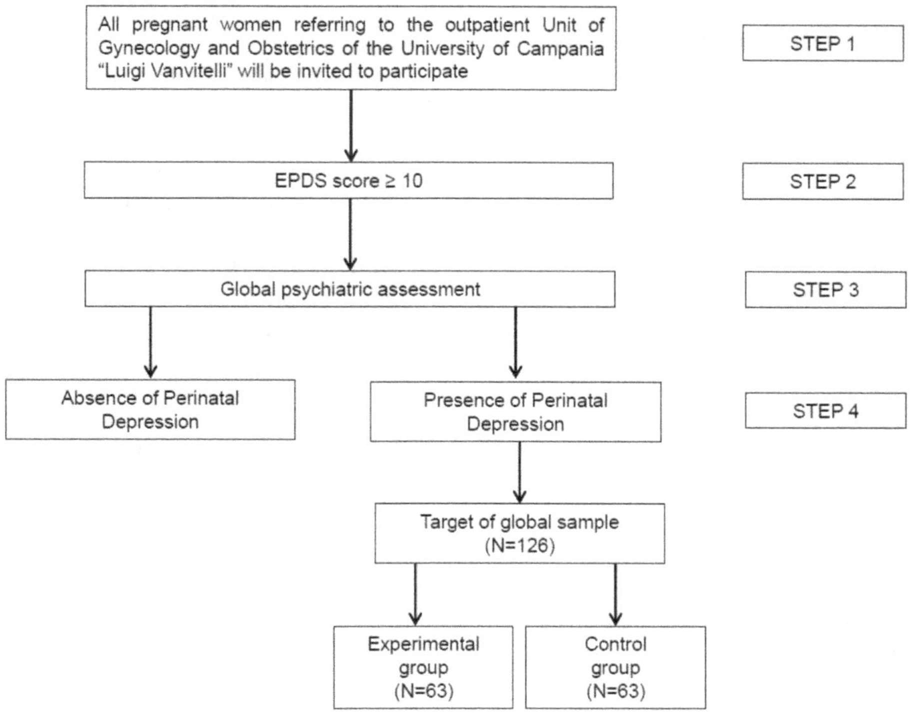

FIGURE 1 | Multi-step recruitment procedure.

etc.) and on the importance to early detect such signs. In particular, patients are requested to identify, with the support of the mental health professional, their own warning signs and to report them on the "Schedule on early warning signs." Strategies for preventing or managing crises are discussed and reported in the same schedule.

4) Management of suicidal behaviors. This module is focused on suicidal risk and on the identification of warning suicidal signs. During this module, an *ad-hoc* schedule is provided to participants and family members in order to define a plan to be used in case of necessity.
5) Communication skills sessions are focused on teaching strategies on how to express pleasant or unpleasant feelings, and on how to improve active listening. This module includes the use of role-plays and case vignettes, based on the personal experience of the patients and their family members.
6) Problem solving skills. The last session is focused on teaching problem-solving techniques. Participants are invited to define a problem in their daily routine and to list all potential strategies to solve it. During the session, participants are guided by mental health professional to develop a plan for solving the problem and discuss possible advantages and disadvantages of each possible solution.

Each session lasts about 90 min. Moreover, two or more booster sessions are planned, if needed. Sessions are developed in order to stimulate discussion and interaction among participants. Site and frequency of sessions can be adapted to families' needs and mental health professionals' duties and workloads. The intervention will be carried out at the local mental health center and provided by trained mental health professionals, the time to complete all modules will be between 42 and 60 days. An *ad-hoc* manual has been developed by the research group in order to ensure treatment fidelity. Leaflets and other written materials will be given to patients and family members, when relevant (**Table 1**).

Control Intervention

Patients allocated in the control intervention will receive the best treatment option (BTO) according to the NICE guidelines (62). At each assessment point, the BTO will be documented through the use of the Pattern of Care Schedule (PCS), an *ad-hoc* schedule filled in by the researcher together with the treating psychiatrist. PCS aims to collect all the information related to the treatments received by the patient. Moreover, patients will continue to be in contact with the treating psychiatrist and whether necessary will receive psychological counseling, both individual, or familiar.

TRAINING OF MENTAL HEALTH PROFESSIONALS

Three mental health professionals (at least one will be a psychiatrist) will receive an *ad-hoc* training course for the provision of the experimental intervention. Supervision meetings will be organized during the study period in order to ensure fidelity to the procedure.

TABLE 1 | Characteristics of the interventions.

PSYCHOEDUCATIONAL FAMILY INTERVENTION
Uni-familiar psychoeducational intervention, scheduled every 7–10 days. It consists of six modules: • Individual and family assessment • Information on the clinical and epidemiological characteristics of the disorder • Early warning signs • Management of suicidal behaviors • Communication skills • Problem solving skills Each session lasts about 90 min. Moreover, two or more booster sessions will be planned, if needed. Sessions are developed in order to stimulate discussion and interaction among participants. Leaflets and other written materials will be given to patients and family members when relevant.
BEST TREATMENT OPTION (BTO)
Provided according to the NICE guidelines • Persistent subthreshold depressive symptoms/ mild to moderate depression: self-help and psychological counseling • History of severe depression who initially presents with mild depression: pharmacological treatment • Moderate or severe depression: high intensity psychological intervention, or pharmacological treatments, or an integration of both interventions.

ETHICAL ISSUES

This study is being conducted in accordance with globally accepted standards of good clinical practice, in agreement with the Declaration of Helsinki and with national and local regulations. The study investigators ensure that all mental health professionals involved in the study are qualified and informed about the protocol, interventions, and trial-related duties. The study protocol has been submitted to the Ethical Review Board of the University of Campania "Luigi Vanvitelli."

ASSESSMENT TIME AND INSTRUMENTS

Researchers participating to the study are blinded to patient allocation. All patients are assessed at the following time points: baseline (T0); 3 months post-randomization (T1); 6 months post-randomization (T2); 9 months post-randomization (T3); 12 months post-randomization (T4) (**Table 2**).

The following questionnaires and schedules will be used during the study:

1. The Edinburgh Postnatal Depression Scale (EPDS) (64) is a simple and short 10-items self-report screening questionnaire initially developed for use in postnatal women to improve detection of postnatal depression. The EPDS allows health professionals to detect women who might need help and require a referral for a full diagnostic assessment. EPDS has satisfactory sensitivity and specificity values and it is also sensitive to changes in severity of depression over time. For the purpose of the present study, the cut-off threshold has been set at ≥ 10 (66). In validation studies, different cut-off points have been found due to clinical, social, cultural and economic diversities (70). The cut-off score for possible depression (i.e., a positive screening result) is $\geq$13 points but, as suggested by Hewitt et al. (71), a cut-off score $\geq$ 10 can be used in order to identify patients with both major or minor depression. Moreover, given the observed variability in the performance of the test, the screening procedure could produce both false positives and negatives (72). Therefore, it is essential that this screening tool is complemented by the clinical judgment (73).
2. The Hamilton Depression Rating Scale (HAM-D) (74) is a 17-items questionnaire used to rate the severity of depressive symptoms such as low mood, insomnia, agitation, anxiety and weight loss. The interview and scoring take about 15 min. The score for each item ranges from 0 (not present) to 4 (extreme severity).
3. The Hamilton Anxiety Rating Scale (HAM-A) (75) is a 14-items questionnaire developed to measure the severity of anxiety symptoms, both psychic anxiety (mental agitation and psychological distress) and somatic anxiety (physical complaints related to anxiety). The score for each item ranges from 0 (not present) to 4 (extreme severity).
4. The Global Assessment of Functioning (GAF) (76) is a 100-point rating scale assessing social, occupational, and psychological functioning of adults, with higher scores indicating better level of functioning.
5. The Clinical Global Impression (CGI) (77) scale measures illness severity (CGI-S), global change (CGI-C) and therapeutic response. The CGI-S is rated on a 7-point scale, from 1 (normal) to 7 (the most severely ill patients). The CGI-C scores range from 1 (very much improved) to 7 (very much worse). Treatment response ratings should take into account both the therapeutic efficacy and the treatment-related adverse events, and range from 0 (marked improvement and no side-effects) to 4 (unchanged or worse, and side-effects outweigh the therapeutic effects). Each component of the CGI is rated separately; the instrument does not provide a global score.
6. The Manchester Short Assessment of Quality of Life (MANSA) (78) is a 17-item questionnaire assessing quality of life focusing on satisfaction in twelve aspects of life. For twelve items, the satisfaction is rated on 7-point rating scales, ranging from 1 ("could not be worse") to 7 ("could not be better"). For five items, the responses are binary ("yes" or "no"). The total MANSA score is the mean of the Likert-item scores.
7. The Family Assessment Device (FAD) (79), based on the McMaster Model of Family Functioning, consists of 7 subscales on family involvement in patient's care (affective involvement, affective responsiveness, behavioral control, communication, problem solving, and roles and general family functioning). Scores range from 1 ("healthy functioning") to 4 ("unhealthy functioning").
8. The Family Coping Questionnaire (FCQ) (80) is a self-administered 34-items questionnaire, which has shown a good reliability and external validity. Each item is rated on a 4-level scale, from 1 ("never") to 4 ("always"). The items are grouped into the following 11 subscales: information on patient's illness; positive communication toward the

TABLE 2 | Assessment tools adopted in the study's protocol.

	Screening phase	T0 (baseline)	T1 (month 3)	T2 (month 6)	T3 (month 9)	T4 (month 12)
ASSESSMENT INSTRUMENT						
Edinburgh Postnatal Depression Scale (EPDS)	x					
Hamilton Depression Rating Scale (HAM-D)		x	x	x	x	x
Hamilton Anxiety Rating Scale (HAM-A)		x	x	x	x	x
Global Assessment of Functioning (GAF)		x	x	x	x	x
Clinical Global Impression (CGI)		x	x	x	x	x
Manchester Short Assessment of Quality of Life (MANSA)		x	x	x	x	x
Family Assessment Device (FAD)		x	x	x	x	x
Family Coping Questionnaire (FCQ)		x	x	x	x	x
Socio-demographic schedule		x	x	x	x	x
Pattern of Care Schedule (PCS)		x	x	x	x	x

patient; relatives' maintenance of social interests; patient's involvement in social activities; talking with friends about the patient's condition; coercion; avoidance; resignation; use of alcohol and drugs; collusion; search for spiritual help. The FCQ is widely used for the assessment of coping strategies among relatives of people with severe mental disorders (81, 82).

9. The Pattern of Care Schedule (PCS) (80), a 40-item questionnaire on pharmacological and non-pharmacological treatments as well as on health care access made by the patient. It is compiled by the researcher in collaboration with the patient. If information is inadequate, or if the researcher is not sure about patients' reliability, other sources (e.g., treating physician, relatives, etc.) can be consulted. During the study period, the treating clinician will continue to provide the usual treatment to patient, and–if necessary–to change or adjust the pharmacological regimen. This schedule is used in order to record pharmacological treatments and doses, psychotherapeutic and psychosocial interventions (type of intervention, number of sessions) provided to patients in order to document the BTO.

BASELINE ASSESSMENTS

At baseline the following information will be collected: (1) sociodemographic data (age, nationality, educational level, marital status, employment status, number of family members, duration of the illness, time in charge at the mental health center (months), number of (voluntary and involuntary) hospitalizations, suicide attempts (numbers); (2) clinical features related to pregnancy (gestational period, previous pregnancies, *in vitro* fertilization, clinical conditions of the fetus, and the pregnant); (3) social context, such as relationship with the partner, family conflicts, socio-economic stressors, history of any psychiatric disorder (**Table 3**).

TABLE 3 | Baseline assessments.

Sociodemographic data	Clinical features related to pregnancy	Social context
• Age	• Gestational period	• Relationship with the partner
• Nationality	• Previous pregnancies	• Family conflicts
• Educational level	• *In vitro* fertilization	• Socio-economic stressors
• Marital status	• Clinical conditions of the fetus and the pregnant	• History of any mental disorder
• Employment status		
• Number of family members		
• Duration of the illness		
• Time in charge at the mental health center		
• Number of hospitalizations		
• Suicide attempts		

STATISTICAL ANALYSES

Power Analysis

In order to assess the efficacy of the experimental intervention, a power analysis was performed. As reported by Sockol et al. (83), available psychosocial interventions for perinatal depression have been found to have an overall effect size of 0.65. Therefore, the sample size has been defined selecting 0.65 as desired level of effect size, an α error set at 0.05 and power set at 0.95. Therefore, the total sample will consist of 126 patients, allocated with a 1:1 ratio to the experimental or to the control group (**Figure 1**).

Data Analysis

Differences in socio-demographic and clinical characteristics, such as severity of depressive and anxiety symptoms, quality of life, trimester of pregnancy, and personal functioning between the two groups will be evaluated using Chi-square or T-test for independent samples, as appropriate. Differences in coping strategies and in family accommodation reported by relatives will be evaluated with the same tests.

In order to assess the efficacy of the experimental intervention, a linear multivariable regression model will be implemented, using as main outcome the score at HAM-D at 3 months post-randomization. Moreover, several confounding variables (such as age, marital status, familiarity for mental disorders, peer support, previous pregnancy, etc.) will be entered in the model. Furthermore, predictors of response at the end of the intervention will be identified.

"Response" is generally defined as a 50% decrease in scores on Hamilton Depression Rating Scale (HAMD) (74). In this protocol, we will consider the score at the 3-month HAM-D compared with the baseline score. Therefore, the continuous variable "3-month HAM-D score" will be transformed in a binary variable (1 = response; 0 = absence of response), and it will be entered in a logistic regression multivariate model in order to identify possible predictors of positive response to the experimental intervention.

In order to evaluate differences in relatives' coping strategies according to patients' clinical features and type of relationship with the patient, a two-level model with fixed independent variables and random intercept, using a maximum likelihood estimation, will be performed. The mean score at the subscales of the FCQ will be entered in the model, adding covariates step by step in order to identify the model with indexes of best fit. The final model will be selected according to the−2 loglikelihood value, and the model with the lowest value will be choose. Estimate, standard error, 95% confidence interval, and P-values will be calculated.

The level of significance will be set at $p < 0.05$. All analyses will be performed using the Statistical Package for Social Science software (SPSS), version 18.0 (SPSS).

STEPWISE PROCEDURE

From month 1 to 6, the following phases have been carried out: (1) development of the work plan for data collection; (2) training course for mental health professionals on the interventions; (3) training course for researchers on assessment tools. From month 7 to 12, patients' recruitment will be implemented. From month 7 to 18, interventions will be provided to participating patients. From month 7 to 20, patients' follow-up assessments are being made. From month 20 to 24, statistical analyses will be performed as well as findings will be disseminated through scientific papers, posters and conference participation. A specific plan for dissemination will be developed, including institutional newsletters, press and media release, flyers, training course throughout the national context in order to promote the implementation of the intervention on a large scale. Moreover, users and carers will be involved in the process of dissemination organizing thematic conferences for presenting the characteristics of the intervention.

The stepwise procedure is summarized in **Figure 2**.

ANTICIPATED RESULTS

Primary Outcome

The severity of depressive symptoms, evaluating at the HAM-D, has been selected as primary outcome since it is a reliable index and it has already been used in previous studies on the efficacy of psychosocial interventions (84). In particular, the primary outcome is the reduction of at least 50% of the HAM-D scoring at 3 months post-randomization (T1). The work hypothesis is that BTO plus experimental intervention will be

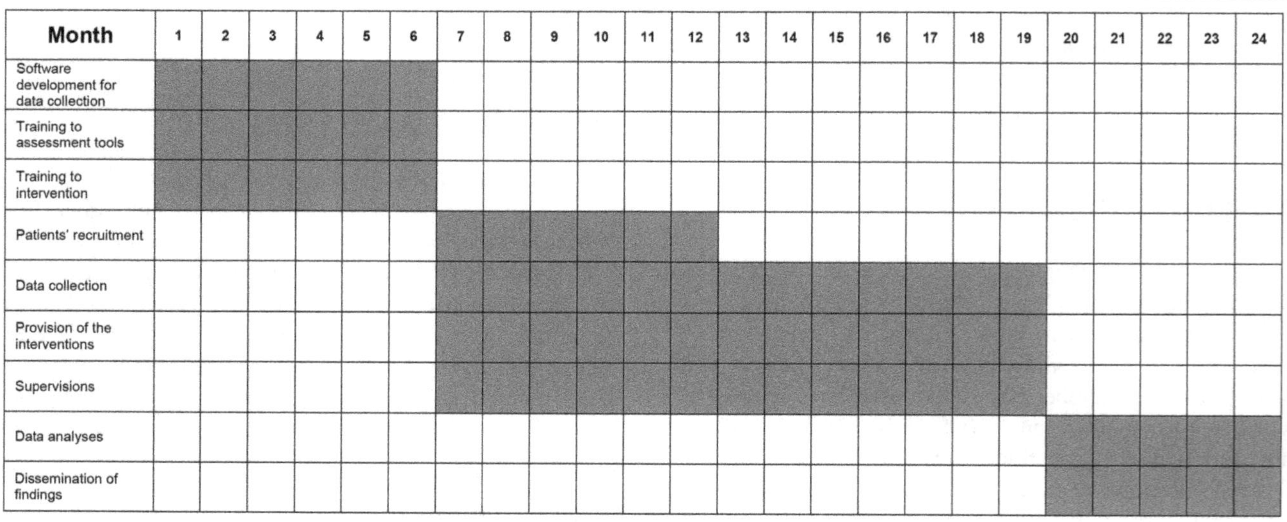

FIGURE 2 | Stepwise procedure.

more effective than the BTO alone in reducing the severity of depressive symptomatology.

Secondary Outcome

The secondary outcomes include an improvement in the severity of anxiety symptoms (evaluating at the HAM-A), of global functioning and personal functioning (evaluated at the CGI and at the GAF, respectively), an improvement in family members' coping strategies (i.e., an improvement in "problem-oriented" strategies reduction); in the level of quality of life (evaluated at the MANSA) and of family functioning.

DISCUSSION

Pregnancy is a stressful period for women, which can be further complicated by an early postnatal hospital discharge (85, 86). Risk factors for PD include previous mental disorders, low socioeconomic status, being a single mother, general life stress (12), unwanted and unplanned pregnancies (22), conflicts with the partner, lack of support, limited information, and stigma (87).

Despite many scientific associations and task forces, including the United States' Preventive Services Task Force (USPSTF) (88), the National Institute for Health and Care Excellence (62), the Canadian Task Force on Preventive Health Care (CTFPHC) (89) and the American College of Obstetricians and Gynecologists (68), have highlighted the importance of developing screening and treating programs for PD, there are still many unsolved issues, such as efficacy and the availability of those programs, whose efficacy has been demonstrated by RCTs.

One of the main strengths of our study is represented by the adaption of a well-known family psychoeducational model to the treatment of perinatal depression. In particular, the Falloon psychoeducational intervention was developed for the community management of schizophrenia (63, 90) and has been subsequently adapted to the management of major depression (59, 91) and bipolar disorder (57, 92–94). Perinatal depression may represent an ideal target for this kind of interventions, since it is highly dependent from stressful life events and from family context. Moreover, peripartum is a period of women's life in which pharmacological treatments should be used very cautiously and only in a limited situations. Another strength of our study is the rigorous methodology adopted, which will allow us to understand the impact of the experimental intervention on patient's outcome through a randomized controlled approach. Moreover, the main outcome is the reduction of depressive symptoms at 3-months after randomization. This is an ambitious outcome, since many confounding variables can impact on it. In particular, in some cases the childbirth represents itself an event associated with a reduction of depressive symptoms (95), thus biasing the effectiveness of the experimental intervention. Moreover, other contextual factors (such as support by family members, changes in the daily routine following the childbirth, or starting a pharmacological treatment) can have an impact on the long-term outcome. We aim to control for such variables using a statistical procedure, in order to accommodate for the impact of all these confounding variables.

Furthermore, the postnatal psychoeducation programme is suitable for clinical use as it is relatively brief and can be delivered by postnatal unit nurses and midwives after a short period of training.

Another strength of this study is the use of the EPDS as screening measure, which will allow comparisons with data from other international studies.

In order to detect patients affected by both major and minor depression, the cut-off at EPDS of $\geq$10 has been selected (71) and it will have to be complemented by the clinical judgment (96).

The assessment tools have been selected on the basis of their wide use in clinical practice and in clinical trials (84). Therefore, the adoption of these instruments will give us the opportunity to compare our findings with those of other previous studies. Moreover, the HAM-A and HAM-D are well-known, validated, reliable, and easy to use scales, and have been selected in order to not overburden the researchers and mental health professionals involved in the study with a specific training on the use of assessment tools (84).

Our study has some limitations. The first is the fact that the study will be carried out in one center only, with a consequent reduced generalizability of findings. However, this can be considered as a pilot study representing the basis for a larger multicentric study that our research group is planning.

Another possible limitation is the exclusion from the study of women with psychotic disorders or women with depressive disorders before pregnancy. This methodological choice was due to the need to assess and treat only patients with an onset of depression during pregnancy. Another possible limitation is the lack of a standardized pharmacological treatment for women that will be recruited for the RCT phase. Despite a standardized pharmacological treatment could be useful to assess more precisely the efficacy of the experimental psychoeducational intervention, we decided not to standardize the pharmacological treatment in order to treat women with PD under ordinary conditions. In any case, the pharmacological management of pregnant women will follow the NICE guidelines (62).

CONCLUSIONS

Perinatal depression represents a serious threat for mental health, also considering the detrimental consequences for children. Therefore, it is an ethical imperative to identify new strategies for adequately treat such conditions and reduce the long-term negative impact on the mothers as well as their babies and family members. We hope that the study we will carry on will help to improve the clinical, psychosocial, and family management of perinatal depression.

AUTHOR CONTRIBUTIONS

LS, VC, ML, MT, GS, and AF designed the study and wrote the protocol. AF, VDV, ML, and LS organized the training and supervision for mental health professionals. ADC, GF, VC, FZ, and VG performed the literature search. GS developed the plan of statistical analyses. LS, AF, MT, and ML coordinated the study.

REFERENCES

1. Friedrich MJ. Depression is the leading cause of disability around the world. *JAMA* (2017) 317:1517. doi: 10.1001/jama.2017.3826
2. Fiorillo A, Carpiniello B, De Giorgi S, La Pia S, Maina G, Sampogna G, et al. Assessment and management of cognitive and psychosocial dysfunctions in patients with major depressive disorder: a clinical review. *Front Psychiatry* (2018) 9:493. doi: 10.3389/fpsyt.2018.00493
3. Woody CA, Ferrari AJ, Siskind DJ, Whiteford HA, Harris MG. A systematic review and meta-regression of the prevalence and incidence of perinatal depression. *J Affect Disord.* (2017) 219:86–92. doi: 10.1016/j.jad.2017.05.003
4. Kingston D, Heaman M, Fell D, Dzakpasu S, Chalmers B. Factors associated with perceived stress and stressful life events in pregnant women: findings from the Canadian maternity experiences survey. *Matern Child Health J.* (2012) 16:158–68. doi: 10.1007/s10995-010-0732-2
5. Herrman H. Improving the mental health of women and girls: psychiatrists as partners for change. *World Psychiatry* (2016) 15:190–1. doi: 10.1002/wps.20316
6. Bauer A, Knapp M, Parsonage M. Lifetime costs of perinatal anxiety and depression. *J Affect Disord.* (2016) 192:83–90. doi: 10.1016/j.jad.2015.12.005
7. Pompili M, Fiorillo A. Editorial: unmet needs in modern psychiatry. *CNS Neurol Disord Drug Targets* (2017) 16:857. doi: 10.2174/187152731608180119110219
8. Susser E, Keyes K, Mascayano F. Healthy pregnancy and prevention of psychosis. *World Psychiatry* (2018) 17:357–8. doi: 10.1002/wps.20554
9. Grigoriadis S, Vonder Porten EH, Mamisashvili L, Tomlinson G, Dennis CL, Koren G, et al. The impact of maternal depression during pregnancy on perinatal outcomes: a systematic review and meta-analysis. *J Clin Psychiatry* (2013) 74:e321–41. doi: 10.4088/JCP.12r07968
10. Leis JA, Heron J, Stuart EA, Mendelson T. Associations between maternal mental health and child emotional and behavioral problems: does prenatal mental health matter? *J Abnorm Child Psychol.* (2014) 42:161–71. doi: 10.1007/s10802-013-9766-4
11. Alhusen JL, Hayat MJ, Gross D. A longitudinal study of maternal attachment and infant developmental outcomes. *Arch Womens Ment Health* (2013) 16:521–9. doi: 10.1007/s00737-013-0357-8
12. Sandman CA, Davis EP, Buss C, Glynn LM. Exposure to prenatal psychobiological stress exerts programming influences on the mother and her fetus. *Neuroendocrinology* (2012) 95:7–21. doi: 10.1159/000327017
13. Cicchetti D, Doyle C. Child maltreatment, attachment and psychopathology: mediating relations. *World Psychiatry* (2016) 15:89–90. doi: 10.1002/wps.20337
14. Morgan C, Gayer-Anderson C. Childhood adversities and psychosis: evidence, challenges, implications. *World Psychiatry* (2016) 15:93–102. doi: 10.1002/wps.20330
15. Yehuda R, Lehrner A. Intergenerational transmission of trauma effects: putative role of epigenetic mechanisms. *World Psychiatry* (2018) 17:243–57. doi: 10.1002/wps.20568
16. Pugliese V, Bruni A, Carbone EA, Calabrò G, Cerminara G, Sampogna G, et al. Maternal stress, prenatal medical illnesses and obstetric complications: risk factors for schizophrenia spectrum disorder, bipolar disorder and major depressive disorder. *Psychiatry Res.* (2018) 13:23–30. doi: 10.1016/j.psychres.2018.11.023
17. Lancaster CA, Gold KJ, Flynn HA, Yoo H, Marcus SM, Davis MM. Risk factors for depressive symptoms during pregnancy: a systematic review. *Am J Obstet Gynecol.* (2010) 202:5–14. doi: 10.1016/j.ajog.2009.09.007
18. Patel V, Burns JK, Dhingra M, Tarver L, Kohrt BA, Lund C. Income inequality and depression: a systematic review and meta-analysis of the association and a scoping review of mechanisms. *World Psychiatry* (2018) 17:76–89. doi: 10.1002/wps.20492
19. Luciano M, Sampogna G, Del Vecchio V, Giacco D, Mulè A, de Rosa C, et al. The family in Italy: cultural changes and implications for treatment. *Int Rev Psychiatry* (2012) 24:149–56. doi: 10.3109/09540261.2012.656306
20. Alhasanat-Khalil D, Fry-McComish J, Dayton C, Benkert R, Yarandi H, Giurgescu C. Acculturative stress and lack of social support predict postpartum depression among U.S. immigrant women of Arabic descent. *Arch Psychiatr Nurs.* (2018) 32:530–5. doi: 10.1016/j.apnu.2018.02.005
21. Southwick SM, Sippel L, Krystal J, Charney D, Mayes L, Pietrzak R. Why are some individuals more resilient than others: the role of social support. *World Psychiatry* (2016) 15:77–9. doi: 10.1002/wps.20282
22. Koleva H, Stuart S, O'Hara MW, Bowman-Reif J. Risk factors for depressive symptoms during pregnancy. *Arch Womens Ment Health* (2011) 14:99–105. doi: 10.1007/s00737-010-0184-0
23. Meltzer-Brody S. New insights into perinatal depression: pathogenesis and treatment during pregnancy and postpartum. *Dialogues Clin Neurosci.* (2011) 13:89–100.
24. Dennis CL, Dowswell T. Psychosocial and psychological interventions for preventing postpartum depression. *Cochrane Database Syst Rev.* (2013) 2:CD001134. doi: 10.1002/14651858.CD001134.pub3
25. Zlotnick C, Tzilos G, Miller I, Seifer R, Stout R. Randomized controlled trial to prevent postpartum depression in mothers on public assistance. *J Affect Disord.* (2016) 189:263–8. doi: 10.1016/j.jad.2015.09.059
26. Sockol LE. A systematic review of the efficacy of cognitive behavioral therapy for treating and preventing perinatal depression. *J Affect Disord.* (2015) 177:7–21. doi: 10.1016/j.jad.2015.01.052
27. Ormel J, Cuijpers P, Jorm AF, Schoevers R. Prevention of depression will only succeed when it is structurally embedded and targets big determinants. *World Psychiatry* (2019) 18:111–2. doi: 10.1002/wps.20580
28. Falah-Hassani K, Shiri R, Dennis CL. Prevalence and risk factors for comorbid postpartum depressive symptomatology and anxiety. *J Affect Disord.* (2016) 198:142–7. doi: 10.1016/j.jad.2016.03.010
29. Reck C, Stehle E, Reinig K, Mundt C. Maternity blues as a predictor of DSM-IV depression and anxiety disorders in the first three months postpartum. *J Affect Disord.* (2009) 113:77–87. doi: 10.1016/j.jad.2008.05.003
30. Mauri M, Oppo A, Montagnani MS, Borri C, Banti S, Camilleri V, et al. Beyond "postpartum depressions": specific anxiety diagnoses during pregnancy predict different outcomes: results from PND-ReScU. *J Affect Disord.* (2010) 127:177–84. doi: 10.1016/j.jad.2010.05.015
31. Stewart DE, Vigod S. Postpartum depression. *N Engl J Med.* (2016) 375:2177–86. doi: 10.1056/NEJMcp1607649
32. Santos H, Tan X, Salomon R. Heterogeneity in perinatal depression: how far have we come? A systematic review. *Arch Womens Ment Health* (2017) 20:11–23. doi: 10.1007/s00737-016-0691-8
33. Chaudron LH, Wisner KL. Perinatal depression screening: let's not throw the baby out with the bath water! *J Psychosom Res.* (2014) 76:489–91. doi: 10.1016/j.jpsychores.2014.03.011
34. Reynolds CF, Patel V. Screening for depression: the global mental health context. *World Psychiatry* (2017) 16:316–7. doi: 10.1002/wps.20459
35. Thombs BD, Arthurs E, Coronado-Montoya S, Roseman M, Delisle VC, Leavens A, et al. Depression screening and patient outcomes in pregnancy or postpartum: a systematic review. J *Psychosom Res.* (2014) 76:433–46. doi: 10.1016/j.jpsychores.2014.01.006
36. Gemmill AW, Leigh B, Ericksen J, Milgrom J. A survey of the clinical acceptability of screening for postnatal depression in depressed and non-depressed women. *BMC Public Health* (2006) 6:211. doi: 10.1186/1471-2458-6-211
37. National Collaborating Centre for Mental Health. *Antenatal and Postnatal Mental Health: Clinical Management and Service Guidance: Updated edition.* London: National Institute for Health and Clinical Excellence: Guidance (2014).
38. American College of Obstetricians and Gynecologists. Committee on obstetric practice. committee opinion no. 453: screening for depression during and after pregnancy. *Obstet Gynecol.* (2010) 115:394–5. doi: 10.1097/AOG.0b013e3181d035aa
39. Earls MF, Committee on Psychosocial Aspects of Child and Family Health American Academy of Pediatrics. Incorporating recognition and management of perinatal and postpartum depression into pediatric practice. *Pediatrics* (2010) 126:1032–9. doi: 10.1542/peds.2010-2348
40. Molenaar NM, Kamperman AM, Boyce P, Bergink V. Guidelines on treatment of perinatal depression with antidepressants: an international review. *Aust N Z J Psychiatry* (2018) 52:320–7. doi: 10.1177/0004867418762057
41. Tosato S, Albert U, Tomassi S, Iasevoli F, Carmassi C, Ferrari S, et al. A systematized review of atypical antipsychotics in pregnant women: balancing between risks of untreated illness and risks of drug-related adverse effects. *J Clin Psychiatry* (2017) 78:e477–89. doi: 10.4088/JCP.15r10483

42. Dell'Osso B, Albert U, Atti AR, Carmassi C, Carrà G, Cosci F, et al. Bridging the gap between education and appropriate use of benzodiazepines in psychiatric clinical practice. *Neuropsychiatr Dis Treat.* (2015) 30:1885–909. doi: 10.2147/NDT.S83130
43. Cuijpers P, Cristea IA, Karyotaki E, Reijnders M, Huibers MJ. How effective are cognitive behavior therapies for major depression and anxiety disorders? A meta-analytic update of the evidence. *World Psychiatry* (2016) 15:245–58. doi: 10.1002/wps.20346
44. Cuijpers P, van Straten A, Andersson G, van Oppen P. Psychotherapy for depression in adults: a meta-analysis of comparative outcome studies. *J Consult Clin Psychol.* (2008) 76:909–22. doi: 10.1037/a0013075
45. Hayes SC, Hofmann SG. The third wave of cognitive behavioral therapy and the rise of process-based care. *World Psychiatry* (2017) 16:245–6. doi: 10.1002/wps.20442
46. Stowe ZN, Casarella J, Landry J, Nemeroff CB. Sertraline in the treatment of women with postpartum major depression. *Depression* (1995) 3:49–55. doi: 10.1002/depr.3050030109
47. Cohen LS, Viguera AC, Bouffard SM, Nonacs RM, Morabito C, Collins MH, et al. Venlafaxine in the treatment of postpartum depression. *J Clin Psychiatry* (2001) 62:592–6. doi: 10.4088/JCP.v62n0803
48. Suri R, Burt VK, Altshuler LL. Nefazodone for the treatment of postpartum depression. *Arch Womens Ment Health* (2005) 8:55–6. doi: 10.1007/s00737-005-0071-2
49. Suri R, Burt VK, Altshuler LL, Zuckerbrow-Miller J, Fairbanks L. Fluvoxamine for postpartum depression. *Am J Psychiatry* (2001) 158:1739–40. doi: 10.1176/appi.ajp.158.10.1739
50. Nonacs RM, Soares CN, Viguera AC, Pearson K, Poitras JR, Cohen LS. Bupropion SR for the treatment of postpartum depression: a pilot study. *Int J Neuropsychopharmacol.* (2005) 8:445–9. doi: 10.1017/S1461145705005079
51. Steinert T. Chance of response to an antidepressant: what should we say to the patient? *World Psychiatry* (2018) 17:114–5. doi: 10.1002/wps.20511
52. van Schaik DJ, Klijn AF, van Hout HP, van Marwijk HW, Beekman AT, de Haan M, et al. Patients' preferences in the treatment of depressive disorder in primary care. *Gen Hosp Psychiatry* (2004) 26:184–9. doi: 10.1016/j.genhosppsych.2003.12.001
53. Dennis CL. Psychosocial interventions for the treatment of perinatal depression. *Best Pract Res Clin Obstet Gynaecol.* (2014) 28:97–111. doi: 10.1016/j.bpobgyn.2013.08.008
54. Honey KL, Bennett P, Morgan M. A brief psycho-educational group intervention for postnatal depression. *Br J Clin Psychol.* (2002) 41:405–9. doi: 10.1348/014466502760387515
55. Gureje O, Oladeji BD, Araya R, Montgomery AA, Kola L, Kirmayer L, et al. Expanding care for perinatal women with depression (EXPONATE): study protocol for a randomized controlled trial of an intervention package for perinatal depression in primary care. *BMC Psychiatry* (2015) 15:136. doi: 10.1186/s12888-015-0537-3
56. Donker T, Griffiths KM, Cuijpers P, Christensen H. Psychoeducation for depression, anxiety and psychological distress: a meta-analysis. *BMC Med.* (2009) 7:79. doi: 10.1186/1741-7015-7-79
57. Fiorillo A, Del Vecchio V, Luciano M, Sampogna G, Sbordone D, Catapano F, et al. Feasibility of a psychoeducational family intervention for people with bipolar I disorder and their relatives: results from an Italian real-world multicentre study. *J Affect Disord.* (2016) 190:657–62. doi: 10.1016/j.jad.2015.10.060
58. Pharoah F, Mari J, Rathbone J, Wong W. Family intervention for schizophrenia. *Cochrane Database Syst Rev.* (2010) 12:CD000088. doi: 10.1002/14651858.CD000088.pub3
59. Shimazu K, Shimodera S, Mino Y, Nishida A, Kamimura N, Sawada K, et al. Family psychoeducation for major depression: randomised controlled trial. *Br J Psychiatry* (2011) 198:385–90. doi: 10.1192/bjp.bp.110.078626
60. Baruah U, Pandian RD, Narayanaswamy JC, Bada Math S, Kandavel T, Reddy YCJ. A randomized controlled study of brief family-based intervention in obsessive compulsive disorder. *J Affect Disord.* (2018) 225:137–46. doi: 10.1016/j.jad.2017.08.014
61. Spettigue W, Maras D, Obeid N, Henderson KA, Buchholz A, Gomez R, et al. A psycho-education intervention for parents of adolescents with eating disorders: a randomized controlled trial. *Eat Disord.* (2015) 23:60–75. doi: 10.1080/10640266.2014.940790
62. National Collaborating Centre for Mental Health. *Antenatal and Postnatal Mental Health: Clinical Management and Service Guidance: Updated edition.* London: National Institute for Health and Clinical Excellence: Guidance (2014).
63. Falloon IRH. *Family Management of Schizophrenia: A Controlled Study of Clinical, Social, Family and Economic Benefits.* Baltimore, MD: John Hopkins University Press (1985).
64. Cox JL, Holden JM, Sagovsky R. Detection of postnatal depression. Development of the 10-item edinburgh postnatal depression scale. *Br J Psychiatry* (1987) 150:782–6. doi: 10.1192/bjp.150.6.782
65. Rogers RW. A protection motivation theory of fear appeals and attitude change. *J Psychol.* (1975) 91:93–114. doi: 10.1080/00223980.1975.9915803
66. Miller WR, Rose GR. Toward a theory of motivational interviewing. *Am Psychol.* (2009) 64:527–37. doi: 10.1037/a0016830
67. Hofmann SG, Asnaani A, Vonk IJ, Sawyer AT, Fang A. The efficacy of cognitive behavioral therapy: a review of meta-analyses. *Cognit Ther Res.* (2012) 36:427–40. doi: 10.1007/s10608-012-9476-1
68. American College of Obstetricians and Gynecologists. Screening for perinatal depression. Committee opinion no. 630. *Obstet Gynecol.* (2015) 125:1268–71. doi: 10.1097/01.AOG.0000465192.34779.dc
69. US Preventive services. Available online at: https://www.uspreventiveservicestaskforce.org/Page/Document/draft-recommendation-statement/perinatal-depression-preventive-interventions
70. Bhusal BR, Bhandari N, Chapagai M, Gavidia T. Validating the edinburgh postnatal depression scale as a screening tool for postpartum depression in Kathmandu, Nepal. *Int J Ment Health Syst.* (2016) 10:71. doi: 10.1186/s13033-016-0102-6
71. Hewitt C, Gilbody S, Brealey S, Paulden M, Palmer S, Mann R, et al. Methods to identify postnatal depression in primary care: an integrated evidence synthesis and value of information analysis. *Health Technol Assess.* (2009) 13:1–145, 147–230. doi: 10.3310/hta13360
72. Milgrom J, Gemmill AW. Screening for perinatal depression. *Best Pract Res Clin Obstet Gynaecol.* (2014) 28:13–23. doi: 10.1016/j.bpobgyn.2013.08.014
73. Maj M. "Clinical judgment" and the DSM-5 diagnosis of major depression. *World Psychiatry* (2013) 12:89–91. doi: 10.1002/wps.20049
74. Hamilton M. A rating scale for depression. *J Neurol Neurosurg Psychiatry* (1960) 23:56–62. doi: 10.1136/jnnp.23.1.56
75. Hamilton M. The assessment of anxiety states by rating. *Br J Med Psychol.* (1959) 32:50–5. doi: 10.1111/j.2044-8341.1959.tb00467.x
76. American Psychiatric Association. *Diagnostic and Statistical Manual of Mental Disorders.* 4th Edn. Washington: American Psychiatric Association (1994). p. 34.
77. Guy W. Clinical Global Impressions. In: Guy W, editor. *ECDEU Assessment Manual for Psychopharmacology, revised.* Rockville, MD: National Institute of Mental Health (1976). p. 218–22.
78. Priebe S, Huxley P, Knight S, Evans S. Application and results of the manchester short assessment of quality of life (MANSA). *Int J Soc Psychiatry* (1999) 45:7–12. doi: 10.1177/002076409904500102
79. Epstein NB, Baldwin LM, Bishop DS. The McMaster family assessment device. *J Martial Fam Ther.* (1983) 9:171–80.
80. Sampogna G, Luciano M, Del Vecchio V, Malangone C, De Rosa C, Giallonardo V, et al. The effects of psychoeducational family intervention on coping strategies of relatives of patients with bipolar I disorder: results from a controlled, real-world, multicentric study. *Neuropsychiatr Dis Treat.* (2018) 14:977–89. doi: 10.2147/NDT.S159277
81. Luciano M, Del Vecchio V, Giacco D, De Rosa C, Malangone C, Fiorillo A. A 'family affair'? The impact of family psychoeducational interventions on depression. *Expert Rev Neurother.* (2012) 12:83–91. doi: 10.1586/ern.11.131
82. Magliano L, Orrico A, Fiorillo A, Del Vecchio H, Castiello G, Malangone C, et al. Family burden in bipolar disorders: results from the Italian Mood Disorder Study (IMDS). *Epidemiol Psychiatr Sci.* (2009) 18:137–46. doi: 10.1017/S1121189X00001020
83. Sockol LE, Epperson CN, Barber JP. A meta-analysis of treatments for perinatal depression. *Clin Psychol Rev.* (2011) 31:839–49. doi: 10.1016/j.cpr.2011.03.009
84. Leucht S, Fennema H, Engel R, Kaspers-Janssen M, Lepping P, Szegedi A. What does the HAMD mean? *J Affect Disord.* (2013) 148:243–8. doi: 10.1016/j.jad.2012.12.001

85. Brown SJ, Davey MA, Bruinsma FJ. Women's views and experiences of postnatal hospital care in the victorian survey of recent mothers 2000. *Midwifery* (2005) 21:109–26. doi: 10.1016/j.midw.2004.09.006
86. Fink AM. Early hospital discharge in maternal and newborn care. *J Obstet Gynecol Neonatal Nurs.* (2011) 40:149–56. doi: 10.1111/j.1552-6909.2011.01225.x
87. Rodríguez MA, Valentine J, Ahmed SR, Eisenman DP, Sumner LA, Heilemann MV, et al. Intimate partner violence and maternal depression during the perinatal period: a longitudinal investigation of Latinas. *Violence Against Women* (2010) 16:543–59. doi: 10.1177/1077801210366959
88. Siu AL, US Preventive Services Task Force (USPSTF), Bibbins-Domingo K, Grossman DC, Baumann LC, Davidson KW, et al. Screening for depression in adults: US preventive services task force recommendation statement. *JAMA* (2016) 315:380–7. doi: 10.1001/jama.2015.18392
89. MacMillan HL, Patterson CJ, Wathen CN, The Canadian task force on preventive health care. Screening for depression in primary care: recommendation statement from the canadian task force on preventive health care. *CMAJ* (2005) 172:33–5. doi: 10.1503/cmaj.1030823
90. McFarlane WR. Family interventions for schizophrenia and the psychoses: a review. *Fam Process* (2016) 55:460–82. doi: 10.1111/famp.12235
91. Brady P, Kangas M, McGill K. "Family Matters": a systematic review of the evidence for family psychoeducation for major depressive disorder. *J Marital Fam Ther.* (2017) 43:245–63. doi: 10.1111/jmft.12204
92. Soo SA, Zhang ZW, Khong SJ, Low JEW, Thambyrajah VS, Alhabsyi SHBT, et al. Randomized controlled trials of psychoeducation modalities in the management of bipolar disorder: a systematic review. *J Clin Psychiatry* (2018) 79:17r11750. doi: 10.4088/JCP.17r11750
93. Fiorillo A, Del Vecchio V, Luciano M, Sampogna G, De Rosa C, Malangone C, et al. Efficacy of psychoeducational family intervention for bipolar I disorder: a controlled, multicentric, real-world study. *J Affect Disord.* (2015) 172:291–9. doi: 10.1016/j.jad.2014.10.021
94. Luciano M, Del Vecchio V, Sampogna G, De Rosa C, Fiorillo A. Including family members in psychoeducation for bipolar disorder: is it worth it? *Bipolar Disord.* (2015) 17:458–9. doi: 10.1111/bdi.12298
95. Bell AF, Carter CS, Davis JM, Golding J, Adejumo O, Pyra M, et al. Childbirth and symptoms of postpartum depression and anxiety: a prospective birth cohort study. *Arch Womens Ment Health* (2016) 19:219–27. doi: 10.1007/s00737-015-0555-7
96. Ben-David V, Jonson-Reid M, Tompkins R. Addressing the missing part of evidence-based practice: the importance of respecting clinical judgment in the process of adopting a new screening tool for postpartum depression. *Issues Ment Health Nurs.* (2017) 38:989–95. doi: 10.1080/01612840.2017.1347221

4

Collective Impact on Prevention: Let's Talk about Children Service Model and Decrease in Referrals to Child Protection Services

Mika Niemelä[1,2,3], Hannu Kallunki[4], Jaana Jokinen[5], Sami Räsänen[2], Birkitta Ala-Aho[4], Helinä Hakko[2,3], Tiina Ristikari[6] and Tytti Solantaus[7,8]**

[1] Center for Life Course Health, Research, University of Oulu, Oulu, Finland, [2] Department of Psychiatry, Oulu University Hospital, Oulu, Finland, [3] Research Unit of Clinical Neurosciences, Department of Psychiatry, University of Oulu, Oulu, Finland, [4] Joint Municipal Authority of Wellbeing in Raahe District, Raahe, Finland, [5] Faculty of Social Sciences, University of Lapland, Rovaniemi, Finland, [6] Adolescents and Families Unit, National Institute for Health and Welfare Children, Oulu, Finland, [7] Finnish Association for Mental Health, Helsinki, Finland, [8] Mental Health Unit, National Institute for Health and Welfare, Helsinki, Finland

***Correspondence:**
Mika Niemelä
mika.niemela@oulu.fi
Tytti Solantaus
Tytti.Solantaus@famh.fi

Background: Families with parental mental health issues often have numerous problems needing multilevel measures to address them. The "Let's Talk about Children Service Model (LT-SM)" is a community-based service approach aiming at collectively impacting population needs regarding child protection services. Three municipalities in the Raahe District (RD) of Finland requested implementation of the LT Service Model. This paper describes the model and first results.

Methods: The LT Service Model connects relevant stakeholders with families and their social networks aiming at the shared goal of supporting children's everyday life at home, kindergarten, school, and leisure environments. Parents, teachers, and other caretakers are supported by LT interventions. An infrastructure for collaboration, decision making, monitoring, training, and feedback is established, embracing health, social and educational services, and other stakeholders. Referrals to child protection services were compared with national data before (2009–2013) and after implementation of the LT Service Model (2013–2016). Analyses were conducted using the joinpoint regression method.

Results: There was a significant decrease in the underage population referred to child protection services in RD (AAPC = −6.9; $p = 0.013$) between 2013 and 2016, in contrast with an increased rate nationwide (AAPC = 1.9; $p = 0.020$).

Conclusion: In the LT Service Model, prevention starts in children's everyday life as the uniting, common goal for multiple stakeholders and an integrated service structure is developed to support this effort. The first results are promising, showing an appreciable decrease in referrals to child protection services, although further research with longer follow-up and across other municipalities is needed.

Keywords: collective impact, child protection services, family adversity, Let's Talk about Children intervention, Let's Talk about Children Service Model, parental mental health disorders, prevention

INTRODUCTION

Intergenerational transfer of parental problems and family adversity is an individual, family, and societal concern. In Finland, parental mental health and substance abuse problems, often associated with other adversities, are also major reasons for child protection measures (1). Family adversity, as well as family resilience, is multi-determined and embedded in the social ecology of the family and society (2). Multilevel prevention is necessary (3) and comprehensive approaches are needed to achieve a collective impact on population-level outcomes (4).

The "Let's Talk about Children Service Model (LT-SM)" is a community-based model for promoting child and family well-being and resilience and preventing family and child dysfunction. It is aimed to overcome the fragmentation of services and lack of common goals, which have been major obstacles for integrated approaches in health, social, and educational services (4). The core of LT-SM is supporting children in their everyday life at home, kindergarten, school, and leisure environments (children's developmental contexts). Parental and family problems interfere with everyday routines and interactions with a risk of compromising the child's well-being and development (3). In LT-SM, health and social services, as well as kindergartens, schools, and available non-governmental organizations, commit to a shared goal: to support, in collaboration with others, children's everyday life in all developmental contexts and to build the corresponding service structure.

Within this model, LT interventions (5–8)[1] are used with families; LT is a relational, cognitive, and behavioral intervention approach aiming to support parents, teachers, and other caretakers in their everyday interactions and activities with children. It is used within mental health and substance use services as well as in cases of severe somatic conditions. In kindergartens and schools, LT for Schools and Early Education (mielenterveysseura.fi) is used universally. The focus is to enhance sensitive and supportive interactions with the child as well as mutually supportive parent-teacher relationships based on a shared understanding of the child at home and school. Children participate in this program depending on their age.

LT Intervention 2018 (www.mielenterveysseura.fi) includes two steps. LT-Discussion depicts the child's ordinary day in all developmental contexts and an action plan is made with parents to enhance the identified strengths and to give support in vulnerabilities; this step is performed in one or two semi-structured meetings. When needed, the second step LT-Network meeting is planned with parents and convened to carry out the necessary support with the family's social network, services, and possible others. LT-Network meeting provides a forum for case-based cross-sectoral collaboration, including also the families and their social network.

RD decided to implement LT-SM in 2011 with the purpose to increase family and child well-being indicated by a reduction in referrals to child protection services (9, 10). It was hypothesized that there would be a decrease in the referrals after an initial increase due to revealing latent needs and that this process would take several years to yield results (11).

The present research paper describes LT-SM and findings related to referrals to child protection services. A detailed description of the implementation of this model is beyond the scope of this paper.

RD includes an industrial town and two smaller rural communities consisting of a population of 35,000 inhabitants with 8,300 under-aged children. The unemployment rate was 10% in 2012. Finland has national health and social services that also cover RD.

MATERIALS AND METHODS

Let's Talk About Children Service Model and Its Implementation

Strategy Level

Both administrative and political leaders in the health, social services, and educational sectors committed to implementing LT-SM at the turn of 2011-2012. LT-SM was incorporated into the Plan for Children's Well-being.

Organizational Level

Multiagent management group (MMG)

MMG is needed to run the implementation and develop cross-sectoral collaboration. This group includes leaders from all relevant sectors. One of its main functions is to report the progress and challenges concerning the implementation of LT-SM. Issues that need to be solved are related to subjects such as decision-making, budgeting and allocating resources across sectoral divides, ethical and practical guidelines relating to reporting and monitoring, documenting patient/client/student records, and networking with families.

MMG was founded in RD in early 2013. MMG meets four times a year and also based on ongoing needs.

One contact service (OCS)

OCS coordinates case-based collaboration. It arranges LT-Network meetings with the necessary participants. Therefore, it also encounters challenges in collaboration and reports them to MMG. Functional feedback system allows the organization to learn from experience.

OCS was created in RD in August 2013 and is being run by two social workers. One phone call or email is enough to activate the Service. As the work of this service concerns prevention and resilience, even a timid and isolated child needing a hobby in a poor family is a valid reason for action.

Workforce Capacity

Different levels of the workforce, from administrative leaders to practitioners working with service users, are educated concerning the main principles, and the ethos and praxis of LT interventions and LT-SM. Method training in LT interventions (in a span of 3 days) is organized for those practitioners working with family members. Training trainers (5 days) is organized to ensure the sustainability of the model. A long-term plan for training is prepared to overcome disruptions due to changes in staff.

[1] https://www.copmi.net.au

Method training in LT interventions started in RD in August 2012. In the first round, 30 practitioners coming from health, social services, and educational sectors were trained. Twenty-five of them also participated in the trainer's training. Dr. Niemelä was responsible for this training program.

Between 2012 and 2013, in RD method training included all 220 workers in health and social services and 270 kindergarten teachers and assistants. Within the schools, practically all employees were trained in this industrial town, including 350 teachers, assistants, and student welfare professionals, while in the two rural communities 30 special education teachers and student welfare professionals were trained.

Population-Level Communication

The population was informed about LT-SM and LT interventions through local media and during evening meetings with parents at the schools and kindergartens. Service users received face-to-face information and leaflets.

Implementation of the Model by 2013

By the end of 2013, LT-SM infrastructure was functional and LT intervention was offered to parents at the mental health and substance use services; attention was also provided to parents with severe somatic conditions. In kindergartens, LT interventions with parents were carried out yearly, and biannually in schools.

Data and Statistical Analyses

Data regarding referrals to child welfare services from 2009 to 2016 were obtained from Sotkanet, an Indicator Bank produced by the National Institute for Health and Welfare (THL) (12). The size of the population between zero and 17 years in RD and the whole country was obtained from the PX-Web population database provided by Statistics Finland. No ethical approval was required for using combined data from open-access data sources.

With regards to time trend analyses, a joinpoint regression program and the average annual percentage change (AAPC) method (13, 14) were employed to estimate the percentage rates of the 0- to 17-year-old population referred to child protection services. The AAPC method used the underlying joinpoint regression model to calculate a summary measure above the fixed pre-specified interval. In the current study, the year 2013 was used as a cut-off year regarding the change in trends. Due to the relatively small number of referrals causing a high variability in the rates of the 0 to 17-year-old population referred to child protection services in RD compared to those of the whole country, a 3-year moving average (3-year moving average at the end of time periods) was used for the statistical modeling.

RESULTS

Figure 1 shows the trend in percentage rates of the 0 to 17-year-old population referred to child protection services in RD and in the whole country. The overall test for parallelism revealed a statistically significant difference in trend rates between RD and the whole country ($p = 0.009$). From year 2013 onwards, the rate of the 0 to 17-year-old population referred to child protection

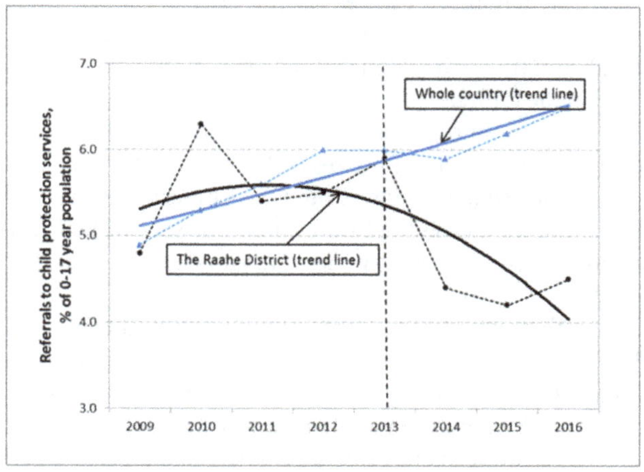

FIGURE 1 | The time trends (solid lines) and the observed percentage rates (dotted lines) of referrals to child protection services among the 0 to 17-year-old population in Raahe District and the whole country. The vertical dotted line indicates the year 2013 from which the Let's Talk about Children Service Model was in the routine use in the services of RD.

services showed a significant decrease in RD (AAPC = −6.9; 95% CI: −10.8,−2.8; $p = 0.013$) compared to an increasing trend in the whole country (AAPC = 1.9; 95% CI: 0.6, 3.3; $p = 0.020$) (AAPC difference = 8.9; 95% CI: 6.2, 11.5; $p < 0.001$). In absolute numbers, during the year 2016, a total of 359 children in RD were referred to child protection services compared to 451 children in 2012, showing a decrease of 25%.

Before the year 2013, the rates had significantly increased in the whole country (AAPC = 4.1; 95% CI: 3.1, 5.2; $p < 0.001$), while no noticeable change was observed in RD (AAPC = −1.5; 95% CI: −4.6, 1.8; $p = 0.373$) (AAPC difference = 5.6; 95% CI: 2.2, 8.9; $p = 0.001$).

DISCUSSION

Let's Talk about Children Model was implemented in RD from 2012 to 2013. We analyzed referrals to child protection services based on the municipal register data and compared them with the national register data from 2009 to 2016. Referrals in RD decreased significantly between 2013 and 2016, while the national data showed a significant increase. We will first discuss the results and then the LT-SM.

The significant decrease in referrals in RD with the launch of LT-SM and the clear departure from the national trend suggest an association between the two. However, possible favorable contextual changes affecting child and family population might also have an impact on this outcome. RD has been an area with high unemployment. However, rather than a decrease, between 2012 and 2016 in RD, there was an increase in unemployment in the general population from 10 to 13%, and among individuals between 18 and 24 years from 14 to 20% (15). Unemployment is known to be a family stressor and related to use of child protection services (16). This was not reflected in the data, which may support the possible preventive impact of LT-SM. Furthermore, there were no other major concurrent projects targeted on families; however, as this was not a randomized controlled study, we cannot make definite causal conclusions. RD will continue to be evaluated to gain a more comprehensive picture in the future.

The decrease in referrals to child protection services suggests that families were getting the needed support before the family situation reached a breaking point. One Contact Service is likely to be crucial for convening LT Network meetings without delay. This might also explain why there was no early increase in the referrals as we expected.

We further hypothesized that the process would take years to yield results, but this was not the case. There are several possible reasons for this, including the expeditious implementation. The leaders of RD were deeply motivated to implement LT-SM and decisions could be made without delay. Training trainers also contributed to the rapid implementation and access to practical work with families.

LT Service Model

LT-SM and its implementation present a novel approach regarding prevention, promotion, and service development. Rather than focusing on individual impact, it aims at the collective impact on population-level outcomes (4). Key aspects of the model are discussed as follows.

First, a commitment from both administrative and political leaders of the model is crucial. The implementation of LT-SM touches all corners of the service system and, through schools and kindergartens, the whole child population and their parents. The role of the Multiagent Management Group is important, which is a decision-making body including leaders from different service sectors. Problems are discussed and successes achieved around the same table.

The core of the Model is the agreement to promote children's well-being in everyday life in all developmental contexts. It is a goal that makes sense and can be scientifically argued and expressed in common language. It is the smallest common denominator for the fragmented services.

It is noteworthy to mention that the starting point for the process is the provision of practical support for children and families. Rather than waiting for the collaborative infrastructure to be developed before the corresponding work with families begins, LT-SM is built up through interaction with the experiences and needs identified in LT interventions with families. The work with families informs the change process and is its generator.

In conclusion, LT-SM recognizes that child and family well-being involves the whole ecological context. Our results are promising, but they are just a starting point from one district. Nevertheless, they encourage the implementation of the model in different types of municipalities and demand research on implementation strategies and impact mechanisms with long-term evaluation.

AUTHOR CONTRIBUTIONS

MN and TS developed the LT-Model and the implementation strategy. MN was responsible for taking the Model into practice and consulting and guiding the implementation process. TS was responsible for negotiating with the Ministries of Health and Social Affairs and Education concerning the needed approvals for the Model and writing up the manuscript with contributions from MN and SR. BA-A and JJ contributed to implementing the Model especially in the child protection and family social services. HK, was the motivational force for the implementation of the Model in Raahe District and instrumental for getting the political support. SR consulted implementation process especially relating to mental health services and made valuable contributions to the manuscript. HH had responsibility of statistical analyses and writing up the data analysis and results section of the manuscript. TR, on the impact of parental illness on children, provided important guidelines for implementing the Model in different services. All authors have approved the final version of the manuscript and agreed to be accountable for all aspects of the work in ensuring that questions related to the accuracy or integrity of any part of the work are appropriately investigated and resolved.

FUNDING

TS has received Eminentia Scholarship 2014 from The Finnish Cultural Foundation.

REFERENCES

1. Heino T, Hyry S, Ikäheimo S, Kuronen M, Rajala R. *Lasten Kodin ulkopuolelle sijoittamisen syyt, Taustat, Palvelut ja Kustannukset. HuosTa-hankkeen (2014–2015) Päätulokset.* Terveyden ja hyvinvoinnin laitos (THL). Raportti3/2016. Helsinki. Available online at: https://thl.fi/documents/2616650/2646346/Lastensuojelu.pdf/e09efa65-c1a3-4e65-8039-6d716e63cdf0
2. Ungar M, Ghazinour M, Richter, J. Annual Research Review: what is resilience within the social ecology of human development? *J Child Psychol Psychiatry* (2013) 54:348–66. doi: 10.1111/jcpp.12025
3. Collishaw S, Hammerton G, Mahedy L, Sellers R, Owen MJ, Craddock N, et al. Mental health resilience in the adolescent offspring of parents with depression: a prospective longitudinal study. *Lancet Psychiatry* (2016) 3:49–57. doi: 10.1016/S2215-0366(15)00358-2
4. Kania J, Kramer M. Collective impact. *Stanford Soc Innov Rev.* (2011) 9:36–41. Available online at: http://ssir.org/articles/entry/collective_impact
5. Toikka S, Solantaus T. The effective family programme II: clinicians' experiences of training in promotive and preventative child mental health methods. *Int J Ment Health Promot.* (2006) 8:4–10. doi: 10.1080/14623730.2006.9721746
6. Solantaus T, Toikka S, Alasuutari M, Beardslee WR, Paavonen EJ. Safety, feasibility and family experiences of preventive interventions for children and families with parental depression. *Int J Ment Health Promot.* (2009) 11:15–24. doi: 10.1080/14623730.2009.9721796
7. Punamäki R, Paavonen J, Toikka S, Solantaus T. Effectiveness of preventive family intervention in improving cognitive attributions among children of depressed parents: a randomized study. *J Fam Psychol.* (2013) 27:683–90. doi: 10.1037/a0033466
8. Solantaus T, Paavonen E, Toikka S, Punamäki R. Preventive interventions in families with parental depression: children's psychosocial symptoms

and prosocial behaviour. *Eur Child Adolesc Psychiatry* (2010) 19:12. doi: 10.1007/s00787-010-0135-3

9. Kallunki H, Niemelä M, Ala-Aho B, Savela S, Pesonen K. Raahen seudulla lapsia ja perheitä tuetaan peruspalvelujen kautta. In: Rimpelä M, Rimpelä M, editors. *Säästöjä Lapsiperheiden Palveluremonteilla. Liiteraportti: Kuntien Kuvaukset Lapsiperheiden Palvelujen Kehittämisestä.* Helsinki: Kunnallisalan kehittämissäätiö (2015). p. 89–96. Available online at: www.kaks.fi/sites/default/files/LIITERAPORTTI_1.pdf
10. Solantaus T, Niemelä M. *Perheterapia* (2016) 32:21–33.
11. Fixsen DL, Blase KA, Naoom SF, Wallace, F. Core Implementation Components. *Res Soc Work Pract.* (2009) 19:531–40. doi: 10.1177/1049731509335549
12. *Sotkanet.fi Statistical Information on Welfare and Health in Finland.* Available online at: https://sotkanet.fi/sotkanet/en/index
13. Jiang Z, Qiu Z, Hatcher J. *Joinpoint Trend Analysis of Cancer Incidence and Mortality Using Alberta data.* Alberta Health Services. Available online at: http://www.cancerview.ca/idc/groups/public/documents/webcontent/csen_cproj_fy0910q3_joinpoint.pdf
14. Kim H, Fay MP, Feuer EJ, Midthune DN. Permutation tests for joinpoint regression with applications to cancer rates. *Stat Med.* (2000) 19:335–51. doi: 10.1002/(SICI)1097-0258(20000215)19:3<335::AID-SIM336>3.0.CO;2-Z
15. PoPSTer. *Pohjois-Pohjanmaan Sosiaali- ja Terveydenhuolto Osana Tulevaisuuden Maakuntaa* (2017). Available online at: https://www.pohjois-pohjanmaa.fi/download/5051/popster-loppuraportti/pdf
16. Brooks-Gunn J, Schneider W, Waldfogel J. The great depression and the risk for child maltreatment. Child *Abuse Neglect.* (2013) 37:721–9. doi: 10.1016/j.chiabu.2013.08.004

5

Improving Identification and Child-Focused Collaborative Care for Children of Parents with a Mental Illness in Tyrol, Austria

Hanna Christiansen[1]*, Annette Bauer[2], Batool Fatima[3], Melinda Goodyear[4], Ingunn Olea Lund[5], Ingrid Zechmeister-Koss[6] and Jean Lillian Paul[7,8]

[1] Department of Clinical Child and Adolescent Psychology, Philipps University Marburg, Marburg, Germany, [2] Personal Social Services Research Unit (PSSRU), London School of Economics and Political Science, London, United Kingdom, [3] Human Development Programme, Aga Khan University, Karachi, Pakistan, [4] School of Rural Health, Monash University, Melbourne, VIC, Australia, [5] The Norwegian Institute of Public Health, Oslo, Norway, [6] Ludwig Boltzmann Institute for Health Technology Assessment, Vienna, Austria, [7] Mental Health Research Program, The Village, Ludwig Boltzmann Gesellschaft, Innsbruck, Austria, [8] Division of Psychiatry I, Department of Psychiatry, Psychotherapy and Psychosomatics, Medical University Innsbruck, Innsbruck, Austria

****Correspondence:***
Hanna Christiansen
christih@staff.uni-marburg.de

Background: Children of parents with a mental illness (COPMI) are more likely to experience negative long-term adversities. However, interventions to support their needs early can significantly enhance adjustment and reduce negative outcomes. Approximately one in four children currently lives with a parent with mental illness worldwide. The lifelong impact for individuals, governments, and broader society is likely to be substantial. There are significant workforce barriers to the early identification of COPMI and addressing their needs, particularly within the adult mental health care system. The current study aims to reduce such barriers and to improve identification of COPMI in the current health care systems.

Objectives: The project "The Village" is a multidisciplinary health and social care policy intervention and seeks to improve child development and well-being outcomes for children of parents with a diagnosed mental illness. This will be achieved through the co-development, implementation, and evaluation of a practice approach to the early identification and collaborative care for COPMI, through establishing child-focused support networks. This will be done with open innovation science (OIS) approaches engaging the public in Tyrol, a geographical region of Austria, throughout 4 years. As part of the co-development process, we will work with stakeholders to co-develop the practice approaches based on evidence-based approaches and determine the most appropriate study design to evaluate those, as well as the implementation processes we will undertake.

Methods: The project is underpinned by theories from different disciplines (i.e., public health, psychology, sociology, linguistics, economic sciences) as well as drawing on different approaches (i.e., co-development, implementation science, symbolic interactionism, and realist evaluation). It is based on the seven content work packages (WPs): 1) management, 2) focusing on children and methods to understand their "voice,"

3) scoping, 4) co-development, 5) implementation, 6) evaluating the practice approaches, and 7) knowledge dissemination. "Scoping" will involve exploring the existing evidence, practice, and current state of identification and collaborative care in Tyrol, Austria. "Co-development" involves the co-design of practice approaches to identify and support children in partnership with key stakeholders and service providers working in Tyrol. The "implementation" of practice approaches will be based on the results of the co-development phase and will involve working with organizations to develop support strategies that draw on known organizational drivers from the field of implementation science to support the rollout of the practice approaches. In "Evaluation" we will follow principles of a realist approach; this includes developing program theories and logic models for the practice approaches. Those will set out the outcomes hypothesized to achieve and the processes that are expected to lead to those changes. This will refer to changes in children, parents, and practitioners. We expect that the main focus will be on measuring child quality of life and mental health outcomes, and outcomes that are on the path to those (such as social support needs, resilience, mental health literacy, stigma, and help-seeking behavior) as well as costs. The "child voice" WP focuses on children's perceptions and needs as the importance of "assent" and support of children to develop their own "voice" in health care is increasingly recognized within child health research. The "dissemination" step focuses on reaching a broad public audience of different stakeholders, researchers, and families involved.

Discussion: The research project aims to directly improve identification and support of vulnerable children across selected regions in Tyrol, Austria, and by doing so, improve the health and well-being of future generations, through breaking the cycle of intergenerational transfer of adverse childhood experiences.

Keywords: children of parents with mental illness, practice approach, implementation, participatory co-design, realist approach, symbolic interactionism, open innovation in science

INTRODUCTION

It is estimated that 50% to 66% of people with serious mental illness are living with one or more children (1), and that approximately 25% of children live with a parent who has a mental illness (2–6). Having a parent with a severe mental illness (SMI) has been associated with adverse child development outcomes, which can have long-lasting effects throughout a child's life including multiple physical and mental health problems (3, 7–10); lower academic achievement (11, 12); and reduced employment opportunities (13). While most studies on COPMI have been carried out in the United States, United Kingdom, and Australia, there is now also evidence from a German national mental health survey showing that parental mental illness is associated with increased risk of mental health problems in children and adolescents (14). A community study found that children of parents with SMI carry a higher risk of developing mental disorders compared to children of parents with mild to moderate mental illness (3). Thus, children of parents with a mental illness (COPMI) are more likely to present as the next generation of people living with SMI and who will use mental health services (10). Further, studies show the overrepresentation of this population in child community mental health services: 48–79% of the children using community mental health services had a parent with a mental illness (15–17). This transgenerational transmission of mental disorders (TTMD) is associated with high costs: In the United Kingdom, the estimated costs of adverse child impact linked to maternal mental illness during the perinatal period alone is £5.8 billion per year (18, 19). The risks associated with the TTMD could result in impaired parent–child interactions, genetic and pregnancy risks, emotion regulation deficits, individual vulnerabilities such as difficult child temperament, stress reactivity, cognitive skills, as well as social environmental factors such as school/work environments and social support. These risk factors are summarized in the Hosman et al. (20) model of the TTMD, though as yet we know currently of only one study testing this model (21).

The treatment of the parental disorder is associated with improved mental health and well-being in COPMI (22–27), though overall there are only a few studies on such effects (25, 28). These studies typically target the same disorder in children and parents, e.g., depressive symptoms in the offspring of parents with depression. However, such a specific transmission of disorders is not typical, as the outcomes often follow a *multifinality* pathway (20) with children of parents with depression developing various kinds of disorders (10, 29). A meta-analysis with nine studies on the effects of psychological treatment of maternal depression on children's psychopathology resulted in an overall moderate effect size, with a Hedge's g = .40 (28). An earlier meta-analysis on preventive interventions for COPMI demonstrated a significant relative risk reduction of 40% in the same disorder as their parent, and overall small effect for children's internalizing (Hedge's g = -.22) and externalizing (Hedge's g = -.16) symptoms (30). The most recent and comprehensive meta-analysis on preventive interventions for COPMI (31) resulted in effect sizes similar to those of Cuijpers et al. (28) for young children, and overall smaller effects for older children that equal those of Siegenthaler et al. (30). Different longitudinal studies on parental anxiety and depressive disorders present heterogeneous effects of parental treatment on children. A 6-year prospective longitudinal study on the effects of parental panic treatment demonstrated that parental treatment is a significant predictor of children's anxiety symptoms (25). The Sequenced Treatment Alternatives to Relieve Depression (STAR*D) Child study is designed to examine the association between maternal remission from depression and children's functioning and psychopathology. The study demonstrates differential effects on child psychopathology in early, late, and nonremitting mothers, with early remission being associated with reduced child externalizing problems (27); similar results have been obtained in another large longitudinal study (22). Thus, overall positive parental treatment effects are associated with reduced psychopathology of the children, though changes in important markers such as well-being, or for children that have not developed psychopathology symptoms yet, are missing.

A major barrier for such positive effects of the parental treatment is the lack of identification of children in families with mental illness. A recent review identified only nine studies systematically assessing whether adult mental health patients admitted to either in- or outpatient care had children or not, and revealed a substantial number of patients that were either not asked about parental status or where this was not documented in patient files (32). The same holds for child and adolescent mental health services (CAMHS) that do not systematically assess the health status of the parents of children and youth in treatment (17). Many systemic barriers exist preventing the early identification of COPMI in adult mental health services including a lack of skill and knowledge of practitioners to talk about parenting, lack of collaboration between the different services involved (i.e., adult and child mental health), individualized funding and treatment focused models of care that limit a family focus in treatment, and a reluctance by parents to talk about their children for fear of child removal into care (33–35).

Hence, according to the review by Maciejewski et al. (36), we are currently lacking opportunities for early identification and thus preventive interventions for COPMI due to adult mental health services neglecting the impact of the TTMD by not asking about parents and children. Developing opportunities or practices that help integrate a focus on intergenerational impacts of mental illness in adult mental health in ways that manage these systemic barriers are considered to be essential (37).

Interestingly, other disciplines have realized the importance of such early identification, especially pediatric primary care (38). As up to 15% of mothers and 7% of fathers suffer from postpartum depression (PPD) (39), they suggest PPD screening in pediatric primary care in order to identify and treat parents and to prevent negative PPD impact on the children, as this has been associated with a high risk of developmental delays and behavior problems (38). This study thus further highlights the necessity of strong collaborative care that, in practice, is rare and challenging between relevant disciplines (40, 41). Currently, this lack of collaboration leads to a lack of identification and thus missed prevention opportunities.

Another significant barrier is the current lack of collaboration itself. Current research suggests a lack of collaboration between different sectors that may impact COPMI—such as adult psychiatry/psychotherapy, child and adolescent psychiatry/psychotherapy, youth welfare agencies, pediatrics, gynecology, as well as family and social services. Instead these sectors offer individualized services that neglect the family as a whole, and the opportunity to capitalize on coordinated services is lost (42, 43). Thus, services that are in touch with families where a parent has a mental illness do not connect and miss chances that might improve overall family and especially child functioning and well-being (33, 40). Even in countries that have taken legislative steps to improve identification of children in families with mental illness, such effective collaboration is still scarce (44). As a result, COPMI often remain invisible, and their needs may be unmet, as their "voice" usually remains unheard (45).

Our project "The Village" has been designed to address these barriers to the care of COPMI through utilizing an open innovation approach (46–48) to design and trial evidence-informed practice approaches in adult mental health and other family support services using principles of symbolic interactionism, realist evaluation, participatory co-design, and knowledge of translation to practice implementation strategies from the field of implementation science (for elaboration on those methods, see below).

The current study has two major objectives: in our model region in Tyrol, Austria, we will 1) facilitate identification of COPMI with a *Sensitive Screening* (SENSE); and 2) establish a *Collaborative Village Approach* (CVA) that will enhance the formal and informal support opportunities for children. The project will be carried out with a focus on understanding children's experiences, challenges, and opportunities to support a child-focused SENSE and CVA, the child's voice. The project aims to ultimately improve child development and well-being outcomes for children and families.

METHODS

The project will be carried through seven work packages to scope, co-design, implement, and evaluate the practice approaches (see **Figure 1**).

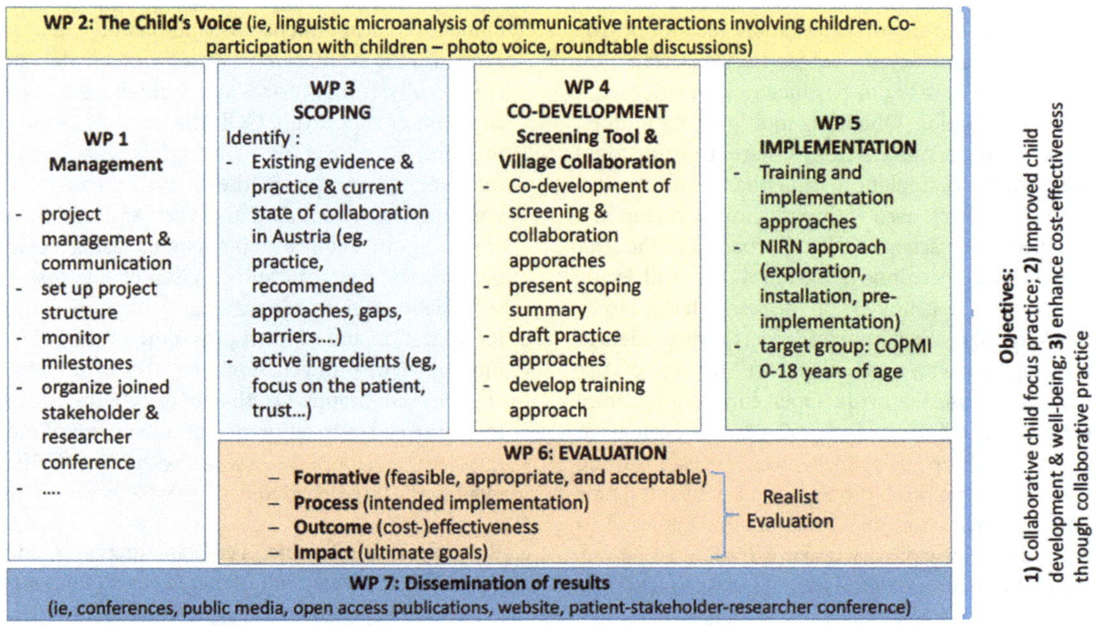

FIGURE 1 | Objectives and work packages (WP) of "The Village."

Design and Theoretical Framework

The project is underpinned by the theories from implementation science (49), a realist evaluation approach (50), and symbolic interactionism (51, 52).

Installing any new practice in routine care is difficult. Many gaps exist, particularly in mental health services, between what is known to be effective evidence-based practice and the translation of these practices into routine care (53). To help move beyond a "train and hope" strategy for workforce development, working with ways to address the systemic barriers within and across services that prevent practice change is a particular focus of implementation science, particularly for practice approaches that aim to address the intergenerational impact of mental illness in families (37). According to the National Implementation Research Network, implementation is defined as a specified set of activities or strategies designed to put into practice an evidence-based program or activity into routine use within specific settings (54). The field of implementation science acknowledges the need to focus on the feasibility and acceptability of new "intervention"/ practice change, in order to facilitate practice change. The principles of co-development and co-design approaches that aim to work alongside key stakeholders in applied settings to co-create and adapt the evidence-based practice with local contingencies in mind, particularly in complex health environments, are one such approach drawn from implementation science to address the gap from research to practice (55).

A realist approach toward evaluation is a theory-driven type of evaluation that is particularly suitable for the examination of complex programs in the health and social care field. It advocates the investigation of theoretical assumptions underpinning a program and whether those are responsible for changes that may occur. The aim of each realist evaluation is to provide a detailed description and analysis of contexts, assumed causal origins, and mechanisms that, in turn, affect the outcome of an intervention (56). Realist evaluation is based on the theory of critical realism as proposed by Archer et al. (57). According to this underpinning theory, the potential mechanisms of causation reside both in the individual actors as well as in society and are real and present even when not active and may or may not be observable when actualized. Realist evaluation is thus different from traditional evaluations that focus on overall effectiveness in that it provides a basis to describe how and why a complex intervention works or does not work (56). Both empirical qualitative and quantitative data will be used to examine not only whether the practice approaches were (cost-) effective but also possible processes and contextual factors that influenced outcomes (or costs).

The theoretical framework of symbolic interactionism is based upon the epistemology of constructionism and refers to the belief that meaning and knowledge are constructed and maintained through social interactions; there is no one truth to be discovered, but many depending on the way in which the question is asked, approached, and analyzed (51, 52). As such, it is important to continuously gather data and perspectives of multiple stakeholders throughout the Village project that provide feedback into the project design. Such an approach focuses on the importance of language and interactions in shaping how people make sense of themselves and their social world (58). Given the stigma experienced by people and families impacted by mental illness, along with the inherent sensitivities of trying to find and support children in this situation, examining the social and interactional nature of experiences is particularly relevant for this study. Research using symbolic interactionism values multiple data sources, commonly obtained through qualitative approaches, and perspectives in order to continuously build and reflect the social interaction of interest. Aligned with this theory, we undertake a period of exploration (scoping). The co-developed approach also acknowledges the importance of collecting multiple views in order to produce new practices that will more likely fit the situation. Obtaining multiple data sources, such as interviews or observations from different perspectives or media, known as data triangulation, can enhance interpretive rigor, a valuable quality check used within qualitative research.

With an open innovation science (OIS) approach, i.e., the strategic use of the public to increase innovation (46, 47), we will decide together with the relevant stakeholders on the research steps to be taken and consult monthly with a group of "experts by experience" (young adults with a parent with a mental illness). Our project's use of OIS will be internally assessed by the Open Innovation Centre at the Ludwig Boltzmann Gesellschaft using novel evaluation criteria based on opening up disciplinary boundaries, fostering public engagement in the research process, and establishing new forms of stakeholder interaction and collaboration that lead to interdisciplinary and transdisciplinary research (59).

The processes of this methodological framework as well as their linkage are described in detail in the work packages "scoping," "co-development," "implementation," and "evaluation" (see below).

The other three work packages of the Village describe the overall management, dissemination of research findings, and our central overarching focus of the project on capturing the "child's voice."

Scoping

Drawing on implementation science, in a staged model of organizational change, scoping (known as the exploration stage) is a critical first step needed to understand the contextual factors shaping existing practice and practice challenges that need to be addressed in the implementation of practice approaches for the translation to routine care (60). This initial step will therefore generate the knowledge and conceptual frameworks to be informed and to be tested in the co-development, implementation, and evaluation of the project. This will include summaries of evidence and draft logic models that inform the development of the two practice approaches, SENSE and CVA. Scoping will be supported by the knowledge generated on conceptualizations of the child's voice (described below).

Evidence will be collected through reviews, and OIS principles such as stakeholder views; sharing and exchanging will be applied to understand and describe 1) current practice, recommended practice, and gaps in relation to the identification of COPMI as well as in relation to current and recommended collaborative care that puts the child at the center of attention ("child's voice"); 2) the (unmet) needs for COPMI; 3) what works for whom and when, what is cost-effective, and what are the mechanisms (active ingredients); and 4) contextual factors that can inform the development of logic models and the development of approaches.

As this work is underpinned by the theoretical framework of symbolic interactionism (51, 52), it is essential to gather perspectives of multiple stakeholders to inform co-development and implementation.

Particular pieces of work to address the scoping objectives will be conducted, using varied techniques:

- mapping of existing Tyrolean support structures and epidemiological dimensions, and mental health service use;
- semistructured interviews with Tyrolean stakeholders in the community, from services and families, to analyze the current situation of supporting COPMIs, existing needs, and barriers in Tyrol;
- mapping of key topics in the COPMI research field to identify what topics are studied together and which are not (and what the current research focus is) using co-word analysis, bibliometric coupling, and co-citation analysis;
- systematic review identifying facilitators and barriers in identification and support provision for COPMI;
- interviews with international experts who have attempted to change adult mental health care to be family-focused in order to improve identification of children at risk of mental illness;
- review of collaborative practice within the COPMI setting to identify the "active ingredients" or what has been shown to work.

The results from the Tyrolean mapping and situational analysis are currently summarized in a separate paper (61). Our preliminary evidence suggests that a variety of services are available both for parents who have a mental illness as well as for families and individual family members. However, services do not address the needs of COPMIs specifically and lack coordination across sectors. Findings further indicate that there is awareness of the problems related to COPMIs at all levels, but there is a lack of installed support processes to meet their needs.

Finally, initial logic models will be drafted in line with a realist approach (50). This work will inform the co-development process where the logic model will be developed further and agreed upon with stakeholders, and the co-creation of new practice approaches with stakeholders that draw on the evidence base for SENSE and CVA.

Co-development

One key element of this research project is that it follows OIS principles (46). This includes the co-development of the practice approaches for SENSE and CVA (informed by knowledge generated during the scoping in the form of initial logic models and the research literature) with local stakeholders and the training and implementation support for the application of these co-created practice approaches into routine care. Furthermore, stakeholders will be involved in decisions about key indicators and (outcome) measures and study design for the evaluation of the practice approaches.

A series of design workshops with stakeholders representing key service providers from the Tyrol region will be held monthly over a 6-month period to draw on the evidence and logic models developed in the earlier stages and existing practice wisdom of key stakeholders to co-develop the components of the two practice approaches (SENSE and CVA). Key stakeholders include leadership representation from psychiatric/psychotherapeutic and social care services across the region supporting adults and/or children, with a mix of professional background, and include people with lived experience of parenting with a mental illness or being an adult child of a parent with mental illness. Consultation will also occur with COPMI (the beneficiaries) acting in an advisory capacity. A training concept and training materials as well as feasibility and implementation indicators will also be prepared with the input of key stakeholders to support the implementation of the practice approaches in their respective contexts. To date, four out of six workshops have been held and draft models for SENSE and CVA for the Tyrolean region are already available. A preliminary Theory of Change model was presented to the workshop participants, which was based upon initial logic models, literature, and data collected during the scoping phase (see **Figure 2**). All workshops will be recorded, transcribed, and analyzed. Additional data will be collected *via* participant observation and by holding a focus group after the final workshop. Qualitative methods will be applied to analyze the data collected to measure the impact and process undertaken during this co-development phase. Core themes will be identified (based on a content analysis), clustered, and critically analyzed (62).

Implementation of the Practice Approaches (SENSE and CVA)

The objective of this step of the project is to implement the key practice approaches and position the evaluation of the impact into the applied settings decided on in the co-development stage. This stage of the project will draw on best practice evidence using known facilitative implementation drivers (49) to support organizational change to embed the 1) SENSE and 2) CVA approaches into selected Tyrolian study sites. Implementation drivers (also known as core components) are a key focus of implementation of the new practice approaches to ensure that the project

- develops, improves, and sustains the ability of selected sites to deliver the new practice approaches and
- creates an enabling positive organizational context that can support and sustain the operation of the new practice over time (49).

Implementation drivers are activities and processes for building the capacity and infrastructure of an organization to influence a program's success and are the "engine of change" needed to initiate and support changes to achieve positive outcomes for children, families, and community (49).

Underpinning these drivers is the level of Program Acceptance and Program Buy-in by staff, including managers and leadership, to the new practice approaches. When attention and action are paid to these key drivers, we are much more likely to see the practice approaches implemented as designed, resulting in change to practice and therefore improvements in family outcomes.

The evidence-based implementation framework will inform the project from the scoping through to the evaluation phase. Implementation is concerned with the use of strategies to adopt, integrate, and use evidence-based interventions/practices to change practice patterns within specific settings. This approach will utilize the NIRN implementation framework developed by the National Implementation Research Network (49) (exploration, installation, implementation), and undertake a series of activities across the entire project that will attempt to understand the context of implementation (the scoping of current practice and existing barriers at selected sites), to design a feasible approach that fits to the context (the co-development approach), to help prepare the environment, to train dedicated staff, and to coach the practice of the approach at selected sites. This implementation phase will also monitor the uptake and address issues with the on-going implementation of the approach at sites participating in the evaluation.

Evaluation

The main objective of the evaluation is to generate knowledge as to whether SENSE and CVA were implemented successfully and whether they were (cost-) effective. More specifically, the objective is to understand feasibility and acceptability of the practice changes, with a focus on the co-developed nature of the process, and on mechanisms and contextual factors; changes in outcomes (i.e., child quality of life and psychopathology, or outcomes that are expected to be on the path to child quality of life and mental health improvements, such as social support, mental health literacy, stigma, confidence); and changes in service use for COPMI and their family. We will also seek to capture impact at the wider system level. We will need to agree on outcomes with stakeholders, but at the moment, according to our current theory of change (**Figure 2**), we will measure mental health literacy, stigma, help seeking, quality of life, and psychopathology.

Evaluation of SENSE and CVA will follow principles of the realist approach, which is particularly suitable for complex interventions, and takes into account the mechanisms and conditions for change (50). Generation of the logic models will inform the framework of evaluation. Planning for process evaluation will start during scoping and co-development and inform modifications before full implementation of the practice approaches. Indicators will include a number of professionals trained, parents screened and children identified, children or families referred, collaborative "Village" meetings held, as well as awareness and behavior change in professionals. Knowledge generated about program theories (e.g., in the form of logic models) during scoping and co-development will inform the evaluation of outcomes and costs. Outcomes, resource use, as well as views and experiences will be captured at baseline and 6- and 12-month follow-up (i.e., after baseline) to assess changes for children and parents. Evaluation parameters and measures will be agreed upon during the scoping and co-developing phase. Personnel at study sites will be trained in the recruitment of study participants and practice approaches during the implementation phase. The cost-effectiveness analysis (in the form of cost-consequences analysis) will examine direct and indirect costs from a public sector as well as a societal perspective, and compare them against outcomes. Statistical analysis will be carried out to examine the causality of SENSE or CVA on outcomes and service use (and costs). The choice of statistical method will depend on the final choice of the study design.

Understanding the "Child's Voice"

Each of the steps outlined above will be influenced by an overarching focus on capturing the child's voice in the research undertaken. The project will explore and identify the concept

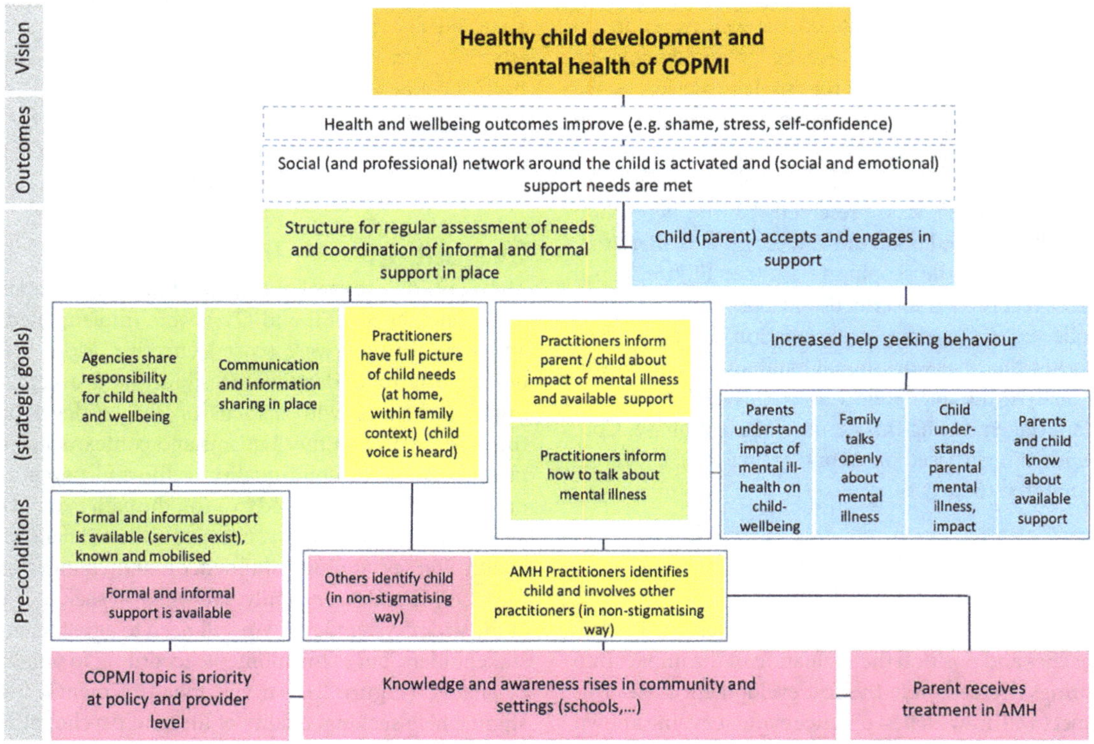

FIGURE 2 | Preliminary theory of change. Green boxes refer to the CVA approach; yellow boxes to SENSE; pink boxes refer to general elements; and blue ones to the family. AMH = Adult Mental Health; COPMI = Children of Parents with a Mental Illness.

of the "child's voice" in COPMI health settings, and knowledge produced will inform the overall research process, particularly in the co-development, implementation, and evaluation. This part of the project will identify how children currently, and wish to, participate in discussions about their needs, from the perspective of the child, service providers, and parents. It will uphold the project's underpinning philosophy to hold the child at the center of their care, and to listen and support them in identifying their own formal and informal support network. It will provide opportunities to educate professionals in the implementation step in appropriate ways to engage and support COPMI to become more communicatively active in conversations with adults about their needs in the evaluation step.

Focus groups and interviews primarily conducted for scoping and co-development will include questions that will address the topic of "child's voice" and communication between children and service providers [c.f. Ref. (63) for an example of methodological approaches]. This work will support the International Charter for Human Values in Healthcare—Compassion, Respect for Persons, Commitment to Integrity and Ethical Practice, Commitment to Excellence, and Justice in Healthcare. It will also draw upon research regarding health care communication with vulnerable people, such as those with disabilities or individuals from migrant populations, in which traditional patient–doctor power balances are amplified, as is the case with doctor–child interactions.

Through close analysis of naturally occurring health care interactions and analysis of stakeholder perspectives, this work aims to understand and improve the nature and possibilities of children's interactive participation in conversations about their needs and concerns. This work spans across the project and makes use of and informs data collected in the other work packages. A series of sociological and linguistic micro-analyses will be performed across collected data sets. Additional data collection will include (audio or video) recordings of health care encounters with children, as determined through consultation with stakeholders in scoping and co-development. This part has already started as we record communications between health care professionals and children. A total of 40 interactions will be recorded. For comparison purposes, those include interactions between health care professionals and children in need of psychotherapeutic/psychiatric treatment as well as interactions between adult health care professionals that treat the parents and their children. We will also investigate current practice (i.e., case meetings) to determine how others do and can speak for the child if they are unable or not present.

The communicative effectiveness of SENSE and CVA to listen to the child's voice and address their needs will be evaluated once this phase of the project starts through recording observations and will also inform and utilize the evaluation. Discourse analytic techniques will be applied, such as Conversation Analysis (CA), pragmatics, and interactional sociolinguistics, to analyze interviews, focus groups, and naturally occurring interactions, which will provide opportunities to educate professionals in this field.

Dissemination

The objectives of the dissemination focus are based on OIS (46–48): (1) to gain ownership and buy-in for the research among stakeholders throughout the different research phases and (2) to achieve impact at an individual, community, regional, and (inter-) national level. This includes impact in regard to research, practice, and policy. All communication and dissemination will be designed sensitively, with the aim to reduce stigma as a relevant barrier to the realization of the project (45).

Communication and dissemination will be an ongoing process from start to end of the research. This includes identifying organizations and representatives of those who will be part of the project; relevant stakeholders will be recruited into advisory and steering groups; a series of open-day forums will be organized throughout the project to which a wide range of stakeholders will be invited. This will include families, service managers, politicians, researchers, commissioners, and practitioners (including clinicians, social workers, school teachers). We inform about upcoming events and provide information and material for all events already having taken place (https://village.lbg.ac.at/news). Events will inform stakeholders about the research and include educational components; for example, keynote speakers might talk about the latest evidence and good practice; policymakers and influencers (including patient and professional associations) will be engaged; partnerships will be built and managed with organizations and projects that have similar aims and work with similar target groups such as early interventions that target families with newborns to support them and promote healthy child development; and formal collaboration agreements will be established. Our first two formal events for stakeholders were held in Innsbruck in June and September 2018, including the project inauguration ("Kick off") and the first of our annual "General Assemblies." These events are an opportunity to present updates to our official and unofficial stakeholders, receive feedback on design and findings, promote the project to policymakers and people working with children in Tyrol, and raise awareness in a sensitive approach that aims to reduce stigma surrounding mental health. Ongoing information is made available *via* our Village research project website (http://village.lbg.ac.at). A range of innovative communication tools (e.g., video, infographics; see: https://www.youtube.com/watch?time_continue=64&v=XHBv7ebFkWU) will be developed, which will be disseminated together with research reports throughout the project to promote the research aims, methods, and findings. Peer-reviewed papers will be produced and published in scientific journals, and a joint researcher–stakeholder conference is planned at the end of the project to communicate findings to the general public.

Analytical Strategy

As outlined in our theoretical framework, as well as in the detailed descriptions of the different work packages, the Village intervention differs substantially from traditional RCTs or other traditional scientific approaches. Although this may bring several risks to the project, it provides a significant opportunity to understand and implement practice approaches that address the local needs in Tyrol. Currently, in Austria, as well as the other German-speaking countries Switzerland and Germany, there are no sustainable structures for COPMI. The Village aims at understanding the currently available structures and how to improve and connect them in order to achieve an improved identification of COPMI with our SENSE approach, as well as improved care with the CVA approach. For this, we will use the tools provided within our theoretical approaches. As those strongly depend on OIS and stakeholder participation, those will be developed and decided on interactively and in collaboration. We thus cannot provide a fixed analytical strategy, as this is work in progress. We have, however, done some preliminary sample size calculations to determine numbers needed to treat to observe change (calculations were performed using the "n4means" function from the R package "CRTSize"; http://r-project.org). As outlined in the Introduction, we can expect small to moderate effects (31). As there are currently no studies on COPMI and the SENSE and CVA approaches, we assume at best small effects. Depending on the number of clusters (i.e., participating sites), the number of participants to be included varies largely. For instance, if we assume a small effect (Cohen's d = 0.1) of our CVA approach as well as clusters participating in Tyrol with an intraclass correlation of 0.01 with $\alpha = 0.05$ (two-sided), $1\text{-}\beta = 0.8$ in a parallel-group cluster-randomized trial, we would need 3,420 participants in 342 clusters (cluster size m = 10). **Tables 1 to 3** provide information on the number of participants to be included for different cluster sizes. However, those numbers depend on whom we will include at what stage with what

TABLE 1 | Required total sample size of clusters and patients to demonstrate an effect of Cohen's d = 0.1/0.2, assuming an **ICC of 0.1** in a parallel-group cluster-randomized trial with respect to cluster size m.

Cluster size m	Cohen's d = 0.1		Cohen's d = 0.2	
	Number of required clusters	Number of required patients	Number of required clusters	Number of required patients
10	596	5,960	150	1,500
20	456	9,120	114	2,280
50	370	18,500	92	4,600
100	342	34,200	86	8,600
500	320	160,000	80	40,000
1,000	316	316,000	80	80,000
2,000	316	632,000	78	156,000
5,000	314	1,570,000	78	390,000

$\alpha = 0.05$ (two-sided), $1\text{-}\beta = 0.8$, ICC = 0.1.

TABLE 2 | Required total sample size of clusters and patients to demonstrate an effect of Cohen's d = 0.1/0.2, assuming an **ICC of 0.05** in a parallel-group cluster-randomized trial with respect to cluster size m.

Cluster size m	Cohen's d = 0.1		Cohen's d = 0.2	
	Number of required clusters	Number of required patients	Number of required clusters	Number of required patients
10	456	4,560	114	1,140
20	306	6,120	76	1,520
50	216	10,800	56	2,800
100	186	18,600	48	4,800
500	162	81,000	42	21,000
1,000	160	160,000	42	42,000
2,000	158	316,000	42	84,000
5,000	158	790,000	42	210,000

α = 0.05 (two-sided), 1-β = 0.8, ICC = 0.05.

TABLE 3 | Required total sample size of clusters and patients to demonstrate an effect of Cohen's d = 0.1/0.2, assuming an **ICC of 0.01** in a parallel-group cluster-randomized trial with respect to cluster size m.

Cluster size m	Cohen's d = 0.1		Cohen's d = 0.2	
	Number of required clusters	Number of required patients	Number of required clusters	Number of required patients
10	342	3,420	86	860
20	186	3,720	48	960
50	94	4,700	26	1,300
100	62	6,200	18	1,800
500	40	20,000	12	6,000
1,000	36	36,000	10	10,000
2,000	34	68,000	10	20,000
5,000	34	170,000	10	50,000

α = 0.05 (two-sided), 1-β = 0.8, ICC = 0.01. Calculations were performed using the "n4means" function from the R package "CRTSize" (http://r-project.org).

expected effect. They are thus currently only an orientation. The same holds true for potential outcome measures. There are measurements often used in the research of COPMI, such as the psychopathology screening instrument, the Strengths and Difficulties Questionnaire (3), or measures on child-well-being (64), but based on our theoretical framework and as laid out above, we decided to actively involve the relevant stakeholders in this process and give them a voice in our research.

Potential primary and secondary outcome measures might include well-being and psychopathology outcomes for children, improvements in family functioning and social support, and process measures of feasibility and acceptability of the new practice approaches in chosen sites. Barriers and facilitators to service change will also be an important indicator of the co-development and implementation processes of this study. We will also have a focus on measurement of the co-development process and satisfaction with outcomes achieved, as well as documenting the implementation drivers and program adaptation needed to translate the co-designed practice approaches into routine care.

For all activities, we ensure performance according to the Declaration of Helsinki and its later amendments and will obtain approval from the relevant Human Research Ethics Committees (see Ethics Statement). Within the scoping project, we have already performed interviews with relevant stakeholders that are currently analyzed. We have obtained ethical approval for the local scoping interviews and development process measures from the Human Research Ethics Committee of Monash University Melbourne, Australia. In addition, internal approval from the London School of Economics, London, UK for the international interviews is undertaken as part of the scoping stage. Once the recruitment of participants starts, we will beforehand obtain ethical approval from Innsbruck Medical University to ensure accordance with national Austrian guidelines.

Implications

COPMI are a highly vulnerable group that are still neglected in the health setting in general and the (adult) mental health setting specifically (15, 17, 32) and thus prone to the TTMD (20).

"The Village" aims to change the invisibility of this vulnerable group due to lack of identification and collaborative care in the model region of Tyrol, Austria. To achieve this, we follow a robust collaborative approach based on child voice and OIS principles involving beneficiaries, relevant stakeholders, and policymakers as outlined in the different phases of the project. In the end, this project will have informed and instigated a low-threshold, nonstigmatizing collaborative care system for COPMI in Tyrol, Austria, which efficiently and effectively integrates services and support from the perspective of the child. Accordingly, practitioners and other front-line staff working with children and adults will know how to sensitively identify families with mental illnesses, and how to carry out sensitive screenings (SENSE) to identify COPMI. They will know when additional services are required. If so, they will be able to put the child's voice at the center and carry out sensitive, low-threshold interventions, based on the child's and family's needs. This is expected to improve child development and quality-of-life outcomes and reduce the risk for the development of mental illness in the children themselves, promoting children's quality of life (65–67). Further, such a best-practice model will be capacity building, providing the evidence for upscaling the practice approaches to other regions of Austria and countries with similar practice challenges. A range of materials about the evidence-informed approaches (SENSE, CVA), and the resource impact of scaling those up, as well as implementation and dissemination strategies will have been made available.

Impact on service users: The project seeks to improve child development and quality of life for a population that is often invisible, i.e., COPMI are affected by multiple disadvantages, and often not known to services until presenting with their own problems later during child- or adulthood (42, 43). The project will improve the child's situation by providing access to a strengthened social support network that supports their emotional, practical, and social needs (45). Although not a specific aim of the project, children will benefit from destigmatized services that put the child at the center of support. This will likely lead to sustainable changes in the child's life and have positive effects on long-term outcomes that reach into adulthood, such as school performance, employment, and mental health.

Impact on policy, practice, and research: The project will test an innovative whole-system approach in an Austrian region. Based on the findings, a training approach, tools, and implementation support package will be developed that (if the project proves cost-effective) would allow scaling up the approach at a national level and may assist practice internationally that seeks to provide holistic care to COPMI. The evaluation can inform a resource impact analysis, which will provide an estimate of the costs to the government (and society) if the approach was to be rolled out more widely. Findings will be disseminated through a number of research outputs. The use of the stakeholders and the media to promote the project will be maximized throughout the project using an OIS design, to increase awareness of the importance of supporting COPMI and ways that this can be done. The message will be that many people in the community can support COPMI. By working with stakeholders, such as patient associations, local community leaders, and health and social care professionals, throughout the entire research project period, knowledge about mental illness in parents and its impact on child health and development will be disseminated. Throughout and toward the end of the project, project stakeholders will be invited to knowledge exchange events, where project progress and results are presented in informal, accessible language.

Through the co-developed research process, the capacity of stakeholders will be built to improve not only their collaborative- and child-centered approaches, but also their evaluation of practice. This includes an increased capacity to collect and analyze data on process, costs, and outcomes to reflect on their practice approaches. This can inform a long-term approach to generating evidence in this area.

Economic impact: Economic analysis will estimate the cost-effectiveness from the perspective of government and society. This will include the costs of informal care that occur when children look after their mentally ill parents, as well as other costs that should be included when planning public services (e.g., out-of-pocket expenditure to families and potential long-term costs if children are removed). In Austria, knowledge of the (cost-) effectiveness is currently not well utilized to inform the planning of services. The research team will work with policy stakeholders and support them in translating the research findings into practice.

Methodological Considerations

"The Village" is a multidimensional project that involves a range of potential risks. Examples of risks include not finding appropriate study sites; too many tasks for the 4-year time period; the unwillingness of stakeholders to be engaged; lack of practice change and fidelity in delivery; and delivering a local project through a multinational team. However, the project includes significant preparatory steps to scope potential study sites, to engage key stakeholders, to co-develop feasible practice approaches, and to use the latest thinking in implementation science to address these potential risks. The project officially started in February 2018 with an initial kick-off event in June 2018. For this kick-off, people with lived experience as well as the range of relevant stakeholders were invited and actively participated in the event. This resulted in positive feedback (https://science.orf.at/stories/2921593/), already suggestive of a high acceptance of and high involvement in "The Village" in Tyrol, Austria.

Finally, the research team will take substantial steps in planning for early identification and mitigation of risks and has indeed started taking some of those steps.

CONCLUSION

The research project aims to directly improve identification and support of vulnerable children across selected regions in Austria, and by doing so, improve the health and well-being of future Austrian generations while breaking the cycle of intergenerational transfer of adverse childhood experiences. The described project underwent a rigorous public review process (https://ois.lbg.ac.at/en/methods-projects/crowdsourcing-research-questions-in-science) with different stakeholders as well as people with lived experience and scientific experts of the field having reviewed our proposal (https://ois.lbg.ac.at/en/methods-projects/ideas-lab). This ensures high acceptance and most likely high probability of implementation of our approach, a highly relevant fact for sustained impact. Further, the research group is genuinely interdisciplinary with researchers from public health, (clinical) psychology, economics, linguistics, and implementation sciences thus combining not only different expertise but also perspectives that are crucial concerning cooperation and collaboration. We believe that the research findings from the described public health intervention will also be relevant for health care providers and policymakers in other countries, and the international research community.

ETHICS STATEMENT

The study is performed according to the Declaration of Helsinki and its later amendments and was approved by the Human Research Ethics Committee of Monash University Melbourne, Australia, in addition to internal approval from the London School of Economics, London, UK. Local human research ethics in Austria will be obtained as appropriate. Written informed consent will be obtained from all study participants. If participants are underage, they will be informed about the study and their written informed consent will be accompanied by the written informed consent of their legal guardians.

AUTHOR CONTRIBUTIONS

HC wrote a first draft of the manuscript. AB, BF, MG, IL, IZ, and JP reviewed and commented the version. HC and JP revised the commented version, which was reviewed again by all coauthors.

FUNDING

"The Village" is a research project funded by the Austrian Federal Ministry of Health–Science and Research through the Open Innovation in Science Centre at the Ludwig Boltzmann Gesellschaft GmbH, hosted at the Medical University of Innsbruck, with the collaboration of Co-Investigator institutions.

ACKNOWLEDGMENTS

The study is supported by expertise from Prof. Lesley Stirling (linguistics) and Prof. Geoff Wong (realist approach). The authors would like to acknowledge the support of Dr. Raphaela Kaisler, the program relationship manager, as well as the project steering committee: Prof. Alex Hofer, Director, Medical University Innsbruck, Department of Psychiatry, Psychotherapy and Psychosomatics, Division of Psychiatry I; and Dr. Lucia Malfent, Operations Manager, Open Innovation in Science Centre, Ludwig Boltzmann Gesellschaft GmBH. The authors would also like to acknowledge the work and contributions of the Innsbruck "Village team": Rosanna Buchauer, Daniel Purtscheller, Franziska Huck, Lisa Dobener, Julia Kapferer, Elena Seis, Anna-Elena Pinggera, Johanna Krönner, and Marie Niederleithinger.

REFERENCES

1. Bee P, Bower P, Byford S, Churchill R, Calam R, Stallard P, et al. The clinical effectiveness, cost-effectiveness and acceptability of community-based interventions aimed at improving or maintaining quality of life in children of parents with serious mental illness: a systematic review. *Health Technol Assess (Winchester, England)* (2014) 18(8):1–250. doi: 10.3310/hta18080
2. Fraser C, James EL, Anderson K, Lloyd D, Judd F. Intervention programs for children of parents with a mental illness: a critical review. *Int J Ment Health Promot* (2006) 8:9–20. doi: 10.1080/14623730.2006.9721897
3. Maybery D, Reupert A, Goodyear M, Ritchie R, Brann P. Investigating the strengths and difficulties of children from families with a parental mental illness. *Aust E J Adv Ment Health* (2009) 8(2):1–10. doi: 10.5172/jamh.8.2.165
4. Ostman M, Hansson L. Children in families with a severely mentally ill member. Prevalence and needs for support. *Soc Psychiatry Psychiatr Epidemiol* (2002) 37(5):243–8. doi: 10.1007/s00127-002-0540-0
5. Pretis M, Dimova A. Vulnerable children of mentally ill parents: towards evidence-based support for improving resilience. *Support Learn* (2008) 23:152–9. doi: 10.1111/j.1467-9604.2008.00386.x
6. Test MA, Burke SS, Wallisch LS. Gender differences of young adults with schizophrenic disorders in community care. *Schizophr Bull* (1990) 16(2):331–44. doi: 10.1093/schbul/16.2.331
7. Goodman SH, Rouse MH, Connell AM, Broth MR, Hall CM, Heyward D. Maternal depression and child psychopathology: a meta-analytic review. *Clin Child Fam Psychol Rev* (2011) 14(1):1–27. doi: 10.1007/s10567-010-0080-1
8. Goodman SH, Gotlib IH. Risk for psychopathology in the children of depressed mothers: a developmental model for understanding mechanisms of transmission. *Psychol Rev* (1999) 106(3):458–90. doi: 10.1037/0033-295X.106.3.458
9. McLaughlin KA, Gadermann AM, Hwang I, Sampson NA, Al-Hamzawi A, Andrade LH, et al. Parent psychopathology and offspring mental disorders: results from the WHO World Mental Health Surveys. *Br J Psychiatry* (2012) 200(4):290–9. doi: 10.1192/bjp.bp.111.101253
10. Van Santvoort F, Hosman CMH, Janssens JMAM, van Doesum KTM, Reupert A, van Loon LMA. The impact of various parental mental disorders on children's diagnoses: a systematic review. *Clin Child Fam Psychol Rev* (2015) 18(4):281–99. doi: 10.1007/s10567-015-0191-9
11. Berg L, Bäck K, Vinnerljung B, Hjern A. Parental alcohol-related disorders and school performance in 16-year-olds-a Swedish national cohort study. *Addiction (Abingdon, England)* (2016) 111(10):1795–1803. doi: 10.1111/add.13454
12. Kersten-Alvarez LE, Hosman CMH, Riksen-Walraven JM, van Doesum, KTM, Smeekens S, et al. Early school outcomes for children of postpartum depressed mothers: comparison with a community sample. *Child Psychiatry Hum Dev* (2012) 43(2):201–18. doi: 10.1007/s10578-011-0257-y
13. Christoffersen MN, Soothill K. The long-term consequences of parental alcohol abuse: a cohort study of children in Denmark. *J Subst Abuse Treat* (2003) 25(2):107–16. doi: 10.1016/S0740-5472(03)00116-8
14. Wille N, Bettge S, Ravens-Sieberer U. Risk and protective factors for children's and adolescents' mental health: results of the BELLA study. *Eur Child Adolesc Psychiatry* (2008) 17 Suppl 1:133–47. doi: 10.1007/s00787-008-1015-y
15. Gatsou L, Yates S, Hussain S, Barrett M, Gangavati S, Ghafoor R. Parental mental illness: incidence, assessment and practice. *Ment Health Pract* (2016) 19(5):25–7. doi: 10.7748/mhp.19.5.25.s18
16. Mattejat F, Remschmidt H. The children of mentally ill parents. *Dtsch Ärztebl Int* (2008) 105(23):413–8. doi: 10.3238/arztebl.2008.0413
17. Naughton MFA, Maybery DJ, Goodyear M. Prevalence of mental illness within families in a regional child-focussed mental health service. *Int J Ment Health Nurs* (2018) 27(2):901–10. doi: 10.1111/inm.12386
18. Bauer A, Knapp M, Parsonage M. Lifetime costs of perinatal anxiety and depression. *J Affect Disord* (2016) 192:83–90. doi: 10.1016/j.jad.2015.12.005
19. Bauer A, Parsonage M, Knapp M, Iemmi V, Adelaja. B. *Costs of perinatal mental health problems.* London: London School of Economics and Political Science and Centre for Mental Health (2014).
20. Hosman CMH, van Doesum KTM, van Santvoort F. Prevention of emotional problems and psychiatric risks in children of parents with a mental illness in the Netherlands: I. The scientific basis to a comprehensive approach. *Aust E J Adv Ment Health* (2009) 8(3):250–63. Retrieved from http://amh.e-contentmanagement.com/archives/vol/8/issue/3/article/3514/prevention-of-emotioanl-problems-and-psychiatric. doi: 10.5172/jamh.8.3.250
21. Stracke M, Gilbert K, Kieser M, Klose C, Krisam J, Ebert DD, et al. COMPARE family (children of mentally ill parents at risk evaluation): a study protocol for a preventive intervention for children of mentally ill parents (Triple P, evidence-based program that enhances parentings skills, in

addition to gold-standard CBT with the mentally ill parent) in a multicenter RCT—part II. *Front Psychiatry* (2019) 10:281. doi: 10.3389/fpsyt.2019.00054
22. Garber J, Ciesla JA, McCauley E, Diamond G, Schloredt KA. Remission of depression in parents: links to healthy functioning in their children. *Child Dev* (2011) 82(1):226–43. doi: 10.1111/j.1467-8624.2010.01552.x
23. Pilowsky DJ, Wickramaratne P, Talati A, Tang M, Hughes CW, Garber J, et al. Children of depressed mothers 1 year after the initiation of maternal treatment: findings from the STAR*D-Child Study. *Am J Psychiatry* (2008) 165(9):1136–47. doi: 10.1176/appi.ajp.2008.07081286
24. Pilowsky DJ, Wickramaratne P, Poh E, Hernandez M, Batten LA, Flament MF, et al. Psychopathology and functioning among children of treated depressed fathers and mothers. *J Affect Disord* (2014) 164:107–11. doi: 10.1016/j.jad.2014.04.012
25. Schneider S, In-Albon T, Nuendel B, Margraf J. Parental panic treatment reduces children's long-term psychopathology: a prospective longitudinal study. *Psychother Psychosom* (2013) 82(5):346–8. doi: 10.1159/000350448
26. Weissman MM, Pilowsky DJ, Wickramaratne PJ, Talati A, Wisniewski SR, Fava M, et al. Remissions in maternal depression and child psychopathology: a STAR*D-child report. *JAMA* (2006) 295(12):1389–98. doi: 10.1001/jama.295.12.1389
27. Wickramaratne P, Gameroff MJ, Pilowsky DJ, Hughes CW, Garber J, Malloy E, et al. Children of depressed mothers 1 year after remission of maternal depression: findings from the STAR*D-Child study. *Am J Psychiatry* (2011) 168(6):593–602. doi: 10.1176/appi.ajp.2010.10010032
28. Cuijpers P, Weitz E, Karyotaki E, Garber J, Andersson G. The effects of psychological treatment of maternal depression on children and parental functioning: a meta-analysis. *Eur Child Adolesc Psychiatry* (2015) 24(2):237–45. doi: 10.1007/s00787-014-0660-6
29. Kendler KS, Aggen SH, Knudsen GP, Røysamb E, Neale MC, Reichborn-Kjennerud T. The structure of genetic and environmental risk factors for syndromal and subsyndromal common DSM-IV axis I and all axis II disorders. *Am J Psychiatry* (2011) 168(1):29–39. doi: 10.1176/appi.ajp.2010.10030340
30. Siegenthaler E, Munder T, Egger M. Effect of preventive interventions in mentally ill parents on the mental health of the offspring: systematic review and meta-analysis. *J Am Acad Child Adolesc Psychiatry* (2012) 51(1):8. doi: 10.1016/j.jaac.2011.10.018
31. Thanhäuser M, Lemmer G, Girolamo G, Christiansen H. Do preventive interventions for children of mentally ill parents work? Results of a systematic review and meta-analysis. *Curr Opin Psychiatry* (2017) 30(4):283–99. doi: 10.1097/YCO.0000000000000342
32. Maybery D, Reupert AE. The number of parents who are patients attending adult psychiatric services. *Curr Opin Psychiatry* (2018) 31(4):358–62. doi: 10.1097/YCO.0000000000000427
33. Goodyear M, Hill T-L, Allchin B, McCormick F, Hine R, Cuff R, et al. Standards of practice for the adult mental health workforce: meeting the needs of families where a parent has a mental illness. *Int J Ment Health Nurs* (2015) 24(2):169–80. doi: 10.1111/inm.12120
34. Maybery D, Reupert A. Workforce capacity to respond to children whose parents have a mental illness. *Aust N Z J Psychiatry* (2006) 40(8):657–64. doi: 10.1080/j.1440-1614.2006.01865.x
35. Montgomery P, Mossey S, Bailey P, Forchuk C. Mothers with serious mental illness: their experience of "hitting bottom". *ISRN Nurs* (2011) 2011:708318. doi: 10.5402/2011/708318
36. Maciejewski D, Hillegers M, Penninx B. Offspring of parents with mood disorders: time for more transgenerational research, screening and preventive intervention for this high-risk population. *Curr Opin Psychiatry* (2018) 31(4):349–57. doi: 10.1097/YCO.0000000000000423
37. Goodyear M, McDonald M, Doussa H, Cuff R, Dunlop B. Meeting the intergenerational needs of families where a parent has a mental illness. *J Parent Fam Ment Health* (2018) 3(2):e1011. doi: 10.7191/parentandfamily.1011
38. Gilbert AL, Balio C, Bauer NS. Making the legal and ethical case for universal screening for postpartum mood and anxiety disorders in pediatric primary care. *Curr Prob Pediatr Adolesc Health Care* (2017) 47(10):267–77. doi: 10.1016/j.cppeds.2017.08.001
39. Anding JE, Rohrle B, Grieshop M, Schucking B, Christiansen H. Couple comorbidity and correlates of postnatal depressive symptoms in mothers and fathers in the first two weeks following delivery. *J Affect Disord* (2016) 190:300–9. doi: 10.1016/j.jad.2015.10.033
40. Goodyear M, Obradovic A, Allchin B, Cuff R, McCormick F, Cosgriff C. Building capacity for cross-sectorial approaches to the care of families where a parent has a mental illness. *Adv Ment Health* (2015) 13(2):153–64. doi: 10.1080/18387357.2015.1063972
41. Laletas S, Reupert A, Goodyear M. "What do we do? This is not our area". Child care providers' experiences when working with families and preschool children living with parental mental illness. *Child Youth Serv Rev* (2017) 74:71–9. doi: 10.1016/j.childyouth.2017.01.024
42. Clemens V, Berthold O, Fegert JM, Kölch M. Kinder psychisch erkrankter Eltern: Auch ein Thema im Rahmen des Kinderschutzes [Children of mentally ill parents: also a topic in the context of child protection]. *Der Nervenarzt* (2018)89:1262 . doi: 10.1007/s00115-018-0561-x
43. Wahl P, Bruland D, Bauer U, Okan O, Lenz A. What are the family needs when a parent has mental health problems? Evidence from a systematic literature review. *J Child Adolesc Psychiatr Nurs* (2017) 30(1):54–66. doi: 10.1111/jcap.12171
44. Lauritzen C, Reedtz C, van Doesum KTM, Martinussen M. Implementing new routines in adult mental health care to identify and support children of mentally ill parents. *BMC Health Serv Res* (2014) 14:58. doi: 10.1186/1472-6963-14-58
45. Gladstone BM, Boydell KM, Seeman MV, McKeever PD. Children's experiences of parental mental illness: a literature review. *Early Interv Psychiatry* (2011) 5(4):271–89. doi: 10.1111/j.1751-7893.2011.00287.x
46. Afuah A, Tucci CL. Crowdsourcing as a solution to distant search. *Acad Manage Rev* (2012) 37(3):355–75. doi: 10.5465/amr.2010.0146
47. Bayley J, Phipps D. Real impact. In: *Impact literacy workbook*. United Kingdom: Emerald Publishing Limited (2018). Retrieved from www.emeraldgrouppublishing.com/tk/RealWorldImpact.
48. Wagner CS, Jonkers K. Open countries have strong science. *Nature* (2017) 550(7674):32–3. doi: 10.1038/550032a
49. Fixsen DL, Naoom SF, Blasé KA, Friedman RM, Wallace F. *Implementation research: a synthesis of the literature*. Tampa, FL: University of South Florida, Louis de la Parte Florida Mental Health Institute, The National Implementation Research Network (2005). http://nirn.fmhi.usf.edu/resources/detail.cfm?resourceID=31.
50. Pawson R, Tilley N. *Realist evaluation*. London: Sage Publications (1997).
51. Berger PL, Luckmann T. *The social construction of reality: a treatise in the sociology of knowledge (Repr. in Penguin Books)*. London: Penguin (1991).
52. Blumer H. *Symbolic interactionism: perspective and method*. New Jersey: Prentice-Hall Inc. (1969).
53. Proctor EK, Landsverk J, Aarons G, Chambers D, Glisson C, Mittman B. Implementation research in mental health services: an emerging science with conceptual, methodological, and training challenges. *Adm Policy Ment Health* (2009) 36(1):24–34. doi: 10.1007/s10488-008-0197-4
54. National Implementation Research Network. Consensus statement on evidence-based programs and cultural competence (2003). https://nirn.fpg.unc.edu/sites/nirn.fpg.unc.edu/files/resources/NIRN-ConsensusStatementOnEBPAndCultural-07-2003.pdf
55. Greenhalgh T, Jackson C, Shaw S, Janamian T. Achieving research impact through co-creation in community-based health services: literature review and case study. *Milbank Q* (2016) 94(2):392–429. doi: 10.1111/1468-0009.12197
56. Byng R, Norman I, Redfern S. Using realistic evaluation to evaluate a practice-level intervention to improve primary healthcare for patients with long-term mental illness. *Evaluation* (2016) 11(1):69–93. doi: 10.1177/1356389005053198
57. Archer M, Bhaskar R, Collier A, Lawson T, Norrie A. *Critical realism: essential readings*. London: Routledge (1998).
58. Morris CW ed. *Works of George Herbert Mead: Vol. 3. The philosophy of the act*. Chicago, IL, London: University of Chicago Press (1972).
59. Kaisler R, Paul J. Evidence-based practice and polices for impact on mental health of children and adolescents. *J Res Technol Policy Eval* (2019) 48. doi: 10.3389/fpsyt.2019.00233
60. Damschroder LJ, Aron DC, Keith RE, Kirsh SR, Alexander JA, Lowery JC. Fostering implementation of health services research findings into practice: a consolidated framework for advancing implementation science. *Implement Sci* (2009) 4:50. doi: 10.1186/1748-5908-4-50
61. Zechmeister-Koss I, Goodyear M, Paul J. Supporting children who have a parent with a mental illness in Tyrol: a multi-perspective needs-analysis for developing improved practice approaches. (In Preparation).

62. Elo S, Kyngäs H. The qualitative content analysis process. *J Adv Nurs* (2008) 62(1):107–15. doi: 10.1111/j.1365-2648.2007.04569.x
63. Taylor S, Haase-Casanovas S, Weaver T, Kidd J, Garralda EM. Child involvement in the paediatric consultation: a qualitative study of children and carers' views. *Child Care Health Dev* (2010) 36(5):678–85. doi: 10.1111/j.1365-2214.2010.01076.x
64. The KIDSCREEN Group Europe. *The KIDSCREEN Questionnaires—quality of life questionnaires for children and adolescents.* In: *Handbook.* Lengerich: Pabst Science Publishers (2006).
65. Beardslee WR, Brent DA, Weersing VR, Clarke GN, Porta G, Hollon SD, et al. Prevention of depression in at-risk adolescents: longer-term effects. *JAMA Psychiatry* (2013) 70(11):1161–70. doi: 10.1001/jamapsychiatry.2013.295
66. Beardslee WR, Gladstone TR. Prevention of childhood depression: recent findings and future prospects. *Biol Psychiatry* (2001) 49(12):1101–10. doi: 10.1016/S0006-3223(01)01126-X
67. Beardslee WR, Gladstone TRG, Wright EJ, Cooper AB. A family-based approach to the prevention of depressive symptoms in children at risk: evidence of parental and child change. *Pediatrics* (2011) 112(2):e119–e131. doi: 10.1542/peds.112.2.e119

6

Developing an Intervention to Improve the Health Related Quality of Life in Children and Young People with Serious Parental Mental Illness

Judith Gellatly[1,2], Penny Bee[2], Adekeye Kolade[1], Diane Hunter[3], Lina Gega[4], Craig Callender[5], Holly Hope[1] and Kathryn M. Abel[1,6]*

[1] Faculty of Biology, Medicine and Health, Centre for Women's Mental Health, Manchester Academic Health Science Centre, The University of Manchester, Manchester, United Kingdom, [2] Division of Nursing, Faculty of Biology, Medicine and Health, Manchester Academic Health Science Centre, School of Health Sciences, The University of Manchester, Manchester, United Kingdom, [3] NSPCC, London, United Kingdom, [4] Department of Health Sciences, Hull York Medical School, University of York, York, United Kingdom, [5] St. Nicholas Hospital, Northumberland Tyne and Wear NHS Foundation Trust, Newcastle upon Tyne, United Kingdom, [6] Greater Manchester Mental Health NHS Foundation Trust, Manchester, United Kingdom

***Correspondence:**
Judith Gellatly
judith.l.gellatly@manchester.ac.uk

Introduction: Children and adolescents living with parental mental illness (CAPRI) are at increased risk of behavioral, social and educational difficulties, mental and physical health problems and have poorer quality of life (QoL). Adverse outcomes can extend into adulthood but are not inevitable. Recent policy and stakeholder consultation recognize the urgent need for interventions that extend beyond objective, service-led measures of health. Systematic evidence synthesis has demonstrated a lack of evidence-based interventions for enhancing holistic, child-centered outcomes. We aimed to co-develop a manualised, community-based intervention to improve QoL in CAPRI. Precedence was given to the QoL domains that were prioritized by stakeholders and deemed feasible to modify within a health and social care context. We describe here the modeling phase of developing the intervention emphasizing co-production activities with CAPRI, their families and professionals who support them.

Methods: Semi-structured interviews and focus groups with CAPRI (n = 14), parents (n = 7), and professionals from health, social and educational sectors (n = 31) in the UK. Topic guides qualitatively explored participants prior experiences, unmet needs, perceived barriers and facilitators to receiving/delivering support, and their ideals for a new intervention. Findings were synthesized with existing research evidence and presented to a mixed panel of clinical academics and health and social care professionals. A consensus exercise was used to identify the preferred structure, format and content of the manualised intervention.

Results: An 8-week group intervention for 6–16 year olds and their parents, called Young SMILES, has been co-developed along with associated training materials for facilitators. Each session addresses an identified need, but is underpinned by cross-cutting themes pertaining to mental health literacy, parent-child communication, and problem solving skills. Sessions are delivered by two trained facilitators and held in accessible and acceptable community locations weekly for 2 h.

Conclusion: Young SMILES captures a broad age range and level of need for CAPRI and can be evaluated with quantifiable child-centered outcomes. In line with current policy directives, this is the first UK-based, multi-context intervention to improve QoL in this population. Implementation and referral mechanisms are currently being evaluated in a multi-site feasibility trial.

Keywords: co-production, children, young people, serious mental illness, parents, intervention, health-related quality of life

INTRODUCTION

Children and adolescents living with parental mental illness (CAPRI) are poorly provided for in current social care and educational settings (1, 2). Children and young people (CYP) growing up in families affected by parental mental health disorders have an elevated risk of physical health (3–5) and mental ill health (6, 7), attention or educational difficulties (1, 8, 9) and emotional and behavioral problems (10–12). They may be more socially isolated (13), and some will experience neglect (14), family separation (15), or social care involvement (16). Longer term outcomes for these children extend into adulthood and include chronic psychological difficulties, social and occupational dysfunction and substance misuse (17).

Risk of adverse outcomes is of increasing public health concern. Population estimates from the United States, Sweden and Australia suggest that between 38 and 50% of women with serious mental illness (SMI) will be mothers and approximately 25% of men with SMI will be fathers (18). In the UK (and Sweden) 1 in 4 children at any time are living with parental mental illness and, by 16 years of age, with over 50% of children will have experienced parental mental disorder of a severity sufficient to present to services.

Adverse outcomes are not inevitable and the impact of parental mental illness on children's outcomes is modifiable. Data suggests that at least half of all children with a parent with mental illness may not experience any psychiatric symptoms (19), and only a small proportion will access mental health services (10). Individual and family resilience can be heavily determined by an ability to find positive meaning in challenging events, to recognize a need to change social interactions or environmental conditions, and the increased availability of health-sustaining resources. Thus, how a parent or child makes sense of their experiences of mental illness may be as, if not more, important than the actual experience itself.

There is a growing literature exploring community-based interventions for CAPRI which has been comprehensively reviewed (20). Traditionally, parents have been considered the primary change agent for their children and parent-centered interventions have been evaluated for secondary effects on child outcomes. Quantified outcomes have primarily been behavioral or psychological in origin, and mediated by improved parenting or enhanced parental health (11, 21). Meta-analysis suggests that such parent-centered interventions are of variable quality and reliability (20).

Increasingly child and family-based approaches are permeating research arenas and these interventions offer an alternative and promising avenue for change. Child-centered interventions seek to establish the child as the major change agent. Research and consultation has suggested that children often have a different view of their situation, and a different idea of what would help compared to parents or mental health workers (19, 22). A philosophical shift away from "children as patients" has led to clinical, therapeutic interventions being replaced by more strength-based approaches. Peer support interventions have been advocated as a possible means by which to provide respite and reduce the isolation for CAPRI but are often not standardized or time bounded to a degree that facilities their roll-out or implementation across resource-constrained services. Additional work is needed to agree intervention priorities, identify the most likely active ingredients, and deliver these in the most cost and time efficient format.

In evaluating adult and services, focus has moved from simply the absence of disease to a more holistic approach, recognizing that improving the QoL, and specifically health-related QoL (HRQoL) as has great significance (23). QoL concerns how an individual perceives their own well-being and life experiences with respect to their personal beliefs, goals and expectations (24). In the context of severe parental mental illness, it can thus be conceptualized as both outcome and a modifier of children's short- and longer-term resiliency.

Multi-dimensional models of QoL reflect the scope and complexity of an individual's QoL judgments and offer a coherent, empirical based framework through which to potentially maximize intervention impact by simultaneously addressing multiple QoL domains. Targeted approaches to modifiable dimensions of QoL have the potential to improve the shorter and longer term availability of internal assets as well as external resources. These combined resources can strengthen protective factors, counteract or moderate risk factors and help to achieve positive adaptation in the face of adverse life experience (25–30). Effective adaptation can in turn, precipitate improved QoL appraisals, creating a positive feedback loop and maximizing return on investment.

Systematic evidence synthesis has demonstrated a striking lack of evidence-based interventions for enhancing holistic, child-centered outcomes. Bee et al. (20) identified only three trials focused on CYP with severe parental mental illness; and none of these explored QoL outcomes of CAPRI. This knowledge provides a compelling argument for a focused exploration of CAPRI need and the theoretical development, delivery and evaluation of novel, effective interventions (2, 20, 31). This paper describes development of a new intervention called Young SMILES [Simplifying Mental Illness and Life Enhancing Skills; (32)]. Development of the intervention was conducted in line with the Medical Research Council (MRC) complex interventions framework. Following identification of existing evidence and theory development, the MRC framework stipulates modeling an intervention by identifying key components of the intervention and its evaluation prior to conducting a feasibility trial (33).

MATERIALS AND METHODS

Co-development of the intervention involved three phases: Phase 1—Needs analysis—review of existing literature and primary qualitative research with stakeholders to identify needs and preferred delivery models; Phase 2—stakeholder consensus—professional synthesis exercise to identify emerging themes and agree provisional content and delivery preferences and; Phase 3—manual development and refinement—locating stakeholder preferences in existing knowledge literature (20) and theory of change involving team work.

A planning group of research team members, including those with clinical and service delivery experience, met face-to-face monthly throughout the project to discuss existing intervention literature and materials, emerging research data and the development of the Young SMILES intervention. Additional remote meetings were held as required for manual development.

The activities and findings from each development activity follow.

Phase 1 Needs Analysis

Existing Literature

The work presented here reports on a commissioned piece of work that aims to shift the spotlight away from the medicalization of CAPRI to focus on the development of a child-centered, community-based intervention to improve quality of life for all children affected by severe parental mental illness.

Literature exploring community-based interventions for CAPRI has been recently and comprehensively reviewed (20). This review, and the intervention resources identified with it, was used as a starting point for intervention development. An existing intervention, The Family SMILES intervention (34), provided a starting template for intervention development. Family SMILES is based on the SMILES programme, a 3-day intervention for Australian CYP aged 8–16 with a parent experiencing mental ill health (35). SMILES has been evaluated positively with respect to improving CYPs knowledge of mental health and coping skills (36).

Family SMILES has been piloted in the UK but not yet rigourously evaluated. FAMILY SMILES takes a deliberately narrow approach; focusing only on CYP at-risk of maltreatment or neglect. The intervention comprised 8 weekly groups: 6–8 CYP sessions; 6 one-to-one weekly sessions with parents; and a final CYP-parent joint session with each family. Its aim was to enhance children's resilience and self-esteem and parents' protective function; and to improve parent-child communication and family relationships. Preliminary evaluation of Family SMILES has highlighted potential benefits for CAPRI in increased social functioning and confidence, reduced social isolation and reduced blame associated with parental illness. For parents, benefits included less distress and unhappiness, a shift of thinking from own needs to those of their children; and for families overall a more relaxed atmosphere, openness about parental mental illness, empathy between CAPRI and parents and shared responsibilities (34).

Agreeing the Working Aim

The working aim, agreed between the research team and the project steering group, was to broaden the scope and content of Family SMILES to make it specific to families whose parents have SMI; to make it applicable to a wider age-range of CAPRI, to align it with NHS priorities and service structures and to make it deliverable in different practice settings by a varied staff skill mix, including NHS and voluntary sector providers. In the context of the UK NHS, our intention was to co-create a child-centered approach with far broader reach (geographical and across ages and needs), with a specific focus on enhancing children's QoL. QoL was defined according to a published, empirically-led model derived specifically for the target population (37). This definition upheld QoL as a multi-dimensional construct comprising of 5 domains spanning emotional, physical and social well-being, family context and experience and children's self-esteem and self-actualization. Precedence was given to three domains identified as priority by stakeholders and potentially capable of being modified via a time bounded health service intervention. These domains comprised emotional and social wellbeing, family experience and self-esteem and actualization. A fourth domain, physical wellbeing was represented as a secondary goal of the intervention and targeted through in-session education.

Within these priorities the importance of improving problem-based coping skills, increasing mental health literacy, and alleviation of parental mental health symptoms were evident.

Recognizing the importance of stakeholders' voices, our explicit intention was to place childrens' needs at the center of the process to create a best evidence, feasible and acceptable intervention to CAPRI improve health-related QoL (2). We used this approach to ensure that a priori beliefs and existing Family SMILES components did not drive our assumptions about what would and would not work for children. To achieve this, we interviewed participants blind to the Family SMILES intervention and explored ways to support CAPRI directly and separately from the experiences and needs of their parents. Despite the incidence rates of mental illness being increased for CAPRI, as a large percentage will not experience mental illness, we anticipated an intervention relevant to all CAPRI.

Primary Research

Stakeholders, including children and adolescents, parents and practitioners from NHS and voluntary settings (including managers), were invited to participate in discussion groups and individual interviews if they preferred. Individual discussion groups were held for each stakeholder group to maximize opportunities for participation. Consent was taken from

TABLE 1 | Stakeholder consultation methods and participants.

	Young People (n = 14)	Parents (n = 7)	Practitioners (n = 31)
Method:			3
Focus Group (number conducted)	2	1	
Interview (number conducted)	2 face-to-face	2 telephone	0
Family SMILES experience (n, %)	Previous experience 6, 43% No previous experience 8, 57%	No previous experience 7, 100%	Previous experience: Voluntary organization A practitioners (10, 32%) No previous experience: Voluntary organization B practitioners (15) and; NHS practitioners (6) (68%)
Gender	9 girls (64%), 5 boys (36%)	7 women (100%)	28 women, 1 man
Age (mean, range)	11, 10–16	41.14, 33–47	
Siblings (n, %)	11, 79%		
Live with parent experiencing SMI (n, %)	13, 93%		
Awareness of parental mental health type (n, %)	10, 71%		
Number of children under 17 years (mean)		2.43	
Time experienced SMI (mean, range)		14, 2–25	
Professional qualifications			Social work, teaching, counseling, clinical psychology, OT, mental health nursing, family therapy
Numbers in managerial position (n, %)			7, 23%

all participants prior to the discussion group/interview commencing. Parents were asked to consent for their child or adolescent taking part. For CYP, parental/guardian consent was required in addition to their assent. All parents/guardians approached agreed for their child to take part. Participation of both CYP and their parent was not necessary, but all were invited. Practitioners in the recruiting sites initiated contact with families and assisted in obtaining consent. Participants were asked to complete a short demographic questionnaire at the beginning of the discussion (separate questionnaires were developed for each stakeholder group). Discussion groups and individual interviews were held at a community location convenient to the participants. Travel expenses were reimbursed and refreshments provided.

Attendees were informed about the aim of the study and the value of their involvement in developing a new intervention to improve the QoL of CAPRI. The terminology used was altered for each stakeholder group to ensure understanding. Semi-structured topic guides explored experiences of previous support, unmet needs, barriers and facilitators to receiving/delivering support, gaps in current care and what an ideal intervention would look like. Interviews and focus groups were audio recorded or notes were taken. For CYP, methods to enhance engagement, such as using post-it notes to provide views anonymously for discussion, emojiis to express feelings about aspects of their ideal intervention and pens to draw were implemented. Data were analyzed using thematic analysis (38).

Interviews and focus groups took place between June and October 2016. Participants were recruited via two different voluntary organization regional branches (A and B) and the NHS (practitioners only). Some had direct experience of Family SMILES. **Table 1** provides an overview of the data collection methods and participant demographics.

Key themes were identified in relation to the purpose and composition of the Young SMILES intervention with comparisons between participant groups recognized. Core content topics or themes identified across all stakeholder groups highlighted that Young SMILES should educate (improve mental health literacy); reduce isolation and support. A theme about delivery preferences was also documented.

The following provides a summary of these findings and evidence of differing viewpoints.

Educative—Improving MH Literacy

Improving mental health literacy was regarded as important by young people and parents; and considered a key element of Young SMILES. This related to one's own understanding but also understanding within the wider society. For parents, lack of understanding of their own problems was acknowledged as having an impact on their views and beliefs about their ability successfully to undertake their role within the family. One parent highlighted the effect that depression can have and how improving their understanding is needed for help seeking.

> *"I understand what depression is now I can see it coming and see it in other people but the very first time you're not sure if it's ... you question yourself a lot. You question whether you're a good mum. Is it really you that's annoying everyone and people pick up on the signs. So at the beginning of the depression it's really understanding that you have got a mental illness yourself and recognizing it and then going to the doctors to do something about it without feeling embarrassed or stupid. That's a really big part of mental health."* (Parent)

There was a general sense, particularly among CYP, that society lacked awareness of what the experience of having a parent with an SMI is like. The negative consequences of this had an effect on their daily lives.

> *"no-one knows what I'm dealing with, they bully me because of my mum, they know I'm a young carer."* (CYP)

Attending school was challenging for many; lack of understanding and awareness of the effects of having a parent with an SMI extended beyond their peer group to their teachers. CYP were eager for changes to occur:

> *"I want them [school] to understand more, what I am as a young carer going through... understanding of why I come in late."* (CYP)

Whilst it was acknowledged that the intervention could not necessarily change society's awareness and perceptions, professional stakeholders recognized the importance of educating children and teachers about their parent's mental illness and saw this as a key element of providing support and overcoming the challenges those children can face:

> *"And that's often leaving children with a lot of space to create their own ideas of what's going on which is often much more frightening in the reality isn't it?"* (NHS practitioner)
> *"it was quite a normal reaction for the children to be able to want to understand their mother's difficulties which had been quite pronounced and defined really."* (NHS practitioner).

Reducing Isolation

As a result of living with a parent experiencing SMI, children reported that they often felt emotionally isolated. These experiences extended to their social lives, where some sacrificed activities for friends to look after their parent(s).

> *"I just can't go out with friends – need to make sure mum is OK first."* (CYP)

Parents acknowledged this was often the experience of their children and that there was often a reversal of roles, with their children taking on responsibilities they felt they shouldn't. This was distressing for parents, who felt a sense of guilt because of their inability to parent:

> *"you're having this problem you cannot get yourself out of, when you look at your children, you cannot help them."* (Parent)
> *"mental health becomes who you are."* (Parent)

Consistent with these experiences, professionals acknowledged the difficulties that CAPRI experience emotionally, highlighting their inability to understand the root cause.

> *"Yeah, they don't understand their own emotions, they don't understand the parents' emotions. They think that their parents' emotions are a reaction to their behavior, which sometimes that is what's going on, and the child takes all the responsibility for that."* (Voluntary organization A practitioner)

It was acknowledged that an intervention focused on children's needs has to negotiate the sensitivity of helping parents understand that their illness and its behaviors may adversely influence their children.

> *"It's that introductory process really, around, not just introducing what [the intervention] is about, but you're introducing the concept that there's some idea that this issue, that this parent has probably been living with for 20 years or more, can potentially impact on their children, and impact on how they are parenting their children."* (Voluntary organization A practitioner)

Support

Practitioners recognized the need to provide support to CYP and parents. For all stakeholders, the value of support on a predominantly emotional, but at times practical level was considered important. The value of providing a group intervention including peers was recognized as a key element. Many saw it as a way of reducing isolation among CYP and parents. Reflecting upon feedback from families they had worked with previously, one practitioner stated:

> *"It's ultimately about I thought it was only us who was struggling. I thought it was only me that at times hates my mum. And from a parent's perspective, I thought it was only me that is really struggling with my teenager, and all those issues. So I think there's also that experience really, about coming together and that mutual support and that I'm not on my own. And that there are similar experiences shared really."* (Voluntary organization B practitioner)

The additional value that involving their parent in an element of the intervention would provide was thought of positively across both sectors, with additional benefits for the family identified:

> *"And I think permission as well, I think permission to have conversations, that families... that they might be thinking of in their heads but not actually have the courage or feel they've got the permissions to have those conversations with each other."* (Voluntary organization B practitioner)

The importance of helping parents to overcome their unwillingness to approach difficulties via a more family or child-centered approach was acknowledged. Practitioners identified that they could play a supportive role to promote parent engagement:

> *"... my experience is often parents don't want you to, or they're maybe a little bit more reluctant, to have children involved say with the family meeting. And children will often be at school when people are calling... I sense there would be a reluctance and so some of the skill is about connecting to parents I think initially and maybe doing some work there about what maybe could be talked about and things and whether they can do some of that and we can support them in doing that."* (NHS Practitioner)

Parents recognized that talking to their children about mental health was challenging; particularly when they were "*really bad*" and that providing their child with the opportunity to speak to other CYP in similar circumstances helped their child to address some of the issues they were facing via different supportive avenues.

> *"It's like when you're talking to your own friends isn't it, you can open to your best friends and your partner, and whatever. But sometimes it's like, well, I can tell her anything but not about the mental health because you don't want them panicking... But when they're together and they've been through the same experiences... they can open up and they can say, my mum's done that. And then your [other parent's child] little one might say, well, my mum does that as well, or, you know, stuff like that, so they're not alone."* (Parent)

CYP and parents valued having the opportunity to have some "respite." Within the discussions it was evident that there were similarities between the views of parents and CYP such as the recognition of the importance of retaining their family unit but subtle differences were identified. CYP expressed a desire to receive support in an environment separate to their parents, for the most part, to discuss the difficulties they were experiencing and they felt being away from parents would make it easier for them to do so and reduce any impact this may have upon their parent:

> *"Or like anything's happening, any bullying or anything like that, if it did happen to me, I'd rather speak to [voluntary organization] about it than my mum because I don't want to put that pressure on my mum and everything... if it's something that's gone on at school or something that's happened, I have to keep it to myself. If I did keep it to myself, I would be okay with it, but then I'd just get a bit worried."* (CYP)
> *"My mum makes me nervous". (CYP)*

Parents mirrored these views, identifying the importance of '*children having a separate opportunity*' (Parent), but also recognized that, at times, their children's sense of responsibility for them was overwhelming and became a barrier to engaging in activities without them:

> *"I think it would be better if the children were separate and they had, like, a little group together and then all together. I know when our [child's name] had a first referral to [the voluntary organization] and she [facilitator] was, like, come with me. I said, she's dead nice. Because I'd spoken to her before and we'd gone through it all. I said, she's dead nice, she's lovely. And our [child's name] usually... if you meet her, she's, like, hello. And she was, like, no mum. And she got hold of my hand, you're coming with me. And I'm, like, are you sure you want me with you?... We're both turning up, she doesn't want to leave me by myself."* (Parent)

Delivery Preferences

For CYP, it was important that they had "*fun*" and that despite Young SMILES being an opportunity to learn more about their parents' mental health, it was vital that did not mirror the school environment, offering an opportunity to learn in non-traditional formats.

> *"Instead of just sitting down and talking... doing an activity... engaging in a different way so it doesn't feel like you are in school." (CYP)*

CYP focused their discussions on activities that could be included to ensure it was "fun." They wanted an opportunity for relevant team building and physical activities and somewhere to share their own experiences. Older children additionally expressed the value of "*anonymous self-expression.*" Whilst they recognized the potential use of technology in the activities included in the Young SMILES sessions, they were reluctant for it to be incorporated because of its potential effect on their ability to engage with others in the group highlighting it was *"anti-social" and reflecting on the impact that involving technology may have upon the intervention:*

> *"It's [technology] wasting our time together." (CYP)*

While parents acknowledged the need for "*fun*" and allowing their children to experience "*childhood*" they focused less on the type of activities they thought Young SMILES should contain; predominantly exploring the potential outcomes that could be achieved for their children such as encouraging independence/increase confidence, educating and normalizing:

> *"Because they kind of have that attachment to us [our children] and that worry, that anxiety. And that's true really, because they don't want it, they're constantly seeing you on the couch, you know. So that time when they are go off [to Young Carers activity] not to worry, because that's what they're there for. So they kind of get used to that, oh mum can be okay when I'm not around."* (Parent)

Practitioners identified that "selling" the intervention was important and, in doing so, they needed to understand what would be attractive to CYP from an individual perspective:

> *"But they would all have their different reasons for coming, won't they? I mean some may come back because they found it was fun, some may come back because they liked the food, some might come back... So everyone's coming from a different angle, young people and even parents. So it's about trying to attract them in some way, and we do that quite well with our activities and stuff, to try and sell it to young people. You think well, I know they like coming because their friend comes, or they like coming because they like that. So they all have different reasons, motivations for coming."* (Voluntary organization B practitioner)

Phase 2: Stakeholder Consensus

As part of our co-development methodology, a stakeholder synthesis day was held. The aim of the synthesis day was to review existing and new research knowledge in order to agree provisional content and delivery preferences for intervention. The synthesis day was open to all individuals currently working with or potentially working with children of parents with severe mental illness in the future. This involved practitioners, academics and managers representing voluntary sector and NHS services attended. During the day, key findings were presented to professional stakeholders alongside existing research. A consensus exercise was used to identify the preferred structure and key components of the finalized intervention, focusing predominantly on implementation and delivery. Tensions between findings and views were explored and acknowledged.

Two qualitative research team members facilitated the day. The aim was to use group consultation to identify agreement and to resolve areas where the evidence was ambiguous or less established. There were three consecutive activities:

1. Listening
2. Identifying gaps and ambiguities
3. Reaching consensus

Nineteen people (9 research team members and 10 non-team individuals) attended the synthesis day. A variety of different professional organizations and roles were represented including those working in academia e.g., health service researchers, psychiatrists, psychologists and a PhD student and voluntary sector organizations e.g., social workers, team managers, business managers and NHS organizations e.g., family therapists, mental health nurses). Attendees were experienced in at least one of the following—working with vulnerable CYP (who may or may not have parents experiencing SMI); working with vulnerable families (where there may or may not be a parent experiencing SMI); working with adults or children with mental health difficulties; or conducting research in the field of adult or CYP mental health.

1. Listening

   Key messages that emerged from existing literature and Phase 1 stakeholder consultation were presented. Attendees were asked to think about what the data implied about what Young SMILES should look like and to make notes that would be useful for activity two.
2. Identifying gaps and ambiguities

   Attendees were asked to reflect on the information from activity one in order to populate a *synthesis matrix*. The matrix aimed to ascertain three areas: intervention format (e.g., content, facilitation, delivery); intervention resources (e.g., training manuals, service resources), and any additional relevant information.

   The two workshop facilitators reviewed the matrix, identifying any contradictory or missing areas. **Table 2** presents a summary of aspects that participants were in agreement about and those where some inconsistencies or evidence gaps were acknowledged.
3. Reaching consensus

   In response to the findings from activity two, attendees in four small multidisciplinary groups were asked to discuss one of the four areas where gaps in the evidence or ambiguities had been identified (detailed in **Table 2**). Participants were told that the aim was to draw upon their own experiences, express their views to the group and listen to those of others to reduce uncertainties and to come to a consensus.

   Summaries of the discussions, including a clear rationale, were fed back verbally to the wider group.

   Following the synthesis day, the planning group consulted with the steering committee and parent representatives prior to finalizing the Young SMILES intervention. The steering committee and parent representatives reviewed and agreed the proposed intervention format, guidance and training materials. Innovation of Theory of Change was used as a guiding methodology for finalizing the change model underpinning the intervention. The intervention was intended to be child-centered and the primary outcome of the intervention, determined a priori at study commissioning stage was enhanced QoL.

TABLE 2 | Summary of the outcome of activity two discussions.

Agreement	Inconsistencies/lacking evidence
Aim: Respite, social networking, accessing help, integrated services/wider engagement [Mental Health Education] **Content:** Safety plan, mental health education, signposting, communication skills, practical support for parents **Who:** Discrete age groups **Where:** Transport **Who:** Support worker for parent **Engagement:** Build trust, consolidate peer support, develop between session resources **Resources:** Assessment is crucial, food **Facilitator training:** Group management skills	1. Intervention resources 2. Delivery format • Group composition • How long and over what time period/legacy 3. School/multi-agency liaison and engagement 4. Measures/legislative frameworks • Assessment • Progress/success

RESULTS

Figure 1 presents the Theory of Change diagram developed as a result of consultation and consensus activities.

Theory of change conceptualizes Young SMILES with respect to the problems faced by CAPRI, Young SMILES inputs and change mechanisms, primary outcome(s) for children and impact upon associated risk of negative outcomes. It additionally takes into account the QoL domains and priorities as determined by CAPRI within previous literature [e.g., (20, 37)]. The change model built on Phase 1 data synthesis and Phase 2 stakeholder consultation and as such was inclusive of multiple perspectives and participants in its design. It required stakeholders to make a distinction between desired and actual outcomes and to identify their desired outcomes before deciding on possible intervention content and processes to achieve those outcomes.

Processes that normalize children's experiences, improve their social and peer support networks and/or enhance their mental health literacy and problem-based coping skills are upheld as important change mechanisms and influenced both the format and content of the Young SMILES intervention. Children's psychological resistance is dependent on these elements to ensure enhanced wellbeing or protection from the impact of potential risk factors by enabling them to gain a better understanding of parental SMI and interact with their family context. Similar priorities have been reported in the literature (39, 40), and empirical work (41). Studies have identified that many CAPRI

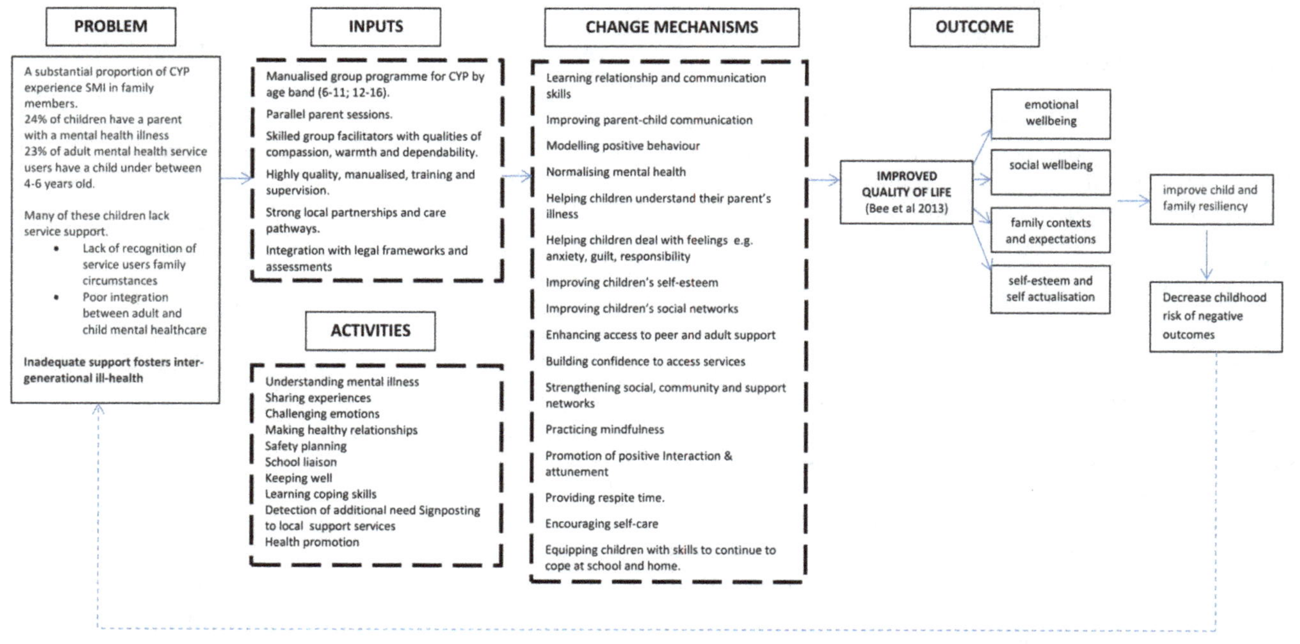

FIGURE 1 | Young SMILES theory of change.

adopt a caring role for this parent(s), a responsibility that can extend to looking after or supporting other family members (42). The importance of Young SMILES including problem-focused approaches to enhance coping strategies was identified as an important element among stakeholders to empower children to maintain their long-term emotional health. The adoption of a group format, and the inclusion of parent sessions, was hypothesized to strengthen children's and young people's support and encourage child-centered developmental opportunities. Establishing and strengthening social networks is recognized as one potentially effective way of enhancing self-management capacity and well-being (43), and positive family and peer interactions are recognized as important contributors to children's QoL (41, 44).

Programme Outline

On establishing the theoretical framework, the planning group finalized the intervention outline and facilitators' manual. Resulting data showed some overlap with Family SMILES such as the involvement of parents, the opportunity to meet other children in similar circumstances and increase knowledge, as well as the need for new components. Integration of these two led to Young SMILES being recognized as separate from, but a derivative of, Family SMILES. It was called Young SMILES in recognition of common components.

Young SMILES is a manualised 8-week group programme for CAPRI designed to work with small groups of children/adolescents: it is recommended that a minimum of 4 to a maximum of 6 children/adolescents are involved per group. Its explicit focus is to improve children's health related QoL. The wide age range of Young SMILES groups is split according to the school the young person attends, either primary (6–11) or secondary (12–16). Each group work session is allocated a 2-h time slot, which includes time for a short break and refreshments (with parents/carers) during and after the group. The structure of each session is presented in **Table 3**.

TABLE 3 | Session structure for CYP and parent sessions.

CPY sessions (week 1–8)	Parent sessions (week 4–8)
• **Welcome:** 10 min • **Warm-up game:** 10 min • **Activity 1:** 10 min • **Made-up family:** 20 min • **Snack break:** 10 min • **Activity 2:** 10 min • **Weekly home activity:** 10 min • **Wind-down game:** 10 min • **Snack and closure:** 30 min	- **Welcome:** 10 min - **Warm-up activity:** 10 min - **Weekly Reflection:** 20 min - **Snack Break:** 10 min - **Feedback from children's sessions:** 20 min - **Wrap-up discussion:** 20 min - **Groups join for end snack:** 30 min

Within each session the following is always covered:

- "Ice-breaker" warm-up activities, including links to previous sessions, to enable the group to recap the main learning points and raise and discuss any issues or questions.
- "Checking in" to identify how things have been since the last session and identifying if any of the CYP need individual time to talk over any particular issues that may have happened since the last session.
- Setting the agenda and objectives for the session—Facilitators set out the session's aims e.g., "today we aim to learn about

managing a crisis: who we can contact in a crisis; how to manage our feelings of fear in times of uncertainty; what to do when we think our parent is going into crisis etc." CYP are given the opportunity to tell the facilitators what they would like to learn or achieve and if they had any anxieties about the session.
- Education and interaction included presentation and discussion of information conveyed via flip charts or drawings, videos, play, creative writing, case studies, and scenarios, all relevant to the learning objectives of the session.
- "Wrapping-up" at the end of the session to elicit feedback on the session, recap on the main learning points, answer questions and agree on activities to be done between sessions and a brief taster of what the next session will cover.
- Getting together as a group for something to eat with in communal space before going home.

At week 4 of the CYP's work group, parallel sessions are offered to the parent/carer who is unwell; and to an additional significant adult in the child's life (identified by the child and their carer) who might attend with the unwell adult, or attend in their place. From week 4 onwards, the CYP and parent groups get together for a snack at the end of the sessions.

Based on stakeholder consultation, we assigned different objectives to each session, but all CYP and parent sessions were underpinned by three emergent themes: mental health literacy, communication and problem-solving skills. Outlined in the facilitator's manual are activities that can be used to achieve the aims of the session. Whilst the overall aims and objectives of each session should not be altered the ways that they can be achieved is flexible to ensure responsiveness to CYP and parent needs. **Figure 2** provides an overview of the structure and aims of each proposed CYP (8) and parent (5) sessions. CYP and parent sessions were delivered by two trained facilitators from the NHS or voluntary organizations and held in accessible and acceptable community locations for 2 h each week.

Intervention Refinement

The final intervention was presented to service users (parents), practitioners and the trial steering committee for feedback and refinement. Positive feedback was received with individuals indicating that it adhered to the aims of the overall feasibility study and was an accurate reflection of what has been identified via exploration of the research evidence and the views of CYP, parents and professionals. Despite this, some practitioners assigned to delivering the intervention requested that additional step-by-step guidance to conduct the in-session activities be provided to improve their understanding and, in some cases, confidence. A more detailed structure for the in-session activities could also support fidelity to the intervention's objectives and consistency of delivery across sites.

DISCUSSION

CAPRI are a growing and vulnerable group of multiply deprived young people whose QoL is compromised significantly (2). Little specific provision is available to meet their needs in current services where the focus has been on the parents. In a wholly novel approach, we undertook a series of consultations, focus groups, and a synthesis workshop with CAPRI themselves, with their parents and a broad range of professional stakeholders involved in the support of CAPRI to co-develop a child-centered QoL intervention. Our intervention development aimed to maximize the involvement of all stakeholder groups at the same time as minimizing burden, but further consultation with CYP in the refinement stages of Young SMILES manual could have been beneficial.

There was consistency and overlap between the perceived needs of the CYP, but parents and professional stakeholders did not appreciate their requirements in detail, nor did they appreciate their need for more basic, quotidian support. Although mental health literacy, communication, and problem solving skills emerged as themes for all, CAPRI were clear in wanting peer-focused help and information to understand and manage their parental illness away from their parents in their own ways and in their own space. The young people described feeling isolated socially and in other ways; as well as lacking support and understanding from teachers and schools with a need for greater recognition about their situation by peers, schools and teachers. It was recognized that helping parents understand how and when their illness and behaviors influenced the lives of their children adversely was important but this communication needed some sensitivity. The consistency between perceived needs amongst stakeholders was inconsistent with previous research (19). This could be as the CYP and parents involved were already engaging with services and as a result may have been more informed about the impact that parental mental health was having within the family. The focus of the questions within focus groups and interviews around what an ideal intervention to meet their needs, rather than focusing solely on what their specific needs are, also may have influenced the commonality of responses.

These insights helped us to create a novel, child-centered intervention to deliver away from parents initially in group-based, peer-focused sessions over 8 weeks. It included valued elements for CAPRI such as fun, creative and physical activities and snack times with parents in the latter half of the intervention weeks. Thus, we were able to prioritize CAPRI needs within the wider context of ensuring the feasibility and acceptability of a multidisciplinary team-developed intervention that integrates best practice from mental health and social care.

Young SMILES may provide opportunity for greater collaboration between NHS and voluntary organizations to support CAPRI and mean individuals in different sectors work together and share their knowledge and expertise to meet the needs of this vulnerable and underserved population. Young SMILES, therefore, optimizes the potential value, impact and

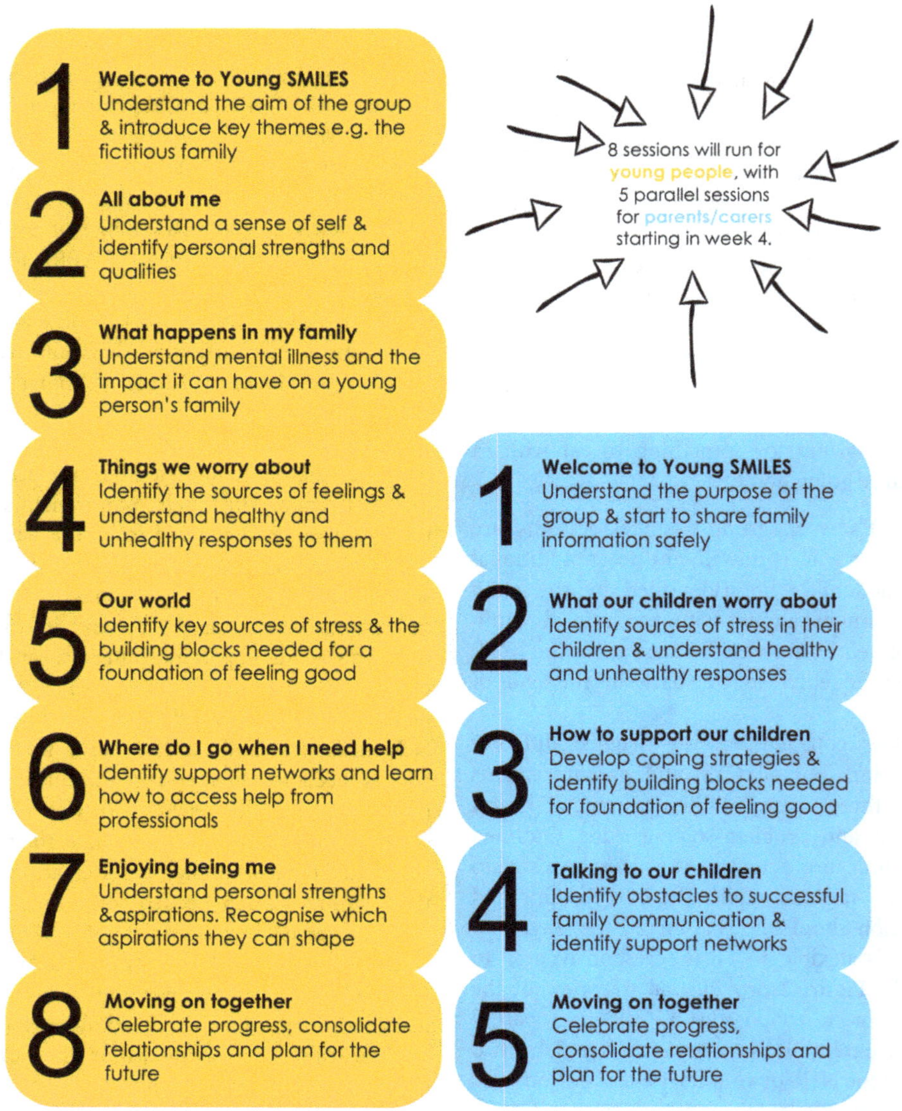
1
Welcome to Young SMILES
Understand the aim of the group & introduce key themes e.g. the fictitious family
2
All about me
Understand a sense of self & identify personal strengths and qualities
3
What happens in my family
Understand mental illness and the impact it can have on a young person's family
4
Things we worry about
Identify the sources of feelings & understand healthy and unhealthy responses to them
5
Our world
Identify key sources of stress & the building blocks needed for a foundation of feeling good
6
Where do I go when I need help
Identify support networks and learn how to access help from professionals
7
Enjoying being me
Understand personal strengths &aspirations. Recognise which aspirations they can shape
8
Moving on together
Celebrate progress, consolidate relationships and plan for the future
8 sessions will run for young people, with 5 parallel sessions for parents/carers starting in week 4.
1
Welcome to Young SMILES
Understand the purpose of the group & start to share family information safely
2
What our children worry about
Identify sources of stress in their children & understand healthy and unhealthy responses
3
How to support our children
Develop coping strategies & identify building blocks needed for foundation of feeling good
4
Talking to our children
Identify obstacles to successful family communication & identify support networks
5
Moving on together
Celebrate progress, consolidate relationships and plan for the future

FIGURE 2 | Young SMILES CYP and parent session overview.

scalability across statutory services none of whom traditionally are not targeting this group which occupies a space between the health and social care interface.

Our future work lies in piloting the broader acceptability and feasibility of the new programme and testing our ability to deliver it to scale within a randomized controlled trial method for future evaluation of clinical and cost effectiveness.

CONCLUSIONS

There is a clear need for a child-centered, specific and focused approach to supporting vulnerable young people living with severe parental mental illness across the UK and globally (2). We have recognized the need to consult closely with children themselves and have co-developed an intervention shaped by their input and understanding with an emphasis on peer support separate to the support their parents receive. Future formal evaluation of Young SMILES will help to consolidate these close links with CAPRI keeping them at the center of solutions to the difficulties they face on a daily basis.

ETHICS STATEMENT

The study was approved by North West - Greater Manchester East Research Ethics Committee (Ref: 16/NW/0207 13th April 2016). Approval was also obtained from Barnardo's Research Ethics Committee (BREC) 26th July 2016. All participants gave written informed consent in accordance with The Declaration of Helsinki.

AUTHOR CONTRIBUTIONS

JG, PB, DH, LG, CC, and KA participated in the development of Young SMILES. JG, PB, and AK analyzed the qualitative data. JG, PB, KA, LG, and HH prepared the manuscript. All the authors read and approved the final manuscript.

FUNDING

This project was funded by the National Institute for Health Research (NIHR) Health Technology Assessment programme (project reference 14/29/01). The views and opinions expressed therein are those of the authors and do not necessarily reflect those of the Health Technology Assessment programme, NIHR, NHS, or the Department of Health.

ACKNOWLEDGMENTS

We would like to thank all the children and young people, parents, practitioners, managers and academics who took part, provided support and contributed to this piece of research. We would also like to thank Caitlin McWilliams for her involvement in the design of the Young SMILES study documentation.

REFERENCES

1. Social Care Institute for Excellence. *Think Child, Think Parent, Think Family: A Guide to Parental Mental Health and Child Welfare SCIE Guide 30.* (2011). Available online at: http://www.scie.org.uk/publications/guides/guide30/index.asp (accessed August 6, 2018).
2. Abel KM, Hope H, Faulds A, Pierce M. Improving the life outcomes of children and adolescents living with parental mental illness. *Br J Psychiatry.* (in press) BJPsych-18-0590.R1.
3. Santos IS, Matijasevich A, Domingues MR, Barros AJ, Barros FC. Long-lasting maternal depression and child growth at 4 years of age: a cohort study. *J Pediatrics.* (2010) 157:401–6. doi: 10.1016/j.jpeds.2010.03.008
4. Giallo R, Bahreinian S, Brown S, Cooklin A, Kingston D, Kozyrskyj A. Maternal depressive symptoms across early childhood and asthma in school children: findings from a Longitudinal Australian Population Based Study. *PLoS ONE.* (2015) 10:e0121459. doi: 10.1371/journal.pone.0121459
5. Letourneau NL, Kozyrskyj AL, Cosic N, Ntanda HN, Anis L, Hart MJ, et al. Maternal sensitivity and social support protect against childhood atopic dermatitis. *Allergy Asthma Clin Immunol.* (2017) 13:26. doi: 10.1186/s13223-017-0199-4
6. Compas BE, Champion JE, Forehand R, Cole DA, Reeslund KL, Fear J, et al. Coping and parenting: mediators of 12-month outcomes of a family group cognitive–behavioral preventive intervention with families of depressed parents. *J Consult Clin Psychol.* (2010) 78:623. doi: 10.1037/a0020459
7. Rasic D, Hajek T, Alda M, Uher R. Risk of mental illness in offspring of parents with schizophrenia, bipolar disorder, and major depressive disorder: a meta-analysis of family high-risk studies. *Schizophr Bull.* (2014) 19:40:28–38. doi: 10.1093/schbul/sbt114
8. Tabak I, Zabłocka-Żytka L, Ryan P, Poma SZ, Joronen K, Viganò G, et al. Needs, expectations and consequences for children growing up in a family where the parent has a mental illness. *Int J Ment Health Nurs.* (2016) 25:319–29. doi: 10.1111/inm.12194
9. Farahati FM, Marcotte DE, Wilcox-Gök V. The effects of parents' psychiatric disorders on children's high school dropout. *Econ Edu Rev.* (2003) 22:167–78. doi: 10.1016/s0272-7757(02)00031-6
10. Dean K, Stevens H, Mortensen PB, Murray RM, Walsh E, Pedersen CB. Full spectrum of psychiatric outcomes among offspring with parental history of mental disorder. *Arch Gen Psychiatry.* (2010) 67:822–9. doi: 10.1001/archgenpsychiatry.2010.86
11. van Santvoort F, Hosman CM, Janssens JM, van Doesum KT, Reupert A, van Loon LM. The impact of various parental mental disorders on children's diagnoses: a systematic review. *Clin Child Fam Psychol Rev.* (2015) 18:281–99. doi: 10.1007/s10567-015-0191-9
12. Siegenthaler E, Munder T, Egger M. Effect of preventive interventions in mentally ill parents on the mental health of the offspring: systematic review and meta-analysis. *J Am Acad Child Adolesc Psychiatry.* (2012) 51:8–17. doi: 10.1016/j.jaac.2011.10.018
13. Breslend NL, Parent J, Forehand R, Peisch V, Compas BE. Children of parents with a history of depression: the impact of a preventive intervention on youth social problems through reductions in internalizing problems. *Dev Psychopathol.* (2019) 31:219–31. doi: 10.1017/S0954579417001821
14. Steer S, Reupert A, Maybery D. Programs for children of parents who have a mental illness: referral and assessment practices "one size fits all"? *Aust Soc Work.* (2011) 64:502–14. doi: 10.1080/0312407x.2011.594901
15. Hall A. Parental psychiatric disorder and the developing child. *Parent Psychiatr Disorder.* (2004) 13:22–49. doi: 10.1017/cbo9780511543838.005
16. Angermeyer MC, Matschinger H. The stigma of mental illness: effects of labelling on public attitudes towards people with mental disorder. *Acta Psychiatr Scandin.* (2003) 108:304–9. doi: 10.1034/j.1600-0447.2003.00150.x
17. Stanley N, Penhale B, Riordan D, Barbour RS, Holden S. Working on the interface: identifying professional responses to families with mental health and childcare needs. *Health Soc Care Commun.* (2003) 11:208–18. doi: 10.1046/j.1365-2524.2003.00428.x
18. Reupert A, Maybery D. What do we know about families where parents have a mental illness? A systematic review. *Child Youth Serv.* (2016) 37:98–111. doi: 10.1080/0145935X.2016.1104037
19. Maybery D, Ling L, Szakacs E, Reupert A. Children of a parent with a mental illness: perspectives on need. *Aust e-J Adv Ment Health.* (2005) 4:78–88. doi: 10.5172/jamh.4.2.78
20. Bee P, Bower P, Byford S, Churchill R, Calam R, Stallard P, et al. The clinical effectiveness, cost-effectiveness and acceptability of community-based interventions aimed at improving or maintaining quality of life in children of parents with serious mental illness: a systematic review. *Health Technol Assessment.* (2014) 18:8. doi: 10.3310/hta18080
21. Bee P. Community preventive interventions for children of parents with serious mental illness: a commentary on the evidence base. *Adv Ment Health.* (2015) 13:165–7. doi: 10.1080/18387357.2015.1066945
22. Cooklin A. Promoting children's resilience to parental mental illness: engaging the child's thinking. *Adv Psychiatr Treatment.* (2013) 19:229–40. doi: 10.1192/apt.bp.111.009050
23. Barry M, Zissi A. Quality of life as an outcome measure in evaluating mental health services: a review of the empirical evidence. *Soc Psychiatr Psychiatr Epidemiol.* (1997) 32:38–47. doi: 10.1007/BF00800666
24. World Health Organization. The World Health Organization Quality of Life assessment (WHOQOL): position paper from the World Health Organization. *Soc Sci Med.* (1995) 41:1403–9. doi: 10.1016/0277-9536(95)00112-K
25. Rethink. *Rethink Policy Statement 43: Rethink's Understanding of Severe Mental Illness.* (2008). Available online at: http://www.rethink.org (accessed December 17, 2012).
26. Reupert A, Maybery D. Families affected by parental mental illness: a multi-perspective account of issues and interventions. *Am J Orthopsychiatr.* (2007) 77:362–9. doi: 10.1037/0002-9432.77.3.362
27. Goodman SH, Rouse MH, Connell AM, Broth MR, Hall CM, Heyward D. Maternal depression and child psychopathology: a meta-analytic review. *Clin Child Fam Psychol Rev.* (2011) 14:1–27. doi: 10.1007/s10567-010-0080-1
28. Beardslee WR, Versage EM, Gladstone TRG. Children of affectively ill parents: a review of the past 10 years. *J Am Acad Child Adolesc Psychiatr.* (1998) 37:1134–41. doi: 10.1097/00004583-199811000-00012

29. Fernbacher S, Goodyear M, Farhall J. Taking a closer look: a cross-sector audit of families where a parent has a mental illness. *Adv Ment Health.* (2009) 8:242–9. doi: 10.5172/jamh.8.3.242
30. Oyserman D, Mowbray CT, Meares PA, Firminger KB. Parenting among mothers with a serious mental illness. *Am J Orthopsychiatr.* (2000) 70:296–315. doi: 10.1037/h0087733
31. Thanhäuser M, Lemmer G, de Girolamo G, Christiansen H. Do preventive interventions for children of mentally ill parents work? Results of a systematic review and meta-analysis. *Curr Opin Psychiatr.* (2017) 30:283–99. doi: 10.1097/YCO.0000000000000342
32. Abel K, Green J, Bower P, Bee P, Wolpert M, Stanley N. *A Community-Based Intervention to Improve Health-Related Quality of Life in Children and Adolescents of Parents with Serious Mental Illness: Feasibility Study.* (2016). Available online at: http://www.nets.nihr.ac.uk/projects/hta/142901
33. Medical Research Council. *A Framework for the Development and Evaluation of RCTs for Complex Interventions to Improve Health.* London: MRC (2000).
34. Margolis R, Fernandes P. *Building Children's Confidence and Improving Parents' Protective Skills: Final Evaluation of the NSPCC Family SMILES Service.* London: NSPCC (2017).
35. Pitman E. *SMILES Program: Simplifying Mental Illness Plus Life Enhancement Skills.* Adelaide: Children of Parents with a Mental Illness (COPMI) (2010).
36. Pitman E, Matthey S. The SMILES program: a group program for children with mentally ill parents or siblings. *Am J Orthopsychiatr.* (2004) 74:383–8. doi: 10.1037/0002-9432.74.3.383
37. Bee P, Berzins K, Calam R, Pryjmachuk S, Abel KM. Defining quality of life in the children of parents with severe mental illness: a preliminary stakeholder-led model. *PLoS ONE.* (2013) 8:e73739. doi: 10.1371/journal.pone.0073739
38. Braun V, Clarke V. Using thematic analysis in psychology. *Qual Res Psychol.* (2006) 3:77–101. doi: 10.1191/1478088706qp063oa
39. Royal College of Psychiatrists. *CR164 Parents as Patients: Supporting the Needs of Patients Who are Parents and Their Children.* (2010). Available online at: http://www.rcpsych.ac.uk/publications/collegereports/cr/cr164.aspx (accessed December 17, 2012).
40. Beresford B, Clarke S, Gridley K, Parker G, Pitman R, Spiers G. *Technical Report for SCIE Research Review on Access, Acceptability and Outcomes of Services/Interventions to Support Parents with Mental Health Problems and their Families.* (2008). York: Social Policy Research Unit, University of York.
41. Gladstone BM, Boydell KM, Seeman MV, McKeever PD. Children's experiences of parental mental illness: a literature review. *Early Interv Psychiatr.* (2011) 5:271–89. doi: 10.1111/j.1751-7893.2011.00287.x
42. Grant G, Repper J, Nolan M. Young people supporting parents with mental health problems: experiences of assessment and support. *Health Soc Care Commun.* (2008) 16:271–81. doi: 10.1111/j.1365-2524.2008.00766.x
43. Reeves D, Blickem C, Vassilev I, Brooks H, Kennedy A, Richardson G. The contribution of social networks to the health and self-management of patients with long-term conditions: a longitudinal study. *PLoS ONE.* (2014) 9:e98340. doi: 10.1371/journal.pone.0098340
44. Crossroads Caring for Carers and The Princess Royal Trust for Carers. *Economic Evaluation of Young Carers' Interventions.* (2008). Available online at: http://static.carers.org/files/finalfinal3-4040.pdf (accessed December 17, 2012).

7

Promotion of Wellbeing for Children of Parents with Mental Illness: A Model Protocol for Research and Intervention

Charlotte Reedtz[1], Karin van Doesum[1,2], Giulia Signorini[3], Camilla Lauritzen[1], Therese van Amelsvoort[4], Floor van Santvoort[5], Allan H. Young[6], Philippe Conus[7], Richard Musil[8], Thomas Schulze[9], Michael Berk[10,11], Argyris Stringaris[12], Geneviève Piché[13] and Giovanni de Girolamo[3]*

[1] RKBU North, Faculty of Health, UiT – Arctic University of Norway, Tromsø, Norway, [2] Team Preventie, Onderzoeker Mindfit, Nijmegen, Netherlands, [3] Unit of Epidemiological and Evaluation Psychiatry, IRCCS Istituto Centro San Giovanni di Dio Fatebenefratelli, Brescia, Italy, [4] Department of Psychiatry and Psychology, Maastricht University, Maastricht, Netherlands, [5] Pluryn/Hoenderloogroep, Research & Development, Nijmegen, Nederlands, [6] Department of Psychological Medicine, Institute of Psychiatry, Psychology and Neuroscience, King's College London and South London and Maudsley NHS Foundation Trust, London, United Kingdom, [7] Service de Psychiatrie Générale, Dép. de Psychiatrie, Centre Hospitalier Universitaire Vaudois (CHUV), Lausanne, Switzerland, [8] Bipolar Disorders and Borderline Personality Disorders Unit, Clinic for Psychiatry and Psychotherapy, LMU Klinikum der Universität München, München, Germany, [9] Institute for Psychiatric Phenomics and Genomics (IPPG), Klinikum der Universität München, München, Germany, [10] IMPACT Strategic Research Centre, School of Medicine, Barwon Health, Deakin University, Melbourne, VIC, Australia, [11] Orygen Youth Health Research Centre and the Centre of Youth Mental Health, The Florey Institute for Neuroscience and Mental Health and the Department of Psychiatry, University of Melbourne, Melbourne, VIC, Australia, [12] Mood and Development Laboratory, Emotion and Development Branch, National Institute of Mental Health, National Institutes of Health, Bethesda, MD, United States, [13] Psychoeducation and Psychology Department, Université du Québec en Outaouais, Gatineau, QC, Canada

***Correspondence:**
Charlotte Reedtz
charlotte.reedtz@uit.no

Background: The main objective of this project is to create a research and intervention model to promote large-scale implementation and evaluations of generic very brief interventions for children of parents with mental disorders (COPMI). Feasible interventions for COPMI aged 0–18 years are highly needed, as this is a large high-risk group in society. Reducing behavioral problems and enhancing wellbeing for families with parents affected by any mental disorder are important preventive initiatives. One key prevention strategy is to reduce the risk and expression of psychopathology in children and to promote wellbeing. The present model protocol offers an intervention for children of parents with mental disorders internationally based on a model already implemented in the Netherlands and Norway.

Methods: Participants will be parents receiving treatment in mental health services in participating countries and their minor children aged 6–18 years. Participants should be randomized into an intervention group or control group. Data should be retrieved from electronic patient journals (demographics, DSM 5/ICD-10, SCID, MINI) as well as from assessment measures administered at baseline and follow-up, including the KIDSCREEN-27, Strengths and Difficulties Questionnaire (SDQ), Parents' Evaluations of Developmental Status (PEDS), Parenting Sense of Competence (PSOC), Resilience Scale for Adolescence (READ), Guilt and Shame Questionnaire for Adolescents of Parents with Mental Illness (GSQ-APMI), Mental Health Literacy Scale, and Parent–Child Communication Scale.

Results: The hypothesis is that there will be improvements of child behavioral and emotional problems, and outcomes in the project will be reported in terms of parent's diagnosis, child behavioral and emotional problems, child wellbeing, family communication and functioning, as well as participants' satisfaction.

Discussion: This multi-site international protocol will focus the attention of European scientific and policy makers toward COPMI. This young segment of the population is presently almost completely neglected in most European health policies, despite having a large burden of disability and being at risk of transgenerational transmission of psychopathology. We will further discuss the feasibility of a very brief intervention aiming at preventing mental disorders in young people.

Keywords: children of parents with mental disorders, mental health care for adults, risk and protective factors, wellbeing, prevention

INTRODUCTION

Mental disorders in parents are a major biological and environmental risk factor to which many young people are exposed. About 15–23% of children live with a parent with a mental disorder worldwide (1, 2). These children are 5.2 times more at risk of depression and 3.7 times more at risk of anxiety disorders compared to their peers (3). Children of parents with mental disorders are also at risk of poorer intellectual and social outcomes (4), affect dysregulation (5), behavioral problems (6), impaired attention, and reduced overall adaptive functioning (7). Research has also shown that children of parents with mental disorders have higher rates of substance abuse and multiple diagnoses (8), as well as a lower occupational status. The transmission of parental psychopathology to children can lead to similar (transgenerational equi-finality) as well as different (transgenerational multi-finality) clinical outcomes than their parent's diagnosis (9–11). The risk factors and adverse outcomes create an amplifying vicious cycle, mandating preventative action (12).

Living with a parent suffering from a mental disorder may imply the exposure to a variety of risk conditions, including: a) an adverse family environment characterized by poor parenting, high stress reactivity, emotional vulnerability, and compromised family functioning; b) experience of guilt, stigma, shame and loneliness, and perceptions of lacking social support and social acceptance; and c) the reversal of care-giving ("parentification") (13). According to Hosman and colleagues (14), the adverse outcomes for these children are the result of a complex interplay between three systemic levels (parent, child, and parent–child relationship) and potential risk factors (such as parents' mental disorder, lack of social support, poor financial conditions, marital discord, etc.). Research has shown that impaired parent–child interaction is the environmental risk factor that explains most variance in child psychological problems (27.2%) (15).

However, through carefully designed interventions addressing this interplay, one can enhance wellbeing for families with parents suffering from a mental disorder. Interventions aiming at reducing the impact of risk factors within the family context and strengthening children's ability to cope are promising, although the results in terms of effect size seem still of limited amplitude. A meta-analysis, from 2012 on 13 trials on preventive interventions for mental disorders in offspring, indicated how the risk of developing parents' mental disorder could be decreased by 40% (16). In a recent meta-analysis, 50 randomized controlled trials on preventive interventions for mental disorders in offspring showed small, but significant effect sizes, stable over 12-month follow-up, for programs enhancing the mother–child interaction (17). Interventions addressing parents and children jointly produced overall larger effects. Nevertheless, the conclusion of this review was that there is a scarcity of high-quality studies that effectively reduce the high risk of COPMI for the development of mental disorders.

Targeting children at risk and approaching them through their parents, rather than waiting until they become adults, will strengthen the reach of youngsters at their most critical point for the onset of mental disorders (18). Some research has explored experiences of youngsters living in these families and their expressed needs (19), and results show that minor children want more information about their parent's disorder and practical support related to coping with the family situation. Moreover, children of parents with a mental disorder should be expected to be as heterogeneous as the group of their parents. In order to understand their life lived experiences and needs, health professionals and social workers therefore need to listen to them. Preventive intervention could provide more complete and effective care provision for parents already in care (20). Including a whole family approach could increase treatment outcomes in adult mental health care as well as patient satisfaction with service providers. For these reasons, healthcare systems seriously need to consider preventive programs for children of mentally ill parents.

As suggested by a pioneering Australian example, it is imperative that such programs are offered to the public once their effectiveness has been established in terms of immediate and long-term outcomes (21), through both quantitative and qualitative data (22). Interventions should be designed to reduce the impact from stress and lack of quality care within the family context (related to poor or absent communication, poor understanding of disorders, insufficient parental care, lack of clinical support, or negative attitudes toward help-seeking, etc.), as well as to strengthening children's ability to cope by informing them of their parents' mental disorder and to supply both emotional and social support.

Inspired by Beardslee and colleagues (23) in the US, various programs have been developed in Australia, Canada, Finland, the Netherlands, and Norway in order to promote youth mental health and reduce risk factors linked to living with parents affected by a mental disorder (24), mostly affective disorders. Family Talk (25) was the first structured family-based preventive intervention, and because of its demonstrated efficacy, this program has been implemented in various countries worldwide (26). As an alternative to family approaches, other programs offer group-based cognitive–behavioral preventive interventions (27) and treatment coordination tailored for individual families (28). Web programs have also been tested. Programs vary in length and include very brief interventions made up of 1–3 sessions (26, 29). Some interventions focus only on parents instead of the whole family (30).

There is a great heterogeneity in the preventive programs for children as well as in their documented efficacy (17, 31). The common component across these preventive initiatives is the provision of psychosocial education on how to cope with parental mental disorder to families and children. However, further evaluation is required to examine what interventions work and for whom (e.g., sample characteristics), and through which mechanisms (e.g., program components and fidelity). Risk screening seems to be necessary to ascertain the type and intensity of support that best meets the risk profiles and needs of individual children and families (16).

At odds with the promising preventive initiatives in this field, many countries in Europe neglect these children's needs or have no structured responses in terms of dedicated mental healthcare pathways or programs. The lack of prevention in many EU countries may stem from culture-mediated lack of consideration of the service users' families (including siblings, partners, and children) in mental healthcare settings, and hence individual- or illness-centered care and treatment models. In addition, specific economic, organizational, and political issues may contribute to the lack of a child focus (i.e., resource distribution may be limited, poor or unavailable protocols for intervention, lack of collaboration between adult mental health services and the rest of the healthcare social care and lack of educational resources).

In 2015, Giovanni de Girolamo, M.D., initiated a joint application for funding from Horizon 2020 named PROCHILD. He created an international consortium with the aim to develop an international multi-site research project to evaluate and compare the effects of a very brief intervention across the nations collaborating in the consortium. The members of the consortium were experienced researchers and clinicians in the field of parental mental disorder and their children. The research and intervention model protocol described in this article is derived out of the PROCHILD protocol.

The aim of the present project is to provide a research and intervention model protocol to evaluate a very brief intervention for children of mentally ill parents adapted for a large-scale implementation. The intervention is based on an existing preventive strategy already adopted in the Netherlands and Norway called the "Child Talks" (29, 32, 33). The intention is to contribute to the current state of the art, by providing a model protocol for a feasible and widely replicable preventive intervention. This is feasible as it makes it possible to:

1. Implement a structured and brief preventive intervention targeted at families with children aged 6–18 years old and one or both parents suffering from mental disorders.
2. Evaluate the efficacy of a very brief intervention compared with treatment as usual.

METHOD

Participants

Participants should be diagnosed parents of minor children aged 6–18 years old where parents are receiving outpatient or inpatient treatment at mental health services for any mental disorders. A total of two to three treatment clinics in each participating country should serve as intervention sites. The minimum final sample size for each experimental condition should be N = 82.

Recruitment

The primary investigator of an international study should establish an international consortium with researchers from the COPMI field represented. Each of the participating researchers should have access to relevant clinical sites *via* university hospitals and clinics. In each country, there should be cluster randomization (site-randomization) of at least two to three participating adult services. Participants should be recruited through adult mental health services where parents are in treatment, inviting patients and their families to take part in the study as part of the treatment offered. Recruitment should be supported by all health care and social workers in each site, and posters and flyers should be available to inform parents. The intervention to be evaluated should be randomly assigned to the experimental or control condition (see **Figure 1** for details).

Inclusion criteria: Families should have at least one parent in treatment for any psychiatric disorder (according to DSM 5 or ICD-10 diagnostic criteria) and at least one child aged 6–18 years.

Exclusion criteria: Parents with current substance or alcohol addiction, who are acutely ill or actively suicidal parents, and parents with serious physical co-morbidities should be excluded, as these families need more intense interventions. Parents who are not able to provide consent/assent due to language or other difficulties and parents with an IQ ≤ 70 or indication of intellectual impairment should be excluded. Exclusion criteria regarding the child(ren) include ongoing psychotherapy and/or pharmacotherapy led by a Child and Adolescent Mental Health Service (CAMHS), as well as children in foster care or custody (even with grandparents).

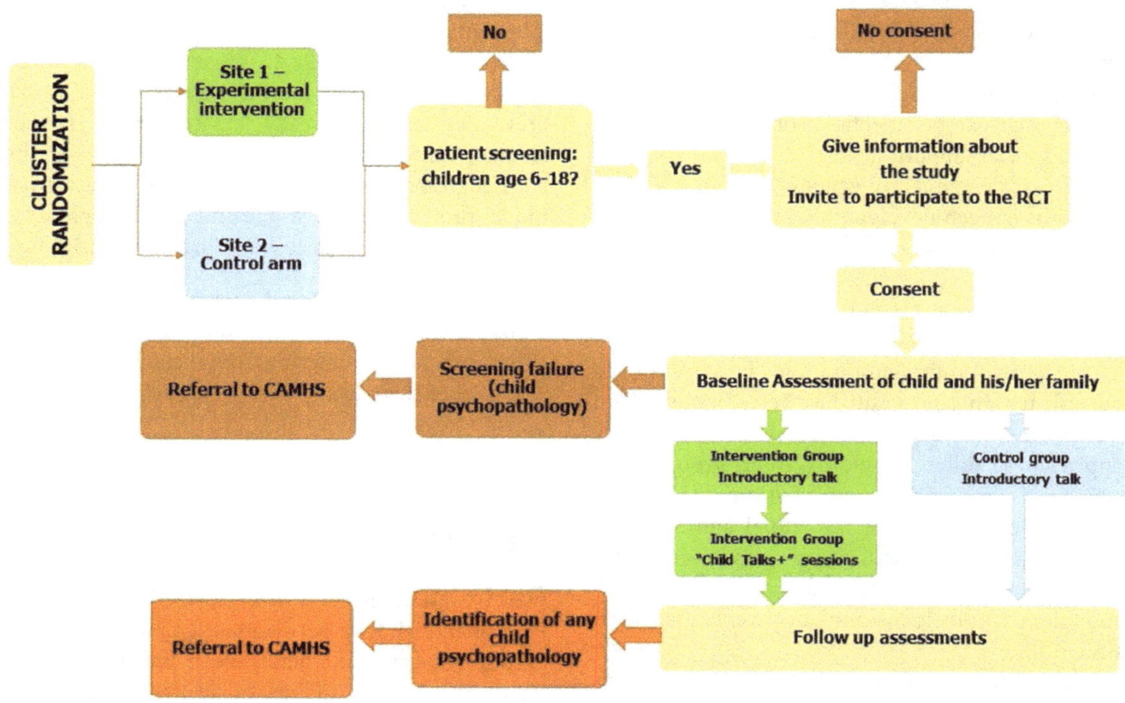

FIGURE 1 | Study design flowchart.

Procedure

A coordinator should explain the study in details to the potential participants and request their consent to contact the rest of the family. Subsequently, consent should be obtained from the participating family members. Participation by the whole family should be encouraged, although intervention can start even when only part of the family (at least one parent and one child) is willing to accept. In order for children (under the age of legal consent) to take part in the study, the parents' consent is required.

Participants should be provided with a calendar-based sessions/assessment schedule and receive reminders for their appointments. For the intervention group, two facilitators (trained in the intervention strategies) should conduct each session. Trained personnel should conduct assessments for all groups.

Design

The design of the research is a cluster-randomized controlled trial evaluating the effects of an improved version of the Child Talk Intervention called Child Talk+. In each country, the participating adult services (clusters) should be randomized into to the following experimental conditions:

Experimental group. After the baseline assessment (T0), recruited patients/families in participating services should be given the manualized "CHILD TALK+" intervention (four weekly 45-minute sessions, with trained facilitators); see **Figure 2** for the outline. After the intervention, assessment should be repeated (T1). Parents and children should be followed up at 6 (T2), 12 (T3), and 18 (T4) months. The contents and language of sessions should be adapted to the type of parental disorder and the age group of the child(ren) (6–12 or 13–18 years).

Control group. After the baseline assessment (T0), participants should receive information session about the mental health of children living with a parent affected by mental disorder, including risk and resiliency factors for the child(ren). The rationale for this experimental condition is that several European countries have policies, which mandates health personnel to identify and provide care for children of parents with mental disorder. A true control condition with no information would force health personnel in such countries to break the laws, and therefore a control condition including information about the risks for the children is necessary to include such countries. After the introductory session, postintervention assessment should be conducted (T1). Participants should be followed up at 6 (T2), 12 (T3), and 18 (T4) months. Support material should be available, but with no active role of facilitators in transferring this information into family practice.

Randomization. Cluster randomization will buffer against contamination effects, and each cluster will only deliver intervention/no intervention representing one experimental condition. The trial should be conducted according to Good Clinical Practice, reported according to CONSORT guidelines, analyzed according to SPIRIT guidelines, and registered at www.clinicaltrials.gov.

Intervention

Child Talks+ is an intervention where the mental health workers talk with the family about the situation of the children and their needs when a parent struggles with mental health issues. This intervention was developed in the Netherlands (32) and has been part of regular practice for two decades there. The updated intervention Child Talk+ comes with a manual that describes the process of carrying out four separate conversations/meetings; two initial conversations/meetings with the patient and possibly his/her partner, followed by two conversations/meetings with the patient (and partner) and the children involved (34).

Meeting 1. The initial meeting is preferably to be conducted with both parents/caregivers. In the beginning of the meeting, the purpose of conversation one should be explained to the parents/caregivers. The mental health workers should talk to the parents about the potential consequences of the mental disorder on their children and the family life. Parents should be given relevant information about the potential impact on the children, and they should be informed about possible protective factors.

Meeting 2. The second meeting is also conducted with both parents/caregivers. The purpose of this meeting is to supervise the parents and inform them about how they can discuss mental disorder at home. Examples on how to address these issues should be given, and the mental health workers should practice with the parents on how to talk to children about mental disorder, for instance, through role-play. At the end of meeting two, preparations for the next meeting should be done together with the parents/caregivers.

Meeting 3. In meeting three, the children also participate, together with the parents. The main purpose of this conversation is to get an overview of how the children are coping with the situation. The children's experiences should be discussed. Another important purpose of this meeting is to give emotional support and to provide information about the parent's mental disorder to the children (by the parents supported by the mental health worker) as prepared in meeting two. If the children have any questions, they should be answered by the parents or the mental health workers.

Meeting 4. The final meeting is with both parents/caregivers and the children if possible. The purpose of this meeting is to sum up and evaluate the previous meetings. Any questions the family may have should be addressed. The possible next steps for the family should also be discussed, and the mental health workers should assist the family in order to seek additional support if necessary. The intervention is illustrated in **Figure 2**.

The intervention allows the parents/patients to describe their children's resources and vulnerability and to participate in planning how they want their child to be informed of the family situation. The intervention includes the children through questions about their understanding and experiences of the family situation, and the children's view of what may improve their situation.

Intervention Integrity

The professionals should follow the manual for the intervention and complete standard checklists (logbook) for each session to ensure this.

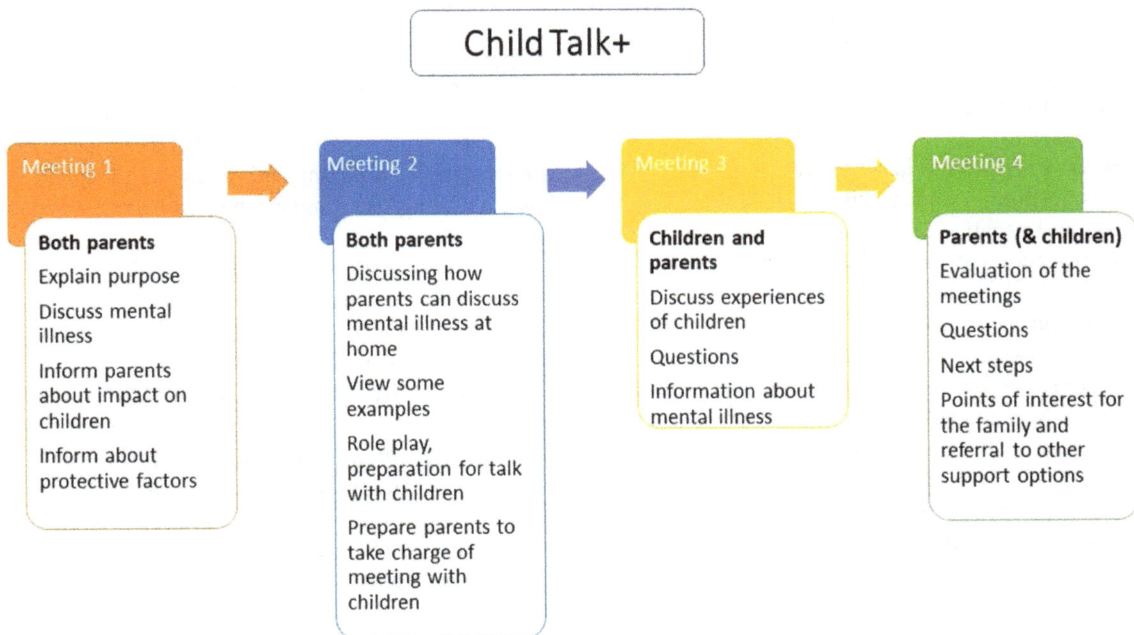

FIGURE 2 | Intervention outline.

Training

Training for facilitators should be provided according to manualized procedures. A set of booklets and slides should be created as consultation materials for both intervention and control conditions.

Measures

Multiple informants, including the children themselves, will contribute to tap a variety of areas at baseline, postintervention, and follow-up assessments. All assessments will be conducted individually with each subject, and these include: child wellbeing, child resilience, feelings of guilt and shame, child problems and development status, parents' evaluations of child developmental status, parent–child communication, child mental health literacy, and parenting competence. The following measures are suggested:

Sociodemographic variables: Parental gender, age, marital state, living situation, education, work, income, as well as parental diagnosis and severity of parental mental disorder. Diagnosis can be retrieved from clinical records. Diagnoses should be based on structured clinical interviews as SCID or MINI (35) and be codified with DMS IV, DSM 5 (36, 37), or ICD-10 (38). Severity of parental mental disorder parent should be retrieved from clinical records or GAF score (36). Children's baseline characteristics should include age, gender, living with mentally ill parent or not, total number of siblings, and educational attainment.

The health-related quality of life (KIDSCREEN-27) (39). The KIDSCREEN-27 is a measure for health-related quality of life for children from 8–18 years of age. It contains 27 items building five subscales: physical wellbeing, psychological wellbeing, autonomy and parents, social support and peers, and school environment. A 5-point Likert response scale is used in all subscales. All scores are reported as T-values, with higher scores indicating higher health-related quality of life. KIDSCREEN-27 was found to be a reliable and valid measure of quality of life in children and adolescents (40). Answering the KIDSCREEN-27 requires 10–15 minutes.

The Resilience Scale for Adolescence (READ) (41). READ is a self-report questionnaire measuring resilience: the ability to handle stress and negative experiences. READ is a 28-item scale with positively formulated items organized in five subscales: personal competence, social competence, social support, family cohesion, and structured style. Statements are answered on a 5-point Likert scale from 1 (completely disagree) to 5 (completely agree). Higher scores indicate higher degrees of protective characteristics associated with resilience within each domain. Subscale scores are summarized into a total score for resilience. It takes 5 minutes to complete the questionnaire. READ shows adequate psychometric properties and promising validity when correlated with measures of mental difficulties (42).

Guilt and Shame Questionnaire for Adolescents of Parents with Mental Illness (GSQ-APMI; 3). This questionnaire includes 10 items, 5 items measuring shame, and 5 measuring guilt. Adolescents are to answer how often they have experienced feelings of guilt and shame, with answers on a 5-point Likert scale from ranging from 0 (never) to 5 (always). Reliability scores were found adequate in a previous study (43).

The Strengths and Difficulties Questionnaire (SDQ) (44). SDQ is a brief behavioral screening questionnaire for children aged 3–16 years old. The scale is composed of 25 items, divided between 5 scales: emotional symptoms, conduct problems, hyperactivity/inattention, peer relationship problems, and prosocial behavior. Statements are answered on a 3-point Likert scale ranging from not true, somewhat true, to certainly true. Reliability scores have been found adequate in previous studies (45).

Parents' Evaluations of Child Developmental Status (PEDS) (46). PEDS is a 10-question measure. The first item is an open-ended question where parents describe any concerns they may have about their children in terms of behavior, learning, and development. In the following eight questions, the parents consider whether they have concerns in each developmental domain, and the final question probes any additional concerns. PEDS determines whether children are at a) high risk for developmental problems, b) moderate risk for developmental and/or mental health problems, c) limited risk but in need of in-office advice, or d) limited/no risk (47). Reliability scores have been found adequate in previous studies.

Parent–Child Communication Scale (48). The Parent–Child Communication Scale consists of one scale for children and one for parents. The child report consists of 10 items measuring children's perceptions of their primary caregiver's openness to communication. Statements are answered on a 5-point Likert scale from 1 ("almost never") to 5 ("almost always"). The parent report reflects the child's perception of the primary caregiver's effort to maintain open communication with him/her. The child communication scale reflects the frequency with which the child communicates his/her feelings and problems with the primary caregiver.

Children's Mental Health Literacy Scale (49). The scale examines children's knowledge of mental disorder, recovery, and stigma. The scale consists of multiple choice questions developed for children of a parent with a mental disorder. The scale is currently being tested and will be ready for dissemination during the next year.

Parenting Sense of Competence (PSOC) (50). The PSOC is a 16-item measure intended to assess parents' beliefs that they are capable of doing a good job parenting their child. It is comprised of two subscales and is rated on a 6-point scale from 1 ("strongly agree") to 6 ("strongly disagree"). The efficacy subscale measures parents perceived competency (e.g., "being a parent is manageable, and my problems are easily solved"), while the satisfaction subscale measures parental satisfaction (e.g., "being a parent makes me tense and anxious"). Research on the PSOC has demonstrated adequate reliability and validity when used with parents of young children (50).

User satisfaction. The satisfaction of healthcare users should be evaluated by a scale tapping into issues related to challenges of being a parent with mental health problems.

Sample Size and Statistical Power

Based on the results in Prchal et al. (51), the delta score, pre-post 4 months, of KIDSCREEN-27 in a single group (similar to an experimental group with four meetings) is equal to 4.28. Therefore, in a precautionary way, we hypothesized a lower difference pre-post of about 2.5 between the experimental group (four meetings) and the control group (one meeting). Considering the longitudinal design of this model study protocol, we hypothesized a preventive correlation between two evaluations (baseline-post treatment) of 0.5 so that the pooled SD of the scores changes will be 4.90. With such data and using a two-tailed paired t-test with confidence level of 95% and a power of 0.8, the estimated sample size is N = 60 for each group (experimental and control group). Considering a drop-out rate of 25%, the minimum sample size is of N = 160 (80 per group). Given that all children of the same sick parent can be involved in the trial, we also have to consider the ICC for the intra-family correlation. Although this ICC is likely to be lower, we hypothesized an ICC of 0.04. The average number of children in European families is quite variable, ranging from 1.2 in Portugal to 2.0 in France (2014 data). Since we also have to account for non-European countries, we hypothesize an average number of children per family of 1.5. The design effect in this case will be 1.02, increasing the sample size to about N = 164 (82 children per group). Finally, this sample size should be adjusted for the multicenter design of the study. DE is defined (52) as: DE = 1+(N/m−1)*ICC, where m is the number of sites, and ICC is the intra-class correlation coefficient (e.g., ICC = 0.03). Therefore, the minimum final sample size for each group will be equal to N = 82*DE.

Statistical Analysis

Group comparisons on demographic variables can be carried out using ANOVA or chi-square tests, depending on whether the variables are continuous or categorical.

We suggest to test three specific questions about group differences over time: 1) Are there any group differences in change from pre- to post-interventions? 2) Are there any group differences in change from pre-intervention to follow-up? And 3) are there any group differences in change from post-intervention to follow-up? Rausch, Maxwell, and Kelley (53) argue that these specific questions should be analyzed using ANCOVA, controlling for the pre-score in all analyses to maximize power. We therefore suggest using ANCOVA and to use the pre-score as covariate in all analyses (53). In order for the ANCOVA to be valid, there should be no treatment group differences on pre-intervention measures. In order to test whether the intervention and control group were different at pre-intervention measures, we suggest using a one-way ANOVA. Effect sizes should be calculated according to suggested methods (54).

Ethical Considerations

Each participating country should apply for ethical approval of the project from their relevant Regional ethics committees. There are several ethical dilemmas, which could be discussed in such application: a) what are the norms to which parents with mental disorders feel obliged to follow, when they try to be good parents; b) how far are they able to follow these norms, or when and why do they fail to follow them; and c) what are the cost of not intervening to stop the transgenerational transfer of mental disorder.

In cases of screening failure due to the child(ren)'s overt psychopathology or in the event that during the trial, or at follow-up assessment, serious concerns about the child(ren)'s psychopathology should emerge; the research team should act according to country-specific guidelines and norms, as agreed with regional ethical committees (i.e., referral to Child and Adolescent Mental Health Services).

Dissemination

Data from projects using the present protocol should be shared and available for researchers *via* accepted data repositories. Principles for storing data in national databases and cross-national exchange should follow relevant laws and guidelines. Results should be published internationally and presented at conferences, as well as disseminated *via* international research groups and collaboratives.

RESULTS

Outcomes should be reported in terms of demographics, parent's diagnosis, child behavioral and emotional problems, child wellbeing, family communication and functioning, as well as user satisfaction. The expectation would be to find greater and more sustained improvements for these outcomes in the intervention group than in the control condition, and test results should be presented.

DISCUSSION

Research projects based on the model study protocol presented in this paper will draw the attention of scientific and political communities toward children of mentally ill parents. This young segment of the population is presently almost completely neglected in most European national health policies, despite carrying the largest burden of disability in this age group. On a daily basis, this population faces social, biological, and environmental risk factors threatening their mental health.

The European context is not homogeneous, but only very few countries (e.g., Netherlands Norway, Sweden, Portugal, and Finland) are currently implementing protocols for children with parents affected by mental disorders. The rest of Europe implements at most, less structured initiatives in a few areas, with no data available in terms of evaluated clinical effectiveness (and costs). A universal approach has never been fully adopted. Thus, our model protocol is consistent and complementary as it aims to implement and test a very brief intervention for children of parents with mental disorders to prevent the onset of mental ill health, reduce disability and symptomatology, and ameliorate developmental disruption. Furthermore, other universal interventions may also be tested using this protocol.

The advance of the current state of the art is twofold. First, for those countries where the intervention has already been implemented, this study will i) offer the chance to test its efficacy through the replication of the results and ii) assess its external validity, exporting the model to other countries. Secondly, countries currently with no structured intervention will be able to implement it in their own health services, testing its efficacy, and evaluating its feasibility. The result of any national or international research projects based on the present model protocol could make a platform for establishing guidelines to be disseminated throughout Europe and beyond. Such guidelines would contribute to: a) recognize the needs of selective prevention initiatives, b) define the minimum requirements in formulating a protocol in each country, and c) ensure greater homogeneity of health policies in Europe and worldwide, regarding prevention and support for all minor children with parents suffering from severe mental disorders.

Improving youth wellbeing and good health is a key issue of current EU and WHO policies. The Child Talk+ intervention is primarily oriented toward promoting positive mental health for young people whose parents suffer from mental disorders. It aims at boosting existing service models. Interventions like this one will create an innovative, evidence-based intervention platform, which will provide a solid basis to improve existing healthcare systems. The present model protocol also opens the possibility to evaluate the sustainability, feasibility, and cost-effectiveness of a very brief intervention in different sites and countries. Results from such projects will inform policy makers and foster decisions that will increase the cost-effectiveness of care, thus improving the therapeutic management of patients with young children and help define preventive strategies for children's wellbeing.

In particular, research projects based on the present model protocol will address the expected impact, as follows:

Improved support and parenting among mentally ill parents. By introducing evidence-based intervention strategies, improving early recognition of children's ill health and malleable risk factors, this RCT will support a family approach in the current adult mental service. The intervention will decrease the potential impact of risk factors related to stressful environmental stimuli within the family, such as poor or absent communication of mental suffering, poor understanding of symptoms or disorders, insufficient parental care, and lack of clinical support or help-seeking. Patients will receive acknowledgement for their parenting role and support in their effort to take good care of their children although they have mental health problems. Its replicability will assist in creating a 21st century clinical framework including neglected children's needs and to promote improved integration of healthcare.

Improved wellbeing among COPMI through supportive interventions that will help them cope with a demanding family environment (created by the fragility and complexity of a parent with mental disorder). This will enhance individual resources to cope with these stressors by providing information about parents' mental disorder and giving families emotional and social support. It will also reduce negative experiences and negative emotions that could lead to feelings of intense discomfort. By limiting the negative effects of prolonged exposure to stress, the medium- and long-term impact will decrease the probability that youngsters' psychological distress leads to mental disorder.

Establish preventative strategies favoring the mental dimension of healthy childhood by allowing youngsters to meet age-specific developmental goals. Research projects based on this model protocol will aid policy makers and service providers at local, national, and international levels concerning the policy, strategic, clinical, and organizational changes needed to ensure appropriate primary and secondary prevention programs. It will also help integrate treatment for this under-served clinical population, promoting the mental and physical dimensions of healthy childhood.

Establish recommendations for the integrated treatment of patients with mental disorders and their children. Research projects based on this model protocol will foster the development of recommendations for training programs targeted at clinicians and allied professionals on how to improve mental health care for patients who are also parents, as well as good collaboration between AMHS and CAMHS. Local variations in service structures, healthcare provision, and clinician training will be taken into account.

AUTHOR CONTRIBUTIONS

All authors have, CR, KD, GS, CL, TA, FS, AY, PC, RM, TS, MB, AS, GP and GG, contributed in the conceptualization of the model protocol with regard to the design and methods, as well as having read and commented on the manuscript text. CR, KD, GS, and CL have put the paper into writing. All authors have approved of the final version of the paper.

ACKNOWLEDGEMENTS

We would like to acknowledge our work institutions which have supported our work on the Horizon 2020 application and the follow up. The views expressed are those of the authors and not necessarily those of our work or funding institutions. The publication charges for this article have been funded by a grant from the publication fund of UiT The Arctic University of Norway.

REFERENCES

1. Leijdesdorff S, Van Doesum K, Popma A, Klaassen R, Van Amelsvoort T. Prevalence of psychopathology in children of parents with mental illness and/or addiction: an up to date narrative review. *CE: Alpana; YCO* (2017) 300412(4):312–17. doi: 10.1097/YCO.0000000000000341
2. Maybery D, Reupert AE. The number of parents who are patients attending adult psychiatric services. *Curr Opin Psychiatry* (2018) 31:358–62. doi: 10.1097/YCO.0000000000000427
3. Havinga PJ, Boschloo L, Bloemen AJ, Nauta MH, de Vries SO, Penninx BW, et al. Doomed for disorder? High incidence of mood and anxiety disorders in offspring of depressed and anxious patients: a prospective cohort study. *J Clin Psychiatry* (2017) 78(1):e8–17. doi: 10.4088/JCP.15m09936
4. Goodman SH, Brumley HE. Schizophrenic and depressed mothers: relational deficits in parenting. *Dev Psychol* (1990) 26(1):31–9. doi: 10.1037//0012-1649.26.1.31
5. Lancaster S. Being There: How parental mental illness can affect children. In: Cowling V, editor. *Children of Parents with Mental Illness.* The Australian Council for Educational Research Ltd (1999).
6. Beck CT. Maternal depression and child behaviour problems: a meta-analysis. *J Adv Nurs.* (1999) 29(3):623–9. doi: 10.1046/j.1365-2648.1999.00943.x

7. Garley D, Gallop R, Johnston N, Pipitone J. Children of the mentally ill: a qualitative focus group approach. *J Psychiatr Ment Health Nurs* (1997) (2), 97–103. doi: 10.1046/j.1365-2850.1997.00036.x
8. Downey G, Coyne JC. Children of depressed parents: an integrative review. *Psychol Bull* (1990) 108(1):50–76.
9. McLaughlin KA, Gadermann AM, Hwang I, Sampson NA, Al-Hamzawi A, Andrade LH, et al. Parent psychopathology and offspring mental disorders: results from the WHO World Mental Health Surveys. *Br J Psychiatry* (2012) 200(4):290–9. doi: 10.1192/bjp.bp.111.101253
10. Van Santvoort F, Hosman CM, Janssens JM, van Doesum KT, Reupert A, van Loon LM. The impact of various parental mental disorders on children's diagnoses: a systematic review. *Clin Child Fam Psychol Rev* (2015) 18(4):281–99. doi: 10.1007/s10567-015-0191-9
11. Hameed MA, Lewis AJ. Offspring of parents with schizophrenia: a systematic review of developmental features across childhood. *Harv Rev Psychiatry* (2016) 24(2):104–17. doi: 10.1097/HRP.0000000000000076
12. Seifer R. Young children with mentally ill parents: resilient developmental systems. In: Luthar SS, editor. Resilience and Vulnerability: Adaptation in the Context of Childhood Adversities. Cambridge University Press (2003). p. 29–49. doi: 10.1017/CBO9780511615788.004
13. Aldridge J, Becker S. Children caring for parents with mental illness: perspectives of young carers, parents and professionals. Bristol: The Policy Press (2003). doi: 10.2307/j.ctt1t89f21
14. Hosman CMH, van Doesum KTM, van Santvoort F. Prevention of emotional problems and psychiatric risks in children of parents with a mental illness in the Netherlands: I. The scientific basis to a comprehensive approach. *Aust e-J Adv Ment Health* (2009) 8(3):250–263. doi: 10.5172/jamh.8.3.250
15. Van Santvoort F. Support groups for children at risk. A study on risk levels and intervention effects in children of mentally ill or addicted parents. In: *Doctoral Thesis*. Radboud University Nijmegen, Nijmegen, NL (2013).
16. Siegenthaler E, Munder T, Egger M. Effect of preventive interventions in mentally ill parents on the mental health of the offspring: systematic review and meta-analysis. *J Am Acad Child Adolesc Psychiatry* (2012) 51(1):8–17.e8. doi: 10.1016/j.jaac.2011.10.018
17. Thanhäuser M, Lemmer G, de Girolamo G, Christiansen H. Do preventive interventions for children of mentally ill parents work?Results of a systematic review and meta-analysis. *Curr Opin Psychiatry* (2017) 30:283–99. doi: 10.1097/YCO.0000000000000342
18. Kim-Cohen J, Caspi A, Moffitt TE, Harrington H, Milne BJ, Poulton R. Prior juvenile diagnoses in adults with mental disorder: developmental follow-back of a prospective-longitudinal cohort. *Arch Gen Psychiatry* (2003) 60(7):709–17. doi: 10.1001/archpsyc.60.7.709
19. Grove C, Reupert A, Maybery D. The perspectives of young people of parents with a mental illness regarding preferred interventions and supports. *J Child Fam Stud* (2016) 25(10):3056–65. doi.org/10.1007/s10826-016-0468-8
20. Luthar SS. Preface. In: Luthar SS, editor. Resilience and vulnerability: adaptation in the context of childhood adversities. Cambridge University Press (2003). doi: 10.1017/CBO9780511615788
21. Australian Infant Child Adolescent and Family Mental Health Association Draft. Principles and Actions for Services and People Working With Children of Parents With A Mental Illness (2003). Australian Infant Child Adolescent and Family Mental Health Association, Stepney, SA.
22. Fraser E, Pakenham KI. Evaluation of a resilience-based intervention for children of parents with mental illness. *Aust N Z J Psychiatry* (2008) 42(12):1041–50. doi: 10.1080/00048670802512065
23. Beardslee WR, Versage EM, Wright EJ, Salt P, Rothberg PC, Drezner K, et al. Examination of preventive interventions for families with depression: evidence of change. *Dev Psychopathol* (1997) 9(1):109–30. doi: 10.1017/S0954579497001090
24. Reupert A, Maybery D, Nicholson J, Göpfert M, Seeman M eds. *Parental psychiatric disorder: distressed parents and their families*. Cambridge: Cambridge University Press (2015). doi: 10.1017/CBO9781107707559
25. Beardslee WR, Solantaus TS, Morgan BS, Gladstone TR, Kowalenko NM. Preventive interventions for children of parents with depression: international perspectives. *Med J Aust* (2013) 199:23–5. doi: 10.5694/mja11.11289
26. Solantaus T, Paavonen EJ, Toikka S, Punamäki RL. Preventive interventions in families with parental depression: children's psychosocial symptoms and prosocial behaviour. *Eur Child Adolesc Psychiatry* (2010) 19(12):883–92. doi: 10.1007/s00787-010-0135-3
27. Compas BE, Forehand R, Keller G, Champion JE, Rakow A, Reeslund KL, et al. Randomized controlled trial of a family cognitive-behavioral preventive intervention for children of depressed parents. *J Consult Clin Psychol* (2009) 77(6):1007–20. doi: 10.1037/a0016930
28. Nicholson J, Albert K, Gershenson B, Williams V, Biebel K. Family options for parents with mental illnesses: a developmental, mixed methods pilot study. *Psychiatr Rehabil J* (2009) 33(2):106–14. doi: 10.2975/33.2.2009.106.114
29. Van Doesum KT, Hosman CM. Prevention of emotional problems and psychiatric risks in children of parents with a mental illness in the Netherlands: II. Interventions. *Adv Ment Health* (2009) 8(3):264–76. doi: 10.5172/jamh.8.3.264
30. Schrank B, Moran K, Borghi C, Priebe S. How to support patients with severe mental illness in their parenting role with children aged over 1 year? A systematic review of interventions. *Soc Psychiatry Psychiatr Epidemiol* (2015) 50(12):1765–83. doi: 10.1007/s00127-015-1069-3
31. Bee P, Bower P, Byford S, Churchill R, Calam R, Stallard P, et al. The clinical effectiveness, cost-effectiveness and acceptability of community-based interventions aimed at improving or maintaining quality of life in children of parents with serious mental illness: a systematic review. *Health Technol Assess* (2014) 18(8):1–250. doi: 10.3310/hta18080
32. Van Doesum KTM, Koster C. *KOPP Praten met ouders kinderen: Handleiding preventieve huisbezoeken voor ouders met psychiatrische problemen en hun kinderen (Manual Child Talks)*. Deventer, the Netherlands: Dimence, Community Mental Health Center (2008).
33. Reedtz C, Lauritzen C, van Doesum K. Evaluating workforce developments to support children of mentally ill parents: implementing new interventions in the adult mental healthcare in Northern Norway. *BMJ Open* (2012) 2(3). doi: 10.1136/bmjopen-2011-000709
34. Van Doesum KTM, Reedtz C, Lauritzen (2019). Child Talks+: Manual. Edited by The Arctic university of Norway, UiT. Manuscript in preparation.
35. Sheehan DV, Lecrubier Y, Sheehan KH, Amorim P, Janavs J, Weiller E, et al. The Mini-International Neuropsychiatric Interview (M.I.N.I.): the development and validation of a structured diagnostic psychiatric interview for DSM-IV and ICD-10. *J Clin Psychiatry* (1998) 59 Suppl 20(22–33):34–57.
36. American Psychiatric Association (2000). *Diagnostic and statistical manual of mental disorders*, 4th ed, Washington, DC: American Psychiatric Association.
37. American Psychiatric Association. *Diagnostic and statistical manual of mental disorders*. 5th ed. Washington, DC (2013). doi: 10.1176/appi.books.9780890425596
38. World Health Organization. *International statistical classification of diseases and related health problems*. Geneva: World Health Organization (2010).
39. The Kidscreen Group Europe. The KIDSCREEN Questionnaires. In: *Quality of Life Questionnaires for Children and Adolescents*. Pabst Science Publishers (2006).
40. Ravens-Sieberer U, Auquier P, Erhart M, Gosch A, Rajmil L, Bruil J, et al. The KIDSCREEN-27 quality of life measures for children and adolescents: psychometric results from a cross-cultural survey in 13 European countries. *Qual Life Res* (2007) 16(4):1347–56. doi: 10.1007/s11136-007-9240-2
41. Hjemdal O. Measuring protective factors: the development of two resilience scales in Norway. *Child Adolesc Psychiatr Clin N Am* (2007) 16(2):303–21. doi: 10.1016/j.chc.2006.12.003
42. Askeland K, Reedtz C. Måleegenskaper ved den norske versjonen av resilience scale for adolescents (READ). *PsykTestBarn* (2015) 1:3.
43. Bosch A, Van de Ven M, Van Doesum KTM (submitted for publication). Development and Validation of the Guilt and Shame Questionnaire for Adolescents of Parents with a Mental Illness (GSQ-APMI).
44. Goodman A, Goodman R. Strengths and difficulties questionnaire as a dimensional measure of child mental health. *J Am Acad Child Adolesc Psychiatry* (2009) 48(4):400–3. doi: 10.1097/CHI.0b013e3181985068
45. Stone LL, Otten R, Engels RC, Vermulst AA, Janssens JM. Psychometric properties of the parent and teacher versions of the strengths and difficulties questionnaire for 4- to 12-year-olds: a review. *Clin Child Fam Psychol Rev* (2010) 13(3):254–74. doi: 10.1007/s10567-010-0071-2

46. Glascoe FP. Parents' evaluation of developmental status: how well do parents' concerns identify children with behavioral and emotional problems? *Clin Pediatr* (2003) 42:133–8. doi: 10.1177/000992280304200206
47. Glascoe FP. Evidence-based early detection of developmental-behavioral problems in primary care: what to expect and how to do it. *J Pediatr Health Care* (2014) 29(1). doi: 10.1016/j.pedhc.2014.06.005
48. McMahon R, Kim H, Jones K. *Parent-Child Communication, Parent Report (Fast Track Project Technical Report)*. Seattle, WA: University of Washington (1997).
49. Grove C, Riebschleger J, Bosch A, Cavanaugh D, van der Ende PC. Expert views of children's knowledge needs regarding parental mental illness. *Child Youth Serv Rev* (2017) 79:249–55. doi: 10.1016/j.childyouth.2017.06.026
50. Johnston C, Mash EJ. A measure of parenting satisfaction and efficacy. *J Clin Child Psychol* (1989) 18:167–75.
51. Prchal A, Graf A, Bergstraesser E, Landolt MA. A two-session psychological intervention for siblings of pediatric cancer patients: a randomized controlled pilot trial. *Child Adolesc Psychiatry Ment Health* (2012) 11:6(1):3. doi: 10.1186/1753-2000-6-3
52. Vierron E, Giraudeau B. Design effect in multicenter studies: gain or loss of power? *Med Res Methodol* (2009) 9:39. doi: 10.1186/1471-2288-9-39
53. Rausch JR, Maxwell SE, Kelley K. Analytic methods for questions pertaining to a randomized pretest, posttest, follow-up design. *J Clin Child Adolesc Psychol* (2003) 32(3):467–86. doi: 10.1207/S15374424JCCP3203_15
54. Cohen J. *Statistical power analysis for the behavioral sciences*. 2nd ed. Hillsdale, NJ: Lawrence Earlbaum Associates (1988).
55. International Classification of Diseases (ICD). World Health Organization. Retrieved 23 November 2010.
56. Reupert AE, Cuff R, Drost L, Foster K, van Doesum KT, van Santvoort F. Intervention programs for children whose parents have a mental illness: a review. *Med J Aust* (2013), 199(3 Suppl):S18–22. doi: 10.5694/mja11.11145
57. Structured Clinical Interview for DSM-5 (SCID-5). American Psychiatric Association Publishing. Retrieved 29 January 2017.

8

Adult Mental Health Outpatients Who have Minor Children: Prevalence of Parents, Referrals of their Children and Patient Characteristics

Torleif Ruud[1,2], Darryl Maybery[3], Andrea Reupert[4], Bente Weimand[1,5], Kim Foster[6,7], Anne Grant[8], Bjørg Eva Skogøy[9,10] and Solveig O. Ose[11]*

[1] Mental Health Services, Akershus University Hospital, Lørenskog, Norway, [2] Institute of Clinical Medicine, University of Oslo, Oslo, Norway, [3] School of Rural Health, Monash University, Moe, VIC, Australia, [4] Faculty of Education, Monash University, Clayton, VIC, Australia, [5] Faculty of Health Sciences, OsloMet—Oslo Metropolitan University, Oslo, Norway, [6] School of Nursing, Midwifery and Paramedicine, Australian Catholic University, Sydney, NSW, Australia, [7] NorthWestern Mental Health, Parkville, VIC, Australia, [8] School of Nursing and Midwifery, Queens University Belfast, Belfast, United Kingdom, [9] Nordland Hospital Trust, Bodø, Norway, [10] Faculty of Health Sciences, UiT The Arctic University of Norway, Tromsø, Norway, [11] Health Services Research, SINTEF, Trondheim, Norway

***Correspondence:**
Torleif Ruud
torleif.ruud@medisin.uio.no

Background: A strong connection exists between parental mental illness and lifetime mental health risk for their children. Thus, it is important to determine, when parents attend for treatment for their illness, the prevalence and characteristics of parents with a mental illness and identify referral actions for their children. Previous studies indicate that 12–45% of adult mental health service patients are parents with minor children. There is a need for studies with larger sample sizes that investigate the prevalence and characteristics of parents, and factors associated with referral actions for their children.

Method: Data on 23,167 outpatients was drawn from a national census study across 107 Norwegian adult mental health outpatient clinics during 2 weeks in April 2013. Clinicians identified various socio-demographic characteristics of patients who were parents and referral actions for their children.

Results: Eight thousand thirty-five (36%) of outpatients had children under 18 years. Thirty-one percent were provided with referrals for their children and 58% were reported to have children with no need for referral. Three percent were reported to have children with unmet needs who were not referred. There were missing data on children's needs and referral actions for 8% of parents. Patients who care for minor children were more likely to be refugees, and less likely to be single, male, not own a house/apartment, and have a schizophrenia spectrum illness or substance use disorder. Children were more likely to be referred when their parent was single, with no income from paid work, low education, not owning house/apartment, poor family network, long outpatient treatment, and an individual care plan; and less likely for men with a moderate or less severe mental illness. Children were referred to child protection agencies, child and adolescent mental health services and school psychological/pedagogic services.

Discussion: The prevalence of outpatients with children is similar to other studies. Referrals were made for children of one third of outpatients with minor children. Needs and referrals of children was unknown for one in ten outpatients. Mental health outpatient clinics must improve procedures to identify parenting status and ascertain and act on children's needs.

Keywords: prevalence of parents with mental illness, children of parents with mental illness, mental health outpatients, patient characteristics, needs of care, referrals

INTRODUCTION

This paper presents data from a national census of patients in adult mental health outpatient clinics in Norway. It provides prevalence of outpatients who care for children under the age of 18 years, prevalence of parents whose children are considered by clinicians to require further support and are referred to external agencies, and how parents' socio economic and clinical characteristics influence prevalence and type of referrals made by clinicians for the children. This information can be used by policy makers and managers to strengthen policy, as well as to support clinicians to better identify parents, determine their children's needs and refer the children to appropriate services.

Parental mental illness impacts on the functioning of the family unit and poses a risk to the healthy development of children. Compared to other children, those growing up with a parent with a mental illness are at risk of a range of adverse behavioural, developmental and emotional outcomes (1–3). Bell et al. (4) found that children of parents who had been hospitalized for a mental illness were much less likely to be school ready. Difficulties with schooling have also been shown in Sweden where Hjern et al. highlighted that twice as many children whose parents had been hospitalised for a mental illness had lower school results and were not able to start secondary education, compared to children without parental mental illness (5). However, it was also estimated that most of the risk was associated with three contributing social factors (needing social support, low parental education level, parental separation/divorce), or an interaction between parental illness and social problems. Foster et al. (6) identified parental functioning and parental mental illness among risk/protective factors for children according to the child.

Evidence suggests that children whose parents have a mental illness have almost double the chance of developing a mental illness themselves (5, 7). In a Swedish study of 535,000 children up to 30–35 years of age, those who grew up with substance abuse and/or mental illness in the family and who also required social welfare were identified as an extreme high-risk group. This group of children reported considerably higher levels of mortality, mental illness, substance abuse, criminality, and were recipients of social welfare benefits, while having low workforce participation (5). In Norway it is estimated that 25% of mental illnesses among adolescents, and 10% of early death, is associated with parental mental illness (8).

A recent systematic literature review found that between 12 and 45% of all patients attending adult mental services were parents (9). Four studies in the review found prevalence rates from 36 to 38% (10–13), suggesting that a substantial minority (one third) of patients using adult mental health services are parents (9). However, a limitation of these audit-style studies (12, 14) is that they commonly focus on a single regional adult mental health service with modest sample sizes. Other studies have assumed an epidemiological approach that projects findings from a representative sample to approximate the whole population (15) or utilised already collected national data sets (16). In Norway it has been estimated that 23.1% of children have a parent with a moderate or severe mental illness that may affect their daily life (8). Among children born in Sweden 1987–1989, 7.8% of minor children have a parent admitted to hospital due to psychiatric illness and/or substance abuse. Further, a survey from 2007 to 2011 found that parental mental health problems, not sufficiently severe to require hospitalizations, were relatively common, with 18.1% of parents to children aged 10–18 years reporting nervousness, anxiety or worry (5).

To the best of our knowledge only one study has examined whole-of-service data for parental mental health prevalence. In the early 2000s, Maybery et al. (16) found that in one year, 20% of adult mental health patients in the Australian state of Victoria were parents. In a follow up study, the authors examined state-wide adult mental health outpatient data over a 4 years period and found that 19–20% of almost 60,000 outpatients were parents (17). While the study provided valuable prevalence data, it failed to go further and illustrate information about the parents (such as gender, diagnosis) nor about the needs of their children. Consequently, there is a lack of whole of population knowledge about the prevalence of adult patients in mental health or addiction services who are parents caring for children. Such information would provide important data that can be used to inform service policy, intake procedure, and professional development of clinicians.

When assessing the risks to such children, it is essential to obtain information about the parent, including diagnosis, gender, socio economic context, and family networks, as well as other circumstances which may influence children's experiences and outcomes. For example, parents who have an anxiety disorder are less likely to grant their children autonomy and more likely to demonstrate lower levels of sensitivity (18), while children of parents with psychosis might be directly involved in a parent's delusions (19). After controlling for other risk factors at birth, Hammond et al. (20) found that two thirds of infants of mothers with a psychotic disorder were reported to child protection services. This was four times that of infants of mothers without a mental illness. Infants of mothers with a mood disorder were twice as likely to be referred to child protection services compared to infants of mothers without a mental illness.

The family environment, including the presence of marital discord, the presence or absence of the other parent and the availability of social support to the family may also influence the level of risk exposure to the children (21). There are also differences between the experiences and needs of mothers and fathers with a mental illness, in terms of custody arrangements and who they call on for help (22). These family circumstances have important implications for the development of risk-assessment tools and case-related decision making and accordingly need to be identified from the outset.

Other studies have considered parent and family variables when determining prevalence. A 4-year census in one Australian adult mental health service identified that a majority of female outpatients were parents (14). Nearly half were married, with around a third separated or divorced. Approximately half of parents reported a good level of social support. The most prevalent diagnoses were mood and psychotic disorders, followed by anxiety disorders. Approximately 60% of dependent children lived with parents, including 34–56% of children whose parents had a psychotic disorder. Around a third of children were identified as having child protection involvement (14). These findings are broadly consistent with those from another Australian adult cross-sector service census, with the majority of identified parents being female and over half of being single (23). In that audit, the most common parental diagnoses were psychotic and mood disorders, with ~40% of parents living with their children or another family member (23). Both audits however were limited by moderate sample sizes (average yearly sample size around 800 limited to specific catchment areas).

It is important that adult mental health services are responsive to the needs of children in these families, which at a minimum would involve identifying children, assessing their needs, and as required, referring them on to appropriate services (24–26). However, little is known about clinicians' actions in adult mental health outpatient services in relation to detection, follow up and referral of patients' children. Some small-scale qualitative studies (25, 27, 28) have shown that clinicians working in adult mental health services struggle to balance the needs of both parents and children and do not routinely refer children on to appropriate services. However, further research is required to generalise and extend these findings.

Research has clearly demonstrated the benefits of family focused practice for parents with a mental illness, their children and other family members (29, 30). Two controlled trials found that family focused approaches significantly improved mental health outcomes for parents (31, 32). A meta-analysis found that family focused preventive interventions reduced the risk of children developing the same mental illness as their parent by 40% (30). Consequently, to inform mental health service policy and practice it is important to identify the number of outpatients attending adult mental health services who are parents with minor children.

CONTEXT OF THE STUDY

In Norway, specialized mental health services are organised in general hospital services across 19 health trusts. The division of mental health and addiction services in each health trust has inpatient and outpatient services for children and adolescents, adults, and older persons. Community mental health centres for adults include all outpatient mental health clinics, mobile teams, day units and almost half of the mental health inpatient beds in Norway (33–35). Almost all mental health services are public, but a few hospitals and CMHCs are owned by private trusts.

The Norwegian Health Personnel Act of 2010 requires health personnel to ascertain whether a patient has minor children and if so, to record this in their patient record. The law also stipulates that clinicians should talk with the patient about their children's needs and offer to give information and guidance. Within the limits of confidentiality, clinicians might invite children to be involved in conversations about their parents' illness, treatment, and the possibility of visiting the service treating their parent. In addition, the law stipulates that clinicians assess the needs of the children and refer children to relevant services such as child protection agency, CAMHS, educational-psychological services in schools and family counselling offices as required (36).

AIMS AND RESEARCH QUESTIONS

The study aimed to determine the number and characteristics of adult outpatients who care for children under the age of 18, from a national outpatient census in mental health services in Norway. A further aim was to identify the prevalence of outpatients with minor children where the clinician identified a need for referral of children to an external agency.

The paper addresses the following research questions: 1. What is the prevalence of outpatients in adult mental health clinics who care for children under the age of 18 years? 2. What are the socio-demographic and clinical characteristics of these outpatients, compared to outpatients who do not care for minor children (in terms of diagnosis, gender, age, marital status, income, education level, housing, refugee status, and country of birth)? 3. For what prevalence of outpatients with minor children do clinicians identify a need for referral of children to an external agency for children, and what agencies are the children referred to? 4. What patient characteristics are associated with referral of children to external agencies?

MATERIALS AND METHODS

Design

The design of the census was a cross-sectional study of outpatients seen by all outpatient clinics and mobile teams in adult Norwegian mental health services during 2 weeks in April 2013. The census was commissioned and financed by the Norwegian Directorate of Health. The work was undertaken by the SINTEF research foundation. The study was approved by the Regional Committee for Medical and Health Research Ethics (reg.no. 2012/848).

Sample

The sample consisted of data on 23,167 adult outpatients seen by 107 of the 110 mental health outpatient clinics in Norway. The prevalence of outpatients included was 60% based on data from the National Patient Register indicating that the total number of outpatients during the 2 weeks was 38,904. The clinics that did not participate were small and cited a lack of time for not participating; these comprised 1% of all outpatient consultations during the 2 weeks.

Variables

The census form included outpatients' socio-demographic data (gender, age, and marital status, main source of income, highest education, housing situation, refugee status, and country of birth), main mental diagnoses using ICD-10 (for substance use disorders secondary diagnosis is also included, as this is often listed as a secondary diagnosis for patients with both a mental and a substance use disorder), and the following questions about patients' children: (1) Does the patient care for children under 18 years? (yes/no/unknown). (2) If yes, number of children. (3) Have measures been taken to follow up any of the children? (available response being; yes; no and no need to refer; no and a need to refer; unknown). (4) What agencies were children referred to (possible to mark more than one of the listed agencies).

Data Collection

All outpatients who had one or more consultations in 2 weeks (15–28 April 2013) were targeted. Several months prior to the census, service managers and clinicians received information about the census and the data collection procedures. Data were collected on hard copy forms. The clinicians completed one anonymous form for each outpatient. They were encouraged to invite the patients to participate in filling in the form, and 57% of the patients participated. The completed forms were returned to a data collection company, who scanned the forms and delivered data files to the project team.

Data Analyses

Descriptive statistics, chi square testing and logit regressions were computed with STATA 15.

RESULTS

Prevalence of Outpatients Who Care for Children Under the Age of 18

Of the 23,167 registered outpatients, information on gender and children was given for 22,398 (97%) of patients. A total of 8,035 (36%) of these had children under age 18, with 5,729 (71%) being female and 2,306 (29%) male.

Characteristics of Outpatients Who Care for Children Under the Age of 18

Bivariate chi square analyses of associations between the patient characteristics in **Table 1** show significant relationships between a higher prevalence of those caring for children under 18 and most of the variables under investigation: being female, age 30–49 years, higher education, income from paid work, having a spouse/partner, living with spouse/partner, owning a house/apartment, having good networks with family, and friends, fewer consultations since start of treatment, being a refugee, born outside Norway, not living in a large municipality, not having an individual care plan (required for anyone in need of long-term and coordinated services), not being on community treatment order, and having a diagnosis of moderate or less severe mental illness like anxiety disorders and moderate depression. Some of the same patterns are found in a more detailed analysis in **Table 2** with a focus especially on gender and main diagnosis.

In a logistic regression analysis of associations between the odds ratio for caring for children under 18 and the same patient characteristics (**Table 3**), most of the patient characteristics showed a significant association with the same direction as in the bivariate analyses, but with various odds ratios. The significant odds ratios were highest for age groups 30–49 and refugees; and lowest for being single, male, not having own house/apartment, and having a schizophrenia spectrum illness, or substance use disorder.

Prevalence of Outpatients With Minor Children Being Referred

The data on the number of children identified by clinicians to require referral to an external agency is shown in **Table 4**.

The clinicians answered the question on whether measures have been taken for referral for the children for 7,405 (92%) outpatients. Of these, 2,488 (31%) were reported to require referral to an agency. Of the 4,917 (61%) outpatients with children reported as not being referred, 247 (3%) were still reported to need a referral. This indicates that for 34% of the parents a referral of their children was identified as required, that some of these were not referred, and that children of 58% of the parents were reported to not require a referral. The need for referral is unknown for children of 630 (8%) of outpatients with minor children, including those who responded with "Do not know" and those with missing answers. Patients were involved in filling in the form in 61% of cases where the patient was a parent (n = 8,035). Sixty-three percent of female patients contributed to filling in the form compared to 59% of the male patients. If the parent was involved in filling in the form, 2% of the answers regarding measures taken for referrals were "Don't know" compared to 6% if the parent was not involved.

Information on the referral agencies is presented in **Table 5**. Almost half the outpatients with referred children (45%) had children who were referred to child protection agencies, closely followed by child and adolescent mental health services (39%) and educational-psychological services in the school system (35%). The most common combinations of services involved in follow up of the children are adult mental health outpatient clinics together with family counselling agencies (n = 388) or child protection agencies (n = 304).

Characteristics for Outpatients With Minor Children Being Referred

Bivariate chi square analyses of associations between the patient characteristics and whether measures were taken

TABLE 1 | Bivariate analyses of the association between patient characteristics and outpatients (N = 22,847) who care for children under 18.

	No children	Have children	Missing data	Total	% with children	Chi-test (x^2)
Gender						x^2 360.66 (1) $p < 0.001$
Female	8,425	5,729	262	14,416	40	
Male	5,938	2,306	187	8,431	28	
Age group						x^2 4087.50 (6) $p < 0.001$
18–23 years	3,258	249	69	3,576	7	
24–29 years	2,919	1,029	74	4,022	26	
30–39 years	2,603	2.965	81	5,649	53	
40–49 years	1,935	2,666	93	4,694	58	
50–59 years	1,805	765	52	2,622	30	
60–69 years	850	95	20	965	10	
70 years and above	672	59	31	762	8	
Education						x^2 506.11 (2) $p < 0.001$
High education	2,432	2,251	60	4,743	48	
Medium education	6,289	3,597	131	10,017	36	
Low education	5,772	2,267	325	8,364	28	
Main source of income						x^2 784.99 (2) $p < 0.001$
Income from labour	3,164	2,922	77	6,163	48	
Health related benefit	7,762	4,179	175	12,116	35	
Other economic support	3,567	1,014	264	4,845	22	
Marital status						x^2 4533.88 (2) $p < 0.001$
Married/cohabitant/partner	3,712	5,203	106	9,021	58	
Separated/divorced/widower/widow	1,624	1,355	64	3,043	45	
Single/unmarried	9,061	1,466	190	10,717	14	
Household						x^2 4258.02 (2) $p < 0.001$
Alone with or without children	7,033	2,704	172	9,909	28	
Spouse/cohabitant	3,596	5,090	98	8,784	59	
Other household	3,705	201	79	3,985	5	
Accommodation						x^2 2614.39 (3) $p < 0.001$
Own house	5,156	5,306	125	10,587	51	
Rented house/apartment, private market	4,298	1,868	95	6,261	30	
Rented house/apartment, local authorities	1,466	341	27	1,834	19	
Other	3,305	361	72	3,738	10	
Network family						x^2 79.72 (3) $p < 0.001$
Very good	4,169	2,642	113	6,924	39	
Good	6,325	3,561	124	10,010	36	
Poor	1,998	979	43	3,020	33	
Very poor	715	251	30	996	26	
Network friends						x^2 178.45 (3) $p < 0.001$
Very good	3,013	2,078	65	5,156	41	
Good	6,531	3,881	152	10,564	37	
Poor	2,180	996	58	3,234	31	
Very poor	825	238	22	1,085	22	
Number of consultations since start of treatment						x^2 145.81 (7) $p < 0.001$
<3	1,567	847	72	2,486	35	
3–5	1,551	1,009	37	2,597	39	
6–9	1,601	1,007	40	2,648	39	
10–19	2,345	1,381	70	3,796	37	
20–39	2,321	1,355	47	3,723	37	
40–99	2,155	1,204	43	3,402	36	
100–199	1,064	484	28	1,576	31	
200 or more	725	185	12	922	20	

(Continued)

TABLE 1 | Continued

	No children	Have children	Missing data	Total	% with children	Chi-test (x^2)
Asylum seeker						x^2 0.67 (1) $p = 0.4129$
No	14,426	8,071	513	23,010	36	
Yes	67	44	3	114	40	
Refugee						x^2 36.22 (1) $p < 0.001$
No	14,093	7,768	496	22,357	36	
Yes	400	347	20	767	46	
Born outside Norway						x^2 94.51 (1) $p < 0.001$
No	12,973	6,903	466	20,342	35	
Yes	1,520	1,212	50	2,782	44	
Having an individual care plan						x^2 411.4 (1) $p < 0.001$
No	12,329	7,608	471	20,408	38	
Yes	2,164	507	45	2,716	19	
Community treatment order						x^2 193.3 (1) $p < 0.001$
No	13,866	8,019	500	22,385	37	
Yes	627	96	16	739	13	
Living in a large municipality						x^2 244.16(1) $p < 0.001$
No	10,680	6,709	413	17,802	39	
Yes	3,813	1,406	103	5,322	27	
Diagnoses						x^2 1013.38(7) $p < 0.001$
Personality disorders	1,118	640	33	1,791	36	
Substance use disorders (as first or second diagnosis)	1,058	241	27	1,326	19	
Schizophrenia etc.	1,902	295	52	2,249	13	
Affective disorders	3,982	2,690	94	6,766	40	
Anxiety disorders	3,128	2,455	90	5,673	44	
Behavioural syndromes	552	221	14	787	29	
Behavioural and emotional disorders	557	418	16	991	43	
Other mental illness	1,320	619	27	1,966	32	

to refer children are shown in **Table 6**. There are highly significant associations for gender, age group, level of education, main source of income, marital status, type of household, accommodation, networks of family, network of friends, number of consultations since start of treatment, having an individual care plan, being under community treatment order, and main diagnosis. There are no significant associations for the size of the municipalities or for being part of a minority group (asylum seeker, refugee, born outside Norway). The pattern of significant differences shows that many indicators on lower socio-demographic status as well as severe mental illness and substance use disorder are associated with referrals of children.

Results of a logistic regression of the association between patient characteristics and odds ratios for referral of children is shown in **Table 7** for the 6,634 outpatients with non-missing data for the independent variables in the logistic regression and who had children who did or did not receive a referral. The significant odds ratios were highest for age groups 30–59, lower education, being single, not having income from paid work, not owning house/apartment, poor family network, having had many outpatient consultations, and having an individual care plan. The significant odds ratios were lowest for being male and for having moderate or less severe mental illness.

DISCUSSION

In the current study one third of adult outpatients from 107 Norwegian mental health outpatient clinics cared for children under 18 years of age. One third of those parents had children who required a referral, six out of 10 had children not requiring a referral, and for one in 10 parents, the needs of their children was unknown or not reported. Children of three of 10 outpatient parents were reported to have been referred to relevant services. Patient characteristics associated with referral actions for their children were low education, being single, not owning a house/apartment, having a poor family network, having an individual care plan, being female, and having moderate or a less severe mental illness.

Prevalence of Outpatients Who Care for Children Under 18

Thirty-six percent of the outpatients in this study cared for children under 18 years of age. This falls within the range of 36–38% found in four previous studies identified in a systematic review of adult mental health services (9). Importantly, this study is the first of its kind internationally to illustrate "whole of country" population data and represents a significant step forward in parent prevalence statistics. The results provide a

TABLE 2 | Gender, diagnosis and prevalence of outpatients ($N = 8{,}035$) with care for children under 18 among sociodemographic subgroups.

	Number of patients with children	Patients with children (%)	Type of household (%) with or without children			Poor family network (%)	Poor friend network (%)
			Alone	Spouse	Other		
Gender							
Female	5,729	40	41	43	15	17	16
Male	2,306	28	47	31	21	18	24
Diagnoses							
Personality disorders	635	37	49	38	13	30	29
Substance use disorders (as first or second diagnosis)	240	19	61	19	20	27	30
Schizophrenia etc.	293	13	67	14	18	19	29
Affective disorders	2,669	40	42	44	14	16	16
Anxiety disorders	2,429	44	36	49	15	15	15
Behavioural syndromes	219	29	33	37	30	12	13
Behavioural and emotional disorders	412	43	43	36	21	15	13
Other mental illness	613	32	36	37	27	15	18

strong rationale for intake systems to identify parenting status, incorporate parenting roles, and responsibilities in treatment plans, and assess and address the needs of patients' children. Overall, these data confirm that a significant minority of patients in adult mental health services are parents with children under the age of 18.

Characteristics of Outpatients With Care for Minor Children

The results also provide greater certainty about the sociodemographic characteristics of parents and children in mental health services. Sociodemographic patient characteristics associated with higher odds ratios for caring for children under 18 were being age groups 30–49 and refugee, and characteristics associated with lower odds ratios were being male, single, not having own house/apartment, poor network of friends and not living in a large municipality. Forty percent of females and 28% of males cared for minor children. In terms of gender, others have shown somewhat similar results, with between 34 and 59% of all female patients recorded as mothers and 25–39% of all males as fathers (10, 13). A 4-year census in one Australian adult mental health service found nearly half of parents (41.2–45.0%) were married, with around a third (30.8–36.2%) separated or divorced. Approximately half of parents (43.9–52.9%) reported a good level of social support. Having a good level of support and network of friends is important for those with a mental illness and especially for the well-being of parents and children (37). A Norwegian study (38) found that the prevalence of refugees was higher among the outpatients in a mental health clinic than in the population in the catchment area, but still concluded that the outpatient clinic was probably underused by refugees based on much higher self-reported mental health problems among refugees that others in an epidemiological study in the area. The higher odds ratio for refugees being parents in the current study may be due to a higher prevalence of refugees being parents to minors, as shown in **Table 1**.

Clinical patient characteristics associated with lower odds ratio for caring for children under 18 were longer outpatient care, having an individual care plan, and having a severe mental illness or a substance use disorder. These data would indicate that those with a severe illness by and large are not presenting to adult mental health services with children or are not disclosing that they have children. It might also be that those with severe mental illness are more often hospitalized and/or cared for by the community care teams than by mental health outpatient clinics, and that more parents with severe mental illness might have lost custody of their children and have little contact with the children. The fear of the involvement of child protection agency might dissuade patients who have a severe illness from disclosing their parenting status (39) and the data highlighting referral patterns in this study in some ways substantiates these fears.

Forty-four percent of parents were reported to have an anxiety disorder, 40% an affective disorder, 43% a behavioural and emotional disorder, and 37% a personality disorder. In Australia, Fernbacher et al. (23) found that 42% of parents in an outpatient service had schizophrenia, 23% depression, and 13% bipolar disorder. In the 4-year census in one Australian adult psychiatric service (14) the most prevalent diagnoses were mood (35–42%) and psychotic (22–35%) disorders, followed by anxiety (11–20%) disorders. Overall, it appears that many parents in adult mental health services have an affective disorder. This is important information that can be used to inform treatment as well as continued professional development for clinicians regarding family focused practice.

Prevalence of Outpatients With Minor Children Being Referred

For 92% of the outpatients with minor children the clinicians had identified if children required a referral to an external agency, and the need for referral was not ascertained for 8% of outpatients with minor children. Children of 61% of outpatient parents were not considered by clinicians to require a referral, even though

TABLE 3 | Logistic regression of the association between patient characteristics and whether the outpatients ($N = 22{,}847$) care for children under 18.

	Odds ratio	Std. Err.	z	$P > z$	95% Confidence interval	
Gender						
Male	0.676	0.028	−9.37	0.00	0.623	0.734
Age group						
18–23 years	1.000	(base)				
24–29 years	3.029	0.274	12.25	0.00	2.537	3.617
30–39 years	8.114	0.724	23.46	0.00	6.812	9.665
40–49 years	7.821	0.730	22.02	0.00	6.512	9.392
50–59 years	1.666	0.168	5.07	0.00	1.367	2.029
60–69 years	0.349	0.051	−7.21	0.00	0.262	0.464
70 years and above	0.213	0.037	−8.80	0.00	0.151	0.300
Education						
High education	1.000	(base)				
Medium education	1.033	0.050	0.67	0.51	0.939	1.136
Low education	1.167	0.065	2.75	0.01	1.046	1.303
Income						
Income from labour	1.000	(base)				
Health related benefits	0.857	0.039	−3.36	0.00	0.784	0.938
Other economic support	1.062	0.071	0.89	0.37	0.930	1.211
Marital status						
Married/cohabitant/partner	1.000	(base)				
Separated/divorced/widow/widower	0.842	0.117	−1.23	0.22	0.641	1.106
Single/unmarried	0.168	0.023	−12.99	0.00	0.128	0.220
Type of household						
Alone with or without children	1.000	(base)				
Spouse/cohabitant	0.832	0.113	−1.35	0.18	0.637	1.086
Other type of household	0.298	0.031	−11.67	0.00	0.243	0.365
Accommodation						
Own house	1.000	(base)				
Rented house/apartment, private marked	0.647	0.031	−9.10	0.00	0.589	0.710
Rented house/apartment, local authorities	0.564	0.049	−6.60	0.00	0.476	0.669
Other accommodation	0.638	0.058	−4.92	0.00	0.534	0.763
Poor network family	0.906	0.048	−1.88	0.06	0.817	1.004
Poor network friends	0.820	0.043	−3.79	0.00	0.740	0.909
Consultations 20 or more since start	0.870	0.035	−3.49	0.00	0.805	0.941
Refugee	1.399	0.163	2.87	0.00	1.112	1.759
Born outside Norway	1.156	0.074	2.27	0.02	1.020	1.311
Has and Individual care plan	0.731	0.051	−4.53	0.00	0.638	0.837
Community treatment order (CTO)	0.838	0.120	−1.24	0.22	0.633	1.109
Living in large municipality	0.681	0.032	−8.20	0.00	0.622	0.747
Main diagnoses						
Personality disorders	1.000	(base)				
Substance use disorders (as first or second diagnosis)	0.627	0.068	−4.31	0.00	0.507	0.775
Schizophrenia spectrum disorders	0.406	0.041	−8.90	0.00	0.333	0.495
Affective disorders	1.047	0.074	0.65	0.52	0.911	1.204
Anxiety disorders	1.038	0.075	0.52	0.60	0.901	1.197
Behavioural syndromes	0.718	0.088	−2.71	0.01	0.565	0.912
Behavioural and emotional disorders	1.528	0.164	3.95	0.00	1.238	1.886
Other mental illness	1.083	0.101	0.85	0.39	0.902	1.301
Constant	0.712	0.129	−1.88	0.06	0.500	1.015

TABLE 4 | Reported needs and whether measures have been taken to follow up of the children of outpatients ($N = 8,035$) with care for children under 18.

	Number of patients	% of patents
Yes child/ren have needs	2,488	31
No, but have needs	247	3
No, but does not have any needs	4,670	58
Do not know	257	3
No answer	373	5
Number of outpatients with responsibility for children under age 18	8,035	100

TABLE 5 | Prevalence of outpatients ($N = 2,488$) where children are reported to be followed up by various services or agencies for children*.

	Number of patients	% of patients
Child protection agency	1,128	45
Family counselling office	165	7
Educational-psychological service/ school	861	35
Child and adolescent mental health service	975	39
Adult mental health outpatient clinic	83	3
Other	544	22
No answer	46	2

More than one agency may have been marked for each outpatient.

3% of these were still provided with a referral to an external agency. In Norway health personnel are required to ascertain whether a patient has minor children, talk with the patient about their children's needs and offer to give information and guidance. But there are no standard procedures or rules for referral of the patients' children. There may be capacity problem in the child and welfare services, as well as variations in resources and availability of such services. However, as shown in **Table 6**, we did not find significant differences between large and small municipalities in the probability of measures taken to follow up children.

Clinicians' actions did not necessarily align with their stated beliefs, an incongruence that has also been highlighted elsewhere (27). Altogether 34% of outpatients with minor children had children who had been referred. For 58% of outpatients, their children were identified as not requiring any further referral or support. In one Australian audit around a third (28–39%) of all children had been identified as requiring the involvement of child protection services (14), slightly less than what was found in the current study (45%). Both figures however indicate sizable referrals to child protection agencies which highlights the need for collaborative service delivery models but also the important role that child protection plays in the lives of these families.

Given the range of risk and protective factors for these children, not all children whose parent has a mental illness will be adversely affected (40), nor will all children in the same family be affected in the same way. Nonetheless, given the high risks for children associated with parental mental illness it is incumbent on clinicians to provide appropriate assessment and monitor their needs over time. It is not clear from the present study whether clinicians undertake such an assessment or whether, as some studies have shown (27), they did not always acknowledge children's needs and accordingly did not follow through on appropriate referrals. Future open-ended survey responses and/or qualitative research may be needed to identify barriers and facilitators to these clinical decisions. In a Norwegian cross-sectional study including a questionnaire to both patients with children and to clinicians in mental health services, 95% of the clinicians answered that they had talked with the patient about the situation with their children, while 71% of patients said that they had such a conversation with a clinician (41).

Characteristics for Outpatients With Minor Children Being Referred

Sociodemographic patient characteristics associated with higher odds ratio for children being referred were being female, single, low education, not owning a house/apartment, not receiving income from paid work, and a poor family network. Maybery et al. (16) argue that risks for children escalates when the parent is single, without a support network, experiences housing insecurity and lives in poverty. So, it is perhaps not surprising that these children were more likely to be referred than other children. However, the specific reasons for why these children were referred still remains unclear.

Having an individual care plan was associated with higher odds ratio for children being referred, while moderate to less severe mental illness was associated with lower odds ratio for children being referred. Though the odds ratio of children being referred were parents having a moderate to less severe psychiatric illness, the established individual care plan suggests that these are families with multiple problems, with a need for coordinated support. The poorer family network might also be an important explanation for the higher need for other types of support.

For 52% of the patients with minor children, children had been referred to child protection agencies (45%) and family counselling offices (7%). This is not surprising as the sociodemographic characteristics of the patients with children being referred might indicate a need for economic and practical help and social support as well as help to cope with the parental illness. Many children (39%) had been referred to the child- and adolescent services, indicating that the children needed treatment for their own mental and/or behavioral problems.

For one third (35%) of the families, children had been referred to educational-psychological services/school, which confirms the need for support found in a Swedish study. Hjern et al. (5) argue that both parents' illness and substance abuse negatively impact school performance in their children, with social factors also having an important impact, and preventive general interventions in schools should be establish for such children. This would apply to children with parental illness, as well as children with separated/divorced parents or parents with low educational levels.

Some explanatory variables in the logistic regression in **Table 7** are correlated, but not to the extent that this is problematic. The highest correlation is between the variable

TABLE 6 | Bivariate analyses of characteristics of outpatients with children ($N = 8{,}035$)* and whether measures have been taken to follow up their children.

	No follow up	Follow up	Missing	Total	% Follow up	Chi-test (X^2)
Gender						x^2 127.13 (1) $p < 0.001$
Female	3,479	1,977	273	5,729	35	
Male	1,695	511	100	2,306	22	
Age group						x^2 59.88 (6) $p < 0.001$
18–23 years	169	67	11	247	27	
24–29 years	673	305	43	1,021	30	
30–39 years	1,839	959	135	2,933	33	
40–49 years	1,661	847	138	2,646	32	
50–59 years	530	213	21	764	28	
60–69 years	79	11	4	94	12	
70 years and above	55	3	1	59	5	
Education						x^2 148.97 (2) $p < 0.001$
High education	1,631	508	89	2,228	23	
Medium education	2,303	1,111	150	3,564	31	
Low education	1,240	869	134	2,243	39	
Main source of income						x^2 154.09 (2) $p < 0.001$
Income from labour	2,107	658	126	2,891	23	
Health related benefit	2,460	1,494	187	4,141	36	
Other economic support	607	336	60	1,003	33	
Marital status						x^2 197.22 (2) $p < 0.001$
Married/cohabitant/partners	3,587	1,319	250	5,156	26	
Separated/divorced/widower/widow	723	564	51	1,338	42	
Single/unmarried	807	580	66	1,453	40	
Household						x^2 180.19 (2) $p < 0.001$
Alone with or without children	1,472	1,094	110	2,676	41	
Spouse/cohabitant	3,498	1,304	243	5,045	26	
Other household	133	56	8	197	28	
Accommodation						x^2 186.72 (3) $p < 0.001$
Own house	3,621	1,386	247	5,254	26	
Rented house/apartment, private marked	1,044	732	73	1,849	40	
Rented house/apartment, local authorities	149	182	7	338	54	
Other	216	124	17	357	35	
Network family						x^2 100.54 (3) $p < 0.001$
Very good	1,817	685	115	2,617	26	
Good	2,266	1,097	164	3,527	31	
Poor	527	404	36	967	42	
Very poor	129	114	5	248	46	
Network friends						x^2 41.07 (3) $p < 0.001$
Very good	1,430	543	82	2,055	26	
Good	2,430	1,244	173	3,847	32	
Poor	581	359	40	9,80	37	
Very poor	144	83	10	237	35	
Number of consultations since start of treatment						x^2 109.68 (7) $p < 0.001$
Less than 3	578	215	48	841	26	
3–5	684	259	51	994	26	
6–9	670	274	56	1,000	27	
10–19	912	374	78	1,364	27	
20–39	856	435	50	1,341	32	
40–99	720	437	37	1,194	37	
100–199	271	199	11	481	41	
200 or more	80	100	4	184	54	

(Continued)

TABLE 6 | Continued

	No follow up	Follow up	Missing	Total	% Follow Up	Chi-test (X^2)
Asylum seeker						x^2 0.59 (1) $p = 0.4413$
No	5,148	2,472	372	7,992	31	
Yes	26	16	1	43	37	
Refugee						x^2 2.35 (1) $p = 0.1252$
No	4,942	2,395	357	7,694	31	
Yes	232	93	16	341	27	
Born outside Norway						x^2 272 (1) $p = 0.0993$
No	4,427	2,093	316	6,836	31	
Yes	747	395	57	1199	33	
Having an individual care plan						x^2 154.62 (1) $p < 0.001$
No	4,971	2,198	362	7,531	29	
Yes	203	290	11	504	58	
Community treatment order						x^2 13.11 (1) $p < 0.001$
No	5,128	2,441	370	7,939	31	
Yes	46	47	3	96	49	
Living in a large municipality						x^2 0.49(1) $p = 0.4856$
No	4,280	2,042	322	6,644	31	
Yes	894	446	51	1,391	32	
Diagnoses						x^2 107.14(7) $p < 0.001$
Personality disorders	353	261	21	635	41	
Substance use disorders (as first or second diagnosis)	110	119	11	240	50	
Schizophrenia etc.	166	115	12	293	39	
Affective disorders	1,769	785	115	2,669	29	
Anxiety disorders	1,648	661	120	2,429	27	
Behavioural syndromes	152	55	12	219	25	
Behavioural and emotional disorders	235	161	16	412	39	
Other mental illness	385	191	37	613	31	

**Those who receive follow up (n = 2,488) compared to those who do not (n = 5,174) or we do not know (n = 373).*

accommodation and marital status. If accommodation is removed from the regression, the size of the coefficient of marital status is the same as when accommodation is included.

In this study, if the patient did not participate in filling in the form, the question on whether children are referred was more often (6%) answered with unknown compared to if the patient participated in filling in the form (2%). This supports the importance of clinicians involving the patient in assessing the needs of their children.

Strengths and Limitations

A major strength of the study is the large census-level sample from almost all the psychiatric outpatient clinics in one country. As the data was registered on anonymous forms and did not require written consent from the patients, there is no obvious reason to expect that the material is skewed due to subgroups being less reluctant to participate. Some clinicians did however indicate that completing the form was time-consuming and that they did not have time to include all their patients. A limitation is that the clinicians might have only included the less complicated cases to save time. It is also possible that outpatients who missed their appointed consultations were less likely to be included. An important limitation of the study compared with epidemiological studies is that only those who receive treatment were included. The prevalence numbers presented are valid for outpatients in specialist mental health treatment and not for the population suffering from mental illness in general. Finally, the results may not be representative of patients in other types of mental health services and in other countries.

The amount of missing data is a limitation, as is the small amount of information collected regarding patients' children. Information was only collected on whether children were considered to have needs and whether these needs warranted a referral to external agencies. It was not possibility to examine the quality and thoroughness of these assessments. Information was not collected on what children's needs were, nor whether referral actions were appropriate, implemented and ultimately successful at addressing children's needs. Future research could explore these factors.

CONCLUSIONS AND IMPLICATIONS

Conclusions

The prevalence of outpatients in adult psychiatric clinics who care for children under the age of 18 years is 36% in this

TABLE 7 | Logit regression of the association between patient characteristics and whether minor children of outpatients ($N = 6634$)* are being referred.

	Odds ratio	Std. Err.	z	P > z	95% Confidence interval	
Gender (male)	0.466	0.032	−11.060	0.00	0.407	0.533
Age group						
18–23 years	1.000	(base)				
24–29 years	1.316	0.237	1.53	0.13	0.925	1.873
30–39 years	1.986	0.343	3.97	0.00	1.416	2.785
40–49 years	1.952	0.345	3.78	0.00	1.380	2.761
50–59 years	1.702	0.332	2.73	0.01	1.161	2.495
60–69 years	0.449	0.175	−2.05	0.04	0.209	0.966
70 years and above	0.123	0.092	−2.79	0.01	0.028	0.535
High education	1.000	(base)				
Medium education	1.419	0.102	4.87	0.00	1.233	1.634
Low education	1.896	0.156	7.77	0.00	1.613	2.228
Income from labour	1.000	(base)				
Health related benefits	1.376	0.091	4.83	0.00	1.209	1.566
Other economic support	1.361	0.136	3.07	0.00	1.118	1.657
Married/cohabitant/partner	1.000	(base)				
Separated/divorced/widow/widower	2.534	0.512	4.60	0.00	1.705	3.766
Single/unmarried	2.056	0.423	3.51	0.00	1.374	3.076
Alone with or without children	1.000	(base)				
Spouse/cohabitant	1.427	0.284	1.79	0.07	0.966	2.107
Other type of household	0.562	0.125	−2.58	0.01	0.362	0.870
Own house	1.000	(base)				
Rented house/apartment, private marked	1.337	0.097	4.02	0.00	1.161	1.541
Rented house/apartment, local authorities	1.701	0.236	3.83	0.00	1.296	2.232
Other	1.439	0.233	2.25	0.03	1.047	1.978
Poor network family	1.447	0.112	4.79	0.00	1.244	1.683
Poor network friends	1.032	0.083	0.40	0.69	0.882	1.209
Consultations from start: 20 or more	1.281	0.075	4.23	0.00	1.142	1.436
Having an individual care plan	2.232	0.247	7.27	0.00	1.797	2.771
Community treatment order	1.121	0.297	0.43	0.67	0.667	1.884
Main diagnosis						
Personality disorders	1.000	(base)				
Substance use disorders (as first or second diagnosis)	1.306	0.239	1.46	0.14	0.913	1.870
Schizophrenia spectrum disorder	0.857	0.147	−0.90	0.37	0.612	1.198
Affective disorders	0.774	0.080	−2.48	0.01	0.633	0.947
Anxiety disorders	0.684	0.072	−3.64	0.00	0.557	0.839
Behavioural syndromes	0.606	0.116	−2.61	0.01	0.416	0.883
Behavioural and emotional disorders	1.174	0.172	1.09	0.27	0.880	1.565
Other mental illness	1.124	0.155	0.85	0.40	0.858	1.472
Constant	0.099	0.028	−8.05	0.00	0.056	0.174

One thousand twenty-eight patients had missing values for one or more of the variables, see* ***Table 6*.

study of a sample from a national census in Norwegian adult mental health clinics. This provides considerable certainty regarding parent prevalence as the statistics emanate from a whole of country data set. The findings also add important information about the characteristics of higher risk families. Significant odds ratios among psychiatric outpatients being parents with care for minor children were highest for age groups 30–49 and refugees; and lowest for being single, male, not having own house/apartment, and having a schizophrenia spectrum disorder. Of the 92% of the patients with minor children where clinicians had answered whether measures have been taken for referral for the children, 31% were reported to have children having been referred, 58% did not have children requiring a referral, and 3% had children who had not been referred in spite of being identified as requiring a referral. The need for referral was unknown for children of 8% of the outpatients with minor children. The agencies most referred to were child protection agencies (45%), CAMHS

(39%) and educational-psychological services in the school system (35%). The significant odds ratios for having children who required referral to an agency were highest for parents aged 30–59 who were single with low education, not having income from paid work, not owning a house/apartment, poor family network, having had many outpatient consultations, and having an individual care plan. The significant odds ratios were lowest for males and for having moderate or less severe psychiatric illness.

Service and Practice Implications

There are several practice and systems implications for the present results. Given the sizable minority of patients who are parents, adult mental health services require appropriate infrastructure systems and procedures to identify parenting status of patients, including those who may be pregnant. Treatment plans should address needs of parents and their children and include referral of parents and their children to early intervention services as appropriate. Referrals to child protection agencies should be carefully considered, once accurate and sensitive assessments of the family's strengths as well as vulnerabilities are made, including the family's personal and professional networks. Appropriate training could be offered to clinicians in adult mental health outpatient services, with particular attention on how mental illness impacts parenting and the range of services that families may be referred to.

Implications for Research

Future studies need to investigate more broadly the family circumstances for children whose parents have mental illness, the specific actions of clinicians and the outcome of referrals for children. Why clinicians provide referrals for the children of some of their patients, but not others, could be further investigated. The pathways of care, as parents and children navigate various mental health and other systems (including but not limited to adult mental health, child protection services, schools), could be documented to determine what happens for families, areas of duplication/gaps, and outcomes for different family members, over time.

AUTHOR CONTRIBUTIONS

TR, DM, and SO contributed conception and design of the study with input from AR, KF, BW, BS, and AG. SO collected the data, organized the database and performed the statistical analyses. DM and TR wrote the first draft of the manuscript. AR, KF, BW, BS, AG, and SO wrote sections of the manuscript. All authors contributed to manuscript revision, read and approved the submitted version.

REFERENCES

1. Farahati F, Marcotte DE, Wilcox-Gök V. The effects of parents' psychiatric disorders on children's high school dropout. *Econ Educ Rev*. (2003) 22:167–78. doi: 10.1016/S0272-7757(02)00031-6
2. Hosman CMH, van Doesum KTM, van Santvoort F. Prevention of emotional problems and psychiatric risks in children of parents with a mental illness in the Netherlands: I. The scientific basis to a comprehensive approach. *Adv Mental Health*. (2009) 8:250–63. doi: 10.5172/jamh.8.3.250
3. Reupert A, Maybery D. What do we know about families where parents have a mental illness? A systematic review. *Child Youth Serv*. (2016) 37:98–111. doi: 10.1080/0145935X.2016.1104037
4. Bell MF, Bayliss DM, Glauert R, Harrison A, Ohan JL. Children of parents who have been hospitalised with psychiatric disorders are at risk of poor school readiness. *Epidemiol Psychiatr Sci*. (2018). doi: 10.1017/S2045796018000148. [Epub ahead of print].
5. Hjern A, Berg L, Arat A, Klöfvermark J, Manhica H, Rostila M, et al. *Children as Next of Kin in Sweden*. Kalmar (2017).
6. Foster K, O'Brien L, Korhonen T. Developing resilient children and families when parents have mental illness: a family-focused approach. *Int J Ment Health Nurs*. (2012) 21:3–11. doi: 10.1111/j.1447-0349.2011.00754.x
7. Leijdesdorff S, van Doesum K, Popma A, Klaassen R, van Amelsvoort T. Prevalence of psychopathology in children of parents with mental illness and/or addiction: an up to date narrative review. *Curr Opin Psychiatry*. (2017) 30:312–7. doi: 10.1097/YCO.0000000000000341
8. Torvik FA, Rognmo K. *Barn av Foreldre Med Psykiske Lidelser Eller Alkoholmisbruk: Omfang og Konsekvenser*. Oslo: Nasjonalt folkehelseinstitutt (2011).
9. Maybery D, Reupert AE. The number of parents who are patients attending adult psychiatric services. *Curr Opin Psychiatry*. (2018) 31:358–62. doi: 10.1097/YCO.0000000000000427
10. Hearle J, Plant K, Jenner L, Barkla J, McGrath J. A survey of contact with offspring and assistance with child care among parents with psychotic disorder. *Psychiatr Serv*. (1999) 50:1354–6. doi: 10.1176/ps.50.10.1354
11. Gatsou L, Yates S, Hussain S, Barrett M, Gangavati S, Ghafoor R. Parental mental illness: incidence, assessment and practice. *Mental Health Pract*. (2016) 19:25–7. doi: 10.7748/mhp.19.5.25.s18
12. Benders-Hadi N, Barber M, Alexander MJ. Motherhood in women with serious mental illness. *Psychiatr Q*. (2013) 84:65–72. doi: 10.1007/s11126-012-9227-1
13. Ostman M, Eidevall L. Illuminating patients with children up to 18 years of age. A 1-day-inventory study in a psychiatric service. *Nordic J Psychiatry*. (2005) 59:388–92. doi: 10.1080/08039480500330164
14. Howe D, Batchelor S, Bochynska K. Prevalence of parents within an adult mental health service: census results 2008-2011. *Australas Psychiatry*. (2012) 20:413–8. doi: 10.1177/1039856212459583
15. Johnson SE, Lawrence D, Perales F, Baxter J, Zubrick SR. Prevalence of mental disorders among children and adolescents of parents with self-reported mental health problems. *Community Ment Health J*. (2018) 54:884–97. doi: 10.1007/s10597-017-0217-5
16. Maybery DJ, Reupert AE, Patrick K, Goodyear M, Crase L. Prevalence of parental mental illness in Australian families. *Psychiatr Bull*. (2009) 33:22–6. doi: 10.1192/pb.bp.107.018861
17. Maybery D, Nicholson J, Reupert A. Prevalence of families, parents and children living with parental mental illness. In: Reupert A, Maybery D, Nicholson J, Gopfert M, and Seeman M, editor. *Parental Psychiatric Disorder: Distressed Parents and their Families*. 3rd Ed. Cambridge: Cambridge University Press (2015).
18. Pape SE, Collins MP. P01-170 - A systematic literature review of parenting behaviours exhibited by anxious people. *Eur Psychiatry*. (2011) 26(Suppl.1):170. doi: 10.1016/S0924-9338(11)71881-8
19. Campbell L, Hanlon M-C, Poon AWC, Paolini S, Stone M, Galletly C, et al. The experiences of Australian parents with psychosis: The second Australian national survey of psychosis. *Aust N Z J Psychiatry*. (2012) 46:890–900. doi: 10.1177/0004867412455108
20. Hammond I, Eastman AL, Leventhal JM, Putnam-Hornstein E. Maternal mental health disorders and reports to child protective services: a birth cohort study. *Int J Environ Res Public Health*. (2017) 14:E1320. doi: 10.3390/ijerph14111320

21. Nilsson S, Gustafsson L, Nolbris MJ. Young adults' childhood experiences of support when living with a parent with a mental illness. *J Child Health Care.* (2015) 19:444–53. doi: 10.1177/13674935135 19296
22. Reupert A, Maybery D. Fathers' experience of parenting with a mental illness. Families in Society. *J Contemp Soc Serv.* (2009) 90:61–8. doi: 10.1606/1044-3894.3846
23. Fernbacher S, Goodyear M, Farhall J. Taking a closer look: a cross-sector audit of families where a parent has a mental illness. *Aust e J Adv Mental Health.* (2009) 8:242–9. doi: 10.5172/jamh.8.3.242
24. Foster K, Goodyear M, Grant A, Weimand B, Nicholson J. Family-focused practice with EASE: a practice framework for strengthening recovery when parents have mental illness. *Int J Mental Health Nurs.* (2019) 28:351–60. doi: 10.1111/inm.12535
25. Grant A, Reupert A, Maybery D, Goodyear M. Predictors and enablers of mental health nurses' family-focused practice. *Int J Ment Health Nurs.* (2018) 28:140–51. doi: 10.1111/inm.12503
26. Skogøy BE, Sørgaard K, Maybery D, Ruud T, Stavnes K, Kufås E, et al. Hospitals implementing changes in law to protect children of ill parents: a cross-sectional study. *BMC Health Serv Res.* (2018) 18:609. doi: 10.1186/s12913-018-3393-2
27. Tchernegovski P, Hine R, Reupert AE, Maybery DJ. Adult mental health clinicians' perspectives of parents with a mental illness and their children: single and dual focus approaches. *BMC Health Serv Res.* (2018) 18:611. doi: 10.1186/s12913-018-3428-8
28. Tchernegovski P, Reupert A, Maybery D. How do Australian adult mental health clinicians manage the challenges of working with parental mental illness? A phenomenological study. *Child Family Soc Work.* (2018) 23:381–9. doi: 10.1111/cfs.12426
29. Okpokoro U, Adams CE, Sampson S. Family intervention (brief) for schizophrenia. *Cochrane Database Syst Rev.* (2014) CD009802. doi: 10.1002/14651858.CD009802.pub2
30. Siegenthaler E, Munder T, Egger M. Effect of preventive interventions in Mentally Ill parents on the Mental health of the offspring: systemic review and Meta-analysis. *J Am Acad Child Adolesc Psychiatry.* (2012) 51:8–17. doi: 10.1016/j.jaac.2011.10.018
31. Solantaus T, Toikka S, Alasuutari M, Beardslee WR, Paavonen EJ. Safety, Feasibility and family experiences of preventive interventions for children and families with parental depression. *Int J Mental Health Promot.* (2009) 11:15–24. doi: 10.1080/14623730.2009.9721796
32. Solantaus T, Paavonen EJ, Toikka S, Punamäki RL. Preventive interventions in families with parental depression: children's psychosocial symptoms and prosocial behaviour. *Eur Child Adolesc Psychiatry.* (2010): 19:883–92. doi: 10.1007/s00787-010-0135-3
33. Olson PR. *Mental Health Systems Compared. Great Britain, Norway, Canada and the United States.* Springfield, MA: Springfield Charles C Thomas Publishers (2006).
34. Ruud T, Hauff E. Community mental health services in Norway. *Int J Mental Health.* (2003) 31:3–14. doi: 10.1080/00207411.2002.11449568
35. OECD. *OECD Reviews of Health Care Quality: Norway 2014: Raising Standards.* Paris: OECD Publishing (2014).
36. Helse- og omsorgsdepartementet. Ot.prp. nr. 84. *Om lov om Endringar i Helsepersonell Loven m.m. (oppfølging av born som pårørande) [About changes in the Health Personnel Act (Followup of Children as Next of Kin)].* Oslo: Ministry of Health and Care Services (2008-2009).
37. O'Hara MW, Wisner KL. Perinatal mental illness: definition, description and aetiology. *Best Pract Res Clin Obstet Gynaecol.* (2014) 28:3–12. doi: 10.1016/j.bpobgyn.2013.09.002
38. Ayazi T, Bøgwald K-P. Innvandreres bruk av poliklinisk psykiatrisk tjeneste [Minorities' use of outpatient psychiatric services]. *Tidsskr Nor Legeforen.* (2008) 128:162–5.
39. Reupert A, Maybery D, Nicholson J, Gopfert M, Seeman M, editors. *Parental Psychiatric Disorder: Distressed Parents and their Families.* 3rd Ed. Cambridge: Cambridge University Press (2015). doi: 10.1017/CBO9781107707559
40. Gladstone BM, Boydell KM, McKeever P. Recasting research into children's experiences of parental mental illness: Beyond risk and resilience. *Soc Sci Med.* (2006) 62:2540–50. doi: 10.1016/j.socscimed.2005.10.038
41. Ruud T, Birkeland B, Faugli A, Hagen KA, Hellman A, Hilsen M, et al. *Barn som pårørende. Resultater fra en multisenterstudie. Rapport, [Children With Ill Parents. Results From a Multi-Center Study. Report.].* Lørenskog: Akershus universitetssykehus HF (2015).

Children of Mentally Ill Parents at Risk Evaluation (COMPARE): Design and Methods of a Randomized Controlled Multicenter Study—Part I

Hanna Christiansen[1], Corinna Reck[2], Anna-Lena Zietlow[3], Kathleen Otto[4], Ricarda Steinmayr[5], Linda Wirthwein[5], Sarah Weigelt[6], Rudolf Stark[7], David D. Ebert[8], Claudia Buntrock[8], Johannes Krisam[9], Christina Klose[9], Meinhard Kieser[9] and Christina Schwenck[10]*

[1] Department of Clinical Child and Adolescent Psychology, Faculty of Psychology, Philipps University Marburg, Marburg, Germany, [2] Department of Clinical Child and Adolescent Psychology, Faculty of Psychology, Ludwig-Maximilians-University München, Munich, Germany, [3] Center for Psychosocial Medicine, Institute of Medical Psychology, Heidelberg University Hospital, Heidelberg, Germany, [4] Department of Social Psychology, Business and Methods, Faculty of Psychology, Philipps University Marburg, Marburg, Germany, [5] Department of Educational Psychology, Faculty of Education, Psychology, and Sociology, Institute of Psychology, Technical University Dortmund, Dortmund, Germany, [6] Department of Vision, Visual Impairment & Blindness, Faculty of Rehabilitation Science, Technical University Dortmund, Dortmund, Germany, [7] Department of Psychotherapy and Systems Neuroscience, Faculty of Psychology and Sports Science, Justus-Liebig-University Gießen, Gießen, Germany, [8] Department of Clinical Psychology and Psychotherapy, Institute of Psychology, Friedrich-Alexander-University Erlangen-Nürnberg, Erlangen, Germany, [9] Department of Medical Biometry, Institute of Medical Biometry and Informatics, Heidelberg University, Heidelberg, Germany, [10] Department of Special Needs Educational and Clinical Child and Adolescent Psychology, Faculty of Psychology and Sports Science, Justus-Liebig-University Gießen, Gießen, Germany

***Correspondence:**
Hanna Christiansen
christih@staff.uni-marburg.de

Objectives: Mental disorders are frequent, associated with disability-adjusted life years, societal, and economic costs. Children of parents with a mental illness (COPMI) are at an increased risk to develop disorders themselves. The transgenerational transmission of mental disorders has been conceptualized in a model that takes parental and family factors, the social environment (i.e., school, work, and social support), parent-child-interaction and possible child outcomes into account. The goal of the "Children of Mentally Ill Parents At Risk Evaluation" (COMPARE) study will thus be twofold: (1) to establish the efficacy and cost-effectiveness of a high-quality randomized controlled trial (RCT) with the aim of interrupting the intergenerational transmission of mental disorders in COPMI, (2) to test the components of the trans-generational transmission model of mental disorders.

Methods: To implement a randomized controlled trial (RCT: comparison of parental cognitive behavioral therapy/CBT with CBT + Positive Parenting Program) that is flanked by four add-on projects that apply behavioral, psychophysiological, and neuro-imaging methods to examine potential moderators and mediators of risk transmission (projects COMPARE-emotion/-interaction/-work/-school). COMPARE-emotion targets emotion processing and regulation and its impact on the transgenerational disorder transmission; COMPARE-interaction focuses especially on the impact of maternal comorbid diagnoses of depression and anxiety disorders and will concentrate on different pathways of the impact of maternal disorders on socio-emotional and cognitive infant development, such as parent-infant interaction and the infant's stress regulation skills. COMPARE-work analyzes the transmission of strains a person experiences in one area of life to another (i.e., from family to work; spill-over), and how stress and strain are transmitted between individuals (i.e., from parent to child; cross-over). COMPARE-school focuses on the psychosocial adjustment, school performance, and subjective well-being in COPMI compared to an adequate control group of healthy children.

Results: This study protocol reports on the interdisciplinary approach of COMPARE testing the model of the transgenerational transmission of mental disorders.

Conclusion: The combination of applied basic with clinical research will facilitate the examination of specific risk transmission mechanisms, promotion, dissemination and implementation of results into a highly important but largely neglected field.

Clinical Trial Registration: DRKS-ID: DRKS00013516 (German Clinical Trials Register, https://www.drks.de/drks_web/navigate.do?navigationId=trial.HTML&TRIAL_ID=DRKS00013516).

Keywords: children of mentally ill parents, transgenerational transmission, mental disorders, intervention, prevention

INTRODUCTION

Children of Mentally Ill Parents

The German social report of the year 2013 indicates a total of 19 million children/adolescents living in 1.6 million single and 8.1 million dual family households (1). Given the estimated lifetime prevalence rate of 27.4% for mental disorders associated with significant disability-adjusted life years (DALYs) for the age group of 18–65 year olds (2), approximately 25% of the children/adolescents in Germany are living with a mentally ill parent, a percentage resembling international rates (3–7). Having a parent with a mental illness has been associated with multiple psychological and developmental risks for children, such as lower academic achievement (8), increased stress-related somatic health conditions (e.g., higher rates of asthma and other atopic diseases (9), internalizing/externalizing symptoms (10, 11), and the development of severe mental illness (SMI) (12). Our own study of $n = 15.904$ adult patients from three different psychiatric/psychosomatic clinics revealed that 65% of the patients had children and that 73.4% of those parents were currently caring for their children (13). The children of the parents of those three different clinics were already exhibiting symptoms of mental disorders themselves (depending on the sample between 15 and 38.4%), thus providing evidence that the trans-generational transmission of mental disorders (TTMD) is a major risk factor for the development of SMI, as demonstrated in numerous other studies (11, 12, 14–16). Long-term studies have shown that children of parents with a mental illness (COPMI) have a higher life-time risk of developing SMI that ranges between 41 and 77%. However, subclinical symptoms often emerge earlier in life (14, 15). The BELLA study revealed a parental mental illness as a powerful risk factor (OR 2.4) for the development of probable mental health problems in children and adolescents (17). Recent studies have added evidence that offspring with two generations previously affected by SMI are at an even greater risk (18, 19). Thus, COPMI are most likely to constitute the next generation of patients with a mental illness (12) associated with significant DALYs and economic costs (20–22). They therefore constitute an essential target high risk group to be addressed by selective prevention programs (23). This is the aim of the COMPARE-family project (see part II of the study protocol published in this research topic by Stracke et al. (24).

Transgenerational Transmission

A recent meta-analysis of the trans-generational transmission of parental mental disorders on children's symptomatology revealed specific effects of parental disorders on children (12). According to this meta-analysis, both transgenerational concordance (specific parental mental disorders increase children's risk for certain disorders) and multifinality (parental mental disorders increase children's risk for mental disorders in general) are used to define the scope of the child's diagnostic outcomes of a particular parental disorder. The concepts of transgenerational specificity and equifinality, respectively, refer to similarities and differences in parental disorders preceding a child's diagnostic outcome. Multi- and equifinality are more common in children of parents with unipolar and bipolar affective disorders, whereas the risk of children of anxious parents is mainly restricted to develop anxiety disorders. For all children, risk transmission is assumed to be partly specific since studies indicate a strong tendency for children to develop the same disorders as their parents. A meta-analysis ($k = 61$ studies included) of the cross-sectional association between paternal and maternal psychopathology on children's internalizing and externalizing behavior problems further revealed parent-specific gender effects (25). There is a general lack of studies on the specific risk transmissions for the broad range of parental disorders other than affective and anxiety disorders (12) and studies assessing a wider range of parental disorders as well as their effects on the children are missing, as are studies on parental comorbidity. This lack is addressed in the current study, as we will consider a broad range of parental disorders as well as comorbid ones.

A comprehensive model (see **Figure 1**) of the TTMD identifies four major domains [(1) parent, (2) family, (3) child, and (4) social environment] that interact with their respective systems and are influenced by five transmission mechanisms [(1) genetics, (2) prenatal factors, (3) parent-child-interaction, (4) family, and (5) social factors]. Child development over its whole span is considered, as well as the concepts of multi- and equifinality, concordance, and specificity. While there is empirical support for the model's different domains and factors, many research has solely addressed single dimensions (i.e., focusing on family or child factors or on genetics), without taking the whole model into account, which is clearly necessary (for a review of the model components see (13). Furthermore, most of those studies were conducted on individual disorders in parents, and comparative studies on the range of parental disorders and on crucial factors such as parental comorbidities are rare (26) or entirely lacking (12). Moreover, the specific impact of the various moderating and mediating processes between the incidence of mental disorders in parents and their children—such as genetics, epigenetics, stress reactivity, emotion regulation, parenting skills, parent-child-interaction, children's cognitive abilities, family, and environmental influences—as well as their interactions have not been clarified so far. Thus, the aim of the COMPARE consortium with its subprojects COMPARE-family/emotion/interaction/school/work is to test the TTMD model and to simultaneously assess the four major domains as well as the transmission mechanisms. This will enable us to establish specific transmission profiles (equi- vs. multifinality vs. concordance vs. specificity) for a range of parental disorders with/without comorbidities. Furthermore, we will be able to identify risk-profiles for children at high vs. low risk, since studies have shown that not all children will develop disorders themselves (25) although their overall risk is significantly increased (14). This will improve the development of targeted interventions, connecting our first aim with the second one, since the bi-directional influences of interventions on the TTMD as well as specifics of the TTMD on interventions have not been investigated so far.

Summing up, we expect that our study will substantially deepen our knowledge of the relevant risk transmission mechanisms and related child outcomes, as well as markedly improve children's health, by simultaneously assessing the domains and mechanisms of the TTMD model as well as the bi-directional influences of a selective intervention in one study. This paper reports on part I of the overall protocol paper describing the consortium structure with the clinical trial and the four add-on research projects. Part II is the protocol paper of the clinical trial, also published in this research topic (24).

Aims of the Research Consortium

The research consortium "Children Of Mentally Ill Parents At Risk Evaluation" (COMPARE) is a network of researchers that includes disciplines from clinical, work and organizational, developmental, and educational psychology. Using a randomized controlled trial (RCT) and accompanying add-on projects, the COMPARE consortium addresses the following main goals:

1. To establish effects of parental treatment on child outcome [see the protocol on COMPARE-family by Stracke et al. (24) in this Frontiers research topic].
2. To tests the domains of the TTMD model within the RCT.
3. To identify specific transmission mechanisms.

The primary hypotheses of the model testing part of the study are:

COMPARE-family: To test the transgenerational transmission of mental disorders from parents to children. We will establish risk profiles and analyze the transmission pathways of multifinality, equifinality, specificity, and concordance. We further test the effects of parental psychotherapy treatment on the children and whether a training of parenting skills will result in additional effects [for details see (24) in this research topic].

COMPARE-emotion: Emotion processing and emotion regulation demonstrate processes that, on the one hand, are reduced in COPMI compared to children of parents without mental illness. This relationship should be moderated by factors related to the mental diseases of the parents, such as the type of disorder, disease duration, age of the children at disease onset and disease severity. On the other hand, we assume these processes to be influenced by parental treatment and to simultaneously moderate the effectiveness of the intervention. Therefore, the current subproject was designed to (a) compare COPMI with children of parents without mental illness (COPWI) regarding emotion processing (EP) and emotion regulation (ER) skills, (b) to evaluate the impact of EP and ER on treatment outcome, and (c) to assess the effects of different treatments on EP and ER in COPMI.

COMPARE-interaction: Maternal psychopathology, infant stress reactivity, and the quality of the parent-infant interaction at 3–4 months predict infant development at 24 months postpartum, and maternal comorbid depression and anxiety coincide with greater impairment in the infant development at 12, 18, and 24 months than depression alone. Furthermore, it is hypothesized that the parent-infant interaction as well as the infant stress reactivity at 12 months of age mediate the relationship between the maternal psychiatric diagnosis 3–4 months postpartum and infant development (socio-emotional as well as cognitive) at 24 months of age.

COMPARE-work: We expect to observe that mentally ill parents are confronted with more severe working conditions as compared to healthy parents, and that stronger adverse spillover effects of work-based strain toward the family emerge for them. With respect to the transmission of parents' strain to their children, we as well assume that such crossover-effects depend on the parents' health status. Overall, we expect to identify specific patterns with regard to the spillover-crossover effect assuming that the maladaptive cycle leading from the parents' poor working

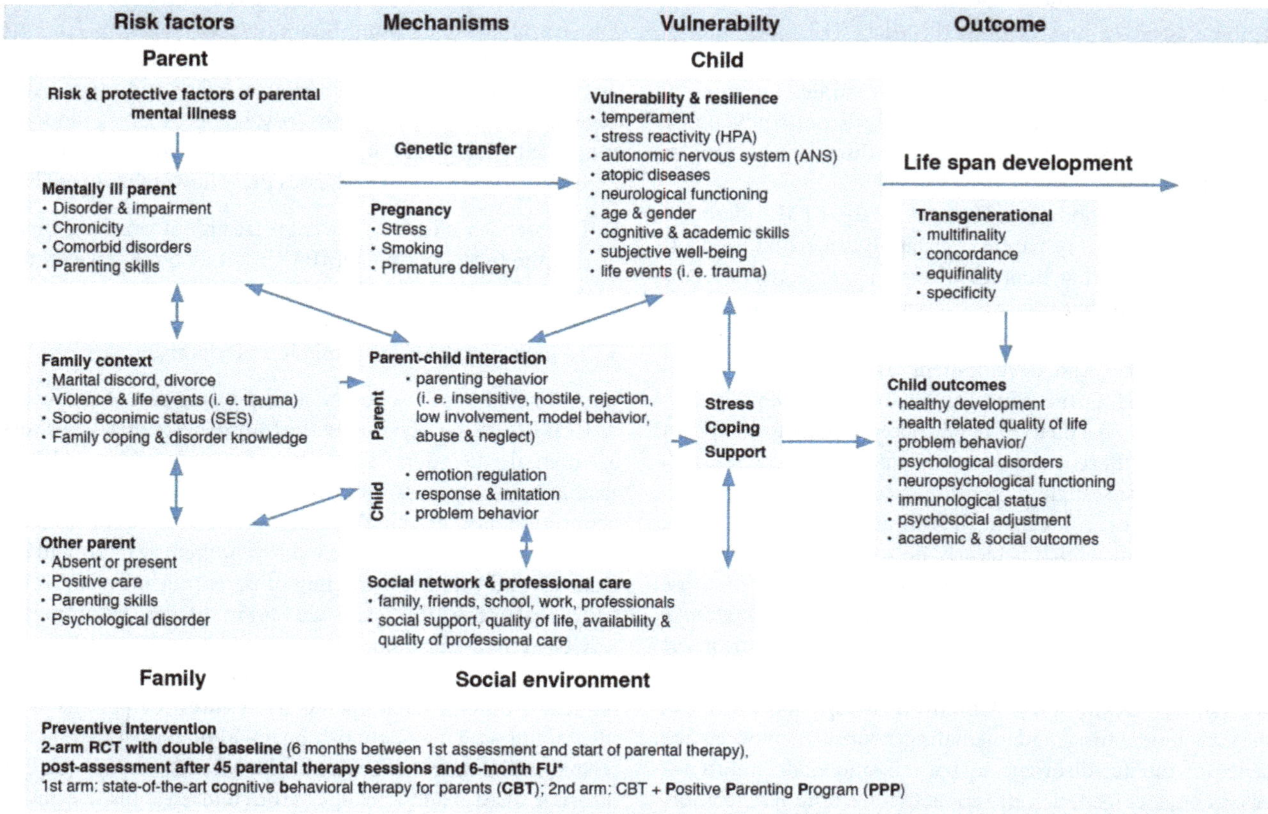

FIGURE 1 | Model of the trans-generational transmission of mental disorders adapted from Hosman et al. (14), p. 253, identifying risk factors, mechanisms, vulnerability, and child outcome. The influence of interventions on the different aspects of the model is an inclusion of the consortium.

conditions (in particular those with a mental illness) via spillover to the family can be interrupted so that no crossover to their children occurs.

COMPARE-school: We expect that COPMI perform poorer on academic achievement scales, display less positive psychosocial adjustment patterns, and suffer from lower general and domain-specific subjective well-being compared to children of mentally healthy parents. Due to the specific parental mental disease and parents' gender, we anticipate identifying different effects in the aforementioned child outcome variables in COPMI.

METHODS

COMPARE-Family: Effects of Parental Psychotherapy and Additional Parent Training on Children

This subproject is central for the entire consortium and planned as a randomized controlled trial establishing the effects of high quality parental therapy (cognitive behavioral therapy/CBT) on the children in comparison to parental CBT and a parent training, the Positive Parenting Program (CBT+PPP). We have chosen CBT for the intervention, as CBT has the soundest evidence base for the psychotherapeutic treatment of mental disorders (72). Studies further demonstrate poorer parenting skills in parents with mental disorders (27–30), and the enhancement of such skills has been a significant mediator in improving child outcomes (31). The Positive Parenting Program (PPP) is a well-established program to enhance parenting skills, and specific effects on child psychopathology could be demonstrated (32, 33). Studies explicitly testing effects of parental treatment in conjunction with parenting skills are lacking so far.

A total of seven university based study sites participates in the RCT and each of them specializes on different mental disorders. We will thus be able not only to address depression and anxiety, but a wider range of disorders such as sleep-wake-, and somatic symptom disorders, obsessive compulsive, trauma and stressor related disorders, eating and personality disorders, bipolar, and schizophrenic disorders. As patients in Germany are required to be abstinent for outpatient psychotherapy, patients with substance use disorders will not be included in the trial.

The structure of the RCT will allow us further (i) to establish effects of the parental disorder(s) with/without comorbidities on children's health; (ii) to establish effects of the different interventions (CBT vs. CBT+PPP) on children's health; (iii) to test assumptions of the TTMD model and bi-directional influences of different treatments on the model; (iv) to analyze specific transmission mechanisms; and (v) to establish risk profiles for children with urgent needs for preventive interventions.

Key inclusion criteria are parents with a mental illness in outpatient treatment caring for a child between 1.5 and 16 years of age. Key exclusion criteria are insufficient German language skills, severe impairment of the children requiring comprehensive treatment.

Description of the Primary Efficacy/Test Accuracy Analysis and Population

The primary analysis is conducted according to the intention-to-treat (ITT) principle and includes all randomized patients. The confirmatory test for treatment group differences between T2 and T3, and T2 and T4 with respect to the primary endpoint each applies linear mixed multi-level model with patients at level 1 and children at level 2, adjusting for center, number of comorbidities, number of children, baseline TRF score at T2, and length of waiting period between T1 and T2 (in weeks). The overall type I error rate is set at 5% (two-sided) and will be controlled by applying the multiple test procedure for hierarchically ordered hypotheses. Effect size assumed for estimation of sample size is set at $d = 0.25$. With a two-sided significance level of $\alpha = 0.05$ and a power of $1-\beta = 0.8$ using a two-sample t-test, 253 patients per group ($n = 506$ total) are required. Taking a drop-out rate of 20% into account, $n = 634$ patients need to be enrolled into the trial. Since it is assumed that parts of the outcome variance can be explained by the inclusion of covariates, the actual power of the analysis by linear mixed multi-level model is expected to be higher than $1-\beta = 0.8$. Sample size calculation was performed using SAS v9.4. For details on COMPARE-family and the full study protocol please refer to Stracke et al. (24) in this research topic.

The projects COMPARE-emotion/interaction/work/school are closely linked to this trial, as the parents of children of COMPARE-family will also be assessed for those subprojects. We will thus gain knowledge on the interaction of therapy effects with the specified TTMD-domains.

COMPARE-Emotion: Emotion Processing and Regulation in Children of Parents With Mental Illness

The TTMD model identifies child factors as one of four major domains of the transmission of parental mental disorders to the child (see above). Therefore, specific characteristics and behavioral traits in the child are likely to raise or lower the risk for a mental disorder in the child of a parent with a mental illness for him- or herself. Emotion processing and emotion regulation have been identified as such factors. Emotion processing (EP) is a broad concept that includes sub-processes of emotion perception, affective stimulus interpretation, and affective reaction to another's emotions. In the current sub-project, we want to focus on (a) emotion recognition, (b) perspective taking, and (c) affective arousal (sympathy vs. personal distress) as a reaction to another person's emotional situation (34). EP aberrations constitute a central characteristic of both individual and a wide range of mental disorders, reflecting a transdiagnostic approach (35–37). Emotion regulation (ER) comprises processes applied by individuals to influence the incidence, kind, intensity, and duration of their emotions as well as their effects on feelings and behaviors (38, 39). Strategies can be adaptive, for example if they increase positive or decrease negative emotions, or be maladaptive, having the opposed effect. Both, EP and ER constitute important skills that are transdiagnostically related to mental disorders. Both skills are affected by parental behavior throughout child development. The research conducted on this topic so far reveals direct and indirect associations between a parental mental illness and aberrant EP or ER in their children. However, no comprehensive study on the impact of the child's EP and ER on the trans-diagnostic trans-generational transmission of mental disorders has been conducted so far, despite the fact that these processes constitute important targets for preventive interventions. Furthermore, the impact of EP and ER on treatment effects has not been studied to date.

To examine these processes, experimental tasks assessing EP and ER will be administered in 200 children of parents participating in the COMPARE-family study [see study by Stracke et al. (24) in this research topic] at the assessment points T1, T3, and T4 of the clinical trial (100 children of parents receiving cognitive behavioral therapy and 100 children of patients additionally receiving the Positive Parenting Program). Furthermore, a sample of 100 children with parents without a history of mental diseases or psychotherapy and no indication of current mental disorders will be assessed with the same tasks at a single measurement point (see **Figure 2**). A version of the Video Sequences Task will measure various aspects of emotion processing including emotion recognition, perspective taking, personal distress, and sympathy. This task has been chosen because of it's high ecological validity. Children are shown short film clips containing scenes with the protagonist conducting a certain basic emotion. Additionally, the morphing task will be adopted to assess emotion recognition with respect to quality and speed. In this task, film clips with neutral faces morphing into affective faces are shown and participants are supposed to press a button as soon as they recognize the emotion. To measure emotion regulation, an emotional Go/Nogo paradigm will be applied. In this task children are supposed to press a button following certain affective stimuli, e.g., happy faces, and inhibit a button press following other stimuli, e.g., sad faces. These two experimental tasks allow for a precise and fine grained assessment of the relevant constructs. Dependent variables include behavioral task performance measures and peripheral physiological activity during the tasks (heart rate variability, skin conductance, and mimicry). Furthermore, questionaires will measure emotion regulation strategies and cognitive and emotional empathy of the children and their parents.

To investigate differences in emotion processing between COPMI and COPWI not manifest in behavioral or physiological measures, patterns of neuronal activity and neuroanatomical connectivity will be compared between subgroups. Especially the amygdala-prefrontal cortex network is assumed to display a specific coordinating role in this context, and different mental disorders in childhood and adolescence have been found to be associated with aberrant amygdala and/or prefrontal cortex activation during EP. Therefore, out of each subgroup 40 participants will be measured with functional magnetic

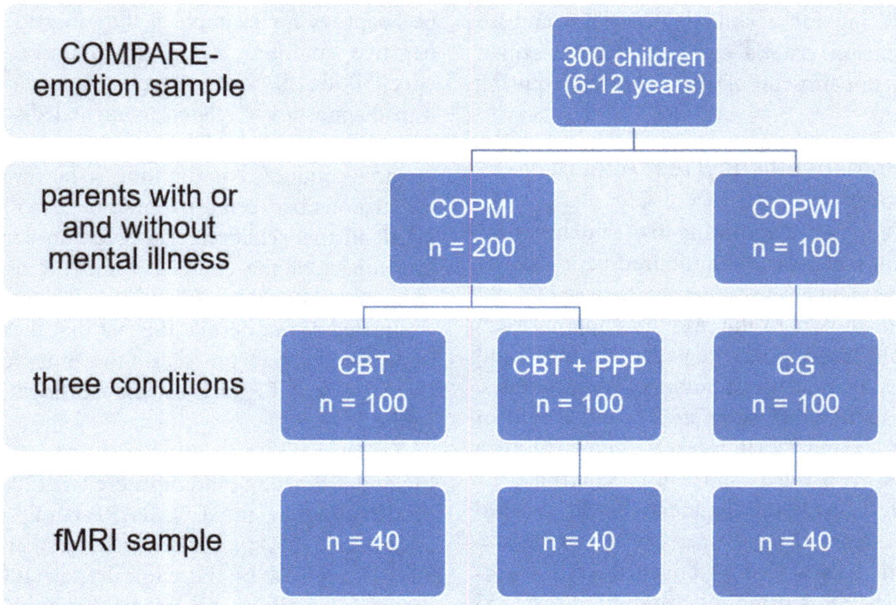

FIGURE 2 | Sample of COMPARE-emotion. fMRI, functional magnetic resonance imaging.

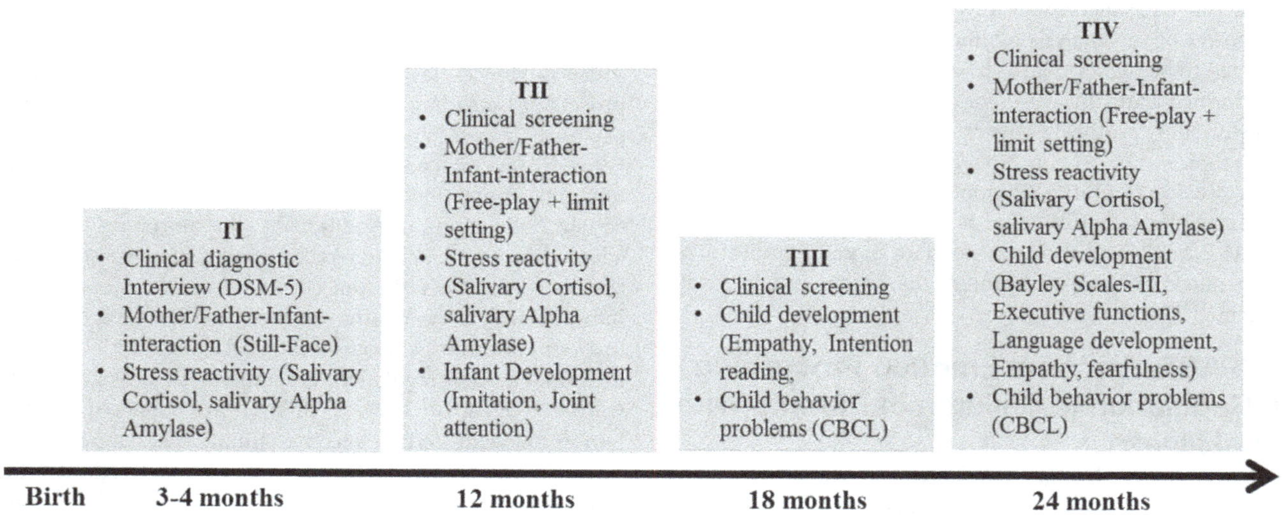

FIGURE 3 | COMPARE-interaction study design.

resonance imaging. A paradigm will be applied that involves processing of emotional faces as well as implicit emotion regulation via emotion labeling. We assume that COPMI will show higher activity in emotion processing brain areas and less habituation of the amygdala than COPWI, in particular if there is no task to perform. When the participants are required to draw attention away from the facial emotional expressions, we additionally expect higher neural costs in the COPMI, especially overactivity in the anterior cingulate cortex. During emotion labeling, COPMI should exhibit less regulatory prefrontal activity than COPWI, i.e., less activity of the ventrolateral prefrontal cortex combined with higher activity in the amygdala and less functional connectivity between both structures. Additional diffusion tensor imaging will be applied to investigate differences in white matter tract integrity in emotion processing networks.

COMPARE-Interaction: Impact of Maternal Comorbid Depression and Anxiety in the Peripartum Period on Infant Development: The Role of Parent-Infant Interaction and Infant Stress Reactivity

The Compare-interaction subproject pursues a developmental approach which aims to identify risk factors for the generational transmission of parental mental health disorders in early childhood as displayed in the TTMD model. This model identifies parent-child interaction as a core mechanism in the transgenerational transmission of parental mental disorders to the child. COMPARE-interaction focuses on the long-term consequences of maternal depressive and comorbid depressive and anxiety disorders during the peripartum period on child development, especially on socio-emotional and cognitive development. Special attention will be paid to the mediational effect of parent-infant interaction and infant stress reactivity on the relationship between the maternal disorder (depressive, comorbid, healthy controls) and infant outcome. Moreover, it will significantly contribute to model testing in the model's following domains: mentally ill parent, family context, other parent, parent-infant interaction, infant outcome. Given the high prevalence of depressive and anxious disorders during the peripartum period and the increased risk for children of depressed and anxious mothers to exhibit adverse developmental problems, further research in this field is urgently needed. The negative impact of depression on infant socio-emotional and cognitive development is well-documented in the literature (40). To date, there are no studies comparing mothers with peripartum depression alone to depressed mothers with comorbid anxiety disorders. As comorbidity is associated with greater impairment and symptom severity related to the primary diagnosis, comorbidity in mothers might raise their offspring's risk of developing internalized disorders even more than has been noted in conjunction with depression alone (41).

N = 168 families (n = 56 per subgroup and n = 84 per study center in Heidelberg and Munich) will be recruited through inpatient and outpatient centers as well as maternity hospitals in Munich and Heidelberg. A drop-out rate of 20% is expected.

This study is designed to assess peripartum depressed mothers with and without comorbid anxiety disorders according to DSM-5, fathers and their infants, as well as a healthy control group at four measurement points over the first 2 years (T1: 3–4 months postpartum, T2: 12 months postpartum, T3: 18 months postpartum, an T4: 24 months postpartum; see **figure 3** for details). Besides the evaluation of parental psychiatric status at all measurement points, parent-infant interaction will be videotaped and coded according to the Coding Infant Behavior Scales (CIB) (42). To determine infant stress-reactivity, cortisol will be extracted from infant saliva, which is collected before (C1), 20 min (C2), and 30 min after the interactional episodes.

At the age of 12 months, declarative and imperative point production and understanding (43), as well as imitation of object-related (44) and intransitive action skills (45) as predictors of later social-cognitive development will be assessed. This will be expanded upon at 18 months by an assessment of empathy (46) and intention reading (47) as milestones of constructive social behavior and mindreading, and at 24 months of empathy, executive functioning (gift delay (48) and reverse categorization (49), language abilities (SET-K (50), and child fearfulness [spider task (51)]. The measurements taken at 24 months will serve as our primary outcome measures for the longitudinal study. Infant socio-emotional development will be rated by mothers, fathers and additional caregivers via the Child Behavior Checklist/Caregiver Teacher Report Form (52, 53) at T3 and T4. Cognitive development will be assessed at T4 using the Bayley Scales of Infant Development-III (54).

This sub-project will yield new insights into the specific effects of maternal depressive and comorbid depressive and anxiety disorders disorders on different aspects of the infant's social and cognitive development, as well as on the interaction mechanisms contributing to this process. We need a deeper understanding of the underlying mediation effects to develop future prevention or intervention approaches, since research on comorbid depressive and anxiety disorders and their impacts on the parent-infant relationship and infant development is still lacking. Therefore, better understanding will enable us to suggest starting points for further research into this area. The multi-perspective approach is novel as we will be analyzing socio-emotional and cognitive parameters together and also include fathers in this study. This is unique as no other research projects have studied these research questions using additional biopsychological measures. Research of this kind is particularly important to help us to better understand adverse developmental pathways and to pave the way for future implementation of prevention and intervention programs.

COMPARE-Work: Parental Work Environment as a Risk Factor: Spillover-Crossover Effects From Parents to Children

Work has a central meaning to our lives: it shapes our identities, offers us social support and appreciation, and helps us to achieve collective goals (55). How important work is and the effects it has on children can be illustrated by the example of being unemployed. Studies indicate that the children of unemployed parents are disadvantaged: their birth weight is lower, they reveal slower growth and have more accidents (56, 57), they exhibit more self-destructive behavior, and that they tend to drop out of school and are more frequently unemployed as adults ["intergenerational unemployment"; (57)]. Similar effects are to be expected if working conditions are detrimental (58); then long-term negative health-effects occur that can spread over to the family and thus be a risk factor for the mental health of children. A negative downward spiral could be activated when parents, because of being emotionally exhausted for example, cannot provide their children any support when doing the homework while their children absorb their parents' work-related worries. Parents' adverse working conditions may have a negative impact on both their children's school performance and mental well-being. To the best of our knowledge, no research so far has attempted to clarify this process.

A first aim of this project is to explore whether mentally ill as compared to healthy parents are confronted with more severe working conditions, namely that they are confronted with more stressors (e.g., time pressure), possess fewer resources (e.g., lack of social support) at their workplaces, and report on a worse career development (e.g., job loss). Across countries findings of the (59), p. 30) revealed that the "average income of people with a moderate mental disorder is around 90% of the total working-age population, and it is 80% or less (...) for those with a severe mental disorder." These statistics suggests that also mentally ill parents face a high unemployment risk or work more frequently in precarious jobs. Moreover, research has identified two different ways in which work demands or strain are carried over: spillover and crossover. Adverse working conditions can strain parents, and such strain is expected to be transferred from the work domain toward the family, rendering it a risk factor for family life (work-family conflicts) and hence for the mental health of children. This "spillover" is the within-person, across-domain transmission of strain from one area of life to another (60). The next step following spillover-processes from work to family is to explore parent-to-child crossover, which has not been studied to date. Crossover represents a phenomenon, where experiences of stress and strain are transmitted between individuals (61). The core assumption is that one's own stress and strain experiences have an impact on others in close surroundings. To clarify the underlying mechanism in the spillover-crossover-process (62), we will try to shed light on the mediators. As proposed in the concept of emotional contagion (63), negative states are transferred easily and automatically. Moreover, crossover can be of cognitive nature through shared social cognition, a factor that can be a source of information to facilitate the interpretation of ambiguous situations. Hence, the way crossover from parents to children works—driven emotionally or cognitively—will also be researched.

In this project, working conditions of parents of children of the RCT [COMPARE-family; see (24) in this research topic] and parents of a representative group of school children not differing in basic demographic variables (assessed together with COMPARE-school) will be compared. We will assess task- and job-related working conditions (e.g., time pressure, autonomy, interruptions at work, and skill utilization) with the Instrument for Stress Oriented Task Analysis [ISTA; (64)] and the Copenhagen Psychosocial Questionnaire [COPSOQ II; (65)]. Further, working conditions on the social level (e.g., social stressors, social support, appreciation) will be explored using well-established measures. To explore spillover, besides working conditions, strain (work-family-conflict, need for recovery) and well-being (life satisfaction, mood, emotional exhaustion) of both groups of parents will be assessed via existing self-report measures. To study crossover, also the children will be investigated regarding their well-being (life satisfaction, mood, emotional exhaustion) and their closeness to their parents. To detect the underyling transmission process, an *ad-hoc* measure that reflects emotional vs. cognitive processes in crossover for children will be developed and pre-tested.

Using the software G-Power and specifying alpha as 5% and statistical power to equal at least 80% and applying MANOVA to test for differences between mentally ill vs. healthy parents' working conditions considering parents' gender, a minimum sample size of 200 parents is suggested. However, to test the more complex models (SEM) detecting the spillover-crossover process, a minimum sample size of 300 parents would be optimal to detect medium-sized effects. As higher attrition rates are not uncommon for longitudinal research in the Occupational Health Psychology field, we plan to contact a total of 887 mothers and/or fathers. Depending on the parents' consent to participate—which we expect to be about 50% (aiming at 450 parents in total)—the exact sample size will be somewhat lower, though.

In sum, this project will deepen our knowledge of the TTMD model. By assessing parental working conditions, an essential element in the TTMD model can be explained. Various stressors and resources in the working context of both mentally ill and healthy parents as well as work-related strain and work-family conflict indicators will be explored, characterizing the aforementioned spillover-crossover process in (all) its complexity.

COMPARE-School: Psychosocial Adjustment, School Performance, and Subjective Well-Being in Children of Mentally Ill Parents

Most studies have focused on the mental health and child psychopathology of COPMI and just a few studies have focused on other relevant child outcomes proposed in the TTMD, such as academic attainment, psychosocial functioning or subjective well-being by investigating an adequate control sample of children with healthy parents [e.g., (66–68)]. One main aim of this subproject is to compare a school control sample to the COMPARE-family intervention groups [see (24) in this research topic]. This control sample will be recruited in elementary and secondary schools during regular school lessons. School children comparable in age to the RCT [COMPARE-family; see (24) in this research topic] will be examined with the same tests as COPMI. All tests will be given during regular school lessons to entire school classes. About $N = 900$ school children will initially be investigated. Within this sample, a propensity score matching [see (73)] will be performed controlling for age, gender, and parental socioeconomic background to obtain a school control cohort comparable to and as large as the COPMI group.

Different indicators of academic achievement will be assessed (standardized achievement tests in reading and mathematics, school grades). Social skills will be measured via self-reports as well as via parental assessments. Subjective well-being will be examined by investigating both cognitive as well as affective variables regarding life as a whole as well as regarding family, school, and peers (69).

Moreover, there is a serious lack of knowledge how parental mental disease affect lower educational attainment. Besides parenting behaviors that are related to child learning (such as homework support) and that in turn affect academic achievement, other mediating child characteristics might also be of influence (e.g., temperament and cognitive abilities). In this context, the child's school values and academic expectations are especially interesting, as research has demonstrated that these variables both differ between children of mentally ill and healthy parents and influence academic achievement (70, 71). Besides other child outcomes such as psychosocial functioning and subjective well-being, especially parenting skills and parenting styles in general might be important process variables.

Research has shown that some COPMI reveal no detrimental outcomes regarding their educational attainment, psychosocial adjustment, or subjective well-being [e.g., (6)]. There is little research to date comparing those children with children suffering from their parent's mental health disorder to identify protective and risk factors. The TTMD model describes various potentially-relevant vulnerability factors such as temperament, cognitive skills or the parenting style and parenting behavior. These vulnerability factors will be additionally examined within COMPARE-school.

Finally, treatment-related changes in educational attainment, psychosocial functioning, and subjective well-being will be examined. The aforementioned outcomes will be assessed at T2 (2nd baseline), T3 (post-test), and T4 (6 months follow-up) in the cohort of COPMI and in the representative control group [for a full description of the RCT-design see (24) in this research topic].

The outcome variables measured in COMPARE-school are closely related to children's health, and provide a holistic perspective onto a child's healthy development. Our project will yield important insights into the specific transmission profiles proposed in the TTMD. In sum, we will contribute to both model testing and the intervention emphasis of the main COMPARE project.

TRANSFER INTO THE ROUTINE PROVIDER SYSTEM

The results of the COMPARE consortium will be made available to the larger scientific community via peer-reviewed publications in scientific journals, presentations at scientific meetings and presentation on the COMPARE website. Partners will be encouraged to publish in "Open Access" journals whenever appropriate, ensuring accessibility to the widest readership worldwide. Throughout the study and beyond, patients, parents, and carers (stakeholder board) will be kept informed about the study through the COMPARE website, flyers, newsletters, and personal contacts. Politicians, public health services, and stakeholders will be informed via teaching seminars and conferences on the background and results of the present study, thus improving public policy and health care decisions whose aim it is to prevent and treat COPMI. Two large health care insurances, the "Allgemeine Ortskrankenkasse/AOK" and "IKK Südwest" have ensured us to disseminate results to their insurance holders. Existing networks (i.e., Kindernetzwerk Deutschland, Diakonisches Werk Baden, unith e. V., BVKJ, DGPS, DGKJP, DGPPN, DGKJ) will be used to disseminate our results to relevant target groups. A joined patient conference on parenting skills is planned. Since all participating Psychology Departments have outpatient departments for children/adolescents and adults and are members of unith e. V. (a collaboration among university-based therapeutic training institutions), the implementation of results in ongoing and future practice is warranted, especially since many of the researchers involved already teach at the respective therapy training institutes and unith e. V. supports this project. The consortium's members also include experts from child and adolescent psychiatry as well as pediatrics, meaning our results will be implemented in those relevant fields as well. As we will be cooperating with a large adult psychiatry institution having many clinics throughout Germany (Schön-Kliniken), our results are certain to be implemented within a major stakeholder. Results will be relevant for and thus included in treatment guidelines as well as in psychology textbooks. Furthermore, as we have included experts from educational psychology will help transfer our findings to educational practice.

DISCUSSION AND LIMITATIONS

COMPARE with its subprojects family, emotion, interaction, work, and school, is the first comprehensive research programme on COMPI in Germany, as to date there is neither standard care nor systematic research with respect to this highly vulnerable group.

The COMPARE-family project is the central RCT testing the effects of high quality parental CBT on the children and whether additional PPP will result in incremental effects above and beyond CBT alone [for details see (24) in this research topic]. Effects of this trial as well as baseline data is informative for the other subprojects, as based on this trial the different domains of the TTMD (influences of emotion processing, parent-child-interaction environmental influences such as work and school) can be tested. So far the TTMD model has not been comprehensively tested.

The COMPARE-emotion subproject focuses on emotion processing and emotion regulation as potential child factors for the transgenerational transmission of mental disorders. Furthermore, these processes will be assessed as predictors and outcome measures for the RCT. Emotion processing and emotion regulation will be assessed with the help of different approaches, comprising behavioral measures, peripheral physiological markers, and neuro-imaging techniques. Thus, we expect to accomplish a comprehensive understanding of relevant child factors that display a significant role in the TTMD model. Moreover, the identification of underlying processes is equivalent to the identification of targets for effective intervention in the future.

The COMPARE-interaction subproject focuses on the long-term consequences of maternal psychopathology during the peripartum period on infant development, especially on socio-emotional and cognitive development. Special attention will be paid to the mediational effect of parent-infant interaction and infant stress reactivity on the relationship between the maternal disorder (depressive, comorbid, healthy controls) and infant outcome. Moreover, it will significantly contribute to the model testing in the model's following domains: mentally ill parent, family context, other parent, parent-infant interaction, infant outcome. This sub-project will yield new insights into the specific effects of maternal mental disorders on different aspects of the infant's social and cognitive development, as well as on the interaction mechanisms contributing to this process. It is of great importance to gain a better understanding of the underlying mediation effects to develop future prevention or intervention approaches, since research on comorbid depressive and anxiety disorders and their impacts on the parent-infant relationship and infant development is still lacking.

COMPARE-work explores the working conditions of mentally ill parents in contrast to those of healthy parents, identifies how these working conditions impact on work-related strain and how this causes strain in family life (work-to-family spillover). The comparison of strain and well-being levels in both groups of parents as well as their children enables us to detect transmission effects (parents-to-children crossover), thereby focusing on the specific transmission mechanisms (mediators), and finally analyzes whether treatment buffers or aggravates the spillover-crossover process (moderators). With respect to the preventive intervention, the consideration of parental work-environments is a significant moderator of therapy outcome. More or less supportive or adverse work-environments can be seen as framing conditions (partly outside the control of a person) shaping the opportunities of a therapeutic intervention at least partly; in particular in such cases where working conditions cause, strengthen or work to maintain mental diseases.

COMPARE-school focuses on different indicators of academic achievement, social functioning, and subjective well-being. A main aim is to compare the children of mentally ill parents with a healthy school control sample in terms of academic and psychosocial outputs and to seek variables that explain those differences. Moreover, we will test whether the specific type of parental mental illness and the mentally ill parent's gender are relevant concerning the aforementioned child outcomes. To create targeted interventions for children suffering from their parent's mental disease, we will additionally focus on those children with a low risk for developing health problems themselves and examine how they differ from those who have mental health problems. This comparison will enable us to explore approaches that can support children suffering from their parent's mental disease. Treatment-related factors in academic and psychosocial outcomes will be examined as well. Taken together, we will examine the theoretical model underlying COMPARE in terms of different outcomes other than psychopathology in COPMI and we will test for intervention effects by taking another adequate control sample into account.

However, there are also some limitations to be considered.

First of all, due to funding decisions, some aspects of the TTMD-model, such as (epi-) genetics and somatic outcomes will not be part of the study. However, if this study proves to be successful in the identification of risk mechanisms, this might provide a strong basis for follow-up (epi-)genetic projects on this topic.

Second, the research programme with a clinical trial at the center [see (24) in this research topic] and the four add-on projects puts high demands on the participating patients and their families that are already under increased stress due to the parental mental illness. On the other hand, the intensive assessment of different areas of life that might be impaired or prove to be associated with resources will substantially increase our knowledge on when to provide which interventions in what areas of life for whom.

ETHICS STATEMENT

The study is carried out according to the Good Clinical Practice (GCP) guidelines, the Declaration of Helsinki and its later supplements and local legal requirements. The lead ethics committee at the department of psychology at Philipps-University Marburg approved the study procedure and all study documents. A positive ethics committee vote is required at a study site, before the inclusion of a first patient at the respective site.

DISSEMINATION

Via peer-reviewed publications in scientific journals, the results of this study will be made available to the scientific community. Using PsychData all primary data will be made available for re- and meta-analyses. Politicians, public health services and stakeholders will be informed throughout the study and beyond, thus, improving public policy and health care decisions concerning preventive interventions and treatments for COPMI.

AUTHOR CONTRIBUTIONS

HC has drafted the main manuscript. CR and A-LZ wrote the section on COMPARE-interaction and commented on the whole manuscript. KO wrote the COMPARE-work section and commented on the whole manuscript. RS and LW wrote the COMPARE-school section and commented on the whole manuscript. SW, RS, and CS wrote the COMPARE-emotion section and commented on the whole manuscript. DE and CB are the study advisories, read the manuscript, and commented. JK, CK, and MK are the trial biometricians, read, and commented on the manuscript.

FUNDING

COMPARE (Children Of Mentally Ill Parents At Risk Evaluation) is a consortium funded by the German Federal Ministry of Education and Research (BMBF). This consortium consist of five projects: P1 clinical trial (Hanna Christiansen, Philipps University Marburg, funding # 01GL1748B), P2 emotion regulation (01GY1748C), P3 mother-infant-interaction (Corinna Reck, Ludwig-Maximilians University Munich, funding # 01GL1748D), P7 cross-over and spill-over effects (Kathleen Otto, Philipps University Marburg, funding # 01GL1748A), P8 psychosocial adjustment, school performance, and subjective well-being (Ricarda Steinmayr and Linda Wirthwein, Technical University Dortmund, funding #01GL1748E). The study programme is performed according to the Declaration of Helsinki and its later amendments and was approved by the Ethics Committee of Philipps University Marburg. The clinical trial has been registered at the German Clinical Trials Register with the DRKS-ID: DRKS00013516.

MEMBERS OF THE CONSORTIUM AND RECRUITING CENTERS

COMPARE-family (P1): Study coordination Marburg: Hanna Christiansen, Kristin Gilbert, Winfried Rief, Markus Stracke.

Data management and biometry Heidelberg: Meinhard Kieser, Christina Klose, Johannes Krisam, Moritz Pohl. Data monitoring Erlangen: Claudia Buntrock, David Daniel Ebert. Recruiting centers: Bochum: Sören Friedrich, Jürgen Margraf, Silvia Schneider; Bielefeld: Angelika Schlarb, Anna-Lena Zurmühlen; Leipzig: Julian Schmitz, Cornelia Exner; Gießen: Pauline Leiders, Arleta Luczejko, Christina Schwenck, Rudolf Stark, Julia Zimmermann; Landau: Jens Heider, Katharina Köck, Annette Schröder. München: Mitho Müller, Corinna Reck, Christian Woll.

COMPARE-emotion (P2): Gießen: Pauline Leiders, Arleta Luczejko, Lena Krüger, Christina Schwenck, Rudolf Stark; Dortmund: Sarah Weigelt, Klara Hagelweide.

COMPARE-interaction (P3): Heidelberg: Nora Nonnenmacher, Anna-Lena Zietlow, Sabine Herpertz; München: Mitho Müller, Corinna Reck, Christian Woll.

COMPARE-work (P7): Marburg: Benjamin Frank, Nathalie Lenninger, Kathleen Otto.

COMPARE-school (P8): Dortmund: Ricarda Steinmayr, Linda Wirthwein.

REFERENCES

1. Datenreport. *Ein Sozialbericht für die Bundesrepublik Deutschland.* (2013). Available online at: https://www.destatis.de/DE/Publikationen/Datenreport/Datenreport.html
2. Wittchen HU, Jacobi F, Rehm J, Gustavsson A, Svensson M, Jönsson B, et al. The size and burden of mental disorders and other disorders of the brain in Europe 2010. *Eur Neuropsychopharmacol.* (2011) 21:655–79. doi: 10.1016/j.euroneuro.2011.07.018
3. Fraser C, James EL, Anderson K, Lloyd D, Judd F. Intervention programs for children of parents with a mental illness: a critical review. *Int J Ment Health Promot.* (2006) 8:9–20. doi: 10.1080/14623730.2006.9721897
4. Maybery D, Reupert A, Goodyear M, Ritchie R, Brann P. Investigating the strenghts and difficulties of children from families with a parental mental illness. *Aust e-J Advancement Ment Health.* (2009) 8:165–74. doi: 10.5172/jamh.8.2.165
5. Ostman M, Hansson L. Children in families with a severely mentally ill member. Prevalence and needs for support. *Soc Psychiatry Psychiatr Epidemiol.* (2002) 37:243–8. doi: 10.1007/s00127-002-0540-0
6. Pretis M, Dimova A. Vulnerable children of mentally ill parents: towards evidence-based support for improving resilience. *Support Learning.* (2008) 23:152–9. doi: 10.1111/j.1467-9604.2008.00386.x
7. Test MA, Burke SS, Wallisch LS. Gender differences of young adults with schizophrenic disorders in community care. *Schizophrenia Bull.* (1990) 16:331–44. doi: 10.1093/schbul/16.2.331
8. Kersten-Alvarez LE, Hosman CMH, Riksen-Walraven JM, van Doesum Karin TM, Smeekens S, Hoefnagels C. Early school outcomes for children of postpartum depressed mothers: comparison with a community sample. *Child Psychiatry Human Dev.* (2012) 43:201–18. doi: 10.1007/s10578-011-0257-y
9. U. S. National Research Council. *Depression in Parents, Parenting, and Children: Opportunities to Improve Identification, Treatment, and Prevention.* Washington, DC: National Academies Press (2009).
10. Goodman SH, Rouse MH, Connell AM, Broth MR, Hall CM, Heyward D. Maternal depression and child psychopathology: a meta-analytic review. *Clin Child Family Psychol Rev.* (2011) 14:1–27. doi: 10.1007/s10567-010-0080-1.
11. Goodman SH, Gotlib IH. Risk for psychopathology in the children of depressed mothers: a developmental model for understanding mechanisms of transmission. *Psychol Rev.* (1999) 106:458–90. doi: 10.1037/0033-295X.106.3.458
12. van Santvoort F, Hosman CM, Janssens JM, van Doesum KT, Reupert A, van Loon LM. The impact of various parental mental disorders on children's diagnoses: a systematic review. *Clin Child Family Psychol Rev.* (2015) 18:281–99. doi: 10.1007/s10567-015-0191-9
13. Christiansen H, Anding J, Donath L. Interventionen für kinder psychisch kranker eltern. In: Kölch M, Ziegenhain U, Fegert JM, editors. *Kinder Psychisch Kranker Eltern: Herausforderungen für Eine Interdisziplinäre Kooperation in Betreuung und Versorgung.* Weinheim und Basel: Beltz Juventa (2014). p. 80–105.
14. Hosman CMH, van Doesum KTM, van Santvoort F. Prevention of emotional problems and psychiatric risks in children of parents with a mental illness in the Netherlands: I. The scientific basis to a comprehensive approach. *Aust e-J Advancement Ment Health.* (2009) 8:250–63. doi: 10.5172/jamh.8.3.250
15. Mattejat F, Remschmidt H. The children of mentally ill parents. *Deutsches Ärzteblatt International.* (2008) 105:413–8. doi: 10.3238/arztebl.2008.0413
16. Schneider S, In-Albon T, Nuendel B, Margraf J. Parental panic treatment reduces children's long-term psychopathology: a prospective longitudinal study. *Psychother Psychosomat.* (2013) 82:346–8. doi: 10.1159/000350448
17. Wille N, Bettge S, Ravens-Sieberer U. Risk and protective factors for children's and adolescents' mental health: results of the BELLA study. *Eur Child Adolescent Psychiatry.* (2008) 17:133–47. doi: 10.1007/s00787-008-1015-y
18. Hancock KJ, Mitrou F, Shipley M, Lawrence D, Zubrick SR. A three generation study of the mental health relationships between grandparents, parents and children. *BMC Psychiatry.* (2013) 13:299. doi: 10.1186/1471-244X-13-299
19. Talati A, Weissman MM, Hamilton SP. Using the high-risk family design to identify biomarkers for major depression. *Philos Transac Roy Soc Lond Ser B Biol Sci.* (2013) 368:20120129. doi: 10.1098/rstb.2012.0129
20. Hakkaart-van Roijen L, Zwirs BWC, Bouwmans C, Tan SS, Schulpen TWJ, Vlasveld L, et al. Societal costs and quality of life of children suffering from attention deficient hyperactivity disorder (ADHD). *Eur Child Adolesc Psychiatry.* (2007) 16:316–26. doi: 10.1007/s00787-007-0603-6
21. Lynch FL, Hornbrook M, Clarke GN, Perrin N, Polen MR, O'Connor E, et al. Cost-effectiveness of an intervention to prevent depression in at-risk teens. *Arch General Psychiatry.* (2005) 62:1241–8. doi: 10.1001/archpsyc.62.11.1241
22. Lynch FL, Clarke GN. Estimating the economic burden of depression in children and adolescents. *Am J Prevent Med.* (2006) 31 (6 Suppl. 1):51. doi: 10.1016/j.amepre.2006.07.001
23. Röhrle B, Christiansen H. Psychische erkrankung eines elternteils. In: Lohaus A, Domsch H, editors. *Psychologische Förder- und Interventionsprogramme für das Kindes- und Jugendalter.* Heidelberg: Springer (2009). p. 259–69. doi: 10.1007/978-3-540-88384-5_19
24. Stracke M, Gilbert K, Kieser M, Klose C, Krisam J, Ebert DD, et al. COMPARE Family (Children of Mentally Ill Parents at Risk Evaluation): a study protocol for a preventive intervention for children of mentally Ill parents (triple P, evidence-based program that enhances parentings skills, in addition to gold-standard CBT with the mentally Ill parent) in a multicenter RCT–part II. *Front Psychiatry.* (2019) 10:54. doi: 10.3389/fpsyt.2019.00054
25. Connell AM, Goodman SH. The association between psychopathology in fathers versus mothers and children's internalizing and externalizing behavior problems: a meta-analysis. *Psychol Bull.* (2002) 128:746–73. doi: 10.1037/0033-2909.128.5.746
26. Lieb R, Isensee B, Höfler M, Pfister H, Wittchen H-U. Parental major depression and the risk of depression and other mental disorders in offspring: a prospective-longitudinal community study. *Arch General Psychiatry.* (2002) 59:365–74. doi: 10.1001/archpsyc.59.4.365
27. Leinonen JA, Solantaus TS, Punamaki R-L. Parental mental health and children's adjustment: the quality of marital interaction and parenting as mediating factors. *J Child Psychol Psychiatry.* (2003) 44:227–41. doi: 10.1111/1469-7610.t01-1-00116
28. Lovejoy MC, Graczyk PA, O'Hare E, Neuman G. Maternal depression and parenting behavior: a meta-analytic review. *Clin Psychol Rev.* (2000) 20:561–92. doi: 10.1016/S0272-7358(98)00100-7
29. Van Loon LMA, Van de Ven MOM, Van Doesum KTM, Witteman CLM, Hosman CMH. The relation between parental mental illness and adolescent mental health: the role of family factors. *J Child Family Stud.* (2014) 23:1201–14. doi: 10.1007/s10826-013-9781-7
30. Wilson S, Durbin CE. Effects of paternal depression on fathers' parenting behaviors: a meta-analytic review. *Clin Psychol Rev.* (2010) 30:167–80. doi: 10.1016/j.cpr.2009.10.007

31. Compas BE, Champion JE, Forehand R, Cole DA, Reeslund KL, Fear J, et al. Coping and parenting: mediators of 12-month outcomes of a family group cognitive-behavioral preventive intervention with families of depressed parents. *J Consult Clin Psychol.* (2010) 78:623–34. doi: 10.1037/a0020459
32. Sanders MR, Kirby JN, Tellegen CL, Day JJ. The Triple P-Positive Parenting Program: a systematic review and meta-analysis of a multi-level system of parenting support. *Clin Psychol Rev.* (2014) 34:337–57. doi: 10.1016/j.cpr.2014.04.003
33. Thomas R, Zimmer-Gembeck MJ. Behavioral outcomes of Parent-Child Interaction Therapy and Triple P-Positive Parenting Program: a review and meta-analysis. *J Abnormal Child Psychol.* (2007) 35:475–95. doi: 10.1007/s10802-007-9104-9
34. Schwenck C, Göhle B, Hauf J, Warnke A, Freitag CM, Schneider W. Cognitive and emotional empathy in typically developing children: the influence of age, gender, and intelligence. *Eur J Dev Psychol.* (2013) 11:63–76. doi: 10.1080/17405629.2013.808994
35. Findlay LC, Girardi A, Coplan RJ. Links between empathy, social behavior, and social understanding in early childhood. *Early Childhood Res Q.* (2006) 21:347–59. doi: 10.1016/j.ecresq.2006.07.009
36. Fossati P. Neural correlates of emotion processing: from emotional to social brain. *Eur Neuropsychopharmacol.* (2012) 22:S487–91. doi: 10.1016/j.euroneuro.2012.07.008
37. Kret ME, Ploeger A. Emotion processing deficits: a liability spectrum providing insight into comorbidity of mental disorders. *Neurosci Biobehav Rev.* (2015) 52:153–71. doi: 10.1016/j.neubiorev.2015.02.011
38. Eisenberg N, Spinrad TL. Emotion-related regulation: sharpening the definition. *Child Dev.* (2004) 75:334–9. doi: 10.1111/j.1467-8624.2004.00674.x
39. Gross JJ. The emerging field of emotion regulation: an integrative review. *Rev General Psychol.* (1998) 2:271–99. doi: 10.1037/1089-2680.2.3.271
40. Kingston D, Tough S. Prenatal and postnatal maternal mental health and school-age child development: a systematic review. *Maternal Child Health J.* (2014) 18:1728–41. doi: 10.1007/s10995-013-1418-3
41. Nomura Y, Warner V, Wickramaratne P. Parents concordant for major depressive disorder and the effect of psychopathology in offspring. *Psychol Med.* (2001) 31:1211–22. doi: 10.1017/S0033291701004585
42. Feldman R. *Coding Interactive Behavior Manual.* Herzliya: Bar-Ilan University (2018).
43. Camaioni L, Perucchini P, Bellagamba F, Colonnesi C. The role of declarative pointing in developing a theory of mind. *Infancy.* (2004) 5:291–308. doi: 10.1207/s15327078in0503_3
44. Goertz C, Knopf M, Kolling T, Frahsek S, Kressley R. Der Frankfurter Imitations-Test für 12 Monate alte Kinder (FIT 12). *Z Entwicklungspsychol Pädagog Psychol.* (2006) 38:88–96. doi: 10.1026/0049-8637.38.2.88
45. Jones SS. Imitation in infancy: the development of mimicry. *Psychol Sci.* (2007) 18:593–9. doi: 10.1111/j.1467-9280.2007.01945.x
46. Paulus M, Kühn-Popp N, Licata M, Sodian B, Meinhardt J. Neural correlates of prosocial behavior in infancy: different neurophysiological mechanisms support the emergence of helping and comforting. *Neuroimage.* (2013) 66:522–30. doi: 10.1016/j.neuroimage.2012.10.041
47. Meltzoff AN. Understanding the intensions of others: re-enactment of intended acts by 18-month-old children. *Annu Prog Child Psychiatry Child Dev.* (1996) 31:838–50.
48. Kochanska G, Murray K, Jacques TY, Koenig AL, Vandegeest KA. Inhibitory control in young children and its role in emerging internalization. *Child Dev.* (1996) 67:490. doi: 10.2307/1131828
49. Carlson SM, Mandell DJ, Williams L. Executive function and theory of mind: stability and prediction from ages 2 to 3. *Dev Psychol.* (2004) 40:1105–22. doi: 10.1037/0012-1649.40.6.1105
50. Grimm H, Aktas M, Frevert S. *Sprachentwicklungstest für Zweijährige Kinder (SETK-2).* Göttingen und Bern: Hogrefe (2000).
51. Liew J, Eisenberg N, Spinrad TL, Eggum ND, Haugen RG, Kupfer A, et al. Physiological regulation and fearfulness as predictors of young children's empathy-related reactions. *Soc Dev.* (2011) 20:111–3. doi: 10.1111/j.1467-9507.2010.00575.x
52. Arbeitsgruppe Deutsche Child Behavior Checklist. *Elternfragebogen für Klein- und Vorschulkinder (CBCL/1 1/2-5).* Köln: Hogrefe publishers (2000a).
53. Arbeitsgruppe Deutsche Child Behavior Checklist. *Fragebogen für Erzieherinnen von Klein- und Vorschulkindern (C-TRF/1,5-5).* Köln: Hogrefe publishers (2000b).
54. Reuner G, Rosenkranz J. *Bayley-III - Bayley Scales of Infant and Toddler Development III: Deutsche Version.* Frankfurt: Pearson Assessment and Information GmbH (2015).
55. Jahoda M. *Wieviel Arbeit Braucht der Mensch? Arbeit und Arbeitslosigkeit im 20. Jahrhundert ([3. Aufl.]).* Weinheim: Beltz (1986).
56. Ström S. Keep out of the reach of children: parental unemployment and children's accident risks in Sweden 1991–1993. *Int J Soc Welfare.* (2002) 11:40–52. doi: 10.1111/1468-2397.00195
57. Ström S. Unemployment and families: a review of research. *Soc Service Rev.* (2003) 77:399–430. doi: 10.1086/375791
58. Otto K, Dalbert C. Are insecure jobs as bad for mental health and occupational commitment as unemployment? Equal threat or downward spiral. *Horizons Psychol.* (2013) 22:27–38. doi: 10.20419/2013.22.375
59. OECD. *Sick on the Job?: Myths and Realities about Mental Health and Work.* Paris: OECD Publishing (2012). doi: 10.1787/9789264124523-en
60. Amstad FT, Meier LL, Fasel U, Elfering A, Semmer NK. A meta-analysis of work-family conflict and various outcomes with a special emphasis on cross-domain versus matching-domain relations. *J Occup Health Psychol.* (2011) 16:151–69. doi: 10.1037/a0022170
61. Bakker AB, Westman M, van Hetty Emmerik IJ. Advancements in crossover theory. *J Manag Psychol.* (2009) 24:206–19. doi: 10.1108/02683940910939304
62. Bakker AB, Demerouti E. The spillover-crossover model. In: Grzywacz JG, Demerouti E, editors. *New Frontiers in Work and Family Research.* Hove: Psychology Press (2013). p. 54–70.
63. Hatfield E, Cacioppo JT, Rapson RL. *Studies in Emotion and Social Interaction.* Cambridge: Cambridge University Press (2003).
64. Semmer NK, Zapf D, Dunckel H. Assessing stress at work: a framework and an instrument. In: Svane O, Johansen C, editors. *Work and Health: Scientific Basis of Progress in the Working Environment.* Luxembourg: Office for Official Publications of the European Communities (1995). p. 105–13.
65. Pejtersen JH, Kristensen TS, Borg V, Bjorner JB. The second version of the Copenhagen Psychosocial Questionnaire. *Scand J Public Health.* (2010) 38:8–24. doi: 10.1177/1403494809349858
66. Augustine JM, Crosnoe R. Mothers' depression and educational attainment and their children's academic trajectories. *J Health Soc Behav.* (2010) 51:274–90. doi: 10.1177/0022146510377757
67. Pearson RM, Bornstein MH, Cordero M, Scerif G, Mahedy L, Evans J, et al. Maternal perinatal mental health and offspring academic achievement at age 16: the mediating role of childhood executive function. *J Child Psychol Psychiatr Allied Disciplines.* (2016) 57:491–501. doi: 10.1111/jcpp.12483
68. Shen H, Magnusson C, Rai D, Lundberg M, Lê-Scherban F, Dalman C, et al. Associations of parental depression with child school performance at age 16 years in Sweden. *JAMA Psychiatry.* (2016) 73:239–46. doi: 10.1001/jamapsychiatry.2015.2917
69. Huebner ES, Laughlin JE, Ash C, Gilman R. Further validation of the multidimensional students' life satisfaction scale. *J Psychoedu Assessment.* (2016) 16:118–34. doi: 10.1177/073428299801600202
70. Nievar MA, Moske AK, Johnson DJ, Chen Q. Parenting practices in preschool leading to later cognitive competence: a family stress model. *Early Edu Dev.* (2014) 25:318–37. doi: 10.1080/10409289.2013.788426
71. Steinmayr R, Spinath B. The importance of motivation as a predictor of school achievement. *Learn Individ Diff.* (2009) 19:80–90. doi: 10.1016/j.lindif.2008.05.004
72. Lambert MJ. Outcome in psychotherapy: the past and important advances. *Psychotherapy.* (2013) 50:42–51. doi: 10.1037/a0030682
73. Stuart EA. Matching methods for causal inference. A review and a look forward. *Stat Sci.* (2010) 25:1–21. doi: 10.1214/09-STS313

10

COMPARE Family (Children of Mentally Ill Parents at Risk Evaluation): A Study Protocol for a Preventive Intervention for Children of Mentally Ill Parents (Triple P, Evidence-Based Program that Enhances Parenting Skills, in Addition to Gold-Standard CBT with the Mentally Ill Parent) in a Multicenter RCT—Part II

Markus Stracke[1], Kristin Gilbert[1], Meinhard Kieser[2], Christina Klose[2], Johannes Krisam[2], David D. Ebert[3,4], Claudia Buntrock[3] and Hanna Christiansen[1]*

[1] Department of Clinical Child and Adolescent Psychology, Philipps University Marburg, Marburg, Germany, [2] Institute of Medical Biometry and Informatics, University of Heidelberg, Heidelberg, Germany, [3] Department of Psychology, Chair for Clinical Psychology and Psychotherapy, Friedrich-Alexander University Erlangen-Nuremberg, Erlangen, Germany, [4] Department of Clinical, Neuro- & Developmental Psychology, Vrije Universiteit Amsterdam, Amsterdam, Netherlands

***Correspondence:**
Markus Stracke
markus.stracke@staff.uni-marburg.de

Background: Mental health problems are highly frequent, as well as being associated with enormous societal and economic costs and significant disability-adjusted life years. Children of parents with a mental illness (COPMI) are at a tremendously increased risk to develop disorders themselves. According to the literature, parental mental disorders launch a wave of risk factors that in turn predict the emergence of psychological problems in the offspring, and effective treatment of the parental disorder has been associated with reduced child psychopathology (launch and grow assumption). Furthermore, studies focusing on parent-child interaction demonstrate generally poorer parenting skills in parents with mental disorders, and the enhancement of such skills has been a significant mediator in improving child outcomes (parenting assumption).

Objective: To implement a preventive intervention for COPMI with the aim of interrupting the transmission of mental disorders in children of a parent with mental disorders. An RCT will compare state-of-the-art cognitive behavioral therapy (CBT) for a parent with mental disorders to CBT plus the Positive Parenting Program (Triple-P), a well-established and evidence-based program that enhances parenting skills.

Methods: A total of 634 patients seeking treatment in 8 outpatient clinics in Germany and their children will be included between January 2018 and April 2021 in the study. We use (clinical) interviews and self- as well as other-report questionnaires to assess the families at four main measurement points [T1: beginning of waiting period for psychotherapy treatment (duration of waiting period depends on usual waiting period in the study center: multiple baselines), T2: begin of parental psychotherapy, T3: post-assessment, T4: 6 months follow-up]. The total observation period will be 39 months. The patients will be randomly assigned to either the control condition (25 to 45 CBT sessions) or the experimental condition (25 to 45 CBT sessions + 10 Triple-P sessions). For evaluating the treatment process, the patients and clinicians will also be assessed after each treatment session. Furthermore, there will be a continuous assessment and report of adverse events during treatment.

Discussion: This trial will be the first ever to address the launch and grow as well as the parenting assumption in one study and to establish effects of the two different interventions on children's health. Our study will also likely be the first one to provide data on the comparative cost-effectiveness and will therefore provide essential information relevant for the potential implementation of such programs. The structure of the RCT will allow us to establish effects of the parental disorder(s) with/without comorbidities on children's health, to test assumptions of the trans-generational transmission model of mental disorders and bi-directional influences of different treatments on the model and to analyze specific transmission mechanisms. A deeper understanding of risk mechanisms will reveal specific transmission profiles that will result in the early detection of and effective reduction in risk factors and thus improve the health of the children at risk.

Ethics: The study is carried out according to the Good Clinical Practice (GCP) guidelines, the Declaration of Helsinki and its later supplements and local legal requirements. The lead ethics committee at the department of psychology at Philipps-University Marburg approved the study procedure and all study documents. A positive ethics committee vote is required at a study site, before the inclusion of a first patient at the respective site.

Dissemination: Via peer-reviewed publications in scientific journals, the results of this study will be made available to the scientific community. Using PsychData all primary data will be made available for re- and meta-analyses. Politicians, public health services, and stakeholders will be informed throughout the study and beyond, thus, improving public policy and health care decisions concerning preventive interventions and treatments for COPMI.

Trial Registration: DRKS-ID: DRKS00013516 (German Clinical Trials Register, https://www.drks.de/drks_web/navigate.do?navigationId=trial.HTML&TRIAL_ID=DRKS00013516)

Keywords: children of mentally ill parents, transgenerational transmission, randomized controlled trial, prevention, intervention, mental disorders, parenting training

INTRODUCTION

Children of mentally ill parents (COPMI) are at a high risk of developing severe mental illness (SMI) themselves and are likely to be the next generation of mentally ill patients (1). There are studies pointing to the fact, that the parental mental disorder launches a wave of risk factors that in turn predict the emergence of psychological problems in the offspring (2). Numerous studies have shown that a parental mental illness is a powerful risk factor for the development of a SMI in children (OR in the BELLA study of 2.4) (1, 3–8). Long-term studies were also able to show that COPMI have a higher life-time risk of developing SMI themselves (ranging from 41 to 77%) with subclinical symptoms emerging earlier and more often (5, 6). The treatment of the parental disorder has been associated with improved outcomes in COPMI (7, 9–13), although there are few studies on such effects (7, 14), and they typically target the same symptoms in the child as the parent's, while such specific transmission of disorders is not typical for COPMI (1). A recent meta-analysis (k = 9) by Cuijpers et al. (14) on the effects of psychological treatment of maternal depression on children's psychopathology resulted in an overall effect-size of g = 0.40. However, the studies included were very heterogeneous (k = 5 targeting women with post-partum depression; k = 4 targeting pregnant women or mothers of young children or mothers of children with psychological/psychiatric problems/disorders), and only 2 studies explicitly applied Cognitive Behavioral Therapy (CBT) as an intervention that resulted in an overall effect of g = 0.31 (14). An earlier meta-analysis by Siegenthaler et al. (15) on preventive interventions for children of mentally ill parents demonstrated a significant relative risk reduction of 40 % for the same disorder as the parents', and overall small effects for children's internalizing (g = −0.22) and externalizing (g = −0.16) symptoms. This analysis included interventions targeting children though and not specifically those that assessed parental psychotherapy effects on their children (15). Our own meta-analysis on preventive interventions for COPMI (16) resulted in effect sizes similar to those of Cuijpers et al. (14) for young (up to 5 years of age) children (g = 0.31), and overall smaller effects for older children (g = 0.14) that equal those of Siegenthaler et al. (15). Different longitudinal studies on parental anxiety and depressive disorders present heterogeneous effects of parental treatment on children. A 6 year prospective longitudinal study on the effects of parental panic treatment demonstrated that parental treatment is a significant predictor of children's anxiety symptoms (d = 0.49–1.09 for different parental psychopathology predictors) (7). The Sequenced Treatment Alternatives to Relieve Depression (STAR*D) Child study was designed to examine the relation between maternal remission from depression and children's functioning and psychopathology. The study demonstrated differential effects on child psychopathology in early, late, and non-remitting mothers, with early remission being associated with reduced child externalizing problems (~5% of Child Behavior Checklist (CBCL) externalizing symptoms explained) (13); similar results have been obtained in another large longitudinal study (9).

Studies focusing on the parent-child interaction tended to demonstrate poorer parenting skills in parents with mental disorders (17–20). The enhancement of such skills has been identified as a significant mediator in improving child outcomes (21). The Positive Parenting Program (Triple P) is a well-established program to enhance parenting skills in parents of children aged 0–16 years (Triple P Kids and Triple P Teens). Universal prevention effects have been established for the Triple P Kids program (22), as well as specific effects for child psychopathology (d = 0.473) (23, 24) that differ for mothers (d = 0.61) and fathers (d = 0.42). The effectiveness of the Triple P Teen program was also shown (25). Studies explicitly testing the parenting assumption in conjunction with the launch and grow assumption are lacking so far.

Regarding psychotherapy research, there have been suggestions that moving from an approach comparing an active treatment with a control group ("does it work?") to one that examines putatively active treatments resulting in relative questions ("which works best?" or "how do the treatments differ?") is advisable. If demand artifacts and differentiating non-specific from specific treatment factors are included, we arrive at this formula: Treatment A = $E + D_T + T_{NS} + T_{S(A)}$ and Treatment B = $E + D_T + T_{NS} + T_{S(B)}$ with E = all extraneous factors; D_T = demand characteristics treatment; T_{NS} = non-specific treatment factors; T_S = characteristic-specific treatment factors. Thus, the relative difference between the two active agents in the proposed study $T_{S(A)}$ = CBT and $T_{S(B)}$ = CBT+PPP estimates how the two treatments differ and enables us to determine relative effects (26). Such head-to-head studies on preventive interventions for COPMI assessing differential effects have been extremely rare; the classic format are "does it work?" studies (15).

Thus, we aim to implement a preventive intervention for COPMI with the aim of interrupting the transmission of mental disorders in children of a parent with a mental disorder. The preventive intervention is planned as a two-arm RCT to establish whether strengthening parenting skills results in incremental COPMI effects above and beyond state-of-the-art CBT for parents. Including an economic evaluation alongside the clinical trial, the results of this study will have an effect on the decision making process on resource allocation for this highly vulnerable group of children of mentally ill parents.

The RCT will thus target the following hypothesis: (1) the treatment of the parental disorder will result in improved child outcome (1st arm: CBT) (2, 7, 12), and (2) the parenting skills of parents with mental illness are impaired and enhancing such skills leads to better child outcomes, thus incremental effects will become apparent in the 2nd arm: CBT+Triple P (17, 18, 20, 27, 28).

Further research questions are: Is the clinical outcome associated with reduced direct medical, direct, and indirect non-medical costs? Are CBT and CBT+PPP associated with improved quality of life for parents and children? Are CBT and CBT+PPP associated with increased psychopathology knowledge of parents and children? Is CBT+PPP associated with higher parenting skills than CBT alone? Are the effects independent of type of diagnosis, comorbid disorders, and psychopharmacology?

METHODS

Design

The planned study is a prospective, multicenter, confirmatory, randomized controlled phase III-trial with two parallel arms comparing the effects of state of the art CBT (control intervention), and CBT + Triple P (experimental intervention) for parents with a mental illness on their children. The study is coordinated by the Department of Psychology, Clinical Child-, and Adolescent Psychology at the Philipps University Marburg (UMR).

After 3 months of study preparation (October–December 2017), a 15 months recruiting period has started in January 2018. The assessment period (first patient in until last patient out) will last for a total of 39 months. Six months are scheduled for data freeze, data cleaning and analysis. Thus, the duration of the whole trial is 48 months (see **Figure 1**).

Using the same instruments (self- and other-report questionnaires as well as (clinical) interviews) each time, patients, and their families will be assessed at four main measurement points (see **Figure 2**): pre-assessment 1 (T1, beginning of waiting period for psychotherapy treatment (duration of waiting period depends on usual waiting period in the study center: multiple baselines), pre-assessment 2, (T2, beginning of parental psychotherapy), post-assessment (T3, after parental psychotherapy), follow-up-assessment (T4, 6 months after parental psychotherapy). Altogether, assessment time comprises between 4 and 5 h for each main assessment (T1, T2, T3, T4) for each family. Patients and therapists are also assessed after each treatment session for treatment fidelity and satisfaction. Every fifth session, the remission status of the patient is also assessed.

Participants

A total of 634 parents with a mental illness (patients) shall be included in the study. The following criteria must be met for patients and their families to be included in the study: (1) patient seeks outpatient psychotherapeutic care, (2) patient currently meets diagnostic criteria for DSM-5 disorder (29), and (3) patient is caring for at least one child between the ages of 1.5–16 years. Patients and their families will not be included in the study if (1) patient is already in psychotherapeutic treatment, (2) patient needs acute inpatient treatment (e.g., acute risk of committing suicide or acute psychosis), (3) all children fulfill criteria for a severe mental illness and are in need of prompt treatment, (4) patient uses benzodiazepines continuously (intermittent drug use less than once every 2 weeks is allowed), or (5) family has insufficient German language skills. No further exclusion criteria will be applied. Hence, we seek to establish effects of parental psychotherapy on children in a naturalistic setting and want to specify the effects of the transgenerational transmission to test the launch and growth assumption. Patients in need of acute inpatient treatment are referred to cooperating hospitals. For children in need of prompt care, treatments are initiated at the study sites or the families are referred to other local specialists/psychiatric hospitals.

The study will be conducted at eight university outpatient clinics throughout Germany: Bielefeld, Bochum, Gießen, Landau, Leipzig, Mainz, Marburg, and Munich. All cooperating sites have established outpatient clinics for research and teaching as well as psychotherapy training institutes and are well-known specialized treatment centers for psychotherapy. The patients are primarily recruited from the university outpatient clinics at each study site. The study centers have continuous experience in conducting psychotherapy studies with recruitment of large patients numbers (30, 31). The patients to be recruited per center and fulfilling all inclusion criteria will be attainable over a 15-month acquisition period at all study sites without the need to change the existing infrastructure. If possible, all children between 1.5 and 16 years of age (at T1) and a partner living together with the family shall be included in the study. A legal guardian not living together with a child can upon request be offered to participate in the study and to complete questionnaires about the respective child. Inclusion only takes place if the family participates voluntarily in the study. There is no compensation for study participation.

Interventions

All patients will receive between 25 (short-term) and 45 (long-term) weekly or bi-weekly sessions of individual state of the art Cognitive Behavioral Therapy (CBT). A high frequency therapy with more than one session per week is also allowed. Depending on the amount and the frequency of therapy sessions, the treatment will usually last between 6 and 12 months. The number of sessions and therapy duration will be documented, thus, allowing us to include therapy duration and number of sessions as a moderating factor in the analyses.

CBT can be considered the current "treatment of choice" for mental disorders in general (32). Central elements are psychoeducation that provides a framework for psychotherapy, cognitive components (i.e., debate of dysfunctional cognitions alias Beck), as well as behavioral interventions (i.e., exposure). As all study sites are outpatient clinics for research and teaching located at university psychology departments, they commit to the highest possible state of the art standard for CBT as outlined in "proceedings in psychotherapy/Fortschritte der Psychotherapie" of which Prof. Rief (Co-PI of COMPARE-family) is an editor (33). As the study shall be conducted as naturalistic as possible and a broad range of disorders shall be included, no specific study manual has been created, rather, the respective therapy manuals of the proceedings in psychotherapy will be used in this study.

Patients randomized to the experimental group will receive 8–10 additional group or individual sessions of the Positive Parenting Program (Triple P) parallel to the last third of the psychotherapy sessions to test whether the enhancement of parenting skills will result in improved child outcome, as suggested in different studies (17, 18, 20, 27, 28), above and beyond parental CBT. Triple P is a well-established, widely used and evidence-based program to enhance parenting skills. The Triple P Kids program can be used in groups or individual sessions with parents of children aged 0–12 years (34, 35) and the Triple P Teens program in groups with parents of children aged 12–16 years (36). The Triple P elements are: (1) promotion of a positive parenting style, (2) promotion of child development, (3) dealing with problem behavior, (4) behavior training sessions (34–36).

Outcomes

Primary Outcome Measure

The primary outcome is the children's pathology according to the [(Caregiver-) Teacher Report Form (C-)TRF, caregiver/teacher version of the Child Behavior Checklist] score between baseline 2 (T2) and post treatment (T3) as well as between T2 and the 6-month follow-up (T4) after end of treatment (37, 38) as the literature shows that mentally ill parents can be biased in rating their children's symptoms (39). Further, teacher ratings have been shown to demonstrate greater predictive validity in the long term ratings (40). In comparison to shorter questionnaires [e.g., Strengths and Difficulties Questionnaire (SDQ) (41)], the CBCL also produces more variance. As the CBCL is used in various studies as a primary outcome measure (15), we will be able to compare our data to a broad range of other results. Further outcome measures are mental disorders according to the Diagnostic Interview of Mental Disorders for parents

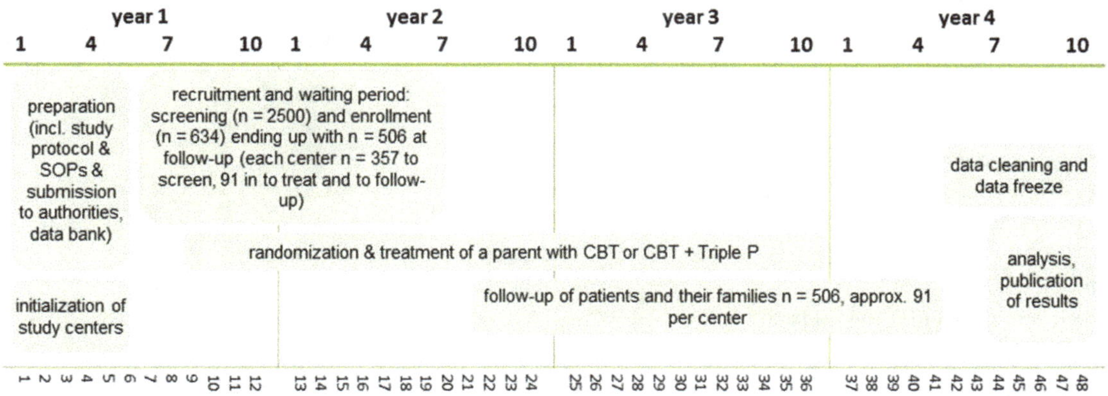

FIGURE 1 | Study design.

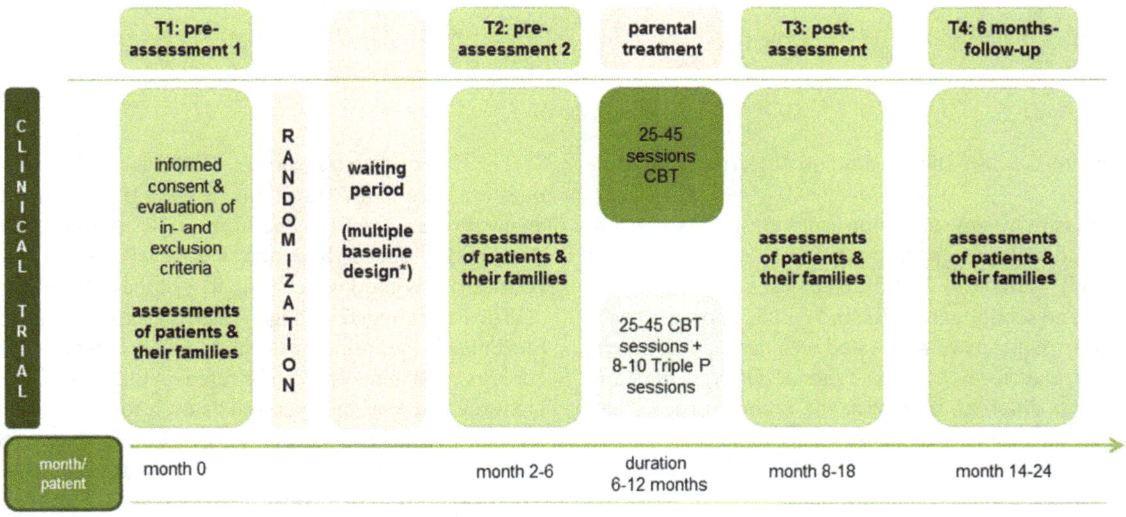

FIGURE 2 | Study assessment points. *Waiting period can vary according to the regular waiting period in the study centers.

and children (DIPS and Kinder-DIPS) (42–44) respectively for children under the age of 6 years the Structured Interview for Preschool Ages (SIVA) (45) and the parent rating of the children's pathology according to the CBCL (for detailed descriptions see below). Thus, we will be able to validate the teacher ratings with the Kinder-DIPS diagnoses and can compare the concordance of the teacher and parent ratings.

Secondary Outcome Measures

Children's and parents dimensional severity index of a broad range of mental disorders according to the DSM-5 based clinical interview (Kinder-)DIPS (42–44) respectively the SIVA (45), parent's psychopathology according to the Brief Symptom Inventory (BSI) (46), personality traits (PID-5-BF) (47), children's psychopathology according to the CBCL-parentversion (37, 38), parenting skills (EFB) (48), parental stress (ESF) (49), children's and parents knowledge about mental disorders [semistructured interview adapted from Beardslee and Röhrle, (50)], direct medical costs and direct and indirect non-medical costs (TiC-P) (51), health-related quality of life in parents [EuroQoL/EQ-5D-5L, AQoL-8D (52, 53)], health-related quality of life in children (KIDSCREEN-10) (54, 55) (for details see **Table 1**).

Instruments

The (Kinder-) DIPS is a diagnostic interview for mental disorders and is available for the diagnoses of mental disorders from age 6 to adulthood according to ICD-10 and DSM-5. The SIVA is a diagnostic interview for mental disorders for preschool ages according to ICD-10 and DC: 0–5. A translation table to DSM-5 diagnoses has been created for this study. For parents we use the DIPS; for their children the Kinder-DIPS or SIVA. Conducting the interviews with the patient takes around 60–90 min as well as the child assessment with the Kinder-DIPS or SIVA for each

TABLE 1 | List of diagnostic domains and measurements.

	Who?	Where?	T1	T2	Intermediate	T3	T4
Eligibility screening	Family	Local	x				
Socio-demographics	Parents	Local	x				
Structured clinical interview with the patient (DIPS)	Patient	Local	x	x		x	x
Structured clinical interview for children (Kinder-DIPS/SIVA)	Parent	Local	x	x		x	x
Brief Symptom Inventory (BSI)	Parents	Online	x	x	x (patient)	x	x
Personality traits (PID-5-BF)	Parents	Online	x	x		x	x
Child Behavior Checklist (CBCL)	Parents	Online	x	x		x	x
(Caregiver-) Teacher Report Form [(C-)TRF, caregiver/teacher version of the CBCL]	Teacher	Online	x	x		x	x
Parenting Skills (EFB)	Parents	Online	x	x		x	x
Parental Stress (ESF)	Parents	Online	x	x		x	x
Knowledge about mental disorders	Parents, children	Local	x	x		x	x
Direct and indirect costs in children and parents (adapted TiC-P)	Parents	Online	x	x		x	x
Health-related quality of life in parents (EuroQoL/EQ-5D-5L, AQoL-8D)	Parents	Online	x	x		x	x
Health-related quality of life in children (KIDSCREEN-10)	Parents, children (>8)	Online	x	x		x	x
(Serious) adverse events	Parents, children	Local		x	x (patient)	x	x
Psychopharmaka and other drugs	Parents, children	Local	x	x	x	x	x
Concomitant interventions	Parents, children	Local	x	x	x	x	x

child. Different studies have shown good quality criteria for these interviews (43, 45).

The Achenbach System of Empirically Based Assessment (ASEBA) (56) consists amongst others of questionnaires for preschool (C-TRF and CBCL 1,5-5, consisting each of 100 problem items) and school-ages (TRF and CBCL, consisting each of 113 problem items). Answers are rated on a three point Likert-scale (0 = Not true to 2 = Very True or Often True) and can be scored on different subscales, the second order scales internalizing problems and externalizing problems as well as on a total problem scale. Studies have reported good to very good internal consistency with $r > 0.86$ for the second order scales and the total problem scale of the preschool age-versions (37) and Cronbach's alpha >0.80 for the second order scales and at least.93 for the total problem scale in the school age-versions (38). In the current study we use the parent (CBCL) and teacher (TRF) ratings of the ASEBA.

The Brief Symptom Inventory (BSI) is a self-report questionnaire consisting of 53 items that are rated on a five point Likert-scale (0 = not at all to 4 = very much). Answers are scored on nine Primary Symptom Dimensions and three Global Indices. Internal consistency with Cronbach's alpha > 0.70 for the subscales and > 0.90 for the Global Indicee GSI is good to very good (46).

The Personality Inventory for DSM-5-Brief Form (PID-5-BF) is a self-report questionnaire assessing 5 personality traits (negative affect, detachment, antagonism, disinhibition, and psychoticism). The 25 items are rated on a 4 point Likert-scale (0 = very false or often false to 3 = very true or often true). An average score for each domain and an overall score can be calculated with higher scores indicating greater dysfunction. The average domain and overall personality dysfunction scores were found to be reliable in the DSM-5 Field Trials (47).

The Elternstressfragebogen (ESF) is a German self-report questionnaire with 38 items assessing parental stress. The answers are rated on the four scales Parental Stress, Role Restriction, Social Support, and Partnership. The internal consistency is good with Cronbach's alpha > 0.76 (49).

The Erziehungsfragebogen (EFB) is the German adaptation of the English Parenting Scale (57). The self-report questionnaire consists of 35 items and can be rated on the scales Overreactivion, Laxness, and Verbosity as well as on a total score. The internal consistencies of the scales Overreaction, Laxness, and the total score is acceptable to good with Cronbach's alpha > 0.74. For Verbosity the internal consistency is lower with Cronbach's alpha > 0.59 (48).

To assess knowledge about mental disorders, a semi structured interview was adapted from Beardslee and Röhrle (50). Domains of the interview are knowledge about mental disorders in general, knowledge about the primary diagnosis of the mentally ill parent, causes of the mental illness, coping with the mental illness and communication. Conducting the interviews separately with all family members over the age of 6 years takes 15 min each.

The questionnaire on healthcare consumption and productivity losses for patients with a Psychiatric disorder (TiC-P) is a comprehensive and widely used self-report questionnaire focusing on establishing direct medical costs and indirect costs (e.g., productivity losses due to absenteeism and presenteeism) (51). The TiC-P is a feasible and reliable instrument for collecting data on medical consumption and productivity losses in patients with common mental health conditions (58). The TiC-P has been previously adapted for use in Germany (59). For this study, we adapted the TiC-P for use in children.

The EQ-5D-5L is a widely used instrument to calculate quality-adjusted life years (QALYs) (52). The EQ-5D-5L comprises 5 items covering 5 domains (mobility, self-care, usual activities, pain/discomfort, and anxiety/depression), each of which is rated as causing "no problems," "slight problems," "moderate problems," "severe problems," and "extreme problems." Theoretically, the EQ-5D-5L generates 3,125 different health states. Preference-based utilities for each of these health states are available for Germany with "full health" and "death" being anchored at 1 and 0, respectively (60).

The Assessment of Quality of Life (AQoL) instruments are health-related multi-attribute utility quality of life instruments. The AQoL is a reliable and valid instrument (53). The AQoL-8D consists of five psycho-social and three physical dimensions. With one exception (dimension "senses"), each of these represents a psychometrically valid sub-scale [e.g., tests indicate they measure a common construct (61)]. Utility scores were obtained by a four-stage methodology (62).

The KIDSCREEN-10 index consists of 10 items each answered on a 5-point Likert scale. The index provides a good discriminatory power along the health-related quality of life trait-continuum. The KIDSCREEN-10 Index shows good psychometric properties (63). Utility scores will be derived by an algorithm for mapping the KIDSCREEN-10 index onto the CHU9D utility scores, a preference-based instrument developed specifically for application in cost-utility analyses (54).

Sample Size

The sample size calculation is based on the primary outcome measure (change in TRF score between T2 and T3) which is hierarchically ranked on top of the multiple testing procedure. Based on the results described above (14, 15, 64), it is assumed that the standardized treatment effect for this outcome expressed by Cohen's d amounts to $d = 0.25$. With a two-sided significance level of $\alpha = 0.05$ and a power of $1-\beta = 0.8$ using a two-sample t-test, 253 patients per group ($n = 506$ in total) are required. Since the primary outcome is measured on the child level and it is possible to enroll multiple children per patient, a hierarchical multi-level model with patients at level 1 and children at level 2 will be fitted. Taking a drop-out rate of 20 % into account, $n = 634$ patients need to be enrolled into the trial in the analysis. This attrition rate is conservative and based on results from the longitudinal STAR*D study that also carried out long-term follow-up assessments (13), as well as on other studies in the field that report even lower attrition rates (65, 66). The problem of attrition and missing values will also be addressed in the analysis by applying the intention-to-treat principle. For missing values, imputation techniques will be applied, thus partly resolving this problem. Since it is assumed that parts of the outcome variance can be explained by the inclusion of covariates, the actual power of the analysis by a linear multi-level model is expected to be higher than $1-\beta = 0.8$. Assuming that the number of children enrolled per patient amounts to 1.5, we expect that $n = 950$ children will participate in the trial. The enrollment of more than one child per patient is expected to yield an additionally increased power. Sample size calculation was performed using SAS v9.4 (SAS Institute, Cary, NC).

Randomization

Patients will be assigned in a 1:1 ratio to either the control intervention (CBT) or the experimental intervention (CBT+Triple P) through a centralized web-based tool (www.randomizer.at). Randomization will be performed stratified by center, comorbidity (yes/no), and total number of children (1/more than 1). To achieve equal group sizes per stratum block randomization will be performed. The block length will be defined by the study biometrician and treated confidentially to prevent selection bias.

Blinding

Assessment interviews will be conducted and analyzed by clinician-raters blinded to the treatment condition. Raters at post and follow-up assessments must not be the therapist of the particular patient being assessed and analyzed.

Statistical Methods

Our primary efficacy analysis will be based on the full analysis set (FAS) according to the intention-to-treat (ITT) principle, reflecting the recommendations given in relevant guidelines (67). The FAS is defined to include all patients enrolled who are assigned to the treatment group they were originally randomized to, regardless of whether they actually underwent the assigned treatment or not. This will be the primary population for evaluating all efficacy endpoints and subject characteristics. Additionally, the per-protocol (PP) population, including all FAS patients with no major protocol deviations, will serve as a secondary analysis population and be used for sensitivity analyses. Before lock of the database, each patient's allocation to the FAS or PP population will be defined in the statistical analysis plan.

The two hypotheses to be assessed in the primary efficacy analysis are ordered hierarchically: In the first step, the null hypothesis H_0^I: $\mu_{CBT+PPP}^{T3-T2} = \mu_{CBT}^{T3-T2}$ for the primary outcome "change in teacher CBCL (Teacher Report Form/TRF) score between T2 and T3" is tested at the two-sided significance level of 5% against the alternative H_1^I: $\mu_{CBT+PPP}^{T3-T2} \neq \mu_{CBT}^{T3-T2}$. If H_0^I can be rejected, the null hypothesis H_0^{II}: $\mu_{CBT+PPP}^{T4-T2} = \mu_{CBT}^{T4-T2}$ for the second primary endpoint "change in TRF score between T2 and T4" is tested at the two-sided level of 5% against its alternative H_1^{II}: $\mu_{CBT+PPP}^{T4-T2} \neq \mu_{CBT}^{T4-T2}$. Application of this multiple test procedure for a priori ordered hypotheses ensures control of the family-wise type I error rate at a level of 5%. The null hypotheses will be assessed using a linear mixed multi-level model with patients at level 1 and children at level 2, adjusting for center, number of comorbidities, number of children, baseline TRF score at T2, and length of waiting period between T1 and T2 (in weeks).

Data missing for the primary outcome variable will be replaced by using multiple imputation (68) which takes the covariates treatment group, center, number of comorbidities, number of children, baseline TRF score at T2, and length of waiting period between T1 and T2 (in weeks) into account by applying the fully conditional specification method (69). This will be realized using the option "FCS" of the SAS "MI" procedure implemented in SAS 9.4. Sensitivity analyses will be performed by applying alternative methods dealing with missing data such as complete case analysis. All secondary outcomes will be evaluated descriptively, and descriptive *p*-values are reported together with 95% confidence intervals for the corresponding effects. Further exploratory analyses will be performed to identify potential prognostic factors (e.g., parental disorder, child psychopathology, socio-economic status) and mediators (e.g., Brief Symptom Inventory/BSI, Parenting Questionnaire/EFB, Parental Stress Inventory/ESF) for an intervention effect. The safety analysis includes calculation of frequencies and rates of adverse and serious adverse events together with 95% confidence intervals. All analyses will be performed with SAS version 9.4 or higher.

The health-economic evaluation will involve a combination of a cost-effectiveness analysis (CEA) and a cost-utility analysis (CUA) (70, 71). The economic evaluation will be done from a societal perspective (all relevant costs) and a public health care perspective (only direct medical costs) within a 6 month time frame. In the CEA, the incremental cost-effectiveness ratio (ICER) will be expressed as the incremental costs per point improvement on the primary clinical outcome (CBCL scores in children; parents' BSI scores). In the CUA, the ICER will be expressed as incremental costs per quality-adjusted life year (QALY) gained as based on the EQ-5D-5L (52, 72) (parents) and KIDSCREEN-10 (63, 73) (children). Sampling uncertainty in the ICER will be handled using non-parametric bootstrapping by resampling patient-level data to generate 2,500 simulations of the ICER. We will bootstrap the SURE model (seemingly unrelated regression equations; sureg command in Stata) to allow for correlated residuals of the cost and effect equations (74). Ninety five percent confidence intervals (CI) will be obtained by the bootstrap acceptability method, since parametric techniques are inappropriate for use on skewed variables and ratios (75).The bootstrapped ICERs will be plotted in a cost-effectiveness plan where the horizontal axis reflects differences in effects and the vertical axis differences in costs. The bootstrapped ICERs will also be shown in a cost-effective acceptability curve disclosing the probability that the intervention is cost-effective for a range of willingness-to-pay ceilings (76). To test the robustness of the base-case findings, a probalistic sensitivity analysis will be done. Several assumptions made in the base-case scenario will be changed to assess their impact on the ICER (e.g., QALY calculation based on AQoL-8D).

DATA MANAGEMENT, MONITORING, AND QUALITY ASSURANCE

Training of Study Personal and Treatment Fidelity

All study personal (assessors, therapists, and supervisors) will be trained before taking part in the study. As all sites are part of associated university training institutes that conform to the highest psychotherapeutic standards. All therapists will receive intense training in CBT for the different disorders. The Triple P institute in Münster, which is the official and certified Triple P institution in Germany, will carry out Triple P training. Trained and certified supervisors will supervise every fourth treatment session at the study sites. At each participating center, a clinical project manager is responsible that the study is conducted in accordance to the procedures outlined in the study protocol. Concerning all information and data collected during the study, all study personal maintain professional secrecy and confidentiality.

After each treatment session, the therapists indicate CBT adherence by rating a checklist extracted from the disorder specific therapy manuals as outlined in the proceedings in psychotherapy (33). Upon termination of a study therapy, a supervisor rates the overall adherence of the therapy based on the adherence checks completed after every session. The adherence rate is documented in the eCRF for further analyzes.

Treatment fidelity/integrity will be analyzed with rating schemes for 5% randomly selected videotaped treatment sessions by the study coordination at the UMR. Before the videotapes are rated; they will be checked for any cues/hints potentially indicating the treatment condition; those will be erased.

Data Collection and Retention

For each included family, a study file will be created at the study site in which all local study documents will be archived. An electronic case report form (eCRF) will be used for the data collection using the secure web based electronic data capture (EDC) tool REDCap (77). The participants complete most of the questionnaires directly in the eCRF. A study staff at each site creates log-in-codes that are handed out to the participants during on site sessions with which the participants (parents, children over the age of 8 years and caregivers/teachers) can log into REDCap to complete the questionnaires at home. The families are asked to fill out the forms independently. The eCRF is programmed to not allow skipping answers to prevent missing data. If questions occur, filling out the eCRF can be paused and continued later on with a trained assessor at a study site. A study staff will enter locally collected data into REDCap preferably on the day of data collection. Upon termination of the study, all local study documents at the study sites will be sent to the UMR where the documents will be digitalized. For supervision and to ensure treatment fidelity, all study sessions will be videotaped. The video data will be stored in encrypted form using VeraCrypt which is useable free of cost under the Apache License 2.0. All videotapes will be send to the study coordination at the UMR and stored there. Upon termination of the study, all video data will be destroyed.

All local study documents are part of the Investigator Site File (ISF) as outlined in section 8 of the ICH Consolidated Guideline which is stored and archived according to the legal retention period. Data quality assessment of the eCRF will be done continuously by the Institute of Medical Biometry and Informatics Heidelberg during the study. Any entry and correction in the EDC system will be documented automatically in an audit file. Completeness, validity, and plausibility of data will be checked in time of data entry (edit-checks) and using validating programs which will generate queries. All assessments and modifications are immediately accessible via web access. The clinical project manager at each study site is also responsible for online transmission of data and site-specific quality assurance. Upon completion of the study, all data will be exported into different data formats for further analyses. The primary data will be made accessible to the public for re- and meta-analyses through PsychData at the Leibniz Institute for Psychology Information (https://www.psychdata.de/). All data will be used in accordance to data protection regulations and the data safety guidelines of the German Psychological Society (DGPs).

Ethical and Legal Aspects

Working with a highly vulnerable group, the procedures set out in this study protocol are designed to ensure that the investigators abide by the principles of the Good Clinical Practice (GCP) guidelines of the International Conference on Harmonization (ICH) and the Declaration of Helsinki and its later supplements. The study will be carried out adhering to local legal requirements. The lead ethics committee at the department of psychology at the UMR has approved the study procedure, study information, and informed consent forms in December 2017 and its subsequent amendments in May and July 2018. A positive ethics committee vote is required at a study site (ethics committees at the departments of psychology at Bielefeld University, Ruhr-University Bochum, Justus Liebig University Giessen, University of Koblenz-Landau, University of Leipzig, Johannes Gutenberg University Mainz, and Ludwig-Maximilians-University Munich), before the inclusion of a first patient at the respective site. At the beginning of the study, patients and their families are informed verbally and written about the aims of the study and the study procedures. All patients and their families (children over 6 years of age) need to provide written informed consent for study participation. For children to participate in the study, written informed consent by all legal guardians is required. Every participant can drop out of the study at any time. All dropouts will be documented in the eCRF.

Pseudonymization

After signing the informed consent, each study participant is assigned a pseudonymized screening-ID. The screening-ID consists of three parts: specific number for the study site, consecutive screening number and individual coding number (1 = patient, 2 = partner, 3, 4, 5 = included children in order of increasing age, X = ex-partner). Members of a family can be recognized by the first two parts of the screening-ID (specific study site number and consecutive screening number).

There is a coding list on paper at each study site on which names and screening-IDs are documented. The coding lists, which are kept locked away, are accessible only to study personal. The lists will be destroyed upon termination of the study but no later than 2021/12/31. After that, all data will be fully anonymized. As long as the coding lists exist, participants can request the deletion, respectively the destruction of all their collected data.

Clinical Monitor

A clinical monitor is responsible for overviewing the implementation of the study in accordance to the ICH-GSP guidelines at the study sites. The clinical monitoring includes pre-study, initiation, intermediate and close-out visits to the study sites. During the site visits, the clinical monitor examines the protocol adherent study implementation, the safety of the patients and the data consistency (e.g., comparison of local study documents and eCRF records).

Data Safety Monitoring Board

An independent Data Safety Monitoring Board (DSMB), consisting of a university professor, which is an expert in the field of the study, and a biometrician, is responsible for monitoring the study as well as assessing the study protocol adherence and the study progress (especially the recruiting plan). The DSMB will be informed about all safety aspects of the study (especially serious adverse events, SAE) and will review them regularly. If necessary, the DSMB will recommend changes to the study protocol or the termination of the study.

DISSEMINATION

The results of this study will be made available to the larger scientific community via peer-reviewed publications in open access scientific journals. Politicians, public health services and stakeholders will be informed through the COMPARE website, conferences, teaching seminars, flyers, newsletters, and personal contacts throughout the study and beyond, thus improving public policy and health care decisions concerning preventive interventions and treatments for COPMI. As all study sites are university based outpatient clinics the implementation of results in ongoing and future practice is ensured.

Upon termination of the study, all primary data will be made available to the scientific community in a completely anonymized manner for re- and meta-analyses using PsychData, a data-sharing platform developed by the Leibniz Institute for Psychology Information (ZPID, https://www.psychdata.de).

DETAILED STUDY PROCEDURE

A detailed flowchart of the study procedure is presented in **Figure 3**.

Pre-assessment T1 and Assessment of Eligibility

After an initial screening of eligibility for an as early and effective as possible selection of patients and their families and a regular intake consultation with the patient in the outpatient clinic, the patients and their families (children over the age of 6 years) are invited to an informational session at the study center. During this session, the families are informed about the study procedure before signing their consent to participate in the study. For pseudonymized data collection, each participant is assigned a Screening-ID. To assess a broad range of DSM-5 based psychological disorders and comorbid ones as well as severity ratings, structured clinical interviews for patients (DIPS), and children (Kinder-DIPS parent version or SIVA) are conducted with the patient respectively a parent (for each child separately). The parent, with whom the Kinder-DIPS/SIVA is conducted, has to be the same for all children of a family at all measurement points. The in- and exclusion criteria are checked on the basis of the information collected during the screening and the diagnoses

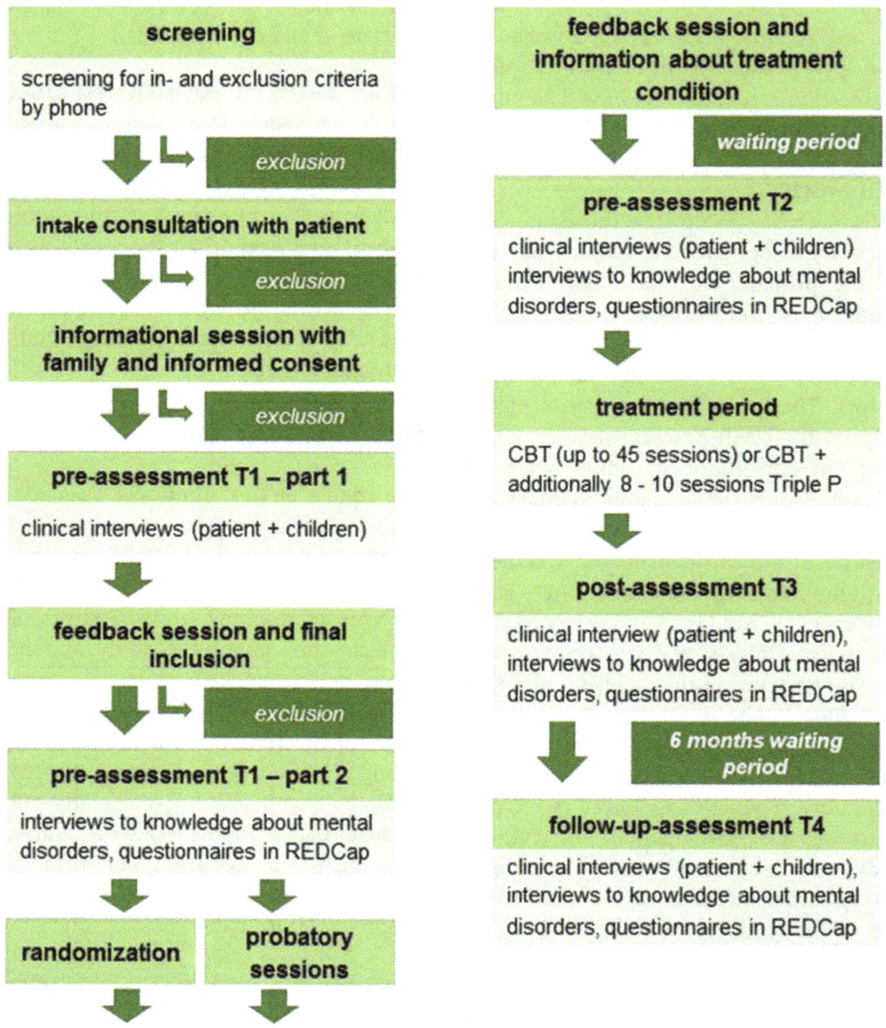

FIGURE 3 | Study flowchart.

based on the clinical interviews. Feedback to diagnoses is given in a separate session. If a patient and its family fulfill all the in- and none of the exclusion criteria, the family is included in the trial and records for the eCRF are created for all the included family members. The family is invited to another session in which interviews about knowledge about mental disorders are conducted with each included family member. After this session codes are handed out with which the family members can log into REDCap at home to complete the questionnaires. Forms with REDCap-codes for the children's caregivers or teachers (one caregiver/teacher for each included child) are also handed out to the family with the request to forward them to the respective caregiver/teachers. There is no reference to the clinical trial of the COMPARE-family project on the caregiver/teacher's form; rather, the questionnaire is generally presented as part of a study at the department of psychology the UMR. After the final inclusion in the study, the randomization to one of the two treatment arms (CBT or CBT+Triple P) takes place. If needed, further probatory sessions can take place at the study centers. In a separate feedback session, the patient is informed about the treatment condition and results of the diagnostic process.

Pre-assessment T2

After the usual waiting period for a psychotherapy treatment in the study centers (waiting period can differ between the study centers depending on their usual waiting periods for a psychotherapy treatment), structured clinical interviews for patients and children are conducted again with the patient respectively the same parent as in T1 (for each child separately). The family is invited to another session in which interviews about knowledge of mental disorders are conducted with each included family member, and codes for logging into REDCap at home to complete the questionnaires are handed out. The forms with REDCap-codes for the children's caregivers/teachers are also handed out to the family with the request to forward them to the respective caregivers/teachers.

Treatment Period

All patients receive between 25 to 45 sessions of individual CBT. Patients allocated to the experimental intervention (CBT+Triple P) receive in addition 8 to 10 group or individual Triple P sessions parallel to the last third of the CBT sessions. After every therapy session, patients, and therapists complete a session-feedback screener including aspects of therapeutic alliance and symptom intensity, as well as on fidelity. (Serious) adverse events [(S)AE] are also assessed after every therapy session with a checklist. If a (S)AE occurs, a report has to be filed and send to the study coordination at the UMR. Every fifth session, the patients are also handed out a code for logging into REDCap at home to complete the BSI to assess remission status (early, late, and non-remitters).

Post-assessment T3

Using the same measurements as in the pre-assessments, the post-assessment is conducted by an assessor who is blind to the treatment condition. Structured clinical interviews for patients and children are conducted again with the patient, respectively the same parent as in T1 (for each child separately). During a separate session, interviews on knowledge about mental disorders are conducted with each included family member separately, (S)AE are assessed for every included family member, and codes for logging into REDCap at home to complete the questionnaires are handed out at the end. The forms with REDCap-codes for the children's caregivers/teachers are also handed out to the family with the request to forward them to the respective caregivers/teachers. If a (S)AE occurs, a report has to be filed and sent to the study coordination at the UMR.

Follow-Up-Assessment T4

After a waiting period of 6 months, the follow-up-assessment is conducted by a blind assessor in the same manner as the post-assessment. The structured clinical interviews for patients and children are conducted again with the patient respectively the same parent as in T1 (for each child separately). In a separate session, knowledge about mental disorders and (S)AE are assessed for each included family member separately. At the end of this session, codes for logging into REDCap at home to complete the questionnaires are handed out. The forms with the code for the children's caregivers/teachers are also handed out to the family with the request to forward them to the respective caregivers/teachers. If a (S)AE occurs, a report has to be filed and sent to the study coordination at the UMR.

DISCUSSION

We expect that in arm I (CBT), the parents will improve through treatment as will their children (2, 7, 12). Since, parenting skills of parents with a mental illness are likely impaired and enhancing such skills leads to better child outcomes (17, 18, 20, 27, 28), we expect that additional incremental effects will become apparent in arm II (CBT+Triple P). We will use the Positive Parenting Program (Triple P) in addition to CBT, as Triple P is an evidence-based, widely used, and well-established program. The positive effects of Triple P have been demonstrated in parents and children (22, 23, 78), although incremental effects above and beyond parental CBT have not been researched in conjunction with COPMI so far.

The established magnitude of this specific incremental effect will result in precise recommendations for this high-risk group that will impact clinical practice (i.e., practice parameters, treatment guidelines). As outlined above, COPMI are most likely to constitute the next generation of patients with a mental illness, and we assume that this intervention will contribute to the prevention of SMI in this specific high-risk group.

As studies so far have focused primarily on specific disorders (e.g., anxiety, depression) and have excluded comorbidities (1, 3), though comorbidities actually occur with the most patients, the COMPARE study will fill this research gap by including a broad range of mental disorders and by not excluding comorbidities. A double baseline measurement with multiple baselines depending on the usual waiting periods in the study centers (T1: 1st assessment of parents and children via clinical interviews and questionnaires; T2: 2nd assessment with the same instruments) will enable us to assess parental disorder effects on the child that can then be related to parental treatment effects (T3: after completion of 25 short-term to 45 long-term sessions of state-of-the-art CBT or CBT+TripleP) for a 6-month follow-up (T4). As there are differential parental psychotherapy effects on children depending on the parental remission status (early, late, and non-remitters), we will also assess such effects (9, 13). By including different therapy durations (short- vs. long-term therapy) we will be able to shed light on treatment duration effects.

Research and Clinical Implications

The RCT is part of the COMPARE consortium [see Christiansen et al. (79) in this research topic] with the subprojects COMPARE-emotion, COMPARE-interaction, COMPARE-work, and COMPARE-school. The findings of the Compare consortium will not only allow for the estimation of parental treatment and parenting skill effects on their children, but also for the novel approach of testing the core assumptions of the transgenerational transmission of mental disorders model (5) comprehensively. The cost-effectiveness and cost-utility analyses from a societal and a health care system perspective will be a basis for negotiations with health care providers, as COPMI at risk can currently not receive professional help, except if they have already developed disorders themselves. The evidence of this trial will hopefully contribute to an understanding of preventing the development of disorders in COMPI to reach this goal. The identification of specific risk profiles will contribute to such an improved understanding and will result in tailored interventions that might either be more preventive or interventive in character, depending on the individual risk.

Limitations

COMPARE-family plans four extensive assessments for all family members as well as up to 55 therapy assessments. Even though the majority of patients has positive attitudes toward extensive diagnostic assessments (80), this might also be a burden on the family, especially as the add-on projects require additional assessments at the same assessment times.

The implementation of a self-wait control design in the RCT was originally planned with a waiting period of 6 months between the first assessment of the patients and their families and the beginning of the therapy. Due to the new psychotherapy guidelines in Germany, that became effective in April 2017, the waiting periods to receive psychotherapy treatment have decreased enormously at the study sites. Although the time span to receive a place in a treatment program can still be up to 9 months, many of the recruiting outpatient clinics have tried to cut those time spans down (e.g., 1–3 months waiting periods). With the original 6 months waiting period, patients wanting to participate in the COMPARE study would consequently have had to wait longer for their psychotherapy treatment than necessary. For the study centers this not only created ethical but also practical issues with interested patients preferring treatments with shorter waiting periods to the participation in COMPARE. With the now implemented multiple baseline design, the waiting period can vary between the study centers depending on the usual waiting periods on-site, therefore not disadvantaging study participants.

The observation period of only 39 months in total is rather short for capturing effects on the prevention of SMI, but due to funding, a longer observation period could not be implemented. For assessing long-term effects, a follow-up study is already planned and all participants are asked permission to be contacted again later on.

The majority of outpatient clinics will most likely treat patients with depressive and affective disorders, a fact possibly hampering the aim of the COMPARE study to cover a broad range of disorders. However, as all outpatient clinics are university-based and all recruiting centers have different research foci, chances are good that the range of disorders will be represented. This will also raise the generalizability of findings.

AUTHOR CONTRIBUTIONS

HC, MS, and KG contributed to conception and design of the study. CB drafted the health economic evaluation study. MK, CK, and JK organized the database and performed the statistical analyses. MS wrote the first draft of the manuscript. All authors contributed to sections of the manuscript, manuscript revision, read, and approved the submitted version.

FUNDING

The study is entirely funded by the Federal Ministry of Education and Research (BMBF) (01GL1748B).

CONSORT CRITERIA

CONSORT Criteria were applied in writing this study protocol.

RECRUITING CENTERS

Members of the recruiting centers are:

Bielefeld: Angelika Schlarb

Bochum: Sören Friedrich, Maike Küppers, Jürgen Margraf, Silvia Schneider, Tobias Teismann

Gießen: Arleta Luczejko, Christina Schwenck, Rudolf Stark, Anett Werner, Julia Zimmermann

Landau: Jens Heider, Katharina Köck, Annette Schröder, Katharina Senger

Leipzig: Cornelia Exner, Julian Schmitz

Mainz: Stella Grau, Stefanie Jungmann, Michael Witthöft

Marburg: Antje Arlt, HC, Julia Fahrer, KG, Winfried Rief, MS

München: Verena Labonte, Corinna Reck, Sophia Wriedt.

REFERENCES

1. van Santvoort F, Hosman CMH, Janssens Jan MAM, van Doesum Karin TM, Reupert A, van Loon Linda MA. The impact of various parental mental disorders on children's diagnoses: a systematic review. *Clin Child Family Psychol Rev.* (2015) 18:281–99. doi: 10.1007/s10567-015-0191-9
2. Garber J, Cole DA. Intergenerational transmission of depression: a launch and grow model of change across adolescence. *Dev Psychopathol.* (2010) 22:819–30. doi: 10.1017/S0954579410000489
3. Christiansen H, Anding J, Donath L. Interventionen für Kinder psychisch kranker Eltern. In: Michael Kölch, Ute Ziegenhain, Jörg M. Fegert editors. *Kinder psychisch kranker Eltern.: Herausforderungen für eine interdisziplinäre Kooperation in Betreuung und Versorgung.* Weinheim; Basel: Beltz Juventa (2014) p. 80–105.
4. Goodman SH, Gotlib IH. Risk for psychopathology in the children of depressed mothers: a developmental model for understanding mechanisms of transmission. *Psychol Rev.* (1999) 106:458–90. doi: 10.1037/0033-295X.106.3.458
5. Hosman CMH, van Doesum KTM, van Santvoort F. Prevention of emotional problems and psychiatric risks in children of parents with a mental illness in the Netherlands: I. The scientific basis to a comprehensive approach. *Austr J Adv Mental Health* (2009) 8:250–63. doi: 10.5172/jamh.8.3.250
6. Mattejat F, Remschmidt H. The children of mentally ill parents. *Deutsches Ärzteblatt Int.* (2008) 105:413–8. doi: 10.3238/arztebl.2008.0413
7. Schneider S, In-Albon T, Nuendel B, Margraf J. Parental panic treatment reduces children's long-term psychopathology: a prospective longitudinal study. *Psychother Psychosomat.* (2013) 82:346–8. doi: 10.1159/000350448
8. Wille N, Bettge S, Ravens-Sieberer U. Risk and protective factors for children's and adolescents' mental health: results of the BELLA study. *Eur Child Adolesc Psychiatry* (2008) 17(Suppl 1):133–47. doi: 10.1007/s00787-008-1015-y
9. Garber J, Ciesla JA, McCauley E, Diamond G, Schloredt KA. Remission of depression in parents: links to healthy functioning in their children. *Child Dev.* (2011) 82:226–43. doi: 10.1111/j.1467-8624.2010.01552.x
10. Pilowsky DJ, Wickramaratne P, Talati A, Tang M, Hughes CW, Garber J, et al. Children of depressed mothers 1 year after the initiation of maternal treatment: findings from the STAR*D-Child Study. *Am J Psychiatry* (2008) 165:1136–47. doi: 10.1176/appi.ajp.2008.07081286
11. Pilowsky DJ, Wickramaratne P, Poh E, Hernandez M, Batten LA, Flament MF, et al. Psychopathology and functioning among children of treated depressed fathers and mothers. *J Affect Disord.* (2014) 164:107–11. doi: 10.1016/j.jad.2014.04.012
12. Weissman MM, Pilowsky DJ, Wickramaratne PJ, Talati A, Wisniewski SR, Fava M, et al. Remissions in maternal depression and child psychopathology: a STAR*D-child report. *JAMA* (2006) 295:1389–98. doi: 10.1001/jama.295.12.1389
13. Wickramaratne P, Gameroff MJ, Pilowsky DJ, Hughes CW, Garber J, Malloy E, et al. Children of depressed mothers 1 year after remission of maternal depression: findings from the STAR*D-Child study. *Am J Psychiatry* (2011) 168:593–602. doi: 10.1176/appi.ajp.2010.10010032
14. Cuijpers P, Weitz E, Karyotaki E, Garber J, Andersson G. The effects of psychological treatment of maternal depression on children and parental

functioning: a meta-analysis. *Eur Child Adolesc Psychiatry* (2015) 24:237–45. doi: 10.1007/s00787-014-0660-6

15. Siegenthaler E, Munder T, Egger M. Effect of preventive interventions in mentally ill parents on the mental health of the offspring: systematic review and meta-analysis. *J Am Acad Child Adolesc Psychiatry* (2012) 51:8. doi: 10.1016/j.jaac.2011.10.018
16. Thanhäuser M, Lemmer G, de Girolamo G, Christiansen H. Do preventive interventions for children of mentally ill parents work? Results of a systematic review and meta-analysis. *Curr Opinion Psychiatry* (2017) 30:283–99. doi: 10.1097/YCO.0000000000000342
17. Leinonen JA, Solantaus TS, Punamaki R-L. Parental mental health and children's adjustment: The quality of marital interaction and parenting as mediating factors. *J Child Psychol Psychiatry* (2003) 44:227–41. doi: 10.1111/1469-7610.t01-1-00116
18. Lovejoy MC, Graczyk PA, O'Hare E, Neuman G. Maternal depression and parenting behavior: a meta-analytic review. *Clin Psychol Rev.* (2000) 20:561–92. doi: 10.1016/S0272-7358(98)00100-7
19. van Loon LMA, van de Ven MOM, van Doesum KTM, Witteman CLM, Hosman CMH. The relation between parental mental illness and adolescent mental health: the role of family factors. *J Child Family Stud.* (2014) 23:1201–14. doi: 10.1007/s10826-013-9781-7
20. Wilson S, Durbin CE. Effects of paternal depression on fathers' parenting behaviors: a meta-analytic review. *Clin Psychol Rev.* (2010) 30:167–80. doi: 10.1016/j.cpr.2009.10.007
21. Compas BE, Champion JE, Forehand R, Cole DA, Reeslund KL, Fear J, et al. Coping and parenting: Mediators of 12-month outcomes of a family group cognitive-behavioral preventive intervention with families of depressed parents. *J Consult Clin Psychol.* (2010) 78:623–34. doi: 10.1037/a0020459
22. Heinrichs N, Kliem S, Hahlweg K. Four-year follow-up of a randomized controlled trial of triple p group for parent and child outcomes. *Prevent Sci.* (2014) 15:233–45. doi: 10.1007/s11121-012-0358-2
23. Sanders MR, Kirby JN, Tellegen CL, Day JJ. The Triple P-Positive Parenting Program: a systematic review and meta-analysis of a multi-level system of parenting support. *Clin Psychol Rev.* (2014) 34:337–57. doi: 10.1016/j.cpr.2014.04.003
24. Thomas R, Zimmer-Gembeck MJ. Behavioral outcomes of Parent-Child Interaction Therapy and Triple P-Positive Parenting Program: a review and meta-analysis. *J Abnormal Child Psychol.* (2007) 35:475–95. doi: 10.1007/s10802-007-9104-9
25. Kliem S, Aurin SS, Kröger C. Zur Wirksamkeit des adoleszenzspezifischen Elterntrainings Group Teen Triple P. *Kindheit Entwicklung* (2014) 23:184–93. doi: 10.1026/0942-5403/a000129
26. Klein DF. Control groups in pharmacotherapy and psychotherapy evaluations. *Prevent Treat.* (1997) 1:1. doi: 10.1037/1522-3736.1.1.11a
27. Barlow J, Coren E. Parent-training programmes for improving maternal psychosocial health. *Cochrane Database Syst Rev.* (2004) 1:CD002020. doi: 10.1002/14651858.CD002020.pub2
28. Parent J, Garai E, Forehand R, Roland E, Potts J, Haker K, et al. Parent mindfulness and child outcome: the roles of parent depressive symptoms and parenting. *Mindfulness* (2011) 1:254–64. doi: 10.1007/s12671-010-0034-1
29. American Psychiatric Association. *Diagnostic and Statistical Manual of Mental Disorders, DSM-5.* 5th edn. Arlington, VA: American Psychiatric Association (2013).
30. Martin A, Rauh E, Fichter M, Rief W. A one-session treatment for patients suffering from medically unexplained symptoms in primary care: a randomized clinical trial. *Psychosomatics* (2007) 48:294–303. doi: 10.1176/appi.psy.48.4.294
31. Rief W, Martin A, Rauh E, Zech T, Bender A. Evaluation of general practitioners' training: how to manage patients with unexplained physical symptoms. *Psychosomatics* (2006) 47:304–11. doi: 10.1176/appi.psy.47.4.304
32. Lambert MJ. Outcome in psychotherapy: the past and important advances. *Psychotherapy* (2013) 50:42–51. doi: 10.1037/a0030682
33. Hahlweg K, Hautzinger M, Margraf J, Rief W (editors). *Fortschritte der Psychotherapie.* Göttingen: Hogrefe (2010). Available online at: https://www.hogrefe.de/shop/fortschritte-der-psychotherapie.html
34. Sanders MR, Markie-Dadds C, Turner KMT. *Trainer-Manual für das Triple P Einzeltraining.* Münster: PAG Institut für Psychologie AG (2006).
35. Turner KMT, Markie-Dadds C, Sanders MR. *Trainermanual für das Triple P Gruppenprogramm* 2nd ed. Münster: PAG Institut für Psychologie AG (2007).
36. Sanders MR, Ralph A. *Trainermanual für das Teen Triple P Gruppenprogramm.* Münster: PAG Institut für Psychologie AG (2006).
37. Achenbach TM, Rescorla LA. *Manual for the ASEBA Preschool Forms and Profiles: An Integrated System of Multi-Informant Assessment; Child Behavior Checklist for Ages 1 1/2-5; Language Development Survey; Caregiver-Teacher Report Form.* Achenbach System of Empirically Based Assessment. Burlington, VT: ASEBA (2000).
38. Döpfner M, Plück J, Kinnen C, and for the Working Group German Child Behavior, Checklist. *CBCL/6-18R, TRF/6-18R, YSR/11-18R Deutsche Schulalter-Formen der Child Behavior Checklist von Thomas M. Achenbach.* Bern: Hogrefe (2014).
39. Maybery D, Reupert A, Goodyear M, Ritchie R, Brann P. Investigating the strenghts and difficulties of children from families with a parental mental illness. *Austr J Adv Mental Health* (2009) 8:1–10. doi: 10.5172/jamh.8.2.165
40. Aitken M, Martinussen R, Tannock R. Incremental validity of teacher and parent symptom and impairment ratings when screening for mental health difficulties. *J Abnormal Child Psychol.* (2017) 45:827–37. doi: 10.1007/s10802-016-0188-y
41. Goodman R. The strengths and difficulties questionnaire: a research note. *J Child Psychol Psychiatry* (1997) 38:581–6. doi: 10.1111/j.1469-7610.1997.tb01545.x
42. Schneider S, Pflug V, Margraf J, In-Albon T. *Kinder-DIPS: Diagnostisches Interview bei Psychischen Störungen im Kindes- und Jugendalter.* Bochum: Forschungs- und Behandlungszentrum für psychische Gesundheit, Ruhr-Universität Bochum (2017).
43. Margraf J, Cwik JC, Pflug V, Schneider S. Strukturierte klinische Interviews zur Erfassung psychischer Störungen über die Lebensspanne. *Zeitschrift Klinische Psychol Psychother.* (2017) 46:176–86. doi: 10.1026/1616-3443/a000430
44. Margraf J, Cwik JC, Suppiger A, Schneider S. *DIPS Open Access: Diagnostic Interview for Mental Disorders.* Bochum: Mental Health Research and Treatment Center, Ruhr-Universität Bochum (2017).
45. Bolten, Equit, von Gontard, In-Albon. *Strukturiertes Interview für das Vorschulalter* (in press).
46. Derogatis LR. *BSI - Brief Symtom Inventory: Manual (1. Auflage).* Deutsche Fassung: Kliem, S. and Brähler, E. Frankfurt am Main: Pearson Deutschland GmbH (2017).
47. Zimmermann J, Altenstein D, Krieger T, Holtforth MG, Pretsch J, Alexopoulos J, et al. The structure and correlates of self-reported DSM-5 maladaptive personality traits: findings from two German-speaking samples. *J Personal Disord.* (2014) 28:518–40. doi: 10.1521/pedi_2014_28_130
48. Naumann S, Bertram H, Kuschel A, Heinrichs N, Hahlweg K, Döpfner M. Der Erziehungsfragebogen (EFB). *Diagnostica* (2010) 56:144–57. doi: 10.1026/0012-1924/a000018
49. Domsch H, Lohaus A. *Elternstressfragebogen (ESF).* Göttingen: Hogrefe (2010).
50. Beardslee WR, Röhrle B (editors). *Hoffnung, Sinn und Kontinuität: Ein Programm für Familien depressiv erkrankter Eltern. Fortschritte der Gemeindepsychologie und Gesundheitsförderung: Vol. 19.* Tübingen: Dgvt-Verl (2009). Available online at: http://www.socialnet.de/rezensionen/isbn.php?isbn=978-3-87159-619-3
51. Hakkaart-van Roijen L, van Straten A, Donker M, Tiemens B. *Handleiding Trimbos/iMTA Questionnaire for Costs associated with Psychiatric illness (TiC-P).* Rotterdam: Erasmus University (2002).
52. Herdman M, Gudex C, Lloyd A, Janssen M, Kind P, Parkin D, et al. Development and preliminary testing of the new five-level version of EQ-5D (EQ-5D-5L). *Qual Life Res.* (2011) 20:1727–36. doi: 10.1007/s11136-011-9903-x
53. Richardson J, Iezzi A, Khan MA, Maxwell A. Validity and reliability of the Assessment of Quality of Life (AQoL)-8D multi-attribute utility instrument. *Patient* (2014) 7:85–96. doi: 10.1007/s40271-013-0036-x
54. Chen G, Stevens K, Rowen D, Ratcliffe J. From KIDSCREEN-10 to CHU9D: creating a unique mapping algorithm for application in economic evaluation. *Health Qual Life Outcomes* (2014) 12:134. doi: 10.1186/s12955-014-0134-z
55. The KIDSCREEN Group Europe. *The KIDSCREEN Questionnaires - Quality of Life Questionnaires for Children and Adolescents. Handbook.* Lengerich: Pabst Science Publishers (2006).

56. Achenbach TM. *The Achenbach System of Empirically Based Assessemnt (ASEBA): Development, Findings, Theory, and Applications.* Burlington, VT: University of Vermont Research Center for Children, Youth, and Families (2009).
57. Arnold DS, O'Leary SG, Wolff LS, Acker MM. The parenting scale: a measure of dysfunctional parenting in discipline situations. *Psychol Assess.* (1993) 5:137–44. doi: 10.1037/1040-3590.5.2.137
58. Bouwmans C, Jong K, de, Timman R, Zijlstra-Vlasveld M, van der Feltz-Cornelis C, Tan Swan S, et al. Feasibility, reliability and validity of a questionnaire on healthcare consumption and productivity loss in patients with a psychiatric disorder (TiC-P). *BMC Health Serv Res.* (2013) 13:217. doi: 10.1186/1472-6963-13-217
59. Buntrock C, Berking M, Smit F, Lehr D, Nobis S, Riper H, et al. Preventing depression in adults with subthreshold depression: health-economic evaluation alongside a pragmatic randomized controlled trial of a web-based intervention. *J Med Internet Res.* (2017) 19:e5. doi: 10.2196/jmir.6587
60. Ludwig K, Graf von der Schulenburg JM, Greiner W. German value set for the EQ-5D-5L. *Pharmacoeconomics* (2018) 36:663–74. doi: 10.1007/s40273-018-0615-8
61. Richardson J, Elsworth G, Iezzi A, Khan MA, Mihalopoulos C, Schweitzer I, et al. *Increasing the Sensitivity of the AQoL Inventory for Evaluation of Interventions Affecting Mental Health.* Research Paper 61. Melbourne: Centre for Health Economics, Monash University (2011).
62. Richardson J, Sinha K, Iezzi A, Khan MA. Modelling utility weights for the Assessment of Quality of Life (AQoL)-8D. *Qual Life Res.* (2014) 23:2395–404. doi: 10.1007/s11136-014-0686-8
63. Ravens-Sieberer U, Erhart M, Rajmil L, Herdman M, Auquier P, Bruil J, et al. Reliability, construct and criterion validity of the KIDSCREEN-10 score: a short measure for children and adolescents' well-being and health-related quality of life. *Qual Life Res.* (2010) 19:1487–500. doi: 10.1007/s11136-010-9706-5
64. Thanhäuser MU. *Wirksamkeit präventiver Interventionen für Kinder psychisch kranker Eltern: Metaanalytische Ergebnisse (Diplomarbeit).* Philipps-Universität Marburg, Marburg (2015).
65. Beardslee WR, Versage EM, Wright EJ, Salt P, Rothberg PC, Drezner K, et al. Examination of preventive interventions for families with depression: evidence of change. *Dev Psychopathol.* (1997) 9:109–30. doi: 10.1017/S0954579497001090
66. Beardslee WR, Brent DA, Weersing VR, Clarke GN, Porta G, Hollon SD, et al. Prevention of depression in at-risk adolescents: longer-term effects. *JAMA Psychiatry* (2013) 70:1161–70. doi: 10.1001/jamapsychiatry.2013.295
67. ICH Harmonised Tripartite Guideline, Statistical principles for clinical trials. International Conference on Harmonisation E9 Expert Working Group. (1999). *Statistics in Medicine.* 18:1905–42.
68. van Buuren S. *Flexible imputation of missing data. Chapman and Hall/CRC interdisciplinary statistics series.* Boca Raton, FL: CRC Press (2012). Available online at: http://search.ebscohost.com/login.aspx?direct=trueandscope=siteanddb=nlebkanddb=nlabkandAN=445864. doi: 10.1201/b11826
69. van Buuren S. Multiple imputation of discrete and continuous data by fully conditional specification. *Stat Methods Med Res.* (2007) 16:219–42. doi: 10.1177/0962280206074463
70. Drummond M, Sculpher M. Common methodological flaws in economic evaluations. *Med Care* (2005) 43(Suppl.):II-5-II-14. doi: 10.1097/01.mlr.0000170001.10393.b7
71. Drummond MF, Sculpher MJ, Torrance GW, O'Brien BJ, Stoddart G. *Cost Methods for the Economic Evaluation of Healthcare Programmes* 3rd ed. Oxford: Oxford University Press (2005).
72. Janssen MF, Pickard AS, Golicki D, Gudex C, Niewada M, Scalone L, et al. Measurement properties of the EQ-5D-5L compared to the EQ-5D-3L across eight patient groups: a multi-country study. *Qual Life Res.* (2013) 22:1717–27. doi: 10.1007/s11136-012-0322-4
73. Erhart M, Ottova V, Gaspar T, Jericek H, Schnohr C, Alikasifoglu M, et al. Measuring mental health and well-being of school-children in 15 European countries using the KIDSCREEN-10 Index. *Int J Public Health* (2009) 54(Suppl 2):160–6. doi: 10.1007/s00038-009-5407-7
74. Willan AR, Briggs AH, Hoch JS. Regression methods for covariate adjustment and subgroup analysis for non-censored cost-effectiveness data. *Health Econom.* (2004) 13:461–75. doi: 10.1002/hec.843
75. Glick HA, Doshi JA, Sonnad SS. *Economic Evaluation in Clinical Trials* 2nd ed. Handbooks in health economic evaluation series (2014). doi: 10.1093/med/9780199685028.001.0001
76. Fenwick E, Claxton K, Sculpher M. Representing uncertainty: the role of cost-effectiveness acceptability curves. *Health Econom.* (2001) 10:779–87. doi: 10.1002/hec.635
77. Harris PA, Taylor R, Thielke R, Payne J, Gonzalez N, Conde JG. Research electronic data capture (REDCap)–a metadata-driven methodology and workflow process for providing translational research informatics support. *J Biomed Inform.* (2009) 42:377–81. doi: 10.1016/j.jbi.2008.08.010
78. Kaminski JW, Valle LA, Filene JH, Boyle CL. A meta-analytic review of components associated with parent training program effectiveness. *J Abnormal Child Psychol.* (2008) 36:567–89. doi: 10.1007/s10802-007-9201-9
79. Christiansen H, Reck C, Zietlow A-L, Otto K, Steinmayr R, Wirthwein L, et al. *Children Of Mentally Ill Parents At Risk Evaluation (COMPARE): Design and Methods of a Randomized Controlled Multicenter Study-Part I* (in review).
80. Suppiger A, In-Albon T, Hendriksen S, Hermann E, Margraf J, Schneider S. Acceptance of structured diagnostic interviews for mental disorders in clinical practice and research settings. *Behav Ther.* (2009) 40:272–9. doi: 10.1016/j.beth.2008.07.002

11

Protective Factors for Early Psychotic Phenomena among Children of Mothers with Psychosis

Simon Riches[1,2], Louise Arseneault[1], Raha Bagher-Niakan[3], Manar Alsultan[3], Eloise Crush[1] and Helen L. Fisher[1]*

[1] *King's College London, Social, Genetic & Developmental Psychiatry Centre, Institute of Psychiatry, Psychology & Neuroscience, London, United Kingdom,* [2] *South London & Maudsley NHS Foundation Trust, London, United Kingdom,* [3] *King's College London, Department of Psychosis Studies, Institute of Psychiatry, Psychology & Neuroscience, London, United Kingdom*

***Correspondence:**
Helen L. Fisher
helen.2.fisher@kcl.ac.uk

Background: Early identification of sub-clinical psychotic experiences in at-risk individuals is vital to prevent the development of psychosis, even before prodromal symptoms emerge. A widely-replicated risk factor is having a family member with psychosis. The Environmental Risk (E-Risk) Longitudinal Twin Study has shown that better cognitive functioning, a stimulating family environment, and a cohesive community, are protective against psychotic experiences among children; while engaging in physical activity, social support, and a cohesive community are protective for adolescents. In the current study we investigate whether these factors also protect against the development of sub-clinical psychotic phenomena among children and adolescents in this cohort who are at high-risk of psychosis by having a mother with psychosis.

Methods: Data were utilized from the E-Risk Longitudinal Twin Study, a nationally-representative cohort of 2,232 twin children born in England and Wales in 1994–1995 followed to age 18. Psychotic phenomena were assessed in private interviews with children at ages 12 and 18, and mothers were interviewed about their own experiences of psychosis when children were aged 10 and 12. Bivariate and multivariate logistic regression analyses explored associations between individual, family, and community-level putative protective factors and absence of age-12 psychotic symptoms and age-18 psychotic experiences in children whose mothers had a diagnosis of a psychosis-spectrum disorder and/or reported psychotic symptoms.

Results: Higher IQ (OR = 0.97, 95% CI 0.94–1.00, P = 0.036) and living in a more socially cohesive neighborhood (OR = 0.88, 95% CI 0.79–0.98, P = 0.023) were independently protective against age-12 psychotic symptoms among children of mothers with psychosis. Higher levels of perceived social support were independently protective against age-18 psychotic experiences among children of mothers with psychosis (OR = 0.92, 95% CI 0.87–0.98, P = 0.006). However, there were no significant interactions between these protective factors and maternal psychosis in relation to an absence of childhood or adolescent psychotic phenomena in the full sample, indicating that protective effects were not specific to this group of high-risk children.

Conclusions: These findings provide preliminary evidence that preventive interventions for early psychotic phenomena could focus on improving cognition, social support, and cohesiveness of the local community. Given scarce resources these might usefully be targeted at high-risk children.

Keywords: child and adolescent mental health, early intervention, familial psychosis, maternal psychosis, prevention, protective factors, psychotic experiences, resilience

INTRODUCTION

Psychotic disorders, especially schizophrenia, are responsible for a substantial proportion of disability worldwide (1), are associated with 10–25 years shorter life expectancy (2), and place a huge burden on families, health services, and society (3–5) Current treatments are unable to provide a cure; therefore, early identification of at-risk individuals may help to prevent the development of psychosis. Interventions in the prodromal stage have yielded some success but often fail to prevent poorer functional outcomes in the longer-term (6). It may therefore be necessary to intervene even earlier, before prodromal symptoms have emerged (7).

One potential target for preventative interventions could be sub-clinical psychotic experiences. These experiences, such as hearing voices, having visions, or feeling extremely paranoid, are relatively common in the general population, especially among young people. A systematic review and meta-analysis of population-based studies concluded that the median prevalence of psychotic symptoms was 17% among children aged 9–12 years, and 7.5% among adolescents aged 13–18 years (8). Early-life psychotic experiences are thought to lie on a continuum with psychotic disorders (9) and have been shown to predict elevated rates of schizophrenia by age 38 (10) and share many of the risk factors commonly associated with psychotic disorders (11). Moreover, these sub-clinical psychotic phenomena have also been shown to increase the risk for other psychiatric disorders (12), suicide attempts (10), and poor functional outcomes (13) in adulthood.

Therefore, one approach to informing early preventive interventions for psychotic disorders and potentially other adverse outcomes is to investigate factors that protect at-risk children and adolescents from developing psychotic experiences. A widely replicated risk factor for psychosis is having a family member with the disorder; for instance, having a parent with schizophrenia increases a child's risk of developing schizophrenia themselves by approximately eight-fold (14). A previous analysis of the Environmental Risk (E-Risk) Longitudinal Twin Study, a nationally-representative general population sample of twins, has shown that children were over twice as likely to report psychotic experiences at age 12 if their mother had experienced a psychosis-spectrum disorder (11). This indicates that young people whose mother has experienced psychosis could be considered a high-risk group for the development of early psychotic phenomena. However, not all offspring of affected mothers developed psychotic experiences (11) and thus it is important to understand what protected these high-risk individuals in order to inform preventive interventions.

In the E-Risk sample, it has previously been shown that, in the context of poly-victimization, having better cognitive functioning, growing up in a happier and more stimulating family environment, and living in a cohesive community, were protective against psychotic experiences among children (15), while engaging in physical activity, social support, and living in a cohesive community were protective for adolescents (16). However, it is also important to determine protective factors for other high-risk groups, such as having a parent with psychosis. Therefore, in the current study we use the E-Risk cohort to investigate whether these factors can also protect against the development of sub-clinical psychotic phenomena among children and adolescents who are at particularly high-risk of psychosis, by virtue of having a mother with a psychotic disorder or psychotic symptoms. We explored whether these factors were protective over and above potential confounding factors, including family socioeconomic status (SES) and other childhood mental health problems, which have previously been shown to be associated with the development of psychotic phenomena (11).

MATERIALS AND METHODS

Participants

Participants were members of the E-Risk Longitudinal Twin Study, which tracks the development of a nationally-representative birth cohort of 2,232 British twin children. The sample was drawn from a larger cohort of twins born in England and Wales in 1994–1995 (17). Full details about the sample are recorded elsewhere (18). Briefly, the E-Risk sample was constructed in 1999–2000, when 1,116 families with same-sex 5-year-old twins (93% of those eligible) participated in home-visit assessments. Families were recruited to represent the UK population of families with new-borns in the 1990s, based on residential location throughout England and Wales and mothers' age. Teenaged mothers with twins were over-selected to replace high-risk families who were selectively lost to the register through non-response. Older mothers having twins via assisted reproduction were under-selected to avoid an excess of well-educated older mothers. E-Risk families are representative of UK households across the spectrum of neighborhood-level deprivation: 25.6% of E-Risk families live in "wealthy achiever" neighborhoods compared to 25.3% of households nation-wide; 5.3 vs. 11.6% live in "urban prosperity" neighborhoods; 29.6 vs. 26.9% live in "comfortably off" neighborhoods; 13.4 vs. 13.9% live in "moderate means" neighborhoods; and 26.1 vs. 20.7%

live in "hard-pressed" neighborhoods (19, 20). E-Risk families under-represent "urban prosperity" neighborhoods because such households are likely to be childless. The sample comprised 56% monozygotic and 44% dizygotic twin pairs, and sex was evenly distributed within zygosity (49% male). All families were English speaking, and the majority (93.7%) were White.

Follow-up home-visits were conducted when children were aged 7, 10, 12, and 18 years (participation rates were 98, 96, 96, and 93%, respectively). Home visits at ages 5, 7, 10, and 12 years included assessments with participants as well as their mother (or primary caretaker); the home visit at age 18 included interviews only with the participants. Each twin participant was assessed by a different interviewer. The average age of the twins at the time of the age 18 assessment was 18.4 years ($SD = 0.36$); all interviews were conducted after the 18th birthday. There were no differences between those who did and did not take part at age 18 in terms of socioeconomic status (SES) assessed when the cohort was initially defined ($\chi^2 = 0.86$, $P = 0.65$), age-5 IQ scores ($t = 0.98$, $P = 0.33$), or age-5 internalizing or externalizing behavior problems ($t = 0.40$, $P = 0.69$ and $t = 0.41$, $P = 0.68$, respectively).

The Joint South London and Maudsley and the Institute of Psychiatry Research Ethics Committee approved each phase of the study. Parents gave informed consent and twins gave assent between 5 and 12 years and then informed consent at age 18.

Measures

Maternal Psychosis-Spectrum Disorder

When children were aged 10, mothers were interviewed using the Diagnostic Interview Schedule (DIS) for DSM-IV (21), which enquires about characteristic symptoms of psychosis: hallucinations, delusions, disorganized speech, grossly disorganized, or catatonic behavior and negative symptoms (avolition, flat affect, alogia). They were asked whether they had experienced these symptoms at any time in their life. The interview ruled out symptoms with plausible explanations and symptoms occurring solely under the influence of alcohol or drugs. Following DSM-IV criteria for schizophrenia, women were classified as having a psychosis-spectrum disorder given the presence of hallucinations plus at least two other symptoms, as well as evidence of social, occupational, or self-care dysfunction (12). The goal was not to diagnose clinical schizophrenia, but to identify women who endorsed impairing psychotic-like experiences and beliefs. Of the 1,060 mothers who completed the DIS, 58 (5.5%) were classified as having a psychosis-spectrum disorder.

Maternal Psychotic Symptoms

When children were aged 12, mothers were interviewed with the Psychosis Screening Questionnaire (PSQ) (22) about psychotic symptoms that they experienced over the past 2 years. The PSQ consists of 6 main items covering symptoms of hypomania, thought insertion, paranoia, strange experiences and hallucinations, and 14 follow-up items. The six main items were all presented first and, if any main items were endorsed, the appropriate follow-up questions were asked. A symptom was considered present if the mother positively endorsed the main item and its follow-up questions. The number of psychotic symptoms was summed and then dichotomized into none vs. 1 or more psychotic symptoms due to the skewed nature of the variable. Of the 1,069 mothers who completed the PSQ, 177 (16.6%) reported one or more psychotic symptoms.

Childhood Psychotic Symptoms

E-Risk families were visited by mental health trainees or professionals when children were aged 12 (11). Each child was privately interviewed about 7 psychotic symptoms pertaining to delusions and hallucinations, with items including "have other people ever read your thoughts?," "have you ever thought you were being followed or spied on?," and "have you ever heard voices that other people cannot hear?." This interview has been described in detail previously (11). The item choice was guided by the Dunedin Study's age-11 interview protocol (12) and an instrument prepared for the Avon Longitudinal Study of Parents and Children (23). Interviewers coded each experience 0, 1, 2 indicating, respectively "not a symptom," "probable symptom," and "definite symptom." A conservative approach was taken in designating a child's report as a symptom. First, the interviewer probed using standard prompts designed to discriminate between experiences that were plausible (e.g., "I was followed by a man after school") and potential symptoms (e.g., "I was followed by an angel who guards my spirit") and wrote down the child's narrative description of the experience. Second, items and interviewer notes were assessed by a psychiatrist expert in schizophrenia, a psychologist expert in interviewing children, and a child and adolescent psychiatrist to verify the validity of the symptoms. Third, because children were twins, experiences limited to the twin experience (e.g., "My twin and I often know what each other are thinking") were coded as "not a symptom." Children were only designated as experiencing psychotic symptoms if they reported at least one definite psychotic symptom. At age 12, 5.9% ($N = 125$) of children reported experiencing psychotic symptoms. This is similar to the prevalence of psychotic symptoms in other community samples of children and adolescents (8, 24–27). Furthermore, our psychotic symptom measure has good construct validity, sharing many of the genetic, social, neurodevelopmental, and behavioral risk factors and correlates as adult schizophrenia (11).

Adolescent Psychotic Phenomena

The present study used two measures of adolescent psychotic phenomena which were both obtained from private interviews when participants were aged 18. The primary outcome was a self-report measure of adolescent psychotic *experiences* which reflects the methodology used by many groups in the psychosis prodromal research field (28). At age 18, each E-Risk participant was privately interviewed by a research worker about 13 psychotic experiences occurring since age 12. Seven items pertained to delusions and hallucinations, which were the same as those used in childhood (see above). This interview has been described in detail previously (11). Six items pertained to unusual experiences, which drew on item pools since formalized in prodromal psychosis instruments including the PRIME-screen and Structured Interview for Prodromal Syndromes (28). These included "I worry that my food may be poisoned" and "My thinking is unusual or frightening." Interviewers coded each item 0, 1, 2 indicating, respectively "not present," "probably present," and "definitely present." All 13 items were summed to create a psychotic experiences scale (range = 0–18, $M = 1.19$, SD = 2.58). Just over 30% of participants had at least one psychotic experience between ages 12 and 18 ($n = 623$, 30.2%). This is similar to the prevalence of self-reported psychotic experiences in other community samples of teenagers and young adults (8, 25).

Clinician-verified adolescent psychotic *symptoms* were also examined as a secondary outcome, using the same methodology as used at age 12 in this cohort (11). Adolescents were only designated as having psychotic *symptoms* if they reported at least one definite and verified symptom. At age 18, 2.9% ($N = 59$) of adolescents reported having one or more psychotic symptoms since age 12. This is somewhat lower than the prevalence of psychotic symptoms in this sample at age 12 (5.9%, $N = 125$), consistent with the attenuation of psychotic symptoms documented from childhood to adulthood (8, 29).

Childhood Protective Factors

Iq

The Wechsler Preschool and Primary Scale of Intelligence Revised (WPSSI; (30) was used to assess IQ at age 5. Children were administered two subtests (Vocabulary and Block Design), and IQ scores were prorated following procedures described previously (31) and then standardized with a mean of 100 and standard deviation of 15.

Atmosphere at home

The creation of the atmosphere at home measure has been previously documented (32). It was derived from the Coder's Impression Inventory, which is based on the Home Observation for Measurement of the Environment (33) and the University of Washington Parenting Clinic Questionnaire (Parent-Child Observations) (34). The Coder's Impression Inventory was rated immediately following the study visit at ages 7 and 10 by interviewers who had undergone 4-day training. This measure comprised items representing the state of the home (e.g., "Are visible rooms of the house clean?"), stimulation (e.g., "Is the children's art displayed in the home?"), happiness (e.g., "Is this a happy home?"), and chaos (e.g., "Is the house chaotic or overly noisy?"). The internal consistency at age 7 was $\alpha = 0.77$ and $\alpha = 0.79$ at age 10. The average of the overall atmosphere at home scores at ages 7 and 10 was used for analysis because they were significantly correlated ($r = 0.64$, $P < 0.001$).

Neighborhood social cohesion

Social cohesion within the neighborhood (35) was assessed when children were aged 5 by asking mothers five questions, including whether their neighborhood was close-knit, whether neighbors shared values, and whether neighbors trusted and got along with each other. A total score was derived by summing the answers to all five questions, with higher scores indicative of greater social cohesion.

Adolescent Protective Factors

Physical activity

At age 18, participants completed the Stanford Brief Activity Survey (SBAS; Stanford University, 2001). The SBAS contains 2 items, the first item relates to the extent of physical activity engaged in at work, school, or college and the second refers to physical activity during leisure time. Both questions were rated on a 5-point scale: inactive, low intensity, moderate intensity, hard intensity, and very hard intensity. The scales were then combined to derive an overall activity measure (36).

Neighborhood social cohesion

Social cohesion in the participants' neighborhoods was estimated via a postal survey sent to residents living alongside E-Risk families when participants were aged 13–14 (37, 38). Survey respondents, who were typically living on the same street or within the same apartment block as the participants in the study, reported on various characteristics of their immediate neighborhood. Five items (each coded 0–4) were assessed by asking residents whether their neighbors shared values and trusted and got along with each other, etc. A total score was derived by summing the answers to all 5 questions with higher scores indicating greater social cohesion.

Social support

Perceived social support was assessed at age 18 using the Multidimensional Scale of Perceived Social Support (MSPSS), which assesses individuals' access to supportive relationships with family, friends, and significant others (39). The 12 items in the MSPSS consist of statements such as "There is a special person who is around when I am in need" and "I can count on my friends when things go wrong." Participants rated these statements as "not true" (0), "somewhat true" (1) or "very true" (2). Scores were summed to produce an overall social support scale with higher scores reflecting greater social support (internal consistency: $\alpha = 0.88$).

Confounding Variables

Family SES was measured via a composite of parental income (total household), education (highest for mother/father), and occupation (highest for mother/father) when children were aged 5 (40). The three SES indicators were highly correlated (r's ranged from 0.57 to 0.68, all p's < 0.05) and loaded significantly onto one latent factor (factor loadings = 0.82, 0.70, and 0.83 for income, education, and occupation, respectively). This latent factor was categorized into tertiles (i.e., low-, medium-, and high-SES). A variable for childhood mental health problems was derived to capture children who met criteria for extreme anxiety, clinically-relevant depression symptoms, attention deficit hyperactivity disorder (ADHD), or conduct disorder by age 12. Anxiety was assessed when children were aged 12, via private interviews using the 10-item version of the Multidimensional Anxiety Scale for Children (MASC) (41). An extreme anxiety group was formed with children who scored at or above the 95th percentile ($N = 129$, 6.1%). Depression symptoms were assessed at age 12 using the Children's Depression Inventory (CDI) (42). Children who scored 20 or more were deemed to have clinically significant depressive symptoms ($N = 74$, 3.5%). ADHD was assessed using the DSM-IV and the requirement of symptom onset prior to age 12 was met if parents or teachers reported more than 2 ADHD symptoms at ages 5, 7, 10, or 12 years. We derived diagnoses of conduct disorder on the basis of mothers' and teachers' reports of children's behavior problems using the Achenbach family of instruments and additional DSM-IV items assessing conduct disorder which have previously been described (32). Conduct disorder was assumed present if it was diagnosed at ages 5, 7, 10, or 12 years. The childhood mental health problems variable was dichotomized to distinguish between the presence of any of the above mental health problems (coded 1) vs. the absence of any age-12 mental health problems (coded as 0), as used previously in this cohort (16).

Statistical Analysis

Analyses were conducted in STATA 15 (Stata-Corp, College Station, TX). Bivariate and multivariate logistic regression analyses were conducted to explore associations between individual, family, and community-level putative protective factors and absence of age-12 and age-18 psychotic phenomena, in the E-Risk sub-sample of children whose mothers had experienced psychosis. Maternal psychosis was defined as either diagnosis of psychosis-spectrum disorder and/or presence of one or more psychotic symptoms to utilize the largest possible group of mothers experiencing psychotic phenomena ($N = 408$).

In phase 1 (age-12 analysis), binary logistic regression analyses were conducted to explore associations between each protective factor (IQ, atmosphere at home, and neighborhood social cohesion), individually and then altogether, and the absence of age-12 psychotic symptoms in the sub-sample of children whose mothers had experienced psychosis. We also tested in the whole sample for interactions between maternal psychosis status and each protective factor to examine whether these factors were specifically protective in relation to having a mother who had experienced psychotic phenomena or were more generally protective.

In phase 2 (age-18 analysis), binary logistic regression analyses were conducted to explore associations between each protective factor (physical activity, neighborhood social cohesion, and perceived social support), individually and then altogether, and the absence of age-18 psychotic experiences in the sub-sample of children whose mothers had experienced psychosis. Interactions between maternal psychosis status and each protective factor were conducted to examine whether these factors were specifically protective in relation to having a mother who had experienced psychotic phenomena. Sensitivity analyses substituting age-18 psychotic experiences with the clinician-verified psychotic symptoms at age 18 were also conducted.

Because each study family contains two children, all statistical analyses were corrected conservatively for the non-independence of twin observations by using tests based on the Huber/White variance estimator (43). All analyses were also adjusted for child's gender and family socio-economic status because these factors have previously been associated with psychosis (44, 45). Age-18 analyses were also adjusted for age-12 psychotic symptoms and childhood mental health problems as these have been shown to predict the occurrence of psychotic phenomena in adolescence (29, 46).

RESULTS

Phase 1: Age-12

Sample

The sample ($N = 2{,}182$) was 51.1% ($N = 1{,}114$) female. Family SES was categorized into low- (33.2%, $N = 724$), medium- (32.8%, $N = 716$), and high-SES (34.0%, $N = 742$). Having a mother with either a diagnosis of psychosis-spectrum disorder or at least one psychotic symptom was associated with an increased likelihood of age-12 psychotic symptoms among their children (OR = 2.14, 95% CI 1.38–3.31, $P = 0.001$).

Associations Between Putative Protective Factors and Absence of Age-12 Psychotic Symptoms Among Mothers With Psychosis

Having a higher IQ, a more positive atmosphere in the home, and residing in a more socially cohesive neighborhood were all found to be significantly protective against age-12 psychotic symptoms among children of mothers who had experienced either psychotic symptoms or had a psychosis-spectrum diagnosis after adjusting for gender and family SES (**Table 1**). When additionally controlling for the other protective factors, higher IQ (OR = 0.97, 95% CI 0.94–1.00, $P = 0.036$) and neighborhood social cohesion (OR = 0.88, 95% CI 0.79–0.98, $P = 0.023$) remained significantly associated with a reduced likelihood of the child having psychotic symptoms, but the association for atmosphere at home became non-significant (OR = 0.96, 95% CI 0.92–1.01, $P = 0.133$).

Interactions Between Maternal Psychosis Status and Protective Factors in the Whole Sample

Mean IQ ($M = 101.1$, SD = 14.8), atmosphere at home ($M = 26.6$, SD = 4.8) and neighborhood social cohesion ($M = 7.8$, SD = 2.6) were highest when neither the child nor mother had symptoms or diagnosis of psychosis. Mean scores were lowest when both mother and child had psychotic symptoms or diagnosis: IQ ($M = 88.9$, SD = 14.6); atmosphere at home ($M = 19.5$, SD = 7.0); neighborhood social cohesion ($M = 5.3$, SD = 3.3). However, none of the interactions between maternal psychosis status and the protective factors were statistically significant (**Table 2**). Indeed, higher average IQ (OR = 0.98, 95% CI 0.96–0.99, $P = 0.002$) and a more positive atmosphere at home (OR = 0.93 95% CI 0.89–0.97, $P = 0.002$) were significantly associated with a reduced likelihood of age-12 psychotic symptoms in children of mothers *without* psychosis, with a non-significant trend for greater neighborhood social cohesion (OR = 0.93, 95% CI 0.85–1.01, $P = 0.071$).

TABLE 1 | Associations between putative protective factors and absence of age-12 psychotic symptoms among children of mothers with diagnosis or symptoms of psychosis.

Putative protective factor	Psychotic symptoms absent $N = 359$	Psychotic symptoms present $N = 40$	Adjusted OR[a]	95% CI	*P*
	M (SD)	*M (SD)*			
IQ	97.84 (14.77)	88.88 (14.58)	0.96	0.94–0.99	0.007
Atmosphere at home	23.32 (6.92)	19.51 (6.96)	0.93	0.89–0.98	0.003
Neighborhood social cohesion	7.14 (3.02)	5.30 (3.28)	0.85	0.76–0.96	0.007

CI, confidence interval; IQ, intelligent quotient; OR, odds ratio; SD, standard deviation.
[a]Adjusted for gender and family socioeconomic status. All analyses account for the non-independence of twin observations.

TABLE 2 | Interactions between maternal psychosis and putative protective factors in relation to the absence of age-12 psychotic symptoms and age-18 psychotic experiences in the whole sample.

Interaction with maternal psychosis	Adjusted OR	95% CI	*P*
AGE-12			
IQ	0.98	0.95–1.01	0.300
Atmosphere at home	1.01	0.96–1.07	0.739
Neighborhood social cohesion	0.92	0.81–1.06	0.247
AGE-18			
Physical activity	1.08	0.87–1.34	0.494
Neighborhood social cohesion	0.86	0.51–1.43	0.553
Social support	1.01	0.94–1.07	0.818

CI, confidence interval; IQ, intelligent quotient; OR, odds ratio. All analyses are adjusted for gender and family socioeconomic status; age-18 analyses are additionally adjusted for age-12 psychotic symptoms and other age-12 mental health problems. All analyses account for the non-independence of twin observations.

Phase 2: Age-18

Sample

The sample ($N = 2{,}041$) was 52.3% ($N = 1{,}067$) female. Family SES was categorized into low- (33.4%, $N = 681$), medium- (33.1%, $N = 675$), and high-SES (33.5%, $N = 685$). Having a mother with either a diagnosis of psychosis-spectrum disorder or at least one psychotic symptom was associated with an increased likelihood of age-18 psychotic experiences among their children (OR = 1.56, 95% CI 1.21–2.01, $P = 0.001$).

Are Protective Factors Associated With an Absence of Age-18 Psychotic Phenomena Among Adolescents Whose Mother has Psychosis?

Greater levels of perceived social support were significantly associated with a reduced likelihood of adolescent psychotic experiences when controlling for all confounders among children of mothers with a psychosis-spectrum disorder or psychotic symptoms (**Table 3**). No associations were evident for physical activity, but there was a non-significant trend for greater neighborhood social cohesion to be associated with a reduced likelihood of adolescent psychotic experiences (OR = 0.67, 95% CI 0.42–1.08, $P = 0.101$). When additionally controlling for the other protective factors, higher levels of perceived social support remained significantly associated with a reduced likelihood of adolescents having psychotic experiences (OR = 0.92, 95% CI 0.87–0.98, $P = 0.006$).

Sensitivity analyses were then conducted substituting the psychotic experiences outcome with the rarer clinician-verified psychotic symptoms at age 18. None of the protective factors were found to be significantly associated with a reduced likelihood of psychotic symptoms being reported at age 18 when controlling for potential confounders among the adolescents whose mothers had psychosis (**Table 4**). However, the effect sizes were similar to those for psychotic experiences, and there was a non-significant trend for greater neighborhood social cohesion to be associated with a reduced likelihood of adolescent psychotic symptoms (OR = 0.62, 95% CI 0.22–1.69, $P = 0.346$).

Are Protective Factors Only Associated With an Absence of Age-18 Psychotic Experiences Among Adolescents Whose Mother has Psychosis?

There were no significant interactions between each of the protective factors and maternal psychosis status in relation to an absence of age-18 psychotic experiences in the full sample (**Table 2**). Indeed, higher levels of perceived social support were also associated with a reduced likelihood of age-18 psychotic experiences in children of mothers *without* psychosis (OR = 0.91, 95% CI 0.89–0.94, $P < 0.001$).

DISCUSSION

Summary of Findings

Higher IQ and greater neighborhood social cohesion were found to be independently protective against the development of age-12 psychotic symptoms among children of mothers with a psychosis-spectrum disorder or psychotic symptoms. At age 18, higher levels of perceived social support were found to be independently protective of psychotic experiences among adolescents of mothers with a psychosis-spectrum disorder or psychotic symptoms. There was a non-significant trend for neighborhood social cohesion to be protective for adolescent psychotic experiences. As none of the interactions between protective factors and maternal psychosis status investigated were found to be significant, this indicates that factors were not specifically protective against psychotic phenomena amongst these high-risk children. Indeed, all of the factors

TABLE 3 | Associations between putative protective factors and absence of age-18 psychotic experiences among children of mothers with a diagnosis or symptoms of psychosis.

Putative protective factor	Psychotic experiences absent $N = 238$	Psychotic experiences present $N = 144$	Adjusted OR[a]	95% CI	P
	M (SD)	M (SD)			
Physical activity	2.71 (1.09)	2.72 (1.09)	1.02	0.83–1.25	0.871
Neighborhood social cohesion	2.24 (0.52)	2.09 (0.50)	0.67	0.42–1.08	0.101
Social support	21.02 (4.55)	18.63 (4.99)	0.92	0.87–0.98	0.006

CI, confidence interval; OR, odds ratio; SD, standard deviation.
[a]Adjusted for gender, family socioeconomic status, age-12 psychotic symptoms, and other age-12 mental health problems. All analyses account for the non-independence of twin observations.

TABLE 4 | Associations between putative protective factors and an absence of age-18 psychotic symptoms among adolescents whose mothers had a psychosis-spectrum disorder or psychotic symptoms.

Putative protective factor	Psychotic symptoms absent $N = 360$	Psychotic symptoms present $N = 22$	Adjusted OR[a]	95% CI	P
	M (SD)	M (SD)			
Physical activity	2.71 (1.08)	2.68 (1.25)	1.00	0.64–1.58	0.991
Neighborhood social cohesion	2.19 (0.50)	2.00 (0.68)	0.62	0.22–1.69	0.346
Social support	20.16 (4.88)	19.36 (4.38)	0.99	0.93–1.07	0.882

CI, confidence interval; M, mean; OR, odds ratio; SD, standard deviation.
[a]Adjusted for gender, family socioeconomic status, age-12 psychotic symptoms, and other age-12 mental health problems. All analyses account for the non-independence of twin observations.

were also found to be protective amongst children and adolescents whose mothers had not experienced psychotic phenomena.

Comparison to Previous Research

Our results are consistent with previous research on the E-Risk study which reported that higher IQ, a more positive atmosphere at home, and greater neighborhood social cohesion were associated with a reduced likelihood of childhood psychotic symptoms in the whole sample and not just in high-risk children exposed to multiple forms of victimization (15). Similarly, previous studies show that possessing a higher IQ is associated with a reduced likelihood of developing psychotic symptoms (47, 48); while lower childhood IQ is associated with a range of mental health problems, including an increased risk of developing schizophrenia, depression and anxiety as an adult (49). Our findings also suggest that high levels of neighborhood social cohesion are independently protective in children with mothers who have either symptoms or a diagnosis of psychosis, and in the whole population. This result is consistent with previous research showing that low levels of social cohesion are associated with greater odds of developing psychotic symptoms (50–52). Additionally, our findings highlight the protective effect of perceived social support in adolescence which is consistent with previous research in E-Risk showing that social support was associated with a reduced likelihood of psychotic experiences among high-risk adolescents who had been poly-victimized (16). A study of clinical-level psychosis also demonstrated the protective nature of social support among high-risk individuals (53).

Strengths and Limitations

Strengths of the study include our novel analysis that examines protective factors for children and adolescents who are at high risk of psychosis by having a mother with a psychotic disorder or psychotic symptoms. Furthermore, our participants were taken from a large, nationally-representative longitudinal cohort study that measured psychotic phenomena at two time-points and enabled us to control for a range of potentially confounding factors. Several limitations warrant consideration. The sample size was relatively small when focusing on children of mothers with psychosis and so we may have lacked statistical power to detect significant effects, especially for the interaction analysis. Moreover, it was not possible to explore protective effects in children who mothers had a diagnosis of psychosis-spectrum disorder separately to those whose mothers had psychotic symptoms due to the small number of children in the former group ($N = 58$). The sample was composed of twins and so we cannot be certain if the findings can be generalized to single children, although the prevalence of childhood and adolescent psychotic phenomena in this study are similar to rates found in singleton samples (8, 25, 27). We limited our analyses to factors that have previously been found to be protective for psychotic phenomena in this cohort and it is possible that a range of other multi-level factors may also be protective. For instance, self-esteem (54), attachment style (55), and positive behavioral support (56). These require further investigation ideally in even larger population-based cohorts. In adolescence several of the measures were assessed at the same time-point and therefore it is not possible to ascertain the direction of the associations found. We did however control for earlier psychopathology, but it would be useful in future to utilize prospective measures, ideally obtained from different informants. Additionally, psychotic phenomena in childhood and adolescence have been associated not only with later development of schizophrenia but also with other mental health problems (10, 12), and thus the findings cannot specifically be generalized to indicate protection against clinically-relevant psychosis. Finally, our analyses focused on psychotic phenomena assessed only at the ages of 12 and 18 so we do not know if the factors analyzed would be protective if symptoms were to develop at other ages in childhood or adolescence, or in adulthood.

Clinical Applications and Future Research

The findings of this study have the potential to inform the focus of interventions to prevent the emergence of early psychotic phenomena and thus ultimately improve the outcomes of high-risk children and adolescents. Intellectual ability, neighborhood social cohesion, and perceptions of social support appear to be key target areas for early intervention. It is possible that possessing a higher IQ may facilitate problem-solving skills, coping strategies in adverse situations, and better self-regulation of emotions, particularly in relation to having a parent with psychosis. Cognitive behavioral therapies are being developed for young people that aim to target and develop skills such as reasoning and emotional coping, as a way of increasing resilience (57). Cognitive remediation therapy is another approach that may offer a way to alleviate cognitive difficulties in young people (58). Additionally, neighborhood support interventions to improve parenting have been demonstrated in a study which found high levels of neighborhood social cohesion were associated with reduced instances of child neglect (59). Such an outcome could occur through alleviating the burden that comes with childcare for mothers with psychosis as neighbors meet the physical and emotional needs of both child and parent. Trust between neighbors may also mean that children approach them for help when they are feeling distressed, providing further adaptive ways of coping (60). Research suggests that when people with early psychosis perceive greater social support, they appear to be more likely to cope with day-to-day stressors (61). Higher levels of social support have been found to correlate with lower levels of positive symptoms and fewer hospitalizations in people with first episode psychosis (62). Therefore, if the current findings are replicated in other cohorts, it would be helpful to investigate whether such interventions might prevent the development of psychotic phenomena in children and adolescents.

CONCLUSIONS

Higher IQ and neighborhood social cohesion were found to be independently associated with a reduced likelihood of age-12 psychotic symptoms among children of mothers with symptoms of psychosis or a psychosis-spectrum diagnosis. Similarly, higher levels of perceived social support were found to be independently protective against adolescent psychotic experiences in this high-risk group. In terms of clinical implications, if replicated, the findings suggest that interventions should be aimed at cultivating these factors for children and adolescents who are considered at-risk by virtue of having a mother with psychosis. All of these factors were also found to be associated with a reduced likelihood of having psychotic phenomena among children whose mother had not experienced psychosis, which suggests that preventative interventions could also be targeted at the general population regardless of risk. These preventative interventions should improve the cohesiveness of a child's community environment, increase their perceptions of social support, and bolster their cognitive functioning. Replication of these findings is required in larger populations, amongst single children, in order to ascertain generalizability and subsequently inform the development and testing of interventions to prevent the emergence of early psychotic phenomena. Ultimately, such preventive strategies may reduce the incidence of psychosis and other mental health problems in adulthood.

AUTHOR CONTRIBUTIONS

HF designed the project and oversaw the analyses and write-up of the manuscript. RB-N, MA, and SR conducted the analyses and wrote the first draft of the manuscript. LA oversaw data collection for the E-Risk Study. All authors critically reviewed and amended the content of the manuscript and approved the final version.

FUNDING

The E-Risk Study is funded by the UK Medical Research Council (G1002190). Additional support was provided by the National Institute of Child Health and Human Development (HD077482); the Jacobs Foundation; the Avielle Foundation; a research grant from the National Society for Prevention of Cruelty to Children (NSPCC) and Economic and Social Research Council (ESRC); a Medical Research Council Studentship to Eloise Crush; and an MQ Fellows Award to HF (MQ14F40). Louise Arseneault is the Mental Health Leadership Fellow for the UK ESRC.

ACKNOWLEDGMENTS

We are grateful to the study mothers and fathers, the twins, and the twins' teachers for their participation. Our thanks to Professors Terrie Moffitt and Avshalom Caspi who founded the E-Risk study, CACI, Inc., and to members of the E-Risk team for their dedication, hard work and insights.

REFERENCES

1. Farooq S, Large M, Nielssen O, Waheed W. The relationship between the duration of untreated psychosis and outcome in low-and-middle income countries: a systematic review and meta analysis. *Schizophr Res.* (2009) 109:15–23. doi: 10.1016/j.schres.2009.01.008
2. Chang C-K, Hayes RD, Perera G, Broadbent MT, Fernandes AC, Lee WE, et al. Life expectancy at birth for people with serious mental illness and other major disorders from a secondary mental health care case register in London. *PLoS ONE* 6:e19590. doi: 10.1371/journal.pone.0019590
3. Costello EJ, Egger H, Angold A. 10-year research update review: the epidemiology of child and adolescent psychiatric disorders: I. Methods and public health burden. *J Am Acad Child Adolesc Psychiatry* (2005) 44:972–86. doi: 10.1097/01.chi.0000172552.41596.6f
4. Boydell J, Onwumere J, Dutta R, Bhavsar V, Hill N, Morgan C, et al. Caregiving in first-episode psychosis: social characteristics associated with perceived 'burden'and associations with compulsory treatment. *Early Interv Psychiatry* (2014) 8:122–9. doi: 10.1111/eip.12041
5. Penttilä M, Jääskeläinen E, Hirvonen N, Isohanni M, Miettunen J. Duration of untreated psychosis as predictor of long-term outcome in schizophrenia: systematic review and meta-analysis. *Br J Psychiatry* (2014) 205:88–94. doi: 10.1192/bjp.bp.113.127753
6. Addington J, Cornblatt BA, Cadenhead KS, Cannon TD, Mcglashan TH, Perkins DO, et al. At clinical high risk for psychosis: outcome for nonconverters. *Am J Psychiatry* (2011) 168:800–5. doi: 10.1176/appi.ajp.2011.10081191
7. Uher R, Cumby J, Mackenzie LE, Morash-Conway J, Glover JM, Aylott A, et al. A familial risk enriched cohort as a platform for testing early interventions to prevent severe mental illness. *BMC Psychiatry* 14:344. doi: 10.1186/s12888-014-0344-2
8. Kelleher I, Connor D, Clarke MC, Devlin N, Harley M, Cannon M. Prevalence of psychotic symptoms in childhood and adolescence: a systematic review and meta-analysis of population-based studies. *Psychol Med.* (2012) 42:1857–63. doi: 10.1017/S0033291711002960
9. van Os J, Linscott RJ, Myin-Germeys I, Delespaul P, Krabbendam L. A systematic review and meta-analysis of the psychosis continuum: evidence for a psychosis proneness–persistence–impairment model of psychotic disorder. *Psychol Med.* (2009) 39:179–95. doi: 10.1017/S0033291708003814
10. Fisher HL, Caspi A, Poulton R, Meier MH, Houts R, Harrington H, et al. Specificity of childhood psychotic symptoms for predicting schizophrenia by 38 years of age: a birth cohort study. *Psychol Med.* (2013) 43:2077–86. doi: 10.1017/S0033291712003091
11. Polanczyk G, Moffitt TE, Arseneault L, Cannon M, Ambler A, Keefe RS, et al. Etiological and clinical features of childhood psychotic symptoms: results from a birth cohort. *Arch Gen Psychiatry* (2010) 67:328–38. doi: 10.1001/archgenpsychiatry.2010.14
12. Poulton R, Caspi A, Moffitt TE, Cannon M, Murray R, Harrington H. Children's self-reported psychotic symptoms and adult schizophreniform disorder: a 15-year longitudinal study. *Arch Gen Psychiatry* (2000) 57:1053–8. doi: 10.1001/archpsyc.57.11.1053
13. Healy C, Campbell D, Coughlan H, Clarke M, Kelleher I, Cannon M. Childhood psychotic experiences are associated with poorer global functioning throughout adolescence and into early adulthood. *Acta Psychiatr Scand.* (2018) 138:26–34. doi: 10.1111/acps.12907
14. Rasic D, Hajek T, Alda M, Uher R. Risk of mental illness in offspring of parents with schizophrenia, bipolar disorder, and major depressive disorder: a meta-analysis of family high-risk studies. *Schizophr Bull.* (2013) 40:28–38. doi: 10.1016/j.comppsych.2013.07.057
15. Crush E, Arseneault L, Jaffee SR, Danese A, Fisher HL. Protective factors for psychotic symptoms among poly-victimized children. *Schizophr Bull.* (2018) 44:691–700. doi: 10.1093/schbul/sbx111
16. Crush E, Arseneault L, Moffitt TE, Danese A, Caspi A, Jaffee SR, et al. Protective factors for psychotic experiences amongst adolescents exposed to multiple forms of victimization. *J Psychiatr Res.* (2018) 104:32–8. doi: 10.1016/j.jpsychires.2018.06.011
17. Trouton A, Spinath FM, Plomin R. Twins early development study (TEDS): a multivariate, longitudinal genetic investigation of language, cognition and behavior problems in childhood. *Twin Res Hum Genet.* (2002) 5:444–8. doi: 10.1375/136905202320906255
18. Moffitt TE, E-Risk Study Team. Teen-aged mothers in contemporary Britain. *J Child Psychol Psychiatry* (2002) 43:727–42. doi: 10.1111/1469-7610.00082
19. Caspi A, Taylor A, Moffitt TE, Plomin R. Neighborhood deprivation affects children's mental health: environmental risks identified in a genetic design. *Psychol Sci.* (2000) 11:338–42. doi: 10.1111/1467-9280.00267
20. CACI. *ACORN User Guide.* London: CACI (2006).
21. Robbins L, Cottler L, Bucholz K, Compton W, North C, Rourke K. *Diagnostic Interview Schedule for DSM-IV (DIS-IV).* St. Louis, MO: Washington University (1995).
22. Bebbington P, Nayani T. The psychosis screening questionnaire. *Int J Methods Psychiatr Res.* (1995) 5:11–9.
23. Schreier A, Wolke D, Thomas K, Horwood J, Hollis C, Gunnell D, et al. Prospective study of peer victimization in childhood and psychotic symptoms in a nonclinical population at age 12 years. *Arch Gen Psychiatry* (2009) 66:527–36. doi: 10.1001/archgenpsychiatry.2009.23
24. Dhossche D, Ferdinand R, Van Der Ende J, Hofstra M, Verhulst F. Diagnostic outcome of self-reported hallucinations in a community sample of adolescents. *Psychol Med.* (2002) 32:619–27. doi: 10.1017/S003329170200555X
25. Yoshizumi T, Murase S, Honjo S, Kaneko H, Murakami T. Hallucinatory experiences in a community sample of Japanese children. *J Am Acad Child Adolesc Psychiatry* (2004) 43:1030–6. doi: 10.1097/01.chi.0000126937.44875.6b
26. Scott J, Chant D, Andrews G, McGrath J. Psychotic-like experiences in the general community: the correlates of CIDI psychosis screen items in an Australian sample. *Psychol Med.* (2006) 36:231–8. doi: 10.1017/S0033291705006392
27. Horwood J, Salvi G, Thomas K, Duffy L, Gunnell D, Hollis C, et al. IQ and non-clinical psychotic symptoms in 12-year-olds: results from the ALSPAC birth cohort. *Br J Psychiatry* (2008) 193:185–91. doi: 10.1192/bjp.bp.108.051904
28. Loewy RL, Pearson R, Vinogradov S, Bearden CE, Cannon TD. Psychosis risk screening with the Prodromal Questionnaire—brief version (PQ-B). *Schizophr Res.* (2011) 129:42–6. doi: 10.1016/j.schres.2011.03.029
29. Zammit S, Kounali D, Cannon M, David AS, Gunnell D, Heron J, et al. Psychotic experiences and psychotic disorders at age 18 in relation to psychotic experiences at age 12 in a longitudinal population-based cohort study. *Am J Psychiatry* (2013) 170:742–50. doi: 10.1176/appi.ajp.2013.12060768
30. Wechsler D. *Wechesler Preschool and Primary Scale of Intelligence-Revised.* WPPSI-R. London: Psychological Corporation (1989).
31. Sattler J. *Assessment of Children: WISC-III and WPPSI-R Supplement.* San Diego, CA: Jerome M. Sattler, Publisher, Inc. (1992).
32. Kim-Cohen J, Caspi A, Taylor A, Williams B, Newcombe R, Craig IW, et al. MAOA, maltreatment, and gene–environment interaction predicting children's mental health: new evidence and a meta-analysis. *Mol Psychiatry* (2006) 11:903–13. doi: 10.1038/sj.mp.4001851
33. Bradley RH, Caldwell BM. Home observation for measurement of the environment: a validation study of screening efficiency. *Am J Ment Def.* (1977) 81:417–20.
34. Webster-Stratton C. Preventing conduct problems in Head Start children: strengthening parenting competencies. *J Consult Clin Psychol.* (1998) 66:715. doi: 10.1037/0022-006X.66.5.715
35. Sampson RJ, Raudenbush SW, Earls F. Neighborhoods and violent crime: a multilevel study of collective efficacy. *Science* (1997) 277:918–24. doi: 10.1126/science.277.5328.918
36. Taylor-Piliae RE, Fair JM, Haskell WL, Varady AN, Iribarren C, Hlatky MA, et al. Validation of the Stanford brief activity survey: examining psychological factors and physical activity levels in older adults. *J Phys Act Health* (2010) 7:87–94. doi: 10.1123/jpah.7.1.87
37. Odgers CL, Moffitt TE, Tach LM, Sampson RJ, Taylor A, Matthews CL, et al. The protective effects of neighborhood collective efficacy on British children growing up in deprivation: a developmental analysis. *Dev Psychol.* (2009) 45:942. doi: 10.1037/a0016162
38. Odgers CL, Caspi A, Bates CJ, Sampson RJ, Moffitt TE. Systematic social observation of children's neighborhoods using Google Street View: a reliable

and cost-effective method. *J Child Psychol Psychiatry* (2012) 53:1009–17. doi: 10.1111/j.1469-7610.2012.02565.x

39. Zimet GD, Powell SS, Farley GK, Werkman S, Berkoff KA. Psychometric characteristics of the multidimensional scale of perceived social support. *J Pers Assess.* (1990) 55:610–7. doi: 10.1080/00223891.1990.9674095
40. Trzesniewski KH, Moffitt TE, Caspi A, Taylor A, Maughan B. Revisiting the association between reading achievement and antisocial behavior: new evidence of an environmental explanation from a twin study. *Child Dev.* (2006) 77:72–88. doi: 10.1111/j.1467-8624.2006.00857.x
41. March JS, Parker JD, Sullivan K, Stallings P, Conners CK. The multidimensional anxiety scale for children (MASC): factor structure, reliability, and validity. *J Am Acad Child Adolesc Psychiatry* (1997) 36:554–65. doi: 10.1097/00004583-199704000-00019
42. Kovacs M. *Children's Depression Inventory.* North Tonawanda, NY: Multi-Health Systems. (1992).
43. Williams RL. A note on robust variance estimation for cluster-correlated data. *Biometrics* (2000) 56:645–6. doi: 10.1111/j.0006-341X.2000.00645.x
44. Byrne M, Agerbo E, Eaton WW, Mortensen PB. Parental socio-economic status and risk of first admission with schizophrenia. *Soc Psychiatry Psychiatr Epidemiol.* (2004) 39:87–96. doi: 10.1007/s00127-004-0715-y
45. Cotton S, Lambert M, Schimmelmann B, Foley D, Morley K, Mcgorry P, et al. Gender differences in premorbid, entry, treatment, and outcome characteristics in a treated epidemiological sample of 661 patients with first episode psychosis. *Schizophr Res.* (2009) 114:17–24. doi: 10.1016/j.schres.2009.07.002
46. Siebald C, Khandaker GM, Zammit S, Lewis G, Jones PB. Association between childhood psychiatric disorders and psychotic experiences in adolescence: a population-based longitudinal study. *Compr Psychiatry* (2016) 69:45–52. doi: 10.1016/j.comppsych.2016.05.004
47. de Nijs J, Zoun K, Investigators G. The association between cognitive deficits and different outcomes of schizophrenia. *Psychiatr Pol.* (2014) 48:1087–104. doi: 10.12740/PP/37438
48. Mollon J, David AS, Zammit S, Lewis G, Reichenberg A. Course of cognitive development from infancy to early adulthood in the psychosis spectrum. *JAMA Psychiatry* (2018) 75:270–9. doi: 10.1001/jamapsychiatry.2017.4327
49. Koenen KC, Moffitt TE, Roberts AL, Martin LT, Kubzansky L, Harrington H, et al. Childhood IQ and adult mental disorders: a test of the cognitive reserve hypothesis. *Am J Psychiatry* (2009) 166:50–7. doi: 10.1176/appi.ajp.2008.08030343
50. Newbury J, Arseneault L, Caspi A, Moffitt TE, Odgers CL, Fisher HL. Why are children in urban neighborhoods at increased risk for psychotic symptoms? Findings from a UK longitudinal cohort study. *Schizophr Bull.* (2016) 42:1372–83. doi: 10.1093/schbul/sbw052
51. Newbury J, Arseneault L, Caspi A, Moffitt TE, Odgers CL, Fisher HL. Cumulative effects of neighborhood social adversity and personal crime victimization on adolescent psychotic experiences. *Schizophr Bull.* (2018) 44:348–58. doi: 10.1093/schbul/sbx060
52. Solmi F, Colman I, Weeks M, Lewis G, Kirkbride JB. Trajectories of neighborhood cohesion in childhood, and psychotic and depressive symptoms at age 13 and 18 years. *J Am Acad Child Adolesc Psychiatry* (2017) 56:570–7. doi: 10.1016/j.jaac.2017.04.003
53. Gayer-Anderson C, Fisher HL, Fearon P, Hutchinson G, Morgan K, Dazzan P, et al. Gender differences in the association between childhood physical and sexual abuse, social support and psychosis. *Soc Psychiatr Psychiatr Epidemiol.* (2015) 50:1489–500. doi: 10.1007/s00127-015-1058-6
54. Pruessner M, Iyer SN, Faridi K, Joober R, Malla AK. Stress and protective factors in individuals at ultra-high risk for psychosis, first episode psychosis and healthy controls. *Schizophr Res.* (2011) 129:29–35. doi: 10.1016/j.schres.2011.03.022
55. Cicchetti D, Rogosch FA, Toth SL. Fostering secure attachment in infants in maltreating families through preventive interventions. *Dev Psychopathol.* (2006) 18:623–49. doi: 10.1017/S0954579406060329
56. Vanderbilt-Adriance E, Shaw DS, Brennan LM, Dishion TJ, Gardner F, Wilson MN. Child, family, and community protective factors in the development of children's early conduct problems. *Fam Relat.* (2015) 64:64–79. doi: 10.1111/fare.12105
57. Ames CS, Jolley S, Laurens KR, Maddox L, Corrigall R, Browning S, et al. Modelling psychosocial influences on the distress and impairment caused by psychotic-like experiences in children and adolescents. *Eur Child Adolesc Psychiatry* (2014) 23:715–22. doi: 10.1007/s00787-013-0500-0
58. Wykes T, Reeder C, Williams C, Corner J, Rice C, Everitt B. Are the effects of cognitive remediation therapy (CRT) durable? Results from an exploratory trial in schizophrenia. *Schizophr Res.* (2003) 61:163–74. doi: 10.1016/S0920-9964(02)00239-6
59. Maguire-Jack K, Showalter K. The protective effect of neighborhood social cohesion in child abuse and neglect. *Child Abuse Negl.* (2016) 52:29–37. doi: 10.1016/j.chiabu.2015.12.011
60. Erdem Ö, Prins RG, Voorham TA, Van Lenthe FJ, Burdorf A. Structural neighbourhood conditions, social cohesion and psychological distress in the Netherlands. *Eur J Public Health* (2015) 25:995–1001. doi: 10.1093/eurpub/ckv120
61. Macdonald EM, Pica S, Mcdonald S, Hayes RL, Baglioni AJ Jr. Stress and coping in early psychosis. Role of symptoms, self-efficacy, and social support in coping with stress. *Br J Psychiatry Suppl.* (1998) 172: 122–7.
62. Norman RM, Malla AK, Manchanda R, Harricharan R, Takhar J, Northcott S. Social support and three-year symptom and admission outcomes for first episode psychosis. *Schizophr Res.* (2005) 80:227–34. doi: 10.1016/j.schres.2005.05.006

12

Using Social Networking Sites in Research: An Emerging Approach to Engaging with Young People Who have a Parent with a Mental Illness and/or Substance Abuse Disorder

*Christine Grové**

Faculty of Education, Monash University, Melbourne, VIC, Australia

***Correspondence:**
Christine Grové
christine.grove@monash.edu

The challenges involved in engaging young people who have a parent with a mental illness in research and in programs are well documented. Social networking sites provide a potentially useful medium to include at-risk youths and their families by removing some accessibility barriers that may prevent engagement and connection with individuals whose parents or family members have a mental illness. This paper examines how social networking sites can be used to recruit youths and/or their families and engage them in research. Applying a case study analysis, the implications of using social media as a tool for recruitment and data collection and the ethical considerations and limitations will be discussed. Results tentatively indicate that social networking sites may be an effective method to engage young people of parents with a mental illness. The study argues for more informed use of social platforms for the translation and dissemination of research and intervention prevention. Overall, this paper will contribute to public mental health practice through guidelines and policy about social media research with at-risk young people and their families.

Keywords: young people with parents with mental illness, social networking sites, mental health practices, recruitment, research with young people, online research methods, youth at risk, research ethics

INTRODUCTION

Young people who have a parent with a mental illness can experience difficulties throughout their lives, sometimes beginning in their early years. These difficulties can impact on the young person's well-being and can lead to their own mental health challenges (1). An epidemiological study suggests that around 21–23% of young people have been found to have, or have had, a parent with a mental illness (2). Research consistently reports higher rates of emotional, behavioral, and developmental difficulties in these youths compared with those in the general community (3), with long-term effects including social and occupational issues (1). They may experience increased rates of psychiatric disorders through an interplay of both genetic and environmental factors (4). Self-harm and suicide rates tend to be higher in these youths (5, 6). The young person may harbor resentment towards the parent (7) as well as experience negative emotions including shame, depressed mood, fear of conflicts, loneliness, feelings of abandonment, anger, or envy of peers (8). It could then be said that young people who have parents with mental illness and/or substance abuse disorders are an at-risk group within society. Despite the risks that the young person with a parent with a mental illness may experience, many demonstrate resilience. Researchers agree that some children with a parent with a mental illness can cope well (9), acquire and practice effective problem-solving skills (10), and access functional social supports external to the family (9). Young people need protective factors, for example, adequate community support and intervention (11) and accurate mental health information (12), to reduce the impact of negative risk factors. In this paper, young people or youths are considered to be aged between 14 and 18 years old.

Children of parents with a mental illness are aware that there are some predictable and unpredictable elements of their parents' behavior, and it is the unpredictable elements that often impact the young person the most (13). Their understanding of parental mental illness changes with age as well as with the amount and type of information about mental health they acquire (14). Slominski (15) measured adult children's perceptions of growing up in a family where a parent was diagnosed with a mental illness. He, too, proposed that it was not only the experiences themselves that shaped the individual but also the way the individual made sense of those experiences. When young people do not receive complete, accurate mental health information, they may come to their own—often inaccurate—conclusions that can exacerbate their fears. A general lack of awareness of their parent's condition may negatively influence the youth's ability to access systems of support. Some young people make attempts to obtain information from the mental health professionals who care for their parents, but many report that they do not get the recognition they feel they deserve, for example, a lack of acknowledgment of the young person's role in caregiving and their need to understand what is happening for their parents and themselves (7, 16).

While extensive research has identified young people's risk of adverse outcomes and the potential for resilience (2, 17), it is challenging to recruit young people and families where a parent has a mental illness in research and into prevention programs (18). The difficulties of engaging with youths from high-risk communities in research may be due to barriers in recruiting vulnerable youths (19, 20). These barriers can include i) insufficient understanding of research (21, 22), ii) mistrust of research (21), iii) stigma associated with participation in clinical research (23), and iv) issues surrounding parental consent (23). There are few papers that outline "adolescent friendly" recruitment strategies that can be employed to overcome barriers to recruitment and effectively engage with at-risk young people in research initiatives (24). A potential way to address these barriers can be to recruit at-risk youths through the mediums in which they connect with most—that is on the Internet *via* social networking sites (25). How social networking sites are used to recruit youths and/or their families and engage them in research should be explored, as well as the potential to use social networking sites for translation and dissemination of accurate public health information. This paper is the first attempt to examine social networking platforms as a potentially useful medium to include at-risk youths and their families by attempting to remove barriers that could prevent access to and involvement of individuals in research.

A TECHNOLOGY-BASED RESPONSE: SOCIAL NETWORKING PLATFORMS AS A POTENTIALLY USEFUL MEDIUM TO INCLUDE AT-RISK YOUTHS AND FAMILIES

Social networking platforms are online communication systems that facilitate community-based contributions, interactions, content sharing, and collaboration in virtual networks *via* social media websites Facebook, Twitter, blogs (i.e., Tumblr), and/or YouTube (26). Social networking sites have potential when recruiting a younger population as well as targeted groups of individuals (24), such as youth with a parent who has a mental illness. For some young people, the Internet is their primary source of information and their main means of communication with the world (25). There has been a large growth of online social connections: Facebook has around 1.59 billion monthly users (Facebook 2018), while on Twitter around 500 million tweets are sent per day (Twitter 2018). Social media is increasingly an information source for youths, where they use websites to learn about the world and themselves and connect with others (27). Young people are more inclined to use social networking sites than older adults (28). As a result of the rise in social media usage, researchers and policymakers have begun to consider how such platforms can be harnessed to support research, share accurate public health messages, and inform robust evidence-based policymaking.

A systematic review of 25 studies that employed Facebook to recruit young people (10–18 years old) found that paying Facebook for advertising about specific research projects was a successful tool for recruiting adolescent participants into mental health research (24). However, the review noted that there have been few studies in which underrepresented or at-risk adolescents have been recruited *via* social media platforms (24). There have been no studies that examine social media use in recruiting children and families where a parent has a mental illness. There is relatively little guidance on using online platforms in social and mental health research. Further research is clearly needed particularly given that social networking sites are considered to be an emerging data collection, recruitment, and research dissemination strategy that is gaining traction in research (25, 26, 29).

Social networking sites can be a useful tool for gathering data, which has the potential to address barriers in research. For example, they can be a platform to deliver health interventions and recruit participants for studies in a cost-effective manner (25, 26, 29). Some of the barriers to recruiting and engaging young people who have a parent with a mental illness in research may be addressed through social platforms. Ongoing discussion about the purpose of social media methods is necessary to identify how social networking sites are applied across individual research studies. This will contribute to the field's understanding of the ways in which these platforms can be used to access at-risk groups in the community (19). There are, however, several factors to consider, such as whether to use social media research as the sole method or in conjunction with other methods, processes of data collection and analysis, ethical implications of consent and privacy, and the presentation of social media research findings. There is a lack of policy and guidelines for using social networking sites in research (19). This paper will apply a case study analysis of a research project that used social media as a strategy to recruit young people who have parents with a mental illness and to translate and disseminate research knowledge.

METHOD AND RESULTS OF CASE STUDY

Stage 1 of the research project was to explore whether a social networking site could be used to recruit and engage with youths whose parents have a mental illness (the focus of this paper). Stage 2 gathered youth people's experiences of help seeking using a mixed methods approach (16). The objective of stage 2 was to identify their expressed preferences for supports (for example, informal supports such as talking to peers or parents) and more formal interventions (such as developed programs). In order to answer this research focus, a self-administered questionnaire followed by individual semi-structured interviews was employed. In total, 173 young people (13–17 years) who have a parent with a mental illness completed a questionnaire and 6 of these participants took part in interviews. Initially, 175 youths were recruited; however, 2 in the sample were male and subsequently removed, leaving the sample of females only. During stage 1 of the study, the social networking site Facebook was used in two ways: i) as a recruitment strategy in response to the research objectives and questions, and ii) as a technology-based mechanism for knowledge translation and dissemination with the aim to provide accurate and helpful information about mental health and support for young people and their families.

Online Research Presence

A Facebook page was created to provide participants with information about the research project (see **Figure 1**). It was titled "Children of Parents with a Mental Illness: Views of Intervention." The main objective of the Facebook research page was to disseminate the online questionnaire, promote awareness of the study, and disseminate public mental health information. Posts made on the Facebook page included information about the research team and project, support services, the latest research about mental health and well-being, and study announcements that included a link to the study questionnaire. On average, the lead researcher made two Facebook posts a week. During the recruitment period, the researcher made 100 Facebook posts, received 75 Facebook followers, and liked 78 organizations relating to young people and mental health. The lead researcher reviewed and approved all wall posts in a timely manner and took them down if inappropriate due to swearing or cursing. The author interacted with other Facebook pages by "liking" the pages of community

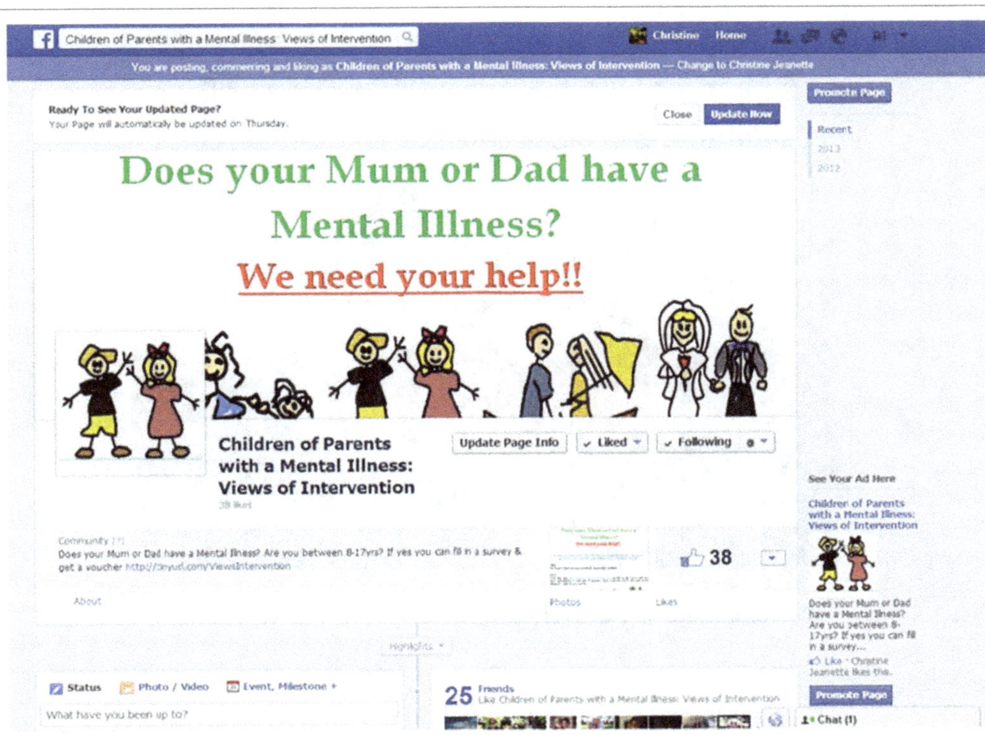

FIGURE 1 | Facebook research page.

organizations. The organizations were found using keyword search terms on the Facebook search engine, such as "children of parents with a mental illness," "young carers," "youth mental health," and "youth well-being." The "About" section on the Facebook research page included detailed information about the study, the researchers' names and affiliations, and links to the researchers' official affiliation website.

Advertising Research on Facebook

The researchers paid for targeted advertising to meet specific criteria. The criteria included the age group of the targeted youths (13–18 years), a specific population (children who have parents with a mental illness), and geographical location (Australia only). The study advertisements were only presented to Facebook users who met the study criteria set by the researchers *via* the Facebook administration page. It was shown to potential participants on their personal Facebook pages *via* their desktop computer and/or mobile device. Advertisements on Facebook must adhere to language and image guidelines. The headline had a limit of 25 characters, and the body text of the advertisement had a limit of 90 characters. Images were required for all advertisements. The study advertisement (see **Figure 2**) was placed on Facebook from August 2013 to February 2014, inviting youths to participate. Those who clicked on the poster were directed to the research explanatory statement at the beginning of the survey on a survey website called Qualtrics. Consent was obtained from the young person when they agreed to complete the questionnaire through an online form at the beginning of the questionnaire. Participants were requested to obtain parental consent before completing the survey; this request was on each page in the survey (e.g., "Ask your parent if you can take part in this study").

A total of 1,382 people clicked on the link to the questionnaire on the advertisement on Facebook. Of those who accessed the website link, 192 provided consent. Of these, 175 met the study inclusion criteria and subsequently completed the questionnaire. No other methods of data collection (such as mail-out surveys) were used. Of the 175 samples, 6 participants agreed to take part in an individual semi-structured telephone interview and were offered a $10 gift voucher upon completion. The study found that the use of social media, specifically Facebook, was a more effective recruitment tool than using traditional methods (such as flyers or mail-out surveys) to recruit young people of parents with a mental illness (12, 16).

Online Snowball Sampling

Snowball sampling occurred online during the recruitment phase of this study. Snowballing transpired when community organizations shared the Facebook research page and the survey on

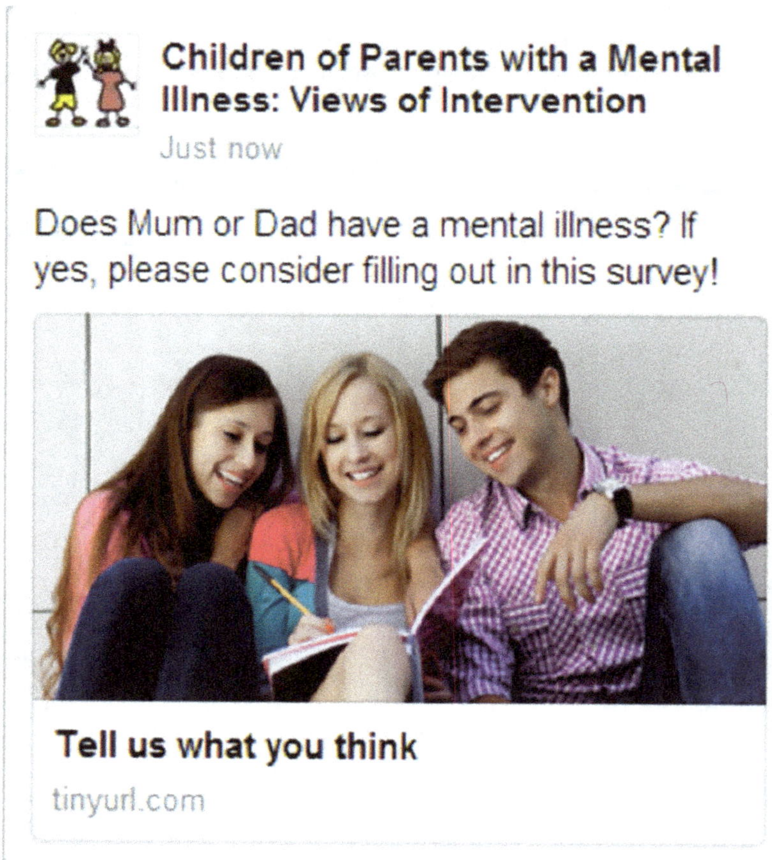
Children of Parents with a Mental Illness: Views of Intervention
Just now
Does Mum or Dad have a mental illness? If yes, please consider filling out in this survey!
Tell us what you think
tinyurl.com

FIGURE 2 | Example of advertisement used.

their websites and social media pages. From there, a snowballing effect occurred: the Facebook research page and posts made by the author were distributed *via* social media through community organization followers (individuals who followed the page of the organization). These were then subsequently shared by individuals on their individual social network site, that is, on blogs, in personal newsletters, and/or on their Twitter/Facebook pages. In addition, online snowball sampling occurred through group and friendship connections between Facebook users, where the study details were shared further.

DISCUSSION

There are benefits and challenges of using social media as a recruitment tool when engaging with vulnerable youths in research. Some benefits include using a platform that is widely interacted with by young people, whereby the research can be shared across many social sites within a young person's network, enabling a questionnaire to be disseminated quickly among many potential participants (30, 31). Amon and colleagues (24) suggest that advertising on social networking sites alongside traditional means of recruitment (i.e., flyers, mail-outs, and telephone calling) could be helpful in accessing larger and more specific groups. Social media presents a fast, affordable method of recruiting study participants for questionnaire research. In the current study, using social media was found to be a successful strategy to recruit a large sample of young people who have parents with a mental illness in a short period of time (16). Clearly, online recruitment for structured questionnaires *via* social media is a feasible and efficient tool that can be used to access at-risk individuals.

The Australian Psychology Society (32) released a national survey examining the impact of technology and social media on the well-being of young people (aged 14–17 years old). The survey found that young people are self-reporting that they use social media for an average of 3.3 h each day, on five or more days of the week. The vast majority of teenagers reported that their screens and social media accounts were a positive part of their lives. Many use social media channels to connect with family and friends and to entertain themselves. Despite social media playing a positive role for most, the high use of social media and technology can have a negative impact on youth self-esteem. Two in three young people feel pressure to look good, and nearly a third of youths have been bullied online (32). Clearly, there are ethical and potential limitations when using social networking platforms in practice or research that should to be taken into account.

Young people and their families from rural or lower socioeconomic status have been found to be more difficult to recruit and engage than those from higher socioeconomic status or from urban areas (33). This may be due, in part, to disadvantages associated with living in these areas that include reduced quality of services (34), but can also be attributed to the challenges that coincide with living in poverty or far from central towns including lack of a reliable telephone service and limited or nonexistent access to the Internet (33). Thus, a possible limitation is that participants recruited through social media may not be representative of the population as not all young people have access to computers or the Internet. Some research suggests that the digital divide is reducing as more individuals are online; however, age is a crucial factor. Nine in 10 people aged between 15 and 54 use the Internet; however, this statistic reduces to 8 in 10 of those aged 55–64 years, and to under 6 in 10 of those over 65 years (35). The age of young people who can be recruited *via* social platforms is limited to those over the age of 13. Due to age restrictions, individuals 13 years and below cannot create a Facebook, YouTube, or Tumblr account.

A challenge of social networking sites is that the participants are not representative of the population. The findings here thus might not be generalizable to the wider population. It could be that the population is not representative because children of parents with a mental illness may search for information elsewhere than on social media platforms. A predominant limitation of social media for collecting data is that it may introduce self-selection bias. Self-selection bias can lead to a sample bias. Self-selected and self-reported data may affect the reliability and validity of results (36). The validity of the completion of the online survey should be considered, as members of social media sites may not be truthful in their responses and/or complete the survey as a "fake" participant. The online identity of a person may not be the same as their real-life identity. Often, social media identities are to a certain extent more "positive." This limitation could be helpful, though, if the research is focused on a particular group that is active on a social media platform, and there is the potential to gather data from participants who may not tend to respond to other types of research methods (37). The anonymous nature of online recruitment can be a challenge in that researchers may not be aware if a young person is upset or triggered by the content in the survey. Researchers are not able to check or provide more information if the youth does not understand the project. The Facebook research page seems to have multiple purposes, which makes it difficult to disentangle to what extent this medium is useful for research participation versus general information versus referral or information to other prevention services. For example, the current case study recruited mainly females; thus, the findings or suggestions here may not be appropriate for the recruitment of males. While Facebook is still one of the most used networks in general, currently among some young persons' Facebook is not their only or main social site they access, when compared to other platforms such as Snapchat, Instagram, or YouTube (38).

Rarely are there papers that include strategies for recruiting at-risk youths (18, 24). Effective recruitment strategies are needed as it is widely recognized that underrepresented adolescents can be challenging to recruit due to barriers that impact their participation. A barrier to youth participation is the way in which at-risk adolescents are recruited. Consent for youths to participate in a study is usually attained from an adult in the young person's life, such as a parent or guardian, known as a "gatekeeper." The parent/guardian is not typically the intended audience for a study directed at youths, yet recruitment strategies are often focused at connecting with the "adult gatekeeper" in order to attain consent for the young person's participation. The challenge in accessing youths *via* a "gatekeeper" is that two sets of individuals are to be recruited for the study and the researchers usually need the parent/guardian to be interested in the research and then the youth. Depending on the study considerations required in recruiting vulnerable youths, such as whether the young person themselves can self-select into a study by providing their own consent, young people can then have "buy in" into a project in that they make the decision to participate in the study. The young person then becomes the "gatekeeper" who chooses to share study information with their parent/guardian, potentially building trust and respect of the young person. This approach respects autonomy and privacy of the young person, who, as noted by the United Nations Rights of the Child under the Convention on the Rights of the Child (39), can decide and choose to take part in matters that directly impact them, and that includes their inclusivity in firstly opting into developmentally appropriate research. A "youth-centered approach" has ethical justification. Some researchers advocate, however, that "adult gatekeepers" are a necessity in that they protect the adolescent from exposure to information that may not be appropriate (40). However, first and foremost, researching alongside at-risk youths requires procedures for the researcher to be aware of, or sensitive about, the "risk status." An understanding and sensitivity is required of researchers regarding the information they are gathering and to be done so in ways that convey respect for the young person and their circumstance, for example, using a non-judgmental attitude, respect of opinions, and collaborative approaches to consult with young people. A paradigm shift is needed for some whereby youths are seen as experts on their lives, where they have the right to share their perspectives and to initially choose to engage in research.

An ethical consideration when removing "adult gatekeepers" is regarding the ability of minors to provide consent. In the study by Grové et al. (16), formal consent was required from youths only and formal consent was not required from the parents. However, youths were invited throughout the online questionnaire to inform their parents of their participation in the study. The young persons were reminded that they did not have to be involved in the research if they chose not to. The gatekeepers were not in the role of insisting or convincing a student to participate in the research project.

Some youths express concern about identifying or sharing their at-risk status, such as being a child of a parent with a mental illness. If youths are recruited in community or public places, such as at school or through an organization, they know, and are fearful others know, they are being sought for a problem or issue and may not indicate their interest. A fear of exposure of their at-risk status and a lack of privacy are a barrier to youths participating. Social networking sites attend to their concern in that they can take part in the research anonymously and privately. Respect for youth privacy and autonomy, again, are key to recruiting and retention (41) whereby youths view the research as "something interesting and not because of a problem." However, anonymity can be a challenge in that researchers may not be aware if a young person is upset or potentially triggered by the content in the survey or if the youth has the language to understand the research. Young people who participate in preventive interventions may not necessarily want to participate in research or vice versa. Social media could help with intervention recruitment and delivery—an area that future research could explore.

Research using social network sites is a relatively new phenomenon. Social networking sites appear to be suited to recruiting a younger population who regularly use these platforms and also may be hard to reach, for example, young people of parents with a mental illness and/or substance abuse disorder (18). More generally, the emerging role of social media in research raises ethical concerns:

- privacy of participants (Are their IP addresses identifying)?,
- ownership of the data gathered (Do the data belong to the third-party website as well as the research team? What is done with these data and who are they shared with)?,
- participants providing informed consent (Is informed consent needed when conducting research studies on public websites and social media platforms and, if so, how should the researchers attain this consent)?, and
- access to participants (Who has access to which participant groups in the community and which participants are being excluded)?.

Research that uses social media platforms may consider guidelines for social networking platforms in research that are specific to their study and its context. The guidelines may outline the benefits and limitations of interacting with social media, including the relevant ethical, legal, and governance issues. The practice guidelines will depend on the sensitivity of the research area and if privacy and confidentiality (or lack of) can be provided to participants. For example, depending on the social media user's privacy settings, posts that they follow, like, or comment on can be seen by others online, creating a digital footprint or trail of interaction. Researchers may also choose to monitor and record the frequency of occurrence of the online snowball sampling strategy to determine its impact.

Researchers may consider whether the method of social media recruitment and dissemination is the appropriate tool to use, with attention to ongoing and regular interactions by the research team of content and public communication within the platform. Given the infancy of social media research, researchers need to make methodological decisions based on previous case study illustrations of research using social media rather than prior personal experience. Social media methods often make use of existing, publicly available data, so the need for participants to complete demographic questions can be reduced. However, existing data may not be accurate and ethical discussions of whether consent should be provided for its use are warranted. Researchers should provide information about their project and the research team publicly, including the research purpose and how the data gathered will be used, stored, and accessed. Ways to protect the interests of vulnerable populations in the community, such as young people who have a parent with a mental illness and/or substance abuse disorder, need to be included in project-specific guidelines. The guidelines may choose to provide suggestions about support, promote help seeking, and disseminate summary information gathered during the study. More research is vital to determine how scholars can use social media to explore participants' understanding, engagement, and active participation in public mental health practice guidelines and policy.

A challenge with some of the research with children of parents with a mental illness could be that many participants are already connected to support networks. Often, they are recruited *via* this connection. Unless the research aims are to examine outside of this network specifically (recruiting external to support networks, in rural areas, or those not accessing support), it can otherwise be challenging to recruit. Using a social networking site (i.e., Facebook) to aid in recruiting participants outside associated, connected networks did help in addressing this bias. However, if researchers are recruiting vulnerable families who may not be connected to support, educational information about supports (i.e., online or telephone counselling services or how to connect with local doctors) should be provided.

CONCLUSION

There are challenges in connecting with and engaging with young people in research, particularly if the young person is considered underrepresented in the community. An untapped approach in attaining youth involvement in research can be through social networking sites. Social networking sites are platforms that young people use directly and regularly, and could be used as a possible recruitment tool depending on the research study objectives. Further research will do well to illustrate the use of social media in research, the risks and benefits, and how efficacious this strategy is in recruiting different at-risk groups of youths.

ETHICS STATEMENT

Ethics for this study was approved through the relevant Monash University committee. Ethical approval number is MUHREC CF13/1766-2013000918. Paid advertising on Facebook was used to recruit participants. Potential participants were shown the information that is on the recruitment poster as an advertisement. The Facebook recruitment advertisement that was shown to potential participants comprised of 1) short title (e.g., "Tell us what you think"), 2) an image (e.g., stock image of young people), and 3) main text, up to 74 characters in length: "Does Mum or Dad have a mental illness? If yes, please consider filling out in this survey!" (See **Figures 1** and **2** for an example of the advertisement used for mobile device and desktop computer). If participants chose to take part in the project, they then clicked the advertisement. This took them directly to the explanatory statement and participant consent forms for participants to take part in the study.

AUTHOR CONTRIBUTIONS

The author developed the conception and design of the research work, conducted the data collection, the data analysis and interpretation, drafted the article, provided critical revision of the article, and examined the final approval of the version to be submitted.

FUNDING

The author declares that the research was conducted in the absence of any specific funding.

ACKNOWLEDGMENTS

The supervision of Professors Andrew Reupert and Daryl Maybery who provided mentorship and guidance during the development of this research is acknowledged.

REFERENCES

1. Reupert A, Maybery D, Nicholson J, Gopfert M, Seeman M. *Parental psychiatric disorder: distressed parents and their families* (Cambridge: Cambridge University Press) (2015). doi: 10.1017/CBO9781107707559
2. Maybery D, Reupert A, Goodyear M, Patrick K, Crase L. Prevalence of children whose parents have a mental illness. *Psychiatr Bull* (2009) 33:22–6. doi: 10.1192/pb.bp.107.018861
3. Duncan G, Browning J. Adult attachment in children raised by parents with schizophrenia. *J Adult Dev* (2009) 16:76–86. doi: 10.1007/s10804-009-9054-2
4. Beardslee WR, Keller MB, Seifer R, Lavori PW, Staley J, Podorefsky D, et al. Prediction of adolescent affective disorder: effects of prior parental affective disorders and child psychopathology. *J Am Acad Child Adolesc Psychiatry* (1996) 35:279–88. doi: 10.1097/00004583-199603000-00008
5. Ferguson B. *Children of parents with mental illness: parental disclosure, children's illness beliefs and the development of a shared understanding of mental illness in the family. [PhD thesis]* (Adelaide: University of Adelaide) (2011).
6. Weitzman M, Rosenthal DG, Liu Y. Paternal depressive symptoms and child behavioral or emotional problems in the United States. *Pediatrics* (2011) 127(6):1126–34. doi: 10.1542/peds.2010-3034
7. Foster K. "You'd think this roller coaster was never going to stop": experiences of adult children of parents with serious mental illness. *J Clin Nurs* (2010) 19:3143–51. doi: 10.1111/j.1365-2702.2010.03293.x
8. Knutsson-Medin L, Edlund B, Ramklint M. Experiences in a group of grown-up children of mentally ill parents. *J Psychiatr Ment Health Nurs* (2007) 14:744–52. doi: 10.1111/j.1365-2850.2007.01181.x
9. Masten AS. *Ordinary magic: resilience in development* (New York, NY: Guilford Press) (2015).
10. Zimmerman MA. Resiliency theory: a strengths-based approach to research and practice for adolescent health. *Health Educ Behav* (2013) 40:381–3. doi: 10.1177/1090198113493782
11. Reupert A, Maybery D, Kowalenko N. Children whose parents have a mental illness: prevalence, need and treatment. *Med J Aust* (2012) 16:7–9. doi: 10.5694/mjao11.11200
12. Grové C, Reupert AE, Maybery D. Gaining knowledge about parental mental illness: how does it empower children? *Child Fam Soc Work* (2015) 20(4):377–86. doi: 10.1111/cfs.12086
13. Mordoch E. How children understand parental mental illness: "You don't get life insurance. What's life insurance?" *J Can Acad Child Adolesc Psychiatry* (2010) 19(1):19–25.
14. Fox C, Buchanan-Barrow E, Barrett M. Children's understanding of mental illness: an exploratory study. *Child Care Health Dev* (2008) 34:10–8. doi: 10.1111/j.1365-2214.2007.00783.x
15. Slominski JL. *The effects of parental mental illness on children: pathways to risk to resilience from infancy to adulthood. [PhD thesis]* (Ann Arbor, MI: University of Michigan) (2010). https://deepblue.lib.umich.edu/handle/2027.42/77750?show=full.

16. Grové C, Reupert A, Maybery D. The perspectives of young people of parents with a mental illness regarding preferred interventions and supports. *J Child Fam Stud* (2016) 25(10):3056–65. doi: 10.1007/s10826-016-0468-8
17. Edwards EP, Eiden RD, Leonard KE. Behaviour problems in 18- to 36-month-old children of alcoholic fathers: secure mother-infant attachment as a protective factor. *Dev Psychopathol* (2006) 18:395–407. doi: 10.1017/S0954579406060214
18. van Doesum KTM, Riebschleger J, Carroll J, Grové C, Lauritzen C, Murdoch E, et al. Successful recruitment strategies for prevention programs targeting children of parents with mental health challenges: an international study. *Child Youth Serv* (2016) 37(2):156–74. doi: 10.1080/0145935X.2016.1104075
19. Steinbeck K, Baur L, Cowell C, Pietrobelli A. Clinical research in adolescents: challenges and opportunities using obesity as a model. *Int J Obes* (2009) 33(1):2–7. doi: 10.1038/ijo.2008.263
20. Smith KL, Straker LM, McManus A, Fenner AA. Barriers and enablers for participation in healthy lifestyle programs by adolescents who are overweight: a qualitative study of the opinions of adolescents, their parents and community stakeholders. *BMC Pediatrics* (2014) 14:53. doi: 10.1186/1471-2431-14-53
21. Baquet, Henderson, Commiskey, Morrow. Clinical trials: the art of enrollment. *Seminars in Oncology Nursing* (2008) 24(4):262–9.
22. Herlihy A, Halliday J, Gillam L. Ethical issues in recruiting prenatally diagnosed adults for research: Klinefelter Syndrome as an example. *Public Health Genomics* (2011) 15(1):31–3.
23. DiClemente R, Ruiz M, Sales J. Barriers to adolescents' participation in HIV biomedical prevention research. *J Acquired Immune Deficiency Syndromes* (2010) 54:S12.
24. Amon KL, Campbell AJ, Hawke C, Steinbeck K. Facebook as a recruitment tool for adolescent health research: a systematic review. *Acad Pediatr* (2014) 14(5):439–47. doi: 10.1016/j.acap.2014.05.049
25. Collin P, Rahilly K, Richardson I, Third A. *The benefits of social networking services: literature review* (Melbourne: Cooperative Research Centre for Young People, Technology and Wellbeing) (2011).
26. Kietzmann JH, Hermkens K, McCarthy IP, Silvestre BS. Social media? Get serious! Understanding the functional building blocks of social media. *Bus Horiz* (2011) 54(3):241–51. doi: 10.1016/j.bushor.2011.01.005
27. Best P, Manktelow R, Taylor B. Online communication, social media and adolescent wellbeing: a systematic narrative review. *Children and Youth Services Review* (2014) 41:27–36. doi: 10.1016/j.childyouth.2014.03.001
28. Khan AS, Rahman AU, Qazi TL. The relationship between internet usage, socioeconomic status, subjective health and social status. *Bus Econ Rev* (2016) 8:67–82. doi: 10.22547/BER/8.SE.5
29. Eytan T, Benabio J, Golla V, Parikh R, Stein S. Social media and the health system. *Perm J* (2011) 15(1):71–4. doi: 10.7812/TPP/10-154
30. Fenner Y, Garland SM, Moore EE, Jayasinghe Y, Fletcher A, Tabrizi SN, et al. Web-based recruiting for health research using a social networking site: an exploratory study. *J Med Intern Res* (2012) 14(1):e20. doi: 10.2196/jmir.1978
31. Yuan P, Bare MG, Johnson MO, Saberi P. Using online social media for recruitment of human immunodeficiency virus-positive participants: a cross-sectional survey. *J Med Intern Res* (2014) 16(5):e117. doi: 10.2196/jmir.3229
32. Australian Psychological Society. *Digital me: a survey exploring the effect of social media and digital technology on Australians' wellbeing* (Melbourne, Vic: Australian Psychological Society) (2017). Accessed March 8, 2019. https://apo.org.au/sites/default/files/resource-files/2017/11/apo-nid118961-1180226.pdf
33. Blitz LV, Kida L, Gresham M, Bronstein LR. Prevention through collaboration: family engagement with rural schools and families living in poverty. *J Contemp Soc Serv* (2013) 94(3):157–65. doi: 10.1606/1044-3894.4306
34. Heinrichs N, Bertram H, Kuschel A, Hahlweg K. Parent recruitment and retention in a universal prevention program for child behavior and emotional problems: barriers to research and program participation. *Prev Sci* (2005) 6(4):275–86. doi: 10.1007/s11121-005-0006-1
35. Australian Bureau of Statistics. *Australian social trends, cat.* (2018). no. 8146.0. Accessed September 10, 2018. http://www.abs.gov.au/ausstats/abs@.nsf/mf/8146.0?OpenDocument
36. Strasser SM, Smith M, Pendrick-Denney D, Boos-Beddington S, Chen K, McCarty F. Feasibility study of social media to reduce intimate partner violence among gay men in Metro Atlanta, Georgia. *West J Emerg Med* (2012) 13(3):298–304. doi: 10.5811/westjem.2012.3.11783.
37. Ruths D, Pfeffer J. Social media for large studies of behavior. *Science* (2014) 346(6213):1063–4. doi: 10.1126/science.346.6213.1063
38. Nielsen Online. 2016 Nielsen social media report. In: *Social studies: a look at the social landscape.* (2016). Accessed 28 February 2019. https://www.nielsen.com/us/en/insights/reports/2017/2016-nielsen-social-media-report.html
39. UN General Assembly, *Convention on the Rights of the Child*, 20 November 1989, United Nations, Treaty Series, vol. 1577, p. 3, available at: https://www.refworld.org/docid/3ae6b38f0.html [accessed 26 April 2019]
40. Collings S, Grace R, Llewellyn G. Negotiating with gatekeepers in research with disadvantaged children: a case study of children of mothers with intellectual disability. *Children & Society* (2016) 30(6);499–509.
41. Fox D, Gottfredson D. Differentiating completers from non-completers of a family-based prevention program. *The Journal of Primary Prevention* (2003) 24:111–24

13

Identification of Children of Parents with Mental Illness: A Necessity to Provide Relevant Support

Charlotte Reedtz[1]*, Camilla Lauritzen[1], Ylva V. Stover[2], Janita L. Freili[2] and Kamilla Rognmo[2]

[1] Regional Centre for Child and Adolescent Mental Health and Child Wellfare, Faculty of Health Sciences, UiT The Arctic University of Norway, Tromsø, Norway,
[2] Institute of Psychology, Faculty of Health Sciences, UiT The Arctic University of Norway, Tromsø, Norway

***Correspondence:**
Charlotte Reedtz
charlotte.reedtz@uit.no

Background: The main objective of this study was to identify and describe core life circumstances of children with mentally ill parents (COPMI) and their parents. Knowledge about COPMI aged 0–17 years is necessary, as assessment of the risk and protective factors in their lives provide solid background for preventive interventions.

Methods: Participants ($N = 422$) were parents of minor children ($N = 589$) receiving treatment in the clinic for psychiatric illness and substance abuse at the University Hospital of Northern Norway. Data was drawn from electronic patient journals.

Results: A total of 286 mothers and 136 fathers participated in the study, and 46.3% were single parents. Parents had 1–7 children ($M = 2.24$; $SD = 1.02$). Most parents had one diagnosis ($n = 311$, 73.7%), and mood disorders was the most frequent type of diagnosis. The largest proportion of parents had serious mental disorders ($n = 185$; 46.0%), and a large proportion of the sample was affected by disorders of moderate severity ($n = 156$; 38.8%). The mean age of the children was 8.6 years (SD = 4.97), and 432 children (74.6%) had one or more siblings. The large majority of children had access to adult resource persons other than the mentally ill parent ($n = 424$; 94%), but 6% of the children ($n = 27$) did not. About three quarters of the children (76.2%, $n = 526$) were living with the mentally ill parent ($n = 401$), and 170 children (32.5%) lived with a single parent with a mental health disorder and siblings, full time or part of the time. The odds that parents had informed their children about the treatment/hospitalization and condition was higher the older the child was ($p < 0.001$), and the youngest children rarely got necessary information about this.

Discussion: Risk and protective factors associated with the children's ages, access to resource persons, information about the parent's health problems and treatment are discussed in relation to different preventive steps for COPMI.

Keywords: parents, mental illness, mental health care services for adults, risk factors, children

INTRODUCTION

Worldwide around onev in five minor children has a parent with a mental illness (1). In Norway it is estimated that 450,000 children have parents with a mental illness or substance use disorders (2). These children are at high risk of developing a mental illness themselves (3).

In a meta-analysis, (4) found that children of parents with a severe mental illness had a 50% chance of developing any mental illness, and 32% chance of developing a severe mental illness.

In Norway, it has been estimated that children of parents with a mental illness (COPMI) have double the risk of both short-term and long-term negative consequences compared to children of parents without mental illnesses (2). Elevated risk has been documented for COPMI across the diagnostic spectrum of mental disorders in parents, including schizophrenia (5) obsessive-compulsive disorder (6), depression (7, 8), substance abuse disorders (9), anxiety disorders (10), bipolar disorder (11), eating disorders (12), personality disorders (13) and suicide (14). The transmission of risk for psychopathology from parents to children is both diagnosis-specific such that children may develop the same mental illness as their parents, and general, such that children are at risk of developing a wide range of disorders (10).

In addition to hereditary components of mental illness enhancing the risk of mental illness among the offspring, parents' symptomatology may also has a social impact and the ways parents interact with their children is therefore highly significant (8). Psychopathology in a parent often impairs parenting skills, the quality of care they provide and the parent-child interaction (15, 16). Such impairments may in turn lead to reduced involvement with the child, as well as insensitivity, hostility, rejection, neglect and potential abuse (17). The failure in one or more aspects of parenting can lead to insecure attachment (18, 19), emotional dysregulation, negative emotionality and pathological coping strategies (17), as well as psychopathology in childhood, adolescence and adulthood (20).

Different characteristics of the parent's psychopathology predict increased risk for the COPMI, including the symptom burden, comorbidity, and the severity and duration of illness. Empirical studies have repeatedly found that there is a greater negative impact on children whose parents have co-morbid disorders and personality disorders, compared to children whose parents have single disorders (21). Comorbid mental disorders in a parent may lead to larger and more long-lasting functional impairments, poorer prognosis and treatment complications (22, 23). Brennan et al. (24) found that children of depressed mothers were at greater risk of developing behavioral problems if the depression was severe, and that severity had a significant relationship to aspects of the children's language development. Although there are several risk factors related to parent's psychopathology, some COPMI are very resilient and are not impacted adversely. To our knowledge, no systematic reviews or meta-analyses have been conducted to quantify resiliency factors, but qualities of child personality and temperament, quality of attachment between the child and primary caregivers, as well as social support in the family and social network, is believed to buffer against adverse outcomes for COPMI.

It seems evident that the child's age is an important factor contributing to the outcomes for children at risk, and that younger children are at higher risk. For 1- and 2-years old children, depression in parents has been associated with impaired cognitive development, more behavioral problems, lower IQ scores in late childhood, as well as elevated rates of affective disorders in adolescence (8, 25).

The family is the core arena of development for children. However, the family situation for COPMI may be characterized by family conflicts, violence and negative life events (17, 26). Research findings have shown that children from conflict-ridden families were viewed less favorably by their peers and had fewer friends (26). In addition, COPMI often have care responsibilities in the household that exceed their emotional and cognitive maturity (27). Therefore, the risk for negative outcomes may be higher for children who live alone with one parent with mental illnesses, compared with those who live with both one parent with a mental illness and one healthy parent. Studies have found that single parents report having more mental health problems and behavioral problems compared with married parents (28). In contrast, the presence of a supportive and caring parent who understands the suffering of the ill parent can act as a buffer against negative child developmental outcomes related to depression in the mother (29).

Social and emotional ties to people outside the family can also moderate the effect of mental illness in parents (30), and the children's social network therefore plays a major protective role. Children benefit from having access to stable, non-familial trusted adults, such as teachers and other educational staff, as well as other adults in the child or parents' social support network and friends (31, 32).

Though impaired parenting as a result of parental psychopathology is a very potent risk factor for the development of emotional and behavioral problems in children, especially in early childhood, key parental functions are also modifiable (15, 16). Siegenthaler et al. (4) reported that family-focused interventions reduced children's risk of acquiring their own mental health problems by 40%. Another recent systematic review and meta-analysis reported small, but significant and lasting effects related to interventions for mothers and infants, as well as for children and adolescents themselves (20). Psycho-education is a common component across programs for COPMI and their families (33). The aim of such efforts is often to strengthen children's knowledge of the parent's psychopathology, as well as to reduce feelings of guilt and shame related to parental psychopathology. In general, research gives some indications that most parents do not speak with their children about mental illness. For example, a British survey showed that 55% of parents without mental illnesses and with children aged 6 to 18 did not talk with their children about mental illnesses.[1] For COPMI, who are exposed to parental mental health symptoms on a daily basis, mental health literacy tend to be low (34), and they do not have access to accurate, non-stigmatized information about mental health disorders and treatments (35). Many COPMI do not seek help, neither from health care providers nor in their own network (36, 37). However, interviews of COPMI indicate that they want to be recognized as full-fledged members of the family by their parent's treatment providers, and to participate in the parent's therapeutic process to gain knowledge about the parent's illness and how to deal with it (36, 38). Many parents

[1] Warren E. New Survey Shows That Mental Health is a "Nonversation" for Parents (2015). Available online at: http://www.time-to-change.org.uk/news/new-survey-shows-mental-health-%E2%80%98nonversation%E2%80%99-parents-0

with mental illness are also concerned about the effects their mental illness may have on their children. They often want help, advice and guidance about how to talk to their children about their troubles.

In spite of this, COPMI receive little attention within mainstream mental health services (1, 34). In Norway, systematic routines for identifying these children did not exist until a few years ago (39). Based on knowledge about the transmission of mental disorders across generations, Norwegian authorities adopted amendments to the Health Personnel Act and Specialized Health Services Act in 2010. These provisions require health personnel in adult mental health services to identify and fulfill the needs of COPMI. It has taken time to implement these legal amendments, and they have thus far not led to satisfactory changes in clinical practice (40, 41). One study showed that 56% of health personnel at a large Norwegian university hospital did not identify patients' children (39), and a 5-years follow-up study showed that 28% of the health personnel in the same clinic still did not identify patients' minor children (42). Another recent Norwegian study showed that only 17% of patients in two psychiatric hospitals were assessed completely with family assessment forms (43). These results indicate that although the law requires identification of COPMI and provision of support in Norway, there has not been sufficient systematic work around implementing new clinical practice related to this issue in adult mental health care. Similar findings were reported in a study from adult mental health services in New Zealand (44).

The lack of identification of COPMI has large implications for public health as it is a core prerequisite to intervene in the high risk group of COPMI. Routine identification of COPMI in adult mental health services will provide necessary information about the children, their family situation and needs, and hence form the basis for provision of necessary family support and necessary professional collaboration across services and service levels in the municipalities where the family lives.

THE NORWEGIAN COPMI PROJECT—THE PRESENT STUDY

The COPMI project is a longitudinal research project in which the goal was to support the implementation of new routines arising from legislative amendments, as well as to evaluate the process of change (45). The project started in 2010, and involves a long-term strategy for changing clinical practice. The clinic initiated new procedures to identify COPMI by the use of *Family Assessment*. The *Family Assessment* form is an intervention for treatment providers to increase the identification of patients' minor children. The form consists of questions that the health personnel were required to collect as a result of legislative changes.

The main objective of the present study was to identify the children and basic life circumstances related to child development in families where the parent has a mental disorder, as well as to discuss how this information may be utilized to plan and strengthen professional collaboration in the provision of relevant support for COPMI.

These research questions were investigated:

(a) What are the demographic (gender, marital status, total number of children), and illness characteristics of the patients?
(b) What characterizes the children's gender, age, number of siblings, day care, and living arrangements, as well as the knowledge provided to them about parental mental illness and access to social supports?
(c) What is the relation between parent's diagnosis and disorder severity, and where the children live?
(d) Which factors influence whether or not the children get information about their parent's psychopathology?

METHODS

Participants

The participants were 422 parents with mental disorders who received treatment at a clinic for psychiatric disorders and substance abuse at the University Hospital of North Norway (UNN). If the parent had more than one child, one assessment form per child was filled out. A total of 581 minor children were assessed.

Data Material

The data consisted of information gathered by health personnel by using an adapted version of the information form "Family Assessment" (45). This is a standardized information form, designed to gather information about the child's gender, age, siblings, parental access, residence, and other caregivers who cared for the child during the parent's illness, as well as where the child was during the day and whether the child had received information about the parent's psychopathology. The form contained two questions about whether or not the children had been given information about the parent's treatment/hospitalization and the parent's condition. The response options for these questions were "yes," "partially," and "no." In addition, ordinary electronic patient journals were assessed to gather information on the patient's gender, marital status, the total number of children, and diagnoses.

Procedure

The information form was implemented as a compulsory routine for all staff in the participating departments and it was integrated in the electronic patient record. Under Norwegian law, collecting this information does not require consent.

The treatment provider filled in the information form in the electronic patient record during the conversation with the parent about the children. The treatment providers were psychologists, specialist psychologists, clinical social workers, clinical social educators, nurses, psychiatric nurses, activity therapists, doctors, psychiatrists, and social workers.

Analysis

All analyses were performed using IBM SPSS Statistics 24. Descriptive frequency analyses were used to describe the sample. A chi-squared test was used to evaluate the relation between the parent's gender, whether the child lived alone with a parent with a mental illness or addiction, who cared for the child during any hospitalization, and whether the child had received information about the parent's illness. A chi-squared test was also used to look at the relationship between family composition and whether the child had other adult resource persons (i.e., the mentally healthy parent, a step parent, teachers, relatives, family friends, and/or neighbors).

Multivariate hierarchical logistic regression analyses were conducted to investigate the odds of having received information about the mental condition of the parent or about the parent being in treatment for children who lived with a single parent with a mental illness compared to other children. Multivariate hierarchical logistic regression analyses were also conducted to examine the relationships between information provided (about the mental condition and treatment), and the children's age, gender, and parental diagnosis. Interaction effects between the parental diagnosis and child age and gender were tested.

In order to compare whether the parent's diagnoses were connected to the various dependent variables (information about the disorder, receiving health care, living arrangements) in logistic regression analyses, the diagnosis variable was re-coded into dummy variables. Diagnoses that belonged to the same chapter in ICD-10 (46) were coded into the same dummy variables. Diagnostic categories with $n < 15$ were excluded in these analyses. This was true for F00–F09 Organic, including symptomatic, mental disorders ($n = 5$), F50–F59 Behavioral syndromes associated with physiological disturbances and physical factors ($n = 5$), F70–F79 Mental retardation ($n = 1$), F80–F89 Disorders of psychological development ($n = 0$), F99 Unspecified mental disorder ($n = 0$), F90–F98 Behavioral and emotional disorders with onset usually occurring in childhood and adolescence ($n = 14$), and R-/Z diagnoses ($n = 11$). In a regression analysis where the children's age was one of the variables, age was categorized in groups. In order to use the variables "has your child received information about your condition?" and "has your child received information about your health care/hospitalization?" as independent variables in a binary logistic regression, these were coded as dichotomous variables, where the response option "partially" was coded as "yes."

The parents' primary diagnoses were categorized by their presumed severity. However, the distinction between serious and milder mental disorders is not firmly established in the discipline. The data set also did not contain information about daily functioning. The divisions used by Kessler et al. (22) was therefore adopted for this purpose, but without the functional goals. The diagnosis was coded as serious if it fulfilled one of the following criteria; assumed disability or significant limitations as a result of illness, drug addiction or if the disorder typically leads to 30 or more days per year in which the person is not able to maintain their roles socially, in the household, as an employee or as a partner. The diagnosis was coded as moderate if it did not meet any of the above criteria, but was considered to have a moderate impact on the aforementioned roles. All other disorders were classified as mild.

Logistic regression was used to examine the relationship between diagnoses and whether or not the child had received information about the parent's treatment and condition. To be able to compare the odds that the child had received information depending on the type of diagnosis, the diagnosis variable was recoded into dummy variables. Diagnoses that belonged to the same chapter in ICD-10 were coded in the same dummy variable, and diagnostic categories with $n < 15$ were excluded in these analyses.

RESULTS

Characteristics of the Parents/Patients

Gender

The sample ($N = 422$) consisted of 286 mothers (67.7%) and 136 fathers (32.3%). The proportion of mothers was significantly larger than the proportion of fathers ($p < 0.001$).

Marital Status

The Family Assessment Form did not distinguish between being married or cohabiting. A total of 105 parents (43.4%,) reported to be married or living together with the other parent, 25 parents (10.3%) were married or living together with the child's step-parent, and 112 parents (46.3%) were single. Information about marital status was provided for 242 parents (57.3%), while for 180 parents (42.7%) information was missing.

Number of Children

Parents ($N = 402$) had between one and seven children ($M = 2.24$; $SD = 1.02$), whereas eight (1.9%) replied that they were expecting children.

The Parents' Diagnoses

The majority of parents had one diagnosis ($n = 311$, 73.7%), and some had two diagnoses ($n = 70$, 16.6%). A small proportion of parents had three diagnoses ($n = 21$; 5.0%), while few had no diagnosis ($n = 20$, 4.7%). The most commonly occurring diagnosis type were mood disorders ($n = 190$, 45%). Individually, the three most common diagnoses were F32.1 Moderate depressive episode ($n = 60$, 10.3%), F33.1 Recurrent depressive disorder, current episode moderate ($n = 53$, 9.1%) and F43.1 Post-traumatic stress disorder ($n = 31$, 5.3%).

Severity of Mental Illness

The largest proportion of parents in the sample had serious mental disorders ($n = 185$; 46.0%), followed by parents with disorders of moderate severity ($n = 156$; 38.8%). Mild mental disorders were the least common ($n = 61$; 15.2%).

Characteristics of COPMI

Gender

The sample consisted of 290 (52.4%) boys and 263 (47.6%) girls. Information on gender was missing for 28 of the children (4.8%).

Age

The children's ages ($N = 543$) were evenly distributed from 0 to 17 years (**Table 1**). The average age was 8.6 years (SD = 4.97). A total of 76 children (14%) were below the age of 2 years old.

TABLE 1 | Child age.

Child age	N	%
1–12 months	24	4.4
1 year	30	5.5
2 years	22	4.1
3 years	30	4.4
4 years	33	6.1
5 years	32	5.9
6 years	22	4.1
7 years	43	7.9
8 years	34	6.3
9 years	20	3.7
10 years	33	6.1
11 years	37	6.8
12 years	39	7.2
13 years	34	6.3
14 years	32	5.9
15 years	25	4.6
16 years	31	5.7
17 years	22	4.1
Total	543	100
Age missing	39	6.7

TABLE 2 | Caregivers when mother/father is receiving treatment/hospitalized.

Caregiver	N	%
Mother	128	29.8
Father	180	41.9
Grandparent/s	24	5.6
Other family member/s	22	5.1
Fosterparent/s	20	4.7
Emergency placement	9	2.1
Stepparent	9	2.1
Friends/others	4	0.9
Child lives alone	3	0.7
Not applicable	31	7.2
Missing	149	25.6

Siblings

A total of 432 children (74.6%) had one or more siblings ($M = 1.25$; $SD = 1.04$), and 382 children (66.0%) had one or more siblings under the age of 18, whereas 93 children (16.1%) had one or more siblings above the age of 18. A total of 147 children (25.4%) had no siblings.

Custody For the Child

A total of 186 children (38.9%) lived with both parents, whereas 83 children lived with each parent in a 50–50% manner. A total of 146 children (30.5%) lived with their mother, and 29 (6.1%) with their father.

Access to Adult Resource Persons

Most parents stated that their children had access to adult resource persons other than the mentally ill parent (n = 424, 94%). A total of 6% of the children (n = 27) did not have this. A chi-squared test was used to see if there was a relationship between being a single parent with a mental illness and whether or not the children had other adult resource persons. The results showed that there was no significant difference; children who lived with a single parent with a mental illness were just as likely to have other close adults as children in homes with two parents, step-parents or other adults.

Care For the Child When the Mother/Father Is in Treatment/Hospitalized

In sum, one or both the parents cared for the child (n = 308; 71.7%) when one of them received treatment/was hospitalized (**Table 2**). The majority of the remaining children were taken care of by other family members. If the father was in treatment/hospitalized, the child's mother cared for the child in 88.8% of the cases, whereas if the mother was hospitalized, the child's father cared for the child in 62.7% of the cases, which was a significant difference ($\chi^2(2, N = 430) = 31.348, p < 0.01$). Children with mentally ill mothers were more likely to be cared for by grandparents, stepparents and other family members (17.1%) than children with mentally ill fathers were (4.2%).

Children Living With Mentally Ill Parent

About three quarters of the children in the sample (76.2%, n = 526) were living with the mentally ill parent. If the patient was the father, a bigger proportion of the children did not live with him (47.3%) than if the patient was the mother (12.6%).

Children Living With a Single Parent With a Mental Illness

A total of 170 of the children (32.5%) lived with a single parent with a mental illness and any siblings, either all the time (n = 91, 17.3%) or part of the time (n = 80, 15.2%). A greater percentage of the children with a mentally ill mother lived alone with her and any siblings, as compared to the children with a mentally ill father, and this difference was significant ($\chi^2(2, N = 526) = 44.547, p < 0.001$).

Children Living Outside the Home

A total of 45 children (7.8%) lived with neither their mother nor their father. The majority of these children either lived in a foster home (n = 21; 46.7%) or in an emergency placement home (n = 9; 20%). The other children (n = 15; 33.3%) lived with grandparents or siblings of the parents.

School and Day Care

Most of the children were at school (n = 304, 67.6%) or in kindergarten (n = 119, 26.4%) during the day. The others were at home (n = 23, 5.1%), in an emergency placement home (n = 3, 0.5%) or in a youth home (n = 1, 0.2%). Among the children who were at home during the day, 14 were under the age of 2 years.

Parent's Diagnosis and Disorder Severity, and Its Relation to Where the Child Lives

Parent's Diagnosis

Logistic regression showed that F10–F19 *Mental and behavioral disorders due to psychoactive substance use* was the only significant diagnostic category that could predict children's living conditions, and the odds that the child *did not* live with the parent was higher for parents with diagnoses in this category ($n = 44$; OR $= 8.7$; $p < 0.001$).

Diagnosis Severity

Logistic regression also showed that the odds that the child did *not* live with the parent was 3.3 times higher for the most severe mental disorders ($p < 0.001$) compared to mild disorders.

Factors That Affect Whether Children or Not Children Are Informed About the Parent's Treatment/Hospitalization and Condition

The parents of a total of 67.8% of children ($N = 395$) were asked "*Does your child know that you receive treatment/does your child know that you are hospitalized*?" Of these, a total of 54.9% ($n = 217$) responded "yes," 6.8% ($n = 27$) answered "partially," and 38.2% ($n = 151$) replied "no."

The question "*Has your child received information about your condition?*" was answered by the parents of a total of 61.6% of the children ($N = 359$). Of these, a total of 44% ($n = 158$) responded "yes," 14.5% ($n = 52$) answered "partially," and 41.5% ($n = 149$) replied "no."

Family Composition

Children who lived with a single parent with a mental illness were more likely to receive information than the children living with both parents. The results from a hierarchical logistic regression showed that if the child lived with a single parent with a mental illness, the odds that the child had been given information about both treatment/hospitalization (**Table 3**) and the condition (**Table 4**) were higher. An analysis of whether there were interaction effects between the parent's gender and marital status in how much information the child received, showed no such interaction.

TABLE 3 | Relation between information provided for the child about parent's treatment/hospitalization and whether the child lives with a single mentally ill parent or not.

	$X^2(2) = 12{,}225, p = < 0.002$		
	OR[a] [95% CI[b]]	Wald	*p*
Part time	1.93 [1.05, 3.56]	4.43	0.035**
Yes	2.55 [1.36, 4.78]	8.60	0.003*

[a]*Odds ratio.*
[b]*Confidence interval.*
**Significant at 0.01 level.*
***Significant at 0.05 level.*

Logistic regression was used to examine the relationship between the information provided and the children's age. The odds that parents had informed their children about the treatment/hospitalization (**Table 5**) and condition (**Table 6**) was higher for each age group ($p < 0.001$); The odds of 15–17-years-olds having received information about the treatment/hospitalization was 43.77 times higher than for 0–2-years-olds, and the odds that they had received information about the condition was 47.78 times higher.

TABLE 4 | Relation between information provided for the child about parent's condition and whether the child lives with a single mentally ill parent or not.

	$X^2(2) = 12{,}663, p = < 0.002$		
	OR[a] [95% CI[b]]	Wald	*p*
Part time	1.73 [0.92, 3.29]	2.88	0.090
Yes	2.87 [1.50, 5.50]	10.13	0.001*

[a]*Odds ratio.*
[b]*Confidence interval.*
**Significant at 0.01 level.*

TABLE 5 | Relation between information provided for the child about parent's treatment/hospitalization and child age.

	$X^2(5) = 96.128, p = < 0.001$		
Child age	OR[a] [95% CI[b]]	Wald	*p*
3–5	5.06 [1.97, 12.98]	11.37	0.001*
6–8	7.93 [3.14, 20.02]	19.19	0.000*
9–11	13.51 [5.19, 35.22]	28.39	0.000*
12–14	29.77 [10.98, 80.70]	44.48	0.000*
15–17	43.77 [14.73, 130.03]	46.27	0.000*

[a]*Odds ratio.*
[b]*Confidence interval.*
**Significant at 0.01 level.*

TABLE 6 | Relation between information provided for the child about parent's condition and child age.

	$X^2(5) = 95.446, p = < 0.001$		
Child age	OR[a] [95% CI[b]]	Wald	*p*
3–5	4.46 [1.51, 13.14]	7.34	0.007**
6–8	9.62 [3.37, 27.44]	17.92	0.000*
9–11	13.37 [4.56, 39.19]	22.34	0.000*
12–14	39.00 [12.75, 119.35]	41.22	0.000*
15–17	47.78 [14.48, 157.65]	40.29	0.000*

[a]*Odds ratio.*
[b]*Confidence interval.*
**Significant at 0.01 level.*
***Significant at 0.05 level.*

TABLE 7 | Relation between information provided for the child about parent's health condition and parent's diagnosis.

		$X^2(5) = 18{,}665, p = 0.002$*		
	N	OR[a] [95% CI[b]]	Wald	*P*
F10–F19 Mental and behavioral disorders due to psychoactive substance use	44	2.56 [0.82, 7.97]	2.62	0.106
F20–F29 Schizophrenia, schizotypal and delusional disorders	59	8.31 [2.75, 25.09]	14.09	0.000
F30–F39 Mood [affective] disorders	268	3.70 [1.62, 8.44]	9.63	0.002
F40–F48 Neurotic, stress-related and somatoform disorders	121	4.62 [1.86, 11.45]	10.93	0.001
F60–F69 Disorders of adult personality and behavior	25	3.65 [1.06, 12.56]	4.22	0.040

[a] *Odds ratio.*
[b] *Confidence interval.*
**Significant at 0.005 level.*

Children's Gender

There were no significant differences between boys and girls in how much information they had received about the parent's treatment/hospitalization and condition.

Parent's Gender

Results from a chi-squared test showed differences between children with mentally ill mothers and children with mentally ill fathers in terms of how much information they had received about the parental illness. There were significant differences based on the parent's gender in how much information the child had received about the treatment/hospitalization (χ^2(2, N = 316) = 8.606, $p < 0.05$). There were also significant differences in whether or not they had received information about the parent's condition (χ^2(2, N = 349) = 10.015, $p < 0.01$). For both variables, the children of mentally ill mothers were more likely to have received information compared to children of mentally ill fathers.

Parent's Diagnosis

The odds ratio that the child received information about the parent *treatment/hospitalization* were highest if the parents had diagnoses from the categories F20–F29 Schizophrenia, schizotypal and delusional disorders (OR = 2.8; $p > 0.05$) (**Table 7**), and F60–F69 Disorders of adult personality and behavior (OR = 3.2; $p = 0.08$). For the diagnostic category F10–F19 Mental and behavioral disorders due to psychoactive substance use, the odds of information being given were nearly halved (OR = 0.5; $p = 0.22$).

The odds ratio that the child received information about the parent's *condition* were highest when the diagnosis fell within F20–F29 Schizophrenia, schizotypal and delusional disorders (OR = 8.3; $p = < 0.0005$) (**Table 8**).

Diagnosis Severity

A multivariate hierarchical logistic regression was used to examine the relationship between the severity of the parent's

TABLE 8 | Relation between information provided for the child about severity of parent's diagnose, child age, child gender and parent's treatment/hospitalization.

	Model 1			Model 2			Model 3			Model 4		
	$X^2(2) = 3.510, p = 0.173$			$X^2(4) = 83.096, p < 0.001$			$X^2(6) = 85.323, p < 0.001$			$X^2(8) = 87.086, p < 0.001$		
	OR[a] [95% CI[b]]	Wald	*p*	OR [95% CI]	Wald	*p*	OR [95% CI]	Wald	*p*	OR [95% CI]	Wald	*p*
Severity: Mild	Reference group											
Severity: Moderate	1.40 [0.74, 2.65]	1.06	0.303	1.51 [0.740, 3.10]	1.28	0.257	0.48 [0.08, 2.72]	0.70	0.404	0.75 [0.10, 5.65]	0.08	0.781
Severity: Severe	1.81 [0.95, 3.45]	3.27	0.071	1.56 [0.85, 3.59]	2.29	0.130	0.99 [0.1, 5.50]	0.00	0.992	1.83 [0.25, 13.51]	0.35	0.553
Child age				1.92 [1.64, 2.25]	63.75	0.000	1.56 [1.05, 2.30]	4.94	0.026	1.60 [1.07, 2.39]	5.29	0.022
Child gender (1 = boy)				1.00 [0.62, 1.61]	0.00	0.998		0.00	0.967	1.93 [0.57, 6.52]	1.12	0.290
Mild*age								2.23	0.327		1.92	0.384
Moderate*age							1.41 [0.88, 2.26]	2.04	0.153	1.37 [0.85, 2.22]	1.66	0.198
Severe*age							1.18 [0.75, 1.85]	0.49	0.486	1.15 [0.72, 1.82]	0.33	0.567
Mild*gender											1.73	0.420
Moderate*gender										0.53 [0.13, 2.21]	0.76	0.385
Severe*gender										0.39 [0.09, 1.60]	1.72	0.190

[a] *Odds ratio.*
[b] *Confidence interval.*

diagnosis (mild, moderate, severe), the child's age and gender, and whether the child had been given information about the treatment/hospitalization (**Table 9**) and the parent's condition (**Table 10**). In the first model, the severity of the diagnosis was added alone, while in model 2 the child's gender and age were added. In the last model, the interaction effects were also examined. The interaction effects were examined in individual analyses. The odds that someone had informed their children about their treatment/hospitalization was greater the more serious the diagnosis was, but this difference was not significant. The odds that someone had informed their children about the parent's condition were also greater the more serious the diagnosis was, but this difference was not significant.

Model 2 shows that the child's age could predict whether the child received information or not, which was also shown in the results of the *t*-test, but no interaction effect was found between diagnosis severity and age of the child (Model 3). The child's gender did not affect the information the child received, and there was no interaction effect between diagnosis severity and the child's gender when it came to whether or not the child had been given information about the parent's treatment/hospitalization or condition.

DISCUSSION

Characteristics of the Patient/Parents

Parenting is challenging in itself, and a large number of studies indicate that parents with mental illnesses struggle more with parenting than parents who does not experience mental illness (16, 47). Nearly half of the patients in this study were single, and this may result in both a greater scope of problems in the parent (28), lower SES (48), and possibly an increased risk of the children developing mental disorders (49). In addition to their parent's mental illness, children who also have been through a divorce between their parents may have experienced a stressful and risk-enhancing transition in their family life, because of conflicts, moving and breaks in family relationships (50).

The largest proportion of the parents with mental illnesses were mothers, which is consistent with findings showing that more women than men seek help for mental health problems (51). Mood disorders, such as different forms of depression were most common in the sample, and the diagnosis F33 Major depressive disorder (recurrent), recurrent, was listed as the second most common illness. Recurrent and chronic disorders have been shown to lead to higher risks for COPMI (52, 53).

Most parents in our study had serious psychiatric disorders, which add to the high risk in these patients' children, as several studies have found a significant relationship between severity and chronicity of the parent's mental illness and the risk of negative outcomes in their children (3). In addition, mental disorders of moderate severity may lead to significant functional decline (2) and develop into more serious disorders over time.

The implications of the findings regarding the patients in this study is that the majority of patients are characterized by factors that predict high risk for their offspring. Therefore, health professionals in the clinic need to implement family support to reduce these risks and prevent developmental problems in

TABLE 9 | Relation between information provided for the child about severity of parent's diagnose, child age, child gender and parent's health condition.

	Model 1			Model 2			Model 3			Model 4		
	$X^2(2) = 5.246, p = 0.073$			$X^2(4) = 88.778, p < 0.001$			$X^2(6) = 92.552, p < 0.001$			$X^2(8) = 95.957, p < 0.001$		
	OR[a] [95% CI[b]]	Wald	*p*	OR [95% CI]	Wald	*p*	OR [95% CI]	Wald	*p*	OR [95% CI]	Wald	*p*
Severity: Mild	Reference group											
Severity: Moderate	1.50 [0.77, 2.91]	1.41	0.235	1.50 [0.70, 3.19]	1.08	0.300	0.29 [0.05, 1.75]	1.83	0.176	0.27 [0.04, 2.01]	1.63	0.202
Severity: Severe	2.12 [1.08, 4.15]	4.75	0.029	1.94 [0.90, 4.19]	2.88	0.090	0.47 [0.08, 2.83]	0.68	0.410	0.69 [0.10, 4.93]	0.14	0.712
Child age				2.05 [1.72, 2.45]	64.36	0.000	1.42 [0.96, 2.10]	3.01	0.083	1.42 [0.96, 2.11]	3.03	0.082
Child gender (1 = boy)				0.97 [0.59, 1.60]	0.02	0.904	0.96 [0.58, 1.60]	0.02	0.880	1.25 [0.37, 4.22]	0.13	0.714
Mild*age								4.06	0.131		4.18	0.123
Moderate*age							1.62 [1.00, 2.63]	3.79	0.052	1.62 [1.00, 2.64]	3.78	0.052
Severe*age							1.51 [0.93, 2.45]	2.82	0.093	1.55 [0.95, 2.52]	3.08	0.079
Mild*gender											0.05	0.188
Moderate*gender										1.19 [0.28, 5.02]	1.31	0.817
Severe*gender										0.43 [0.10, 1.84]	2.81	0.253

[a] *Odds ratio.*
[b] *Confidence interval.*

TABLE 10 | Relation between information provided for the child about severity of parent's condition, child age, child gender.

	Model 1			Model 2			Model 3			Model 4		
	$X^2(2) = 5.246, p = 0.073$			$X^2(4) = 88.778, p < 0.001$			$X^2(6) = 92.552, p < 0.001$			$X^2(8) = 95.957, p < 0.001$		
	OR[a] [95% CI[b]]	Wald	*p*	OR [95% CI]	Wald	*p*	OR [95% CI]	Wald	*p*	OR [95% CI]	Wald	*p*
Severity: Mild	Reference group											
Severity: Moderate	1.50 [0.77, 2.91]	1.41	0.235	1.50 [0.70, 3.19]	1.08	0.300	0.29 [0.05, 1.75]	1.83	0.176	0.27 [0.04, 2.01]	1.63	0.202
Severity: Severe	2.12 [1.08, 4.15]	4.75	0.029	1.94 [0.90, 4.19]	2.88	0.090	0.47 [0.08, 2.83]	0.68	0.410	0.69 [0.10, 4.93]	0.14	0.712
Child age				2.05 [1.72, 2.45]	64.36	0.000	1.42 [0.96, 2.10]	3.01	0.083	1.42 [0.96, 2.11]	3.03	0.082
Child gender (1 = boy)				0.97 [0.59, 1.60]	0.02	0.904	0.96 [0.58, 1.60]	0.02	0.880	1.25 [0.37, 4.22]	0.13	0.714
Mild*age								4.06	0.131		4.18	0.123
Moderate*age							1.62 [1.00, 2.63]	3.79	0.052	1.62 [1.00, 2.64]	3.78	0.052
Severe*age							1.51 [0.93, 2.45]	2.82	0.093	1.55 [0.95, 2.52]	3.08	0.079
Mild*gender											0.05	0.188
Moderate*gender										1.19 [0.28, 5.02]	1.31	0.817
Severe*gender										0.43 [0.10, 1.84]	2.81	0.253

[a]*Odds ratio.*
[b]*Confidence interval.*

the COPMI. Specifically, there is need for interventions which can be tailored to single parents with moderate to severe mood disorders, as well as recurrent disorders. The finding that parents with mental and behavioral disorders due to psychoactive substance use are less likely to have their children at home, also emphasize the need for interventions that suit these families' needs. It seems evident that these parents and their children need support to communicate and engage with each other in safe ways, as well as support if they are moving together again.

The Characteristics of the Children and Their Living Circumstances

One third of the children in this study were 0–5 years old, one third were 7–11 years old and one third were 12–18 years old. Fourteen percent of them were 2 years or younger, and as such within the 1,001 critical days defined by the well-known manifesto "The Importance of the Conception to Age Two Period" from the UK.[2] This manifesto, and others of its kind, highlights the importance of intervening early to enhance the outcomes for children at risk, and this is also a key objective for the development and implementation of interventions in Norway.

It seems fair to assume that most of the children under six in our study probably do not need outpatient help for their own psychological problems yet. However, unless they are identified and can access necessary support and preventive measures by health professionals treating the parent, only some of those who develop social and emotional problems themselves will be reached at a later point in life, and only after the problems have escalated to the point where the child needs to be referred to the specialist health service. This is demonstrated by the national figures for children who receive treatment in Child and adolescent mental health services (CAMHS), where <7% of patients are boys under 7 years, and <5% are girls below the age of seven. Less than 1% of patients in Norwegian CAMHS are under 4 years of age.

At the same time as the youngest children largely do not receive treatment by the mental health services for children and young people, they are especially vulnerable developmentally. Once problems have emerged, they have the worst prognosis and there are relatively few documented effective interventions and measures designed for this age group (4). In this study, no information was collected about how old the child was when the parent's illness was presented. However, recurrent depression was a common disorder in the sample, and for the youngest children, it is therefore reasonable to assume that a large part of their childhood had been affected by the parent's illness. In addition to this, a large majority of COPMI in the present study lived with the ill parent alone, either all the time or part time. As depression is a prevalent disorder in general psychiatric clinics, and has a documented negative effect on parent-child interaction (25), especially for the very youngest (17), feasible interventions for depressed parents of very young children should be a priority in general psychiatric clinics in

[2]Durkan M, Field F, Lamb N, Loughton T. (2016). Available online at: https://www.1001criticaldays.co.uk/sites/default/files/1001%20days_oct16_1st.pdf

Norway. Collaboration between health personnel in adult mental health services and public nurses in local health clinics, as well as preschool teachers in kindergartens seems especially valuable for this group of children.

Positive social bonds between siblings are an important source of protection for children who undergo stressful life events (54). The majority of our sample had one or more siblings. Sibling bonds can be considered especially beneficial for COPMI with siblings who are older than 18 (16.1% in our sample), where the sister or brother can function as a supporting adult (55). At the same time, dysfunctional sibling bonds, which are not uncommon in families with mental illness, may be a burden and can predict a subsequent psychopathology for COPMI (56). This suggests that sibling relationships between COPMI should also be assessed in mental health services for adults. In our sample, 7.5% of the parents had four or more children, and account must be taken of the negative impact that a larger number of children can have on the family economy, thus contributing to the socio-economic risk (57), as well as the increase in parental burden and need for relevant support for patients with more children. Labor and Welfare Services should be a natural collaboration partner for health personnel in adult mental health services in these regards.

The majority of the children had access to adult resource persons other than the parent with mental illness or addictions. It was usually the other parent or extended family who cared for the child when the parent with a mental illness was hospitalized. In addition, most of the children were at school or in kindergarten during the day. Only a small proportion of the children in the sample were at home during the day (5.1%). These findings emphasize how important the extended family, and personnel in kindergartens and schools are as significant others who may support the child's development. However, the provision of necessary information about the risks and protective factors relevant for each COPMI is crucial to motivate and engage the resources that significant others may contribute with. Child protection services (CPS) may intervene in those families where the children do not have access to resource persons beside the mentally ill parent. However, in a recent study we found that personnel in adult mental health services was reluctant to refer families of concern to the CPS (58). In Norway around 80% of the activity in public child protection services constitutes of preventive and compensating interventions. Examples of such interventions are economic support, practical support for parents and children in the home and related to leisure time activities, visitation homes, as well as parent training interventions offering supervision and guidance for parents in need of professional help to change their parenting practices. Barriers to inter-service collaboration based on lack of knowledge about the CPS in adult mental health services has serious consequences for families in need of support and for dissemination of interventions in the communities they live. Results from our research indicate that there is an unresolved potential for inter-service collaboration involving the children of patients with mental health problems. There is a large potential for improvement in the collaboration between adult mental health services and community services for children and their families in Norway.

COPMI's Family Status and Factors Influencing Their Living Arrangements

Several factors were found that had an impact on the children's living arrangements and factors that led to an increased chance that the child did *not* live with the mentally ill parent were: (1) that the parent had serious mental illness, as compared with mild mental illness, (2) that the parent had an addictive disorder, and (3) that the ill parent was the father.

The severity of the diagnosis was a strong predictor and the odds were three times as high that a child did not live with a parent with a serious mental disorder compared to those with mild mental disorders. This is not a surprising finding, as the more serious mental disorders often lead to higher symptom pressure and malfunction, which to a greater extent leads to a risk of negative outcomes for the child. However, about three quarters of the children in our sample lived with the parent with a mental illness, and one third of them lived alone with this parent all the time or part time. These children will be more vulnerable and at a higher risk for developing mental disorders, as compared with those who also lived with a healthy parent (28).

The COPMI whose parents had addictive disorders were distinct from other COPMI, as their odds of not living with the ill parent were many times higher than for the children of parents whose primary diagnose were from the other categories. This was irrespective of the parent's gender. The reason why families and/or professional helpers choose to move children away from addictive parents is probably associated with substance abuse leading to risk in several different areas, in terms of a problematic social network, crime, physical and mental health problems, impulsive absences from the home, financial problems, on top of challenges with interactions when intoxicated.

About half of the children of mentally ill fathers lived with their fathers, while nearly nine out of ten children of mentally ill mothers lived with their mothers. The majority of children who lived with a single parent with a mental illness lived with their mother. In Norway, most children stay with their mother after a divorce between their parents (59), and it is therefore not possible to say whether it is the break-up or the father's illness that explains this. On the other hand, a previous study showed that mental disorders in fathers may reduce the involvement they have with their children (47). Taken together, our findings indicate that interventions supporting parents with severe mental disorders and their minor children, especially mothers, should be implemented. Service collaboration between community and specialist services is needed to target each family's needs in their everyday lives.

Factors Influencing Whether or Not COPMI Learn About Their Parent's Illness

Half of the children in the clinic had received information about the parent's condition and treatment/hospitalization. Four of ten COPMI had *not* received information about the parent's illness. This indicates that the ill parent and health care providers to a large degree do not speak with the children about mental disorders in parents. The reasons for this are most likely multifaceted, but nevertheless, researchers have postulated that a lack of information may result in an elevated risk of negative developmental outcomes and may run counter to the children's own wishes, needs and rights (7, 36, 38).

The following factors increased the likelihood that the children received information about the parent's condition and treatment/hospitalization: (1) that the child was living with a single parent with a mental illness, (2) that the child was an older child/teenager, (3) that the mother was the parent with a mental illness, (5) that the parent's primary diagnosis was a severe mental illness, and specifically (6) that the parent's disorder was a personality disorder, schizophrenia, or other psychotic disorder.

If the child lived alone with a single parent with a mental illness, the odds that the child had received information were significantly higher. Children who lived with a single parent at all times had almost three times the odds of receiving information about the parent's illness, as compared to children from two-parent homes and children who primarily lived with the other, healthy parent. This may imply that the parent with a mental illness or other adults realized that the child's opportunity to understand and handle their situation would depend on having information about the health status of their primary caregiver.

There were large age differences related to whether the children received information, and the odds that the children received information were higher for each year they grew older. The oldest children were far more likely to receive information about the treatment/hospitalization and about the parent's condition compared to the youngest children. Intuitively, this can be interpreted as a result of older children understanding more about the parent's illness, and thus to a greater extent taking the initiative to talk about it. However, studies have shown that few COPMI seek help from health care providers or their social network (34, 36), which may explain the fact that many of the older children in fact had not received information. It may also be the case that adults feel safer talking to children about a parent's illness when the children are more mature and have a more developed language. Although it could be expected that children under 2 years had generally not received information, the results showed that it was only from age 10 that more than half of the children had received information about the parent's illness. However, school-aged children have both the verbal and cognitive ability to understand phenomena, such as mental illness and substance abuse disorders and they will have perceived that their parents have problems of this type. Therefore, the finding that many children did not receive information about the parent's illness at all could be interpreted as a reflection of that parents and health care providers do not know how to talk to the youngest children about mental illness.(3) For the youngest children this may be due to a culture where adults (both parents and health care providers) have a desire to protect the younger children from "bad things." However, younger children will also be affected by the parent's psychopathology, sometimes even more than older children since they are more depending of predictable daily routines and sensitive care. Therefore, they will also need information adjusted to their age and maturity to help them understand the parent's symptoms, as well as how these affects parenting and the daily routines in the family. In circumstances when someone other than the parents need to take care of the child, an explanation for this should also be offered to the child.

Children of mentally ill mothers were more likely to receive information than the children of mentally ill fathers. This may be partly explained by children often having closer emotional ties to mothers than to fathers, that mother-daughter relationships often is characterized by emotional closeness and increased communication (60), as well as the fact that more of the children lived with their mother than their fathers.

More serious disorders were associated with a greater probability that the child had received information. This may be because these disorders to a greater extent lead to functional impairments in parents, which increases the negative impact on the child and thus the necessity of the child receiving information about the condition.

Children of parents with personality disorders, schizophrenia, schizotypal disorder and other paranoid disorders, also had higher odds of receiving information. A possible explanation for this may be related to the parents having such significant functional impairments and behaving so differently that it would be difficult to keep information about this from the children. For example, psychoses and delusions may present in ways that are very frightening for children and thus necessitate an explanation earlier than many other types of disorders. Again, substance abuse disorders differed from other diagnosis as it led to lower odds that the child received information. Substance abuse disorders are subject to great social stigma (61), and this may be part of the reason that parents are strongly motivated to hide their disorder from their children. It may also be the case that these parents are more worried about losing custody of their children, compared to parents with other mental disorders, and as such openness would seem counterproductive. The stigma of substance abuse disorders may also explain why personnel in mental health care services do not inform the children. Unfortunately, there are few interventions available for children whose parents have severe mental illnesses in Norwegian municipalities. Such interventions should be adopted from other countries, translated, and adapted to the Norwegian context, or developed locally. All new practices should be evaluated to gain knowledge about effects and feasibility.

Limitations

The most important limitation in this study is that the information is based on parents' reports. Other sources of information, such as interviews with the children themselves, as well as supplementary information from teachers, nurses and other relatives, would have given a more accurate, detailed, and comprehensive picture of the children's situation. However, gathering information in this way was not within the scope of the quality assurance framework in this study.

Another limitation is associated with the analyses. To be able to perform a binary logistic regression where two information to the children variables were included, the response "partially" was coded as "yes." These analyses must therefore include the caveat that "partially" could mean anything from almost no information to quite a bit information. Moreover, the extent to which the categorization of diagnoses according to ICD chapters reflect patients' symptom pressures and daily functioning is uncertain. Additionally, many of the diagnostic categories did not have a sufficiently large selection to be included in the analyses, and were therefore excluded.

The categorization of diagnoses by severity was done in accordance with Kessler et al. (22) categorization. They included separate functional goals in their study, which was not included in this study. The severity categorization was therefore only based on the diagnoses, and no controls was made for the fact that psychiatric disorders and their outcomes represent a spectrum of outcomes rather than exact functional measurements. There may therefore be limited correspondence between the assumed and actual degree of severity.

CONCLUSION AND IMPLICATIONS FOR FUTURE CLINICAL PRACTICE AND RESEARCH

The need for new measures seem to be especially significant for COPMI aged 0–5, as this group seems to be the most invisible, and most vulnerable group, while at the same time having few services offered. The finding that this group also receive the least information about their parent's psychopathology, legitimize significant concern. Norwegian law requires health care providers to attend to the children's need for follow-up, but also to ensure that the children receive the necessary information. The youngest group of COPMI is an important target group for early interventions, according to both national and international manifestos, and measures should therefore be developed to support these children and their parents.

The finding that only half of the children receive information about the parent's psychopathology clearly demonstrates that mental health services for adults must be enabled to comply with current legislation. Close to a third of the children live alone with a mentally ill parent, and thus may not have daily access to an adult who can compensate for the functional impairment the parent suffers in their everyday life at home. These children will need significant others to support their development. Enhancing inter-service collaboration seems crucial to reduce the risk that COPMI will develop social problems and mental health disorders themselves.

Based on the findings in this study, there seems to be a strong cause for concern about the continued transmission of psychiatric disorders from one generation to the next. Parents need support and help to inform their children about their mental health problems, and this is especially important for parents of young children. The findings in this study demonstrate how identifying COPMI and their living arrangements, can inform mental health workers about which type of support and interventions their patients need the most.

ETHICS STATEMENT

The data drawn from electronic patient journals in this study is information which health personnel is required by law to obtain. The Data Protection Officer at the University Hospital of Northern Norway approved the quality evaluation project.

AUTHOR CONTRIBUTIONS

All authors agree to be accountable for the content of the work. CR and CL designed the project. CR collected the data. Analyses were conducted by KR, YS, JF, and CR. CR drafted the article. All authors participated in the writing of the manuscript.

ACKNOWLEDGMENTS

This article is a part of a large study that was initiated, planned and financed by The Regional Center for Child and Youth Mental Health and Child Welfare (RKBU North) at the Faculty of Health Sciences, UiT—Arctic University of Norway. The study was carried out at the University Hospital of Northern Norway (UNN). The publication charges for this article have been funded by a grant from the publication fund of UiT The Arctic University of Norway.

REFERENCES

1. Mayberry D, Reupert AE. The number of parents who are patients attending adult psychiatric services. *Curr Opin Psychiatry* (2018) 31:358–62. doi: 10.1097/YCO.0000000000000427
2. Torvik FA, Rognmo K. *Barn av foreldre med psykiske lidelser eller alkoholmisbruk: omfang og konsekvenser* (Rapport 2011:4). (2011). Available online at: https://www.fhi.no/globalassets/migrering/dokumenter/pdf/rapport-20114-pdf.pdf
3. Leijdesdorff S, van Doesum K, Pomac A, Klaassen R, van Amelsvoort T. Prevalence of psychopathology in children of parents with mental illness and/or addiction: an up to date narrative review. *Curr Opin Psychiatry* (2017) 30:312–7. doi: 10.1097/YCO.0000000000000341
4. Siegenthaler E, Munder T, Egger M. Effect of preventive interventions mentally ill parents on the mental health of the offspring: systematic review and meta-analysis. *J Am Acad Child Adolesc Psychiatry* (2012) 1:8–17. doi: 10.1016/j.jaac.2011.10.018
5. Hameed MA, Lewis AJ. Offspring of parents with schizophrenia: a systematic review of developmental features across childhood. *Harv Rev Psychiatry* (2016) 24:104–17. doi: 10.1097/HRP.0000000000000076
6. Meier SM, Petersen L, Schendel DE, Mattheisen M, Mortensen PB, Mors O. Obsessive-compulsive disorder and autism spectrum disorders: longitudinal and offspring risk. *PLoS ONE* (2015) 10:e0141703. doi: 10.1371/journal.pone.0141703
7. Beardslee WR, Versage EM, Gladstone TR. Children of affectively ill parents: a review of the past 10 years. *J Am Acad Child Adolesc Psychiatry* (1998) 37:1134–41. doi: 10.1097/00004583-199811000-00012
8. Kowalenko NM, Mares SP, Newman LK, Sved Williams AE, Powrie RM, van Doesum KTM. Family matters: infants, toddlers and preschoolers of parents affected by mental illness. *MJA Open* (2012) 1 Suppl. 1:14–7. doi: 10.5694/mjao11.11285

9. Staton-Tindall M, Sprang G, Clark J, Walker R, Craig CD. Caregiver substance use and child outcomes: a systematic review. *J Soc Work Pract Addict.* (2013) 13:26. doi: 10.1080/1533256X.2013.752272
10. van Santvoort F, Hosman CMH, Janssens JMAM, van Doesum KTM, Reupert A, van Loon LMA. The impact of various parental mental disorders on children's diagnoses: a systematic review. *Clin Child Fam Psychol Rev.* (2015) 18:281–99. doi: 10.1007/s10567-015-0191-9
11. Rasic D, Hajek T, Alda M, Uher R. Risk of mental illness in offspring of parents with schizophrenia, bipolar disorder, and major depressive disorder: a metaanalysis of family high-risk studies. *Schizophr Bull.* (2014) 40:28–38. doi: 10.1093/schbul/sbt114
12. Park RJ, Senior R, Stein A. The offspring of mothers with eating disorders. *Eur Child Adolesc Psychiatry* (2003) 12:110–9. doi: 10.1007/s00787-003-1114-8
13. Barnow S, Spitzer C, Grabe HJ, Kessler C, Freyberger HJ. Individual characteristics, familial experience, and psychopathology in children of mothers with borderline personality disorder. *J Am Acad Child Adolesc Psychiatry* (2006) 45:965–72. doi: 10.1097/01.chi.0000222790.41853.b9
14. Bronisch T, Lieb R. Maternal suicidality and suicide risk in offspring. *Psychiatr Clin North Am.* (2008) 2:213–21. doi: 10.1016/j.psc.2008.01.003
15. van Doesum K, Hosman C. Prevention of emotional problems and psychiatric risks in children of mentally ill parents in the Netherlands: II. Interventions. *Aust e-J Adv Mental Health* (2009) 3:264–76. doi: 10.5172/jamh.8.3.264
16. Morawska A, Winter L, Sanders MR. Parenting knowledge and its role in the prediction of dysfunctional parenting and disruptive child behaviour. *Child Care Health Dev.* (2009) 2:217–26. doi: 10.1111/j.1365-2214.2008.00929.x
17. Hosman CMH, van Doesum KTM, van Santvoort F. Prevention of emotional problems and psychiatric risks in children of parents with a mental illness in the Netherlands: the scientific basis to a comprehensive approach. *Aust e-J Adv Mental Health* (2009) 8:250–63. doi: 10.5172/jamh.8.3.250
18. Cicchetti D, Rogosch FA, Toth SL. Maternal depressive disorder andcontextual risk: Contributions to the development of attachment insecurity and behavior problems in toddlerhood. *Dev Psychopathol.* (1998) 2:83–300.
19. Hipwell AE, Goossens FA, Melhuish EC, Kumar R. Severe maternal psychopathology and infant-mother attachment. *Dev Psychopathol.* (2000) 2:157–75. doi: 10.1017/S0954579400002030
20. Thanhaüser M, Lemmer G, de Girolamo G, Christiansen H. Do preventive interventions for children of mentally ill parents work? Results of a systematic review and meta-analysis. *Curr Opin Psychiatry* (2017) 30:283–99. doi: 10.1097/YCO.0000000000000342
21. van Santvoort F, Hosman CMH, van Doesum KTM, Janssens JMAM. Children of mentally ill parents participating in preventive support groups: parental diagnoses and child risk. *J Child Fam Stud.* (2014) 23:67–75. doi: 10.1007/s10826-012-9686-x
22. Kessler R, Berglund P, Demler O, Jin R, Merikangas KR, Walters EE. Lifetime prevalence and age-onset distributions of DSM-IV disorders in the national comorbidity survey reprication. *JAMA Psychiatry Arch Gen Psychiatry.* (2005) 62:593–602. doi: 10.1001/archpsyc.62.6.593
23. Skodol AE, Grilo CM, Keyes KM, Geier T, Grant BF, Hasin DS. Relationship of personality disorders to the course of major depressive disorder in a nationally representative sample. *Am J Psychiatry* (2011) 3:257–64. doi: 10.1176/appi.ajp.2010.10050695
24. Brennan PA, Hammen C, Andersen MJ, Bor W, Najman JM, Williams GM. Chronicity, severity, and timing of maternal depressive symptoms: relationships with child outcomes at age 5. *Dev Psychol.* (2000) 6:759–66. doi: 10.1037/0012-1649.36.6.759
25. van Doesum KT, Riksen-Walraven JM, Hosman CM, Hoefnagels C. A randomized controlled trial of a home-visiting intervention aimed at preventing relationship problems in depressed mothers and their infants. *Child Dev.* (2008) 79:547–61. doi: 10.1111/j.1467-8624.2008.01142.x
26. Criss MM, Pettit GS, Bates JE, Dodge KA, Lapp AL. Family adversity, positive peer relationships, and children's externalizing behavior: a longitudinal perspective on risk and resilience. *Child Dev.* (2003) 4:1220–37. doi: 10.1111/1467-8624.00468
27. Aldridge J. The experiences of children living with and caring for parents with mental illness. *Child Abuse Rev.* (2006) 15:79–88. doi: 10.1002/car.904
28. DeKlyen M, Brooks-Gunn J, McLanahan S, Knab J. The mental health of married, cohabiting, and non-coresident parents with infants. *Am J Public Health* (2006) 96:1836–41. doi: 10.2105/AJPH.2004.049296
29. Chang JJ, Halpern CT, Kaufman JS. Maternal depressive symptoms, father's involvement, and the trajectories of child problem behaviors in a US national sample. *Arch Pediatr Adolesc Med.* (2007) 7:697–703. doi: 10.1001/archpedi.161.7.697
30. Masten AS, Coatsworth J, Douglas E. The development of competence in favorable and unfavorable environments: lessons from research on successful children. *Am Psychol.* (1998) 53:205–20. doi: 10.1037/0003-066X.53.2.205
31. Fudge E, Mason P. Consulting with young people about service guidelines relating to parental mental illness. *Aust e-J Adv Mental Health* (2004) 2:50–8. doi: 10.5172/jamh.3.2.50
32. Maybery D, Ling L, Szakacs E, Reupert A. Children of a parent with a mental illness: perspectives on need. *Aust e-J Adv Mental Health* (2005) 2:78–88. doi: 10.5172/jamh.4.2.78
33. Reupert A, Cuff R, Drost L, Foster K, van Doesum KTM, van Santvoort F. Intervention programs for children whose parents have a mental illness: a review. *Med J Aust.* (2012) 1:18–22. doi: 10.5694/mjao11.11145
34. Grové C, Riebschleger J, Bosch A, Cavanaugh D, van der Ende PC. Expert views of children's knowledge needs regarding parental mental illness. *Child Youth Serv Rev.* (2017) 1:249–55. doi: 10.1016/j.childyouth.2017.06.026
35. Bilsborrow S. What we want from mental health professionals: "Telling it like it is". In: Reupert A, Mayberry D, Nicholson J, Göpfert M, Seeman MV, editors. *Parental Psychiatric Disorder: Distressed Parents and Their Families*, 3rd ed. Cambridge: Cambridge University Press (2015). p. 16–19.
36. Drost LM, van der Krieke L, Sytema S, Schippers GM. Self-expressed strengths and resources of children of parents with a mental illness: a systematic review. *Int J Ment Health Nurs.* (2016) 2:102–15. doi: 10.1111/inm.12176
37. Grové C, Reupert A, Maybery D. Gaining knowledge about parental mental illness: how does it empower children? *Child Fam Social Work* (2015) 4:377–86. doi: 10.1111/cfs.12086
38. Bee P, Bower P, Byford S, Churchill R, Calam R, Stallard P, et al. The clinical effectiveness, cost effectivenes and acceptability of community-based interventions aimed at improving or maintaining quality of life in children of parents with serious mental illness: a systematic review. *Health Technol Assess.* (2014) 18:1–250. doi: 10.3310/hta18080
39. Lauritzen C, Reedtz C, Van Doesum K, Martinussen M. Factors that may facilitate or hinder a family focus in the treatment of parents with a mental illness. *J Child Fam Stud.* (2015) 24:864–71. doi: 10.1007/s10826-013-9895-y
40. Reedtz C, Mørch L, Lauritzen C. Registreres psykiatriske pasienters barn i elektronisk pasientjournal? *Nordisk Sygeplejeforskning* (2015) 1:36–45.
41. Reedtz C, Lauritzen C. Barn med psykisk syke foreldre: behov for nye rutiner og bedre implementeringsstrategier. *Scand Psychol.* (2015) 2:e10. doi: 10.15714/scandpsychol.2.e10
42. Lauritzen C, Reedtz C, Rognmo C, Nilsen M, Walstad A. Identification and support for children of mentally ill parents: a five year follow-up study of adult mental health services. *Front Psychiatry* (2018) 9:507. doi: 10.3389/fpsyt.2018.00507
43. Lauritzen C, Kolmannskog AB, Iversen A. Family assessment conversations as a tool to support families affected by parental mental illness: a retrospective review of electronic patient journals. *Int J Ment Health Syst.* (2018) 12:18. doi: 10.1186/s13033-018-0199-x
44. Pfeiffenberger AS, D'Souza AJ, Huthwaite MA, Romans SE. The well-being of children of parents with a mental illness: the responsiveness of crisis mental health services in Wellington, New Zealand. *Child Fam Social Work* (2016) 4:600–7. doi: 10.1111/cfs.12186
45. Reedtz C, Lauritzen C, van Doesum KTM. Evaluating workforce developments to support children of mentally ill parents: implementing new interventions in the adult mental healthcare in Northern Norway. *BMJ Open* (2012) 2:709. doi: 10.1136/bmjopen-2011-000709
46. World Health Organisation. (1992). *ICD-10 Classifications of Mental and Behavioural Disorder: Clinical Descriptions and Diagnostic Guidelines.* Geneva: World Health Organisation.
47. Thomas L, Kalucy R. Parents with mental illness: lacking motivation to parent. *Int J Ment Health Nurs.* (2003) 12:153–7. doi: 10.1046/j.1440-0979.2003.00282.x

48. Jackson A, Brooks-Gunn J, Chien-Chung H, Glassman M. Single mothers in low-wage jobs: financial strain, parenting, and preschoolers' outcomes. *Child Dev.* (2000) 71:1409–23. doi: 10.1111/1467-8624.00236
49. Feldman AR, Stiffman AR, Jung KG. *Children at Risk: in the Web of Parental Mental Illness*. London: Rutgers University Press (1987).
50. Kelly JB, Emery RB. Children's adjustment following divorce: risk and resilience perspectives. *Fam Relat.* (2003) 4:352–62. doi: 10.1111/j.1741-3729.2003.00352.x
51. Möller-Leimkühler AM. Barriers to help-seeking by men: a review of sociocultural and clinical literature with particular reference to depression. *J Affect Disord.* (2002) 1–3:1–9. doi: 10.1016/S0165-0327(01)00379-2
52. Ashman SB, Dawson G, Panagiotides H. Trajectories of maternal depression over 7 years: relations with child psychophysiology and behavior and role of contextual risks. *Dev Psychopathol.* (2008) 1:55–77. doi: 10.1017/S0954579408000035
53. Halligan SL, Murray L, Martins C, Cooper PJ. Maternal depression and psychiatric outcomes in adolescent offspring: a 13-year longitudinal study. *J Affect Disord.* (2007) 1–3:145–54. doi: 10.1016/j.jad.2006.06.010
54. Jenkins J, Rasbash J, Leckie G, Gass K, Dunn J. The role of maternal factors in sibling relationship quality: a multilevel study of multiple duads per family. *J Child Psychol Psychiatry* (2011) 6:622–9. doi: 10.1111/j.1469-7610.2011.02484.x
55. Widmer ED, Weiss CC. Do older siblings make a difference? The effects of older sibling support and older sibling adjustment on the adjustment of socially disadvantaged adolescents. *J Res Adolesc.* (2010) 1:1–27. doi: 10.1207/SJRA1001_1
56. Goodwin MP, Roscoe B. Sibling violence and agonistic interactions among middle adolescents. *Adolescence* (1990) 98:451–67. Available online at: https://search.proquest.com/docview/195920977?accountid=17260
57. Benzies K, Mychasiuk R. Fostering family resiliency: a review of the key protective factors. *Child Fam Social Work* (2009) 14:103–14. doi: 10.1111/j.1365-2206.2008.00586.x
58. Lauritzen C, Reedtz C. Adult mental health services and the collaboration with child protection services. *J Hosp Adm.* (2016) 5:72–8. doi: 10.5430/jha.v5n5p72
59. Kitterød RH, Wiik KA. Shared residence among parents living apart in Norway. *Fam Court Rev.* (2017) 4:556–71. doi: 10.1111/fcre.12304
60. Vangelisti, A. L. (2012). *The Routledge Handbook of Family Communication*, 2nd ed. New York, NY: Routledge Handbooks.
61. Barry CL, McGinty EE, Pescosolido BA, Goldman HH. Stigma, discrimination, treatment effectiveness, and policy: public views about drug addiction and mental illness. *Psychiatr Serv.* (2014) 65:1269–72. doi: 10.1176/appi.ps.201400140

14

Mothers with Postpartum Psychiatric Disorders: Proposal for an Adapted Method to Assess Maternal Sensitivity in Interaction with the Child

Christine Heinisch[1†], Mirijam-Griseldis Galeris[1,2†], Sandra Gabler[1], Susanne Simen[3], Juliane Junge-Hoffmeister[4], Judith Fößel[1] and Gottfried Spangler[1]*

[1] Developmental and Educational Psychology, Institute of Psychology, Friedrich-Alexander University Erlangen-Nürnberg, Erlangen, Germany, [2] Department of Paediatric Psychiatry, Psychotherapy and Psychosomatics, Universitätsklinikum Leipzig, Leipzig, Germany, [3] Klinik für Psychiatrie und Psychotherapie, Universitätsklinik der Paracelsus Medizinischen Privatuniversität, Klinikum Nürnberg Süd, Nürnberg, Germany, [4] Klinik für Psychotherapie und Psychosomatik des Universitätsklinikums Carl Gustav Carus der Technischen Universität Dresden, Dresden, Germany

***Correspondence:**
Christine Heinisch
christine.heinisch@fau.de

†These authors have contributed equally to this work.

About 15% of mothers suffer from postpartum psychiatric disorders, such as depression, anxiety, or psychosis. Numerous studies have shown maternal caregiving behavior to be negatively affected under these circumstances. The current study sets out to shed light on specific caregiving behaviors of affected mothers in the context of parental mental illness at an early stage. There are several methods to assess maternal caregiving behavior in terms of sensitivity. However, all of them have limitations regarding the peculiarities of mothers with postpartum disorders, that is, changes in affect regulation, and the early onset of the disorder postpartum. With the current study, we provide an adapted method to assess maternal sensitivity based on methods recently approved in attachment research. Two groups of mothers, who were either healthy or had different postpartum disorders, were recorded on video during interactions with their infants. Behaviors were rated regarding responsiveness, promptness, appropriateness, intrusiveness, and positive and negative affect. A first analysis revealed an increased number of deficits on all subscales in mothers with postpartum psychiatric disorders as compared to healthy mothers. Depressive mothers with a single diagnosis had lower scores in responsiveness, promptness, and appropriateness and higher scores on intrusiveness as compared to those in healthy mothers. Here, maternal behavior appears more parent-centered, whereas affect seemed to be relatively unharmed. Moreover, as compared to healthy mothers, mothers with comorbid depression and anxiety symptomatology achieved lower scores on responsiveness, appropriateness, and positive affect and higher scores on intrusiveness and negative affect. It is suggested, that increased deficits are related to the severity of illness in mothers with comorbidities. Results on promptness indicate that these mothers are still capable of maintaining higher vigilance to infant cues. Variance in maternal behavior was relatively high in clinical mothers, showing that some of them are well capable of behaving in a sensitive manner toward their child. One strength of our adapted method is that particular aspects of sensitive parent–child interactions are assessed separately. This may shed light on specific behavior patterns of different postpartum psychiatric disorders, which may in turn relate to specific child outcomes. The manual is open for usage, while reliability testing is required.

Keywords: maternal sensitivity, postpartum depression (PPD), postpartum anxiety, mother–child interaction, AINSWORTH

THEORETICAL BACKGROUND

Postpartum Mood Swings and Psychiatric Disorders

The birth of a child is typically represented as a fascinating and happy event. In reality though, a few days after child birth, about 40–80% of mothers experience symptoms of depression and emotional lability (1–3). This phenomenon, commonly known as "baby blues," usually declines after a couple of days without psychiatric treatment. Tremendous changes in hormonal levels and psychological difficulties in adapting to the new situation after childbirth are supposed to be responsible for this emotional status (4–7). However, when these symptoms manifest in a mental disorder during pregnancy or postpartum, as it does in 10–15%, treatment is mandatory (8, 9). Maternal risk factors are a history of (familial) psychiatric disorders, sociodemographic variables, such as early motherhood, low income, low educational level, and low social support, as well as experiences of maltreatment during childhood or later life (10–13).

The most common and significant diagnoses of postpartum psychiatric disorders are postpartum depression (14), followed by postpartum anxiety (15, 16), postpartum obsessive–compulsive disorder (OCD) (17), and postpartum psychosis (18). Additional compulsive infant-focused thoughts are common in perinatal mental illness (19). Postpartum diagnoses often appear comorbid [e.g., Refs. (20, 21). In sum, they are comparable to disorders outside the postpartum period that refer to alterations in affect and cognition. However, additional peculiarities are that fears, obsessive thoughts, and sense of guilt focus on the child [e.g., Refs. (22–24)].

Maternal Sensitivity in Mentally Ill Mothers

Various symptoms with postpartum onset interfere with the demands of caring for a child and handling motherhood. Therefore, mothers with postpartum disorders often exhibit specific behavioral restraints during interaction with their infant. More specifically, postnatally depressed mothers, as compared to healthy mothers, show fewer positive caregiving behaviors, less emotional involvement, and less responsiveness when interacting with their children (25). In contrast, anxious mothers show more exaggerated behaviors and increased arousal when interacting with their children (26). Some mothers suffering from compulsive thoughts in terms of harming their child tend to withdraw from interactions as they are afraid to hurt their child (27, 28). In postpartum psychosis, Hornstein and colleagues (29) describe affected mothers as quickly overstrained, emotionally tense, uncoordinated, and sometimes awkwardly moving their infant.

In sum, postpartum psychiatric disorders compromise a mother's ability to interact with her child in a sensitive way, which decreases the quality of the mother–child interaction [e.g., Refs. (25, 26, 30)]. Sensitive parenting behavior means to consider the child's perspective, adequately infer and respond to emotional needs, and provoke positive reciprocity during interaction. Sensitivity itself is defined by the *perception*, *correct interpretation*, and a *prompt* and *adequate* reaction to a child's signals and communication attempts (31). There is evidence that sensitivity is affected in mothers with postpartum disorders. As prior work suggests, there seem to be symptom-specific patterns regarding alterations on different subscales of sensitivity, which are described below.

Responsiveness. The perception and reaction toward the child's signal was found to be lowered and less contingent in mothers with postpartum depression (25, 32–35). Also, maternal trait anxiety reduces responsiveness in healthy mothers (36, 37), whereas, in contrast, clinically anxious mothers show some overactivity (38).

Appropriateness of maternal behavior can be observed if an interaction sequence is "well-rounded" by being supportive and child-centered in an adequate way. Such supportive behavior is reduced in mothers with depressive symptoms (33). Anxious mothers behave less appropriately (39) and are more open to misinterpretations of children's cries, which may then lead to inappropriate reactions (40). Also, repeating sorrowful thoughts can lead to lower structuring during mother–child interactions (26, 41–43). For postpartum psychosis, results regarding the appropriateness of maternal behavior are ambiguous. A recent review postulates that mothers with postpartum psychosis are as likely as postnatally depressed mothers to harm their children (44), whereas Riordan et al. (45) reported observations of greater interaction deficits than those with affective disorders, namely being more remote, insensitive, intrusive and self-absorbed.

Another important component closely related to the concept of sensitivity is *intrusiveness*. Higher scores on this scale are used when the caregiver denies the child's autonomy and acts in a self-centered controlling way. On the other hand, a nonintrusive caregiver considers the child's perspective an important part of its individuality and respects it. Mothers with postpartum depression were found to exhibit behaviors of intrusiveness and withdrawal inconsistently [e.g., Refs. (16, 25)]. Highly anxious mothers show more intrusive behaviors compared to mothers with low anxiety levels [e.g., Refs. (36, 37, 43)] as less support of the infants' autonomy (46). Similarly, at an older age, teenagers with parents suffering from OCD report to be confronted with more controlling behavior and boundaries from their parents (47). Finally, reactions of psychotic mothers toward their children are assumed to be more intense in their intrusive behavior (48).

Several methods used to assess parental interactional behavior emphasize the importance of warmth and positive climate, although these aspects are not included in the original definition of sensitivity. Key aspects of depression are depressed mood and loss of interest. Thus, mothers with this diagnosis often experience blunted emotionality or an increase in negative affect. These emotional characteristics compromise the affective climate during mother–child interactions. More precisely, depression lowers the mothers' capability to flexibly switch between affective states and adjust to their child's altering affective states and needs sensitively (49, 50). Also, increases in hostility and negativity could even be observed in mothers who only exhibit subclinical levels of depression (34, 51). Finally, depressed mothers are described as less warm, more irritable, and lack joy in interacting with their child (35, 52).

Negative affect in mothers with postpartum anxiety disorder reveals itself in stressful and sorrowful behavior (53), increased criticism, and less satisfaction regarding the child's behavior (54, 55). Some studies also describe mothers with postpartum anxiety disorders as less warm and positive in contact with their children, indicated by fewer smiles or positive gestures (46, 54, 56, 57). However, other studies suggest that maternal anxiety may also yield more positive interactions (26) or that maternal affect is at least comparable to healthy mothers (58–60).

The relevance of maternal sensitivity is evidenced by numerous studies that identify this domain of caregiving behavior as an important predictor of the child's attachment (61–66). Indeed, the quality of attachment is highly sensitive to the appropriateness of early experiences (67, 68). In this line, insecure attachment strategies can be viewed as adaptions to less emotionally available or reliable caregivers, which means that they are functional in a given environment (69). Secure attachment relationships, however, provide the child with a range of competencies and have a positive impact on its social and language development (66, 70–72). With regard to maternal depression, a lack of sensitivity can yield insecure attachment, whereas maternal sensitive behavior can buffer negative effects of depression and increase the likelihood of establishing a secure attachment relationship (73, 74). Interventions focusing on improving maternal sensitivity have the potential to increase the offspring's attachment security (75). However, specific associations between certain aspects of sensitivity and child outcome variables are still unknown, which is why more fine-grained analyses on a subscale level are needed. Finally, this may be especially important with regard to behavioral impairments exhibited by mentally ill mothers.

Previous Measures of Maternal Sensitivity

Observational tools to assess maternal behavior in mother–child interactions are numerous (76–79). Most combine scales measuring sensitivity with other observable behaviors like affect or even play and generate an overall score. In the following, we describe the four most influential methods that a) assess parenting behavior in terms of maternal sensitivity and b) have successfully been used to assess predictors of children's attachment security.

First, the Ainsworth Maternal Sensitivity Scale is one of four scales assessing parental behavior (31): Sensitivity versus Insensitivity to the baby's signals, Cooperation versus Interference with baby's ongoing behavior, Physical and Psychological availability versus Ignoring and Neglecting, and Acceptance versus Rejection of the baby's needs. Here, the scale sensitivity turned out to be a key variable because it was found to be correlated to acceptance, cooperation, and availability and to be a reliable predictor of attachment security (61). Affect is considered in the Acceptance versus Rejection Scale because it deals with the balance between the mother's positive and negative feelings about the baby. The Ainsworth Maternal Sensitivity Scale requires the observer to make one global assessment of sensitivity. In further analyses, it has been related to attachment quality and a range of child behavior. It is the origin of other developing measurement tools like the NICHD–Study of Early Child Care Mother–Child Interaction (ECCN) Scale.

Second, the NICHD-ECCN Scale for mothers of children from 6 up to 24 months quantifies different aspects of maternal behavior rated from videotaped dyadic semistructured play interactions. It assesses the following aspects of parenting behavior: *Sensitivity/Responsivity to distress* (adapted from the original Ainsworth Maternal Sensitivity Scale), *Sensitivity/Responsivity to nondistress, Intrusiveness, Detachment, Stimulation of development, Positive regard for the child, Negative regard for the child,* and *Flatness of affect* (80). Even though there are two separate global rating scales measuring maternal sensitivity/responsivity, most studies use a composite measure of overall maternal sensitivity as an indicator of mothers' sensitive behavior [e.g., Ref. (81)]. The NICHD-ECCN sensitivity scales are one of eight widely used observational measures; however, there are indeed a total of 50 measures related to the construct of maternal sensitivity (79). A number of studies have shown that maternal sensitivity measured by the NICHD-ECCN Scale is predictive of different child outcomes, for example, attachment security (82, 83) or cognitive competence (84).

Third, Biringen and colleagues (85–87) developed the emotional availability (EA) Scales. The EA Scales describe the caregiver's ability to perceive and react to both positive and negative emotions, as well as the child's reaction to the caregiver's behavior. It includes a multidimensional set of features (e.g., caregiver's sensitivity, nonhostility, structuring, nonintrusiveness). Moreover, the child's behavior is observed, too. This leads to the evaluation of the affective quality of parent–child relationships from the first weeks of life to adolescence. There is no given structure for the observational situation, and it has been applied in separation–reunion situations (62), still face procedure (88), and structured and semistructured play situations (89, 90).

Fourth, the CARE-Index is a screening tool intended to enable trained professionals to make judgments about the necessity of a family intervention (91). Similar to the EA Scales, the method evaluates the quality of caregiver–infant interaction.

Observational situations are 3 min of play interaction recorded on video under nonthreatening conditions. It is applicable from birth to 15 months and up to 2.5 years when using the toddler form. The coding procedure focuses the observer's attention on seven aspects of the caregiver's and the infant's behaviors, including affect and cognition. For caregivers, these are sensitivity, control, and unresponsiveness. These codes define four patterns of caregivers' interactional behavior. The "sensitive pattern" involves how the caregiver accommodates to the infant's behavior and shares the most commonalities to the concept of sensitivity. The "controlling pattern" identifies behaviors that are either overtly hostile or covertly hostile comparable to intrusiveness and hostility in other scales, whereas the "unresponsive pattern" consists of items describing forms of withdrawal.

Limitations of Existing Methods for Mentally Ill Mothers

With many other methods, but the four named as influential in attachment research, it should be just a matter of choice to evaluate maternal sensitivity in postpartum psychiatric disorders. Indeed, all of them have been in use for clinical research [e.g., Refs. (76, 79] with their strengths and weaknesses. However, to integrate sensitivity research and specific parenting characteristics with postpartum psychiatric disorders, each of the named methods has its own limitations.

First, the onset of postpartum depression starts either already during pregnancy with signs for mental health problems or manifestations of depression and anxiety or immediately after birth or at least very few weeks or months after delivery. In practice, the diagnosis is given with diagnostic criteria until children reach the age of 1, in some hospitals even 2. Here, it is important to note that sensitivity measures vary regarding recommendations on the child's age range: Whereas the scales of Ainsworth, EA, and CARE-Index allow observation from birth on, the NICHD Scale starts from 6 months of age and was not specifically intentionally developed for newborns or younger infants. Moreover, the CARE-Index and the EA Scales measure dyadic interaction, which increases in older infants. This might account for the number of null findings in studies using the EA Scales in depressed and nondepressed mothers (86).

Second, the development from and application with regard to attachment theory and research are different. The CARE-Index and the EA Scales can be regarded as further developments of the Ainsworth sensitivity scales and are both very promising in evaluating the dyadic interaction within the developing attachment relationship because sensitive maternal behavior is related to secure attachment. According to Bowlby (92), attachment to the primary caregiver develops not earlier than after 8 weeks, with increasing differentiation in the second half of the infant's first year and attachment measures are applied with 12–18 months. Because maternal postpartum psychiatric disorders occur within the infant's first year of life, with an onset immediately until 4 weeks after birth, observational measures of attachment security need to be assessed at follow-up. The Ainsworth sensitivity and the NICHD-ECCN scales have been shown to be good predictors for measures of attachment security. Moreover, the latter two are freely available and open to use for everyone. For research, reliability testing is mandatory. Training to learn the manual of the CARE-Index takes about 8 days plus practice and reliability testing. Also, the EA Scales require 1 week with additional training by Biringen, too. Whereas the Ainsworth sensitivity and the NICHD scales are free for usage, the other two are subject to charges.

Another limitation is that the NICHD ECCN sample mostly stems from the middle class. For samples who are at specific risk to show highly dysfunctional parenting behaviors, however, it is necessary to use scales that particularly differentiate behavioral nuances at low levels of parenting competence and that allow to measure distinct impairments of specific aspects of parenting behaviors.

Furthermore, all methods vary with regard to the observational situation. Whereas the Ainsworth Maternal Sensitivity Scale and the EA Scales can be applied in different settings, the CARE-Index favors free-play situations, and the NICHD-ECCN Scale requires semistructured situations like diaper change or feeding situation or in the toddler form a manualized procedure. Also, the required recording length ranges from 3 min (CARE-Index) to 30 min (EA Scales). Regarding the special group of mentally ill mothers, the observational situation must be carefully chosen. It should be easy to implement during daily routine of several treatment institutions. Because those mothers are limited in their capacity to play freely with their children, it must not enforce the feeling of insufficiency.

Next, a crucial diagnostic criterion of postpartum depression is depressed mood and loss of interest, whereas arousal is increased in mothers with postpartum anxiety. Affect measures have been considered in all scales but only to a limited degree: Hostility or warmth is measured in the Ainsworth Maternal Sensitivity and EA scales. The NICHD-ECCN sensitivity composite score includes positive and negative regard of the child for youngest children, with changes in the negative affect scale in the toddler form.

Further considerations refer to how differentiated maternal behavior is measured, which is especially important with regard to mothers' symptom comorbidity. Recent research finds that depression and anxiety during the first 8 weeks postpartum occur simultaneously in 13% of mothers (20). Symptoms of anxiety often come along with symptoms of compulsive behavior (93). Triple comorbidity of depression, anxiety, and posttraumatic stress disorder (PTSD) is relatively rare with a prevalence of 2% to 3% (94). Other comorbidities are not well studied, although they appear in clinical practice. Next to comorbid symptoms, stresses and strains as parenting or childhood stress, immigration history, and maternal vulnerable personality predict higher rates or symptoms (20). A main concern with the recent methods is that behavioral variance caused by comorbidity may not be represented sufficiently because all ratings use sum scores or general ratings. For instance, a mother with depression can partly be responsive and adequate but not prompt, whereas a psychotic mother might act responsive, prompt but not adequate. By using a sum scale of sensitivity, both mothers would receive low scores, but how can one differentiate behavior between these mothers regarding sensitivity? And how can such differences then be related to later child outcome? With the future goal, that is to describe the mother–child interaction in postpartum disorders with the full spectrum of comorbidities and risk factors, a separation of the concept of sensitivity into its original components described by Ainsworth is valuable.

To sum up, we propose an adaptation of the described methods to measure sensitivity to fully represent the spectrum of altered behavior in postpartum psychiatric disorders with all its comorbidities. Our intention was to develop a method that is applicable in a clinical routine setting (e.g., mother–baby unit) with reasonable effort for patients and the therapeutic team. At the same time, it should be usable for scientific purposes. Future scientific questions can then focus on how maternal caregiving behavior differs with regard to different diagnoses while taking into account the high number of comorbidities. It is also of special interest if other risk factors associated with postpartum psychiatric disorders are related to specific deficits, for example, parenting stress, traumatic experiences, or lack of social support. And finally, we aim to relate our findings to specific child outcomes to increase our understanding on symptom-specific effects of alterations in parenting behavior that are related to maternal mental illness.

The present paper describes the development of an adapted measure of maternal caregiving behavior for scientific and clinical use in mothers with postpartum psychiatric disorder. The adapted measure specifically considers the clinical setting, peculiarities of postpartum disorders, and a fine-grained description of maternal behavior. We then present a preliminary pilot implementing the adapted measure on 38 mothers admitted to a mother–baby unit and 35 healthy mothers.

METHOD

Ethics

This study was carried out in accordance with the Declaration of Helsinki and the permission and recommendations of the Ethics Committee of the Friedrich-Alexander University Erlangen Nuremberg and the Ethics Committee of Technical University Dresden (Ethics committee of the FA: 320_15 B, Ethics committee of the TU: EK450 22013). All participants gave written and informed consent. For all data concerning children, written informed consent was obtained from the parents.

The Pilot Project: Video Screening for the Development of the Adapted Sensitivity Scale

Sample

Mentally ill mothers currently attending a video-based interaction therapy in a mother–baby day unit were asked to participate in the study. Video recordings were made on a voluntary basis. Treatment institutions were the Mother-Baby-Day-Unit of the Clinic of Psychiatry and Psychotherapy of the Paracelsus University Clinic Nuremberg Psychiatry in Nuremberg and the Mother-Baby-Day-Unit of the Clinic for Psychotherapy and Psychosomatics of the University Clinic Carl Gustav Carus at the Technical University in Dresden. In these units, mothers spent time from 8 to 16 o'clock each day for an average of 8 weeks, during which they receive a variety of interventions (e.g., group therapy, psychoeducation, personal counseling, and art therapy). A special focus lies in the improvement of mother–child interaction by providing sensitivity training, baby massage, and mother–baby bonding therapy. Video interaction therapy starts soon after the initial assessment with numerous sessions during the whole stay in treatment. In these sessions, mothers watch videotapes of themselves interacting with their infant and get feedback about positive sequences from their therapist. They are then supported by their therapist to enhance such behaviors and integrate them into daily life situations.

The total sample of mothers who agreed to participate in the current study consisted of 102 mothers with postpartum disorders (67 stemming from the Dresden Unit and 35 from the Nuremberg Unit) and of 38 healthy/nonclinical mothers. For mentally ill mothers, the diagnoses were depression, anxiety, compulsive disorder, PTSD, substance abuse {of medium extent [alcohol, tetrahydrocannabinol (THC), or nicotine during pregnancy and continuing]}, bipolar disorder, personality pathology, and/or psychosis (order according to frequency). More than half of the patients had more than one diagnosis.

Clincial diagnoses were based on clinical assessment according to International Statistical Classification of Diseases and Related Health Problems (ICD-10) criteria, video recordings were made by an interaction therapist, and questionnaires were assessed as self-ratings.

Observation of Mother–Child Interaction

Observation and analysis of mother–child interaction were used for the development of the adapted sensitivity scales. Videos were recorded in clinical routine for therapeutic use at the beginning of their therapy. Mothers were instructed to act as normal as during daily routine.

Description of the Adapted Sensitivity Scales for Observation

The method is based on the Ainsworth Maternal Sensitivity Scale (31) and the NICHD-ECCN Scale (80, 84, 95) and was adapted to the survey situation, children's age, and peculiarities of interaction behavior in mothers with postpartum psychiatric disorders. Analysis of video-recorded interactions was done according to the manual attached (see **Supplementary Material**).

With respect to behavioral deficits in mentally ill mothers (as described above), the following scales were defined: caregiver's ***responsiveness, promptness*** of reaction, ***appropriateness*** of the caregiver's reaction, ***intrusiveness*** of the caregiver, and ***negative affect*** and ***positive affect*** toward the child.

The scale ***responsiveness*** refers to whether the mother reacts to the child's signals. Here, given that the child sends a signal, overtly or subtle, the mother needs to signal back that she recognized it. For example, during diaper change, this can be the exchange of a look or comments on what is happening, when the child displays discomfort. ***Promptness*** is defined whether the response occurs immediately, not exceeding 3 s. Otherwise, the child may not relate its own action to the maternal reaction and experience himself as agent of this interaction.

The scale ***appropriateness*** measures whether the mother's reaction fulfills or at least adequately attempts to fulfill the baby's needs presented in the sequence. Generally spoken, this refers to security, warmth, and comfort. An appropriate reaction is well-rounded and children experiencing appropriate behavior are usually less stressed.

These three scales were chosen based on Ainsworth's definition of sensitivity and the NICHD descriptions, whereas both of them use an overall score for all three types of behaviors referred to as "sensitivity."

Intrusiveness measures to what extent the caregiver respects the child's autonomy and accepts its individuality. High intrusiveness indicates low respect of autonomy. Practically, this can often be observed when mothers unclothe their children in an uncomfortable but quick manner, instead of doing so with respect to the child's reaction and by providing guidance through, for example, verbalization. Mothers with postpartum psychiatric disorders have difficulties here because they often seem to follow an adult-centered script and do not seem to be able to take over the child's perspective.

Negative affect is defined as the presence of active expressions of negative affect either verbally, facial, or by hostile actions. Because infants cannot differentiate whether they are the cause for maternal bad mood or whether there are other causes, all kinds of negative affect and hostility are rated. ***Positive affect***, in contrast, is mirrored in the caregiver's joy within the interaction. These scales already existed in the NICHD-ECCN Scale and were modified with special regard to the altered affectivity in psychiatric disorders.

The method and the rating scheme are described at length in the manual at the appendix (compare **Supplementary Material**). We added examples that were found in the videos to the descriptions.

Scales and blinded videos were repeatedly discussed on lab meetings and with trained sensitivity observers. Other scales, as measuring maternal speech or body contact, were rejected during adaptation because they were not directly related to the concept of sensitivity, although many mothers also show deficits here.

In total, six scales were rated on a 9-point scale ranging from one to five with semisteps in between. Defined anchor points are 1, 2, 3, 4, and 5. Low values indicated low characteristics of the regarding scale, whereas high values go along with frequent observation of the behavior in the scale.

Coding of Mother–Child Interaction

Analyses were conducted by five postgraduate psychology students who participated in a seminar on "observational tools to assess baby's signals" and underwent intense reliability training by experienced researchers. Reliability training included reading literature on sensitivity, discussing videos with mother-child interaction and doing pre-ratings to find misperceptions or positive or negative observation bias on a weekly basis for 6 months. They were trained with the help of the manual and an assessment sheet (see the Manual) analyzing the categories: Responsivity, promptness, appropriateness, intrusiveness, and negative and positive affect. Note: Observers who are familiar and reliable with other sensitivity scales should be able to use the method with less intense training.

Raters were blind to diagnoses. All five students were required to become highly reliable, with all $\kappa > 0.85$ before they were allowed to score the videos included in the study. According to McHugh (96), this indicates that interrater reliability is strong to perfect. *Post hoc* calculated interrater reliability (weighted kappa) was based on 17 double-coded video tapes after 6 months. Here, mean reliability was moderate, with $\kappa = 0.73$. All raters showed strong reliability on the scale intrusiveness, $\kappa = 0.85$, whereas on the scale, promptness reliability was lowest and just weak, with $\kappa = 0.59$. Reliability for the other scales were moderate with responsiveness, $\kappa = 0.66$; appropriateness, $\kappa = 0.73$; negative affect; $\kappa = 0.76$; and positive affect, $\kappa = 0.80$.

First Statistical Analyses Comparing Data on Depressed and Anxious Mothers to a Healthy Group

Sample

For the present study, we examined a subset of the clinical sample including 31 mothers from the Nuremberg Unit and seven mothers from the Dresden Unit with postpartum depression and/or anxiety disorder. The clinical sample was recruited consecutively from 2016 to 2018. Infants were healthy as seen by Pediatrics from the hospital. There was a massive reduction of usable videos because during the pilot phase, criteria for the recordings of the videos for scientific usage have been developed.

Videos were excluded if they were <3 min in length (according to the standard CARE-Index procedure), recorded after the third week of admission, the patient presented with three clinical diagnoses on the basis that the underlying disorder was unclear (e.g., depression and anxiety and personality disorder and substance abuse), invisibility of important parts of the interaction, strong sound problems, or lack of questionnaire data.

In contrast, inclusion criteria were a good quality of the video, recording at the beginning of the therapy, and at least one of the diagnoses from the spectrum of depression, anxiety, or compulsive disorder.

The control group was acquired in the area of Erlangen Nuremberg, Germany, and videos were recorded during home visits. The control mothers were recruited *via* flyer or word of mouth and agreed to participate in a home visit, including the recording of a video and assessment of questionnaires. They were paid 20€ and received a small toy for the child.

All mothers were instructed to act as usual during daily routine. All videos included a semistandardized situation, where they changed the diapers of their infant or fed him or her. In addition, parents were asked to play with their infant without instruction.

Questionnaires

Brief Symptom Inventory

The Brief Symptom Inventory (BSI) (97) is a short form of the Symptom Checklist SCL-90-R (98) and aims to assess mental stress of participants within the last 7 days. Participants respond on a 5-step Likert Scale, ranging from 0 ("not at all") to 4 (very heavy) how much they agree to a total of 53 items. The BSI includes nine scales assessing, for example, depression, anxiety, or psychotic experiences. Finally, the global score [Global Severity Index (GSI)] is calculated to assess general mental stress.

In addition, there are three global scores for general mental stress: GSI, intensity [(Positive Symptom Distress Index (PSDI)], and number of reported symptoms [positive symptom total (PST)].

Scores can be transformed into T scores with different norms for academic students or adults in general, as well as men and women. Here, we used T scores for women (nonstudent) to assess the global severity of mental illness. Clinically relevant GSIT scores are above ≥63 (99).

Edinburgh Postnatal Depression Scale

To assess postpartum symptoms of depression, we used the Edinburgh Postnatal Depression Scale (EPDS) (22). The screening instrument includes 10 items asking for the mood of the last 7 days of young mothers. Mothers had to answer on a 4-point Likert (0–3) Scale how much they agreed with each item. Scores were summed up, with 30 as the highest possible value. High values indicate strong symptoms. Mothers with scores of 13 or higher are regarded as likely to suffer from depression. Validation studies (100) reported good sensitivity (79%) and specificity (85%).

Statistics

We used SPSS 25.0 for analysis. To examine differences between group variables, we used *t*-test. Intercorrelation analysis was done by Pearson correlation. Potentially influencing factors, as age of the child or mother, were also controlled by using Pearson correlation. Group comparisons regarding sensitivity were done with multivariate analysis of variance (ANOVA). All *post hoc* pairwise comparisons were performed using LSD. Significance level followed $p \leq 05^*$, $p \leq 0.01^{**}$, $p \leq 0.001^{***}$. **Tables** show means and standard deviations.

RESULTS

Sample Descriptives

Mothers of both groups were at the same age in the beginning of the thirties and had the same, relatively high, educational background (**Table 1**). The sex of the children had a similar ratio in both groups. Children of mentally ill mothers were significantly younger than children of the control group. In the clinical group, the number of participants with at least one close relative (parents or grandparents) who suffered from mental disorders was twice as high as in the control group.

Psychopathology was significantly higher in the clinical group as indicated by measures of the BSI (GSI) and EPDS. In the control group most participants (27 of 35) had scores below 10, while 5 participants had an EPDS score between 10 and 12, indicating a medium degree of postpartum depressive symptoms, and 3 of them had scores above 12 (clinical relevance). In contrast, in the clinical group, almost all mothers (36 of 38) had scores above 12, whereas 2 of them scored between 10 and 12.

Group Comparisons

We used multivariate ANOVA to test if the group of healthy mothers differs in maternal sensitivity significantly from the clinical group. Although not significant ($F_{(6,66)} = 1.690$; $p = 0.137$), results indicate that the clinical group performs poorer in all subscales compared to the healthy control group (**Table 2**). Nonsignificance is typical when the dependent variables are highly correlated (**Table 4**). Further analysis underlines it: extracting promptness as a dependent factor from analysis leads to approaches of significance ($F_{(5,67)} = 2.042$; $p = 0.084$). However, univariate comparisons result in significant effects for each of the dependent measures. Healthy mothers are more responsive, more prompt, and more appropriate than mentally ill mothers. They respect more of the child's autonomy, whereas clinical mothers are more intrusive. Negative affect is lower and positive affect is higher in the healthy group than in the clinical group. Whereas the group of healthy mothers perform in the upper range of the scale (range 3.87–4.33), clinical mothers perform still in a mediocre to upper range (range 3.12–3.88).

TABLE 1 | Demographic data for healthy and clinical mothers.

	Healthy mothers (n = 35) Mean SD	Clinical mothers (n = 38)	
		Mean SD	Significant differences
Maternal age (years)	31.49 ± 4.27	30.02 ± 5.38	n.s.
Education with A Level (%)	62.85	55.26	n.s.
Age of child (weeks)	49.60 ± 25.22	27.75 ± 21.39	$t(71) = 4.002$, $p = 0.000$
Sex of child (boy:girl)	16:19	19:19	
PTs having relatives with psychiatric disorder	11	22	X^2 (1, n = 73) = 5.152, n = 0.023
EPDS (sum)	5.77 ± 3.98	17.32 ± 5.55	$t(70) = -10.097$, $p = 0.000$
BSI (GSI)	46.97 ± 12.03	74.83 ± 7.72	$t(71) = -11.763$, $p = 0.000$

Values indicate means and standard deviations. PTs, participants; EPDS [sum], sum score of the Edinburgh Postnatal Depression Scale; BSI [GSI], Brief Symptom Inventory [Global Severity Index]; n.s., not significant.

TABLE 2 | Comparison of the sensitivity subscales for healthy and clinical mothers.

	Healthy mothers Mean SD	Clinical mothers	
		Mean SD	Significant differences
Responsivity	4.16 ± 0.73	3.67 ± 0.89	$F_{(1,71)}$ = 6.431; p = 0.013
Promptness	4.01 ± 0.66	3.54 ± 0.93	$F_{(1,71)}$ = 6.214; p = 0.015
Appropriateness	3.97 ± 0.86	3.32 ± 1.00	$F_{(1,71)}$ = 8.942; p = 0.004
Intrusiveness	2.13 ± 0.83	2.88 ± 1.15	$F_{(1,71)}$ = 10.203; p = 0.002
Negative affect	1.67 ± 0.69	2.12 ± 0.86	$F_{(1,71)}$ = 5.984; p = 0.017
Positive affect	4.33 ± 0.86	3.85 ± 0.94	$F_{(1,71)}$ = 5.003; p = 0.041

Values indicate means and standard deviation. P values indicate significance from multivariate testing.

TABLE 3 | No correlation of maternal behavior with maternal or child age.

		Maternal age	Child age
	Healthy mothers		
1	Responsivity	−0.078	0.221
2	Promptness	−0.185	0.122
3	Appropriateness	−0.157	0.297
4	Intrusiveness	0.048	−0.154
5	Negative affect	−0.039	0.042
6	Positive affect	0.212	−0.045
	Mothers with PPD		
1	Responsivity	−0.074	0.137
2	Promptness	−0.043	0.084
3	Appropriateness	0.033	0.066
4	Intrusiveness	−0.100	−0.164
5	Hostility	−0.276	−0.320
6	Positive affect	0.230	0.017

Factors Influencing Maternal Sensitivity

We tested for maternal and child age as possible parameters influencing sensitivity. Spearman correlation revealed no significance with these factors for none of the scales neither in the group of healthy nor clinical mothers (compare **Table 3**). For further testing if the difference of child age between the group still affected the results, we included it as a covariate into the analysis. Here, significance was reduced to a trend level in three scales, namely, responsivity ($F_{(1,70)} = 2.820, p = 0.098$), promptness ($F_{(1,70)} = 3.594, p = 0.062$), and negative affect ($F_{(1,70)} = 3.816, p = 0.055$).

Intercorrelations Between the Scales of Sensitivity

As visible in **Table 4**, all scales correlate significantly with each other in the healthy control group (range from $r = 0.934$ to $r = 0.446$) and the clinical group (range from $r = 0.955$ to $r = 0.620$).

Influence of Severity of Symptoms in Mental Illness on Sensitivity

One goal of the development of the adapted method is to analyze sensitivity with respect to specific symptoms of depression to better differentiate between groups of different mental disorders. In the group of healthy mothers, we found mothers who scored subclinical to moderate on depression or EPDS and/or BSI and were clinically conspicuous. We decided not to exclude them from earlier analysis because they were "healthy enough" not to be in treatment. However, in an additional analysis, we put them in a separate group, named "healthy with mild depressive symptoms" (n = 8). Moreover, we separated the group of clinical mothers. Whereas 16 mothers were diagnosed with depression only, 19 mothers had depression and anxiety disorder or compulsive thoughts comorbid. We excluded three mothers because their comorbid diagnosis appeared to raise a personality disorder. The healthy group without depressive symptoms consists of 27 mothers. It is obvious that, with increasing symptoms, EPDS and BSI scores rise (**Table 5**).

We used multivariate analysis to test whether the sensitivity scales differ significantly between the four groups (healthy vs. mild symptoms vs. clinical with depression vs. clinical with depression and comorbidities). Not significantly, but descriptively, with increasing severity, sensitivity gets worse. Healthy but mildly depressed mothers have lower values in sensitivity but not in their affect. Clinically burdened mothers differ significantly in their sensitivity pattern from that of healthy mothers. Whereas mothers with depression respond less, are less prompt, less appropriate, and more intrusive, their affect does not differ significantly from that of healthy mothers. Mothers with additional diagnoses of anxiety are less responsive, less appropriate, and more intrusive and show more negative and less positive affect but are not significantly less prompt.

TABLE 4 | Intercorrelations of maternal sensitivity in the control group (n = 35) (upper values, gray background) and the clinical group (n = 38) (lower values).

Clinical group		Healthy control group					
		1	2	3	4	5	6
1	Responsivity	1	0.934***	0.883***	−0.661***	−0.529***	0.506**
2	Promptness	0.955***	1	0.835***	−0.585***	−0.478**	0.460**
3	Appropriateness	0.826***	0.846***	1	−0.753***	−0.592***	0.594***
4	Intrusiveness	−0.664***	−0.620***	−0.824***	1	0.493**	−0.446**
5	Negative affect	−0.758***	−0.707***	−0.760***	0.742***	1	−0.837***
6	Positive affect	0.694***	0.659***	0.756***	−0.715***	−0.913***	1

*Asterisks label significance (**p ≤ 0.005, ***p ≤ 0.001).*

TABLE 5 | Comparisons of the sensitivity subscales for groups with different degrees of depressive symptoms, ranging from no symptoms to comorbidities.

	Healthy mothers			Clinical mothers			
	No depression	Mild depression		Depression		Depression + anxiety	
	n = 27	n = 8	p	N = 16	p	N = 19	p
EPDS	3.96 ± 2.31	11.87 ± 1.35	0.000	14.87 ± 5.43	0.000	18.61 ± 5.03	0.000
BSI GSI	43.03 ± 7.83	61.50 ± 12.75	0.013	72.81 ± 7.47	0.000	76.89 ± 3.98	0.000
Responsivity	4.24 ± 0.69	3.87 ± 0.79	n.s.	3.65 ± 0.97	0.029	3.73 ± 0.88	0.047
Promptness	4.05 ± 0.62	3.87 ± 0.79	n.s.	3.53 ± 1.04	0.050	3.57 ± 0.91	n.s.
Appropriateness	4.07 ± 0.80	3.62 ± 0.99	n.s.	3.21 ± 1.04	0.006	3.42 ± 1.03	0.025
Intrusiveness	2.02 ± 0.82	2.50 ± 0.75	n.s.	2.88 ± 1.27	0.008	2.79 ± 1.04	0.012
Negative affect	1.67 ± 0.65	1.69 ± 0.84	n.s.	2.00 ± 0.98	n.s.	2.16 ± 0.74	0.048
Positive affect	4.33 ± 0.82	4.31 ± 1.03	n.s.	4.00 ± 1.01	n.s.	3.78 ± 0.85	0.040

Mean and standard deviation. p values belong always to comparisons from the group left to them with healthy mothers without depression.
n.s., not significant. See ref. (24).
EPDS, Edinburgh Postnatal Depression Scale; BSI GSI, brief symptom inventory, global severity index.

DISCUSSION

General Discussion

The present study aimed at adapting observational methods assessing sensitivity in caregivers to a group of mothers with postpartum mental disorders. Therefore, we screened 102 videos of mentally ill mothers interacting with their infants to identify specific parenting behaviors associated with different postpartum mental disorders. These specific behaviors are described in the manual, which can be found in the supplements. With respect to the main deficits of maternal caregiving behavior, we combined different measurement scales for sensitivity. More precisely, with special regard to attachment research, the Ainsworth's Maternal Sensitivity Scale (31) and the NICHD Scale were chosen as a basis for the present method while integrating aspects taken from the EA Scales, the CARE-Index, and from a range of other observational tools focusing on parental behavior (76, 79). This procedure resulted in the examination of responsiveness, promptness, appropriateness, intrusiveness, negative affect, and positive affect. The compilation of these final scales is adapted to the special group of mothers with postpartum disorders because it considers peculiarities regarding the onset of illness, child age, and disorder-related behavior.

In a second step, we used the adapted scales for a preliminary analysis aiming to investigate whether the method is applicable in a clinical group. Therefore, we compared caregiving behavior in a group of mothers at the beginning of treatment in a psychiatric mother–baby unit to that of a group of healthy mothers. Results revealed that mentally ill mothers have difficulties in all aspects of sensitivity, intrusiveness, and affect. Mothers with postpartum psychiatric disorders were found to be less responsive, respond slower, less adequate and to be more intrusive and show more negative and less positive affect toward their children. These findings are not surprising because it has been repeatedly described that postpartum depression can result in tremendous problems regarding mother–child interactions [e.g., Refs. (25, 26, 30, 55, 98)].

A second aim was to see whether assessing different aspects of sensitivity separately would help identify typical behavior patterns of mothers with mental disorders dependent on their diagnosis or other risk factors for altered mother–child interaction. Here, we found that the severity of symptoms is an important factor influencing maternal sensitivity in the present sample. Even in the healthy group, we observed that mild depressive symptoms already reduce sensitivity, however, the effect was rather small. This is in line with recent research showing that subclinical depressive symptoms may increase hostility and negative affect (51) and reduce maternal sensitivity (101). Moreover, we separated the clinical group into those with depression only and those who have an additional diagnosis for anxiety disorder because postpartum depression and postpartum anxiety are frequently comorbid (102, 103). Comparing results to the healthy control group revealed deficits in both groups of mothers with mental illness, but we found different behavioral patterns: In contrast to healthy mothers, those with depression only scored significantly lower on all scales of sensitivity (responsiveness, promptness, appropriateness) and intrusiveness; they did not differ significantly on the affect scales, although values are lower than those in the healthy group. In comparison, mothers with comorbidities of depression and anxiety scored, apart from promptness, significantly lower on all subscales, indicating general deficits in mother–child interaction including own emotion regulation.

The difficulties with sensitivity and intrusiveness in depressive-only mothers have repeatedly been found in earlier studies. Responsiveness, the perception and reaction to a child's signal, has repeatedly been shown to be lower in postpartum depression (25, 32–35). Moreover, maternal responses are less contingent (25) and less appropriate (33). Intrusiveness and withdrawal are reported to appear inconsistently (16, 25), whereas in our study, depressed mothers generally tend to show less respect for child autonomy. Without the investigation of a behavioral pattern, the lack of responsiveness alone may lead to the assumption that signals are not perceived, likely as a result from a cognitive deficit. In combination with measures of lower appropriateness and higher intrusiveness, it can be assumed that mothers ignore their children purposely, followed by a parent-centered response inappropriate to the child's needs. The underlying cognitive process behind this behavior remains unmeasurable, but it seems as if intuitive behavior is disturbed in depressed mothers (97) and that they rather follow a script or external recommendations during interaction. Also, depression worsens the ability to manage changes between affective states, and it is more difficult to adjust to their child's affective states and needs sensitively (49, 50). Interestingly, in our study, maternal depression did not significantly alter affect during mother–child interactions in mothers with depression only, although depressive mood is central in depression. In contrast, Cohn and colleagues (104) argue that negative affect is increased four times in depressed mothers. Also, prior work found mothers with former or postpartum depression to show more negative behaviors as criticizing or destructive reactions and fewer positive behaviors, such as praise or constructive guidance during interaction sequences (105, 106). One reason why we did not find this could be that, in the present sample, the variance in the affect scale is relatively increased in clinical mothers as compared to healthy mothers. This indicates that some of them are well capable of positive interaction with their infants, whereas others are not. Laucht et al. (107) suggest, that, because of some well-functioning, self-control mechanisms, many depressive mothers are capable of acting as nondepressed in contact with their children, warranting a positive child development (107).

As general explanation, the disturbances in altered mother–child interaction are caused or accompanied by altered brain activation. Mothers with postpartum depression have shown weaker activation of reward and motivation areas, such as the thalamus, nucleus accumbens, caudate, and key emotion regulation areas, such as the lateral orbitofrontal cortex (108). Lower responsiveness may be the result when motivation is lowered to increase contentment and infant stimuli do not feel as rewarding for some of them as for healthy mothers.

In our subsample, mothers with depression and anxiety comorbid presented another behavioral pattern. This group showed deficits in all scales, except promptness, which may represent the increase of impairment caused by the double diagnosis.

Earlier findings on maternal anxiety describe mothers as less responsive and withdrawing from interaction, also in trait anxiety of healthy mothers after birth [e.g., Refs. (36, 37)]. More precisely, anxious mothers behave less appropriate (39) and are more exaggerating or overprotective (26, 38). This exaggeration or overprotection, probably caused by the typical higher arousal in anxiety, is mirrored in the "promptness" scale. In our study, we found mothers with comorbid anxiety to have somewhat lowered scores on this scale; however, they did not significantly differ from those of the healthy group. In the face of comorbid anxiety, promptness may be a sign of higher alertness to threatening keys (such as unfamiliar baby signals combined with low maternal self-efficacy). In our, as well as in recent, studies, highly anxious mothers present more intrusive behaviors compared to mothers with low anxiety levels [e.g., Refs. (36, 37, 43)] and support less autonomy (46). They interfere with and try to control the child's behavior (37, 38, 41), often with the objective to be overprotective (53, 109).

The finding that responsiveness, appropriateness, and intrusiveness are worsened in comorbidly ill mothers may reflect a commonality with depressed mothers' behavior, namely, that they act more parent-centered and less intuitive. The constant alertness reflected in the promptness scale could give a hint to their inner conflict between "waiting for signals" and "not being able to react flexible." This conflict is also visible on the affect scale because they show less cheerful play and more negative affect mimically and verbally, more distressed behavior, or emotional flattening. Negative affect in maternal anxiety has been observed through stress and sorrowful behavior (53), increased criticism, and less satisfaction of the child's behavior (54, 55). In our study, we observed lowering of positive affect in depressed and anxious mothers in contrast to some other studies (26, 58–60). Our finding is in line with those studies describing depressed and anxious mothers as generally less warm and positive in contact with their children, indicated by less smiling and positive gestures (46, 54, 56, 57). The lack of joy in the postpartum phase might also have its cause in altered brain processes, namely, that higher levels of anxiety in relation to parenting correlated with reduced activation in the substantia nigra, a region implicated in reward prediction and processing (110). When a child's smile feels less rewarding, experience of joy is probably reduced, too. Consequently, intentions to make the child laugh may be lacking.

In sum, the presented scales successfully identify specific deficits in mother–child interaction of mothers with postpartum psychiatric disorders. It further shows that these deficits differ depending on the diagnosis or comorbidity of mothers and thus provide simplifications for tailored therapeutic intervention. Although for depressed-only mothers, a training on improving appropriate reactions and on understanding of infant's signals and needs might be sufficient, mothers with depression and anxiety comorbidity may need further support in their own emotion regulation. Our method is very detailed, but it is still closely related to the concept of sensitivity. Therefore, it is suited for the investigation of maternal behavior as a predictor of later attachment security.

Limitations

Results of our study are based on a group of healthy mothers and a subgroup of mothers admitted in a psychiatric/psychosomatic Mother-Baby-Day-Unit Nuremberg or Dresden. Healthy and nonhealthy mothers did not differ in their educational degree or age. One limitation was that the children of clinical mothers were younger than those of the control group because of a change of admission requirements in the hospital while the study was still ongoing. However, there was no correlation of the scales with child's age.

Behavioral assessment was located differently for clinical and healthy mothers that may have caused different levels of stress or comfort during observation.

Another limitation of the study is the rather small sample size in the group with comorbidities with respect to the fact that they are diagnosed with different and/or several anxiety disorders. Anxiety disorders manifest in a wide range: generalized anxiety disorder, OCD, panic disorder, and birth-related PTSD. In the postpartum period, sometimes the severity and symptoms do not rise to the level of an anxiety disorder diagnosis (e.g., hypervigilant concerns and attention for the baby, extreme lability, constant worry) but nevertheless can cause significant distress and disturb mother–child interactions (93, 111). Creating further, more clearly defined subgroups would have yielded in too small sample sizes. So, conclusions for different diagnoses of anxiety on sensitivity must be postponed to future studies. Still, the investigation of subgroups and comorbidities remains an important goal for the present method.

Further Thoughts on the Use of the Method in Postpartum Psychiatric Disorders

Intercorrelations

During development of the method, it was noted repeatedly that "responsiveness" and "promptness" correlate highly significantly and were difficult to separate. We thought about combining these two scales again as the NICHD-ECCN Scale does but decided to keep them separate. First, we found "promptness" to differentiate between depressed-only and depressed-anxious mothers, as presented above. Second, during scale adaptation, we often found single videos (psychosis or very severe depression), where the difference was more obvious as responsiveness was very delayed. Third, all scales correlate with each other what is typical in this research sector. All EA Scales (86) correlate with each other, and in the Ainsworth Maternal Sensitivity Scale, the author describes the scale "sensitivity" as a key variable correlating with the other scales. The positive and negative affect scales correlated very high, too, especially in the group of mothers with mental illness. This is likely to represent the emotional flattening of mothers with depression.

Scaling

A related discussion concerns the scaling of the subunits. A rank of 3 (the mean) relates to a mother who behaves a bit more often with good caregiving skills than bad. Healthy mothers rank relatively high (around 4 from 5). Our present clinical subsample ranges from 5 to 2; only in training videos did we find ratings of 1. Why is this so and should we have adapted the scaling? The scale is not conceptualized to separate very good from perfect maternal behavior. With a rank of 4 or 5, we can assume that the behavior in the observed sequence was ideal. It must be noted that the situation was short had only little instruction. A healthy mother often knows how to perform ideally and can act so for a certain amount of time in stress-free situations. Mentally ill mothers are not necessarily "disturbed" in their sensitivity but limited in their capacities (107) and can partly behave normal. Moreover, although the group presented here is severely impaired, the therapeutic staff decided that the child's well-being is not critically endangered. Otherwise, they must have separated mother and child and decided to treat the mother as inpatient first. We believe that, with more demanding observational settings or other types of mental disorder as psychosis, scores will be lower. Methods of stress reduction or increase can change maternal performance, leading to higher variance between mothers.

Suggested Video Length and Observational Situation

In hospital routine, we implemented video observations with a length of 10 min displaying diaper-changing situations and free play. Especially in the group of mentally ill mothers, videos from the beginning of our studies were strikingly shorter. Whereas the CARE-index requires 3 min of observation of mother–child interaction only, the EA Scales (86) recommend analyzing much longer observations, up to 2 h. Both observations pursue different goals, namely, to decide about intervention with the CARE-Index (91) while extracting information about attachment measures with the EA Scales. Therefore, different recording times are reasonable. In our study, we recommend recording times around 10 min and include a semistructured situation and free play. Because attention span is reduced in depression, video observations should reveal deficits in maternal behavior quickly (112, 113), although many are also capable of sustaining normal behavior for a while. To increase motivation for participation and compliance for therapy and science, stress should be as low as possible during recording.

According to our clinical observations, mentally ill mothers seem to lack ideas for interactive play that may evoke feelings of insufficiency in the face of a given play task. If in future studies, higher differences between the groups are favored, stress in observation situation can be increased by using more difficult tasks or observe mothers with siblings (114). Not only attention itself but also divided attention is reduced in depression (112), what should also affect mother–child interaction in more demanding situations. In this sense, it has been shown that contact to a stranger reduces responsivity to child's signals in mothers with social phobia (115).

Future Directions

The present adapted method is useful to measure sensitivity in postpartum psychiatric disorders. Moreover, it should allow testing for relationships to attachment qualities with later strange situation procedures. Still, the next phase of research includes validation work with other observational tools and measures of attachment. Moreover, an extension of the sample with other diagnoses as psychosis and OCDs is planned. Analyses for further understanding of the disorder and its relation to maternal behavior and then child outcome are prospects. Of further importance in the group of mothers with postpartum psychiatric disorders is the interplay of genetic and caregiving influences in the prediction of attachment and further development of the child. It could be shown that higher maternal sensitivity can be a buffer for disorganized attachment in cases of genetic risk (116).

To describe the full spectrum of deficits in mother–child interaction, risk and protection factors for altered sensitivity postpartum psychiatric disorders should be assessed. Own childhood experiences are a crucial factor for the quality of sensitivity, with adverse experiences leading to less sensitivity, whereas positive experiences make warm and sensitive parenting more likely (117, 118). Moreover, experiences of emotional or physical abuse during childhood are predictors for hostile behavior toward her own child (119), as well as for postpartum maternal depression (120). Lack of social support is related to lower sensitivity and responsiveness toward her own children (121, 122) and a key factor for the development of depression (12). Socioeconomic pressure, as low income or unemployment, leads to lower quality in interaction (123) and increases depressive symptoms (12). In contrast, higher education and maternal employment are related to more sensitivity and less control of children (124). For future studies it may be interesting to study those risk and protection factors that play a role in the development of mental health for both parent and child.

ETHICS STATEMENT

This study was carried out in accordance with the Declaration of Helsinki and the permission and recommendations of the Ethics Committee of the Friedrich-Alexander University Erlangen Nuremberg and the Ethics Committee of Technical University Dresden (Ethics committee of the FA: 320_15 B, Ethics committee of the TU: EK450 22013). All participants gave written and informed consent. For all data concerning children, written informed consent was obtained from the parents.

AUTHOR CONTRIBUTIONS

CH and MG designed and conducted the study, created the manual, and wrote the manuscript. SG was involved in study design, setup of the manual, assessment of control group, and editing the manuscript. JJ-H and SS were involved in study design and assessment of the clinical group and editing the manuscript. JF worked on the manual and the introduction. GS was involved in study design, edits on the manual, statistics and edits on the manuscript.

ACKNOWLEDGMENTS

We thank Melanie Tamara Kungl and Jennifer Schneider for editing the manuscript, and Julia Fenkl, Melanie Lindner, Tina Riedl, Sonja Rapp, and Sarah Schwab for observation of mother–child interaction, and Martin Schmucker for help regarding statistics.

REFERENCES

1. Reck C, Stehle E, Reinig K, Mundt C. Maternity blues as a predictor of DSM-IV depression and anxiety disorders in the first three months postpartum. *J Affect Disord* (2009) 113:77–87. doi: 10.1016/j.jad.2008.05.003
2. Oakley A, Chamberlain G. Medical and social factors in postpartum depression. *J Obstet Gynaecol (Lahore)* (1981) 1:182–7. doi: 10.3109/01443618109067376
3. Gonidakis F, Rabavilas AD, Varsou E, Kreatsas G, Christodoulou GN. Maternity blues in Athens, Greece: a study during the first 3 days after delivery. *J Affect Disord* (2007) 99:107–15. doi: 10.1016/j.jad.2006.08.028
4. Seyfried LS, Marcus SM. Postpartum mood disorders. *Int Rev Psychiatry* (2003) 15:231–42. doi: 10.1080/0954026031000136857
5. O'Keane V, Lightman S, Patrick K, Marsh M, Papadopoulos AS, Pawlby S, et al. Changes in the maternal hypothalamic-pituitary-adrenal axis during the early puerperium may be related to the postpartum "blues." *J Neuroendocrinol* (2011) 23:1149–55. doi: 10.1111/j.1365-2826.2011.02139.x
6. Oddo S, Thiel A, Klinger D, Würzburg J, Steetskamp J, Grabmair C, et al. Postpartale depression: Ein interdisziplinärer Therapie-und Forschungsansatz. *J Gynakol Endokrinol* (2009) 2(3):15–21.
7. Harris B, Lovett L, Newcombe RG, Read GF, Walker R, Riad-Fahmy D. Maternity blues and major endocrine changes: cardiff puerperal mood and hormone study II. *BMJ* (1994) 308:949–53. doi: 10.1136/bmj.308.6934.949
8. Munk-Olsen T, Laursen TM, Pedersen CB, Mors O, Mortensen PB. New parents and mental disorders: a population-based register study. *J Am Med Assoc* (2006) 296:2582–9. doi: 10.1001/jama.296.21.2582
9. O'Hara MW, McCabe JE. Postpartum depression: current status and future directions. *Annu Rev Clin Psychol* (2013) 9:379–407. doi: 10.1146/annurev-clinpsy-050212-185612
10. Goyal D, Gay C, Issues KL-WH. *How much does low socioeconomic status increase the risk of prenatal and postpartum depressive symptoms in first-time mothers?* Women's Health Issues (2010) 20(2):96–104. Available at: https://www.sciencedirect.com/science/article/pii/S1049386709001364 [Accessed October 30, 2018]. doi: 10.1016/j.whi.2009.11.003
11. Jones I, Craddock N. Familiality of the puerperal trigger in bipolar disorder: results of a family study. *Am J Psychiatry* (2001) 158:913–7. doi: 10.1176/appi.ajp.158.6.913
12. Martini J, Petzoldt J, Einsle F, Beesdo-Baum K, Höfler M, Wittchen HU. Risk factors and course patterns of anxiety and depressive disorders during pregnancy and after delivery: a prospective-longitudinal study. *J Affect Disord* (2015) 175:385–95. doi: 10.1016/j.jad.2015.01.012
13. Moehler E, Resch F. Infant development and postnatal psychopathology after maternal history of childhood abuse. *Ment Heal* (2017) 13:615–9.
14. Shorey S, Chee CYI, Ng ED, Chan YH, Tam WWS, Chong YS. Prevalence and incidence of postpartum depression among healthy mothers: a systematic review and meta-analysis. *J Psychiatr Res* (2018) 104:235–48. doi: 10.1016/j.jpsychires.2018.08.001
15. Goodman JH, Watson GR, Stubbs B. Anxiety disorders in postpartum women: a systematic review and meta-analysis. *J Affect Disord* (2016) 203:292–331. doi: 10.1016/j.jad.2016.05.033
16. Reck C, Hunt A, Fuchs T, Weiss R, Noon A, Moehler E, et al. Interactive regulation of affect in postpartum depressed mothers and their infants: an overview. *Psychopathology* (2004) 37:272–80. doi: 10.1159/000081983
17. Zambaldi CF, Cantilino A, Montenegro AC, Paes JA, de Albuquerque TLC, Sougey EB. Postpartum obsessive-compulsive disorder: prevalence and clinical characteristics. *Compr Psychiatry* (2009) 50(6):503–9 doi: 10.1016/j.comppsych.2008.11.014
18. VanderKruik R, Barreix M, Chou D, Allen T, Say L, Cohen LS. The global prevalence of postpartum psychosis: a systematic review. *BMC Psychiatry* (2017) 17:272. doi: 10.1186/s12888-017-1427-7
19. Riecher-Rössler A. Was ist postpartale Depression? in Postpartale Depression. Vienna: Springer (2006) pp. 11–20.Available at: https://link.springer.com/content/pdf/10.1007/3-211-29956-4_2.pdf [Accessed October 31, 2018].
20. Falah-Hassani K, Shiri R, Dennis CL. Prevalence and risk factors for comorbid postpartum depressive symptomatology and anxiety. *J Affect Disord* (2016) 198:142–7. doi: 10.1016/j.jad.2016.03.010
21. Sharma V, Khan M, Corpse C, Sharma P. Missed bipolarity and psychiatric comorbidity in women with postpartum depression. *Bipolar Disord* (2008) 10:742–7. doi: 10.1111/j.1399-5618.2008.00606.x
22. Abramowitz JS, Schwartz SA, Moore KM. Obsessional thoughts in postpartum females and their partners: content, severity, and relationship

with depression. *J Clin Psychol Med Settings* (2003) 10:157–64. doi: 10.1023/A:1025454627242

23. Brockington IF, Macdonald E, Wainscott G. Anxiety, obsessions and morbid preoccupations in pregnancy and the puerperium. *Arch Womens Ment Health* (2006) 9:253–63. doi: 10.1007/s00737-006-0134-z
24. Wimmer-Puchinger B, Riecher-Rössler A, editors. (2006). *Postpartale Depression. Springer Science & Business Media.* Available at: https://books.google.de/books?hl=de&lr=&id=VpqWqSLoIlQC&oi=fnd&pg=PA1&dq=Riecher-Rössler,+A.+(2006).+Was+ist+postpartale+Depression%3F+In+Wimmer-Puchinger,+B.+%26++Riecher-Rössler,+A.+Postpartale+Depression.+Von+der+Forschung+zur+Praxis.+(S.11-20).Wien:+S [Accessed October 31, 2018]. doi: 10.1007/3-211-29956-4_2
25. Hoffman Y, Drotar D. The impact of postpartum depressed mood on mother-infant interaction: like mother like baby? *Infant Ment Health J* (1991) 12:65–80. doi: 10.1002/1097-0355(199121)12:1<65::AID-IMHJ2280120107>3.0.CO;2-T
26. Kaitz M, Maytal H, Devor N, Bergman L, Mankuta D. Maternal anxiety, mother–infant interactions, and infants' response to challenge. *Infant Behav Dev* (2010) 33(2):134–48. doi: 10.1016/j.infbeh.2009.12.003
27. Jennings KD, Ross S, Popper S, Elmore M. Thoughts of harming infants in depressed and nondepressed mothers. *J Affect Disord* (1999) 54:21–8. doi: 10.1016/S0165-0327(98)00185-2
28. Sichel DA, Cohen LS, Dimmock JA, Rosenbaum JF. Postpartum obsessive compulsive disorder: a case series. *J Clin Psychiatry* (1993) 54:156–9.
29. Hornstein C, Trautmann-Villalba P, Hohm E, Rave E, Wortmann-Fleischer S, Schwarz M. Maternal bond and mother-child interaction in severe postpartum psychiatric disorders: is there a link? *Arch Womens Ment Health* (2006) 9:279–84. doi: 10.1007/s00737-006-0148-6
30. Persson-Blennow I, Näslund B, McNeil TF, Kaij L, Malmquist-Larsson A. Offspring of women with nonorganic psychosis: mother-infant interaction at three days of age. *Acta Psychiatr Scand* (1984) 70:149–59. doi: 10.1111/j.1600-0447.1986.tb10589.x
31. Ainsworth M. Maternal sensitivity scales: the baltimore longitudinal project. *Power* (1969) 6:1379–88.
32. Forman DR, O'Hara MW, Stuart S, Gorman LL, Larsen KE, Coy KC. Effective treatment for postpartum depression is not sufficient to improve the developing mother–child relationship. *Dev Psychopathol* (2007) 19(2):585–602. doi: 10.1017/S0954579407070289
33. Dix T, Gershoff ET, Meunier LN, Miller PC. The affective structure of supportive parenting: depressive symptoms, immediate emotions, and child-oriented motivation. *Dev Psychol* (2004) 40:1212–27. doi: 10.1037/0012-1649.40.6.1212
34. Murray L, Cooper P, Hipwell A. Mental health of parents caring for infants. *Arch Womens Ment Health* (2003) 6:s71–7. doi: 10.1007/s00737-003-0007-7
35. Lovejoy MC, Graczyk PA, O'Hare E, Neuman G. Maternal depression and parenting behavior. *Clin Psychol Rev* (2000) 20:561–92. doi: 10.1016/S0272-7358(98)00100-7
36. Nicol-Harper R, Harvey AG, Stein A. Interactions between mothers and infants: impact of maternal anxiety. *Infant Behav Dev* (2007) 30:161–7. doi: 10.1016/j.infbeh.2006.08.005
37. Wijnroks L. Maternal recollected anxiety and mother-infant interaction in preterm infants. *Infant Ment Health J* (1999) 20:393–409. doi: 10.1002/(SICI)1097-0355(199924)20:4<393::AID-IMHJ3>3.0.CO;2-I
38. Kaitz M, Maytal H. Interactions between anxious mothers and their infants: an integration of theory and research findings. *Infant Ment Health J* (2005) 26:570–97. doi: 10.1002/imhj.20069
39. Samuel S, Hayton B, Gold I, Feeley N, Carter CS, Zelkowitz P. Maternal mental health moderates the relationship between oxytocin and interactive behavior. *Infant Ment Health J* (2015) 36:415–26. doi: 10.1002/imhj.21521
40. Petzoldt J, Wittchen H-U, Einsle F, Martini J. Maternal anxiety versus depressive disorders: specific relations to infants' crying, feeding and sleeping problems. *Child Care Health Dev* (2016) 42:231–45. doi: 10.1111/cch.12292
41. Künster a. K, Ziegenhain U, Schulze U, Buchheim A, Wietersheim H, Vicari A, et al. Transgenerationale Effekte mütterlicher Angst. *Monatsschrift Kinderheilkd* (2012) 160:982–7. doi: 10.1007/s00112-012-2661-1
42. Stein A, Craske MG, Lehtonen A, Harvey A, Savage-McGlynn E, Davies B, et al. Maternal cognitions and mother-infant interaction in postnatal depression and generalized anxiety disorder. *J Abnorm Psychol* (2012) 121:795–809. doi: 10.1037/a0026847
43. Zelkowitz P, Papageorgiou A, Bardin C, Wang T. Persistent maternal anxiety affects the interaction between mothers and their very low birthweight children at 24 months. *Early Hum Dev* (2009) 85:51–8. doi: 10.1016/j.earlhumdev.2008.06.010
44. Ramsauer B, Achtergarde S. Mothers with acute and chronic postpartum psychoses and impact on the mother-infant interaction. *Schizophr Res* (2018) 197:45–58. doi: 10.1016/j.schres.2018.02.032
45. Riordan D, Appleby L, Faragher B. Mother–infant interaction in post-partum women with schizophrenia and affective disorders. *Psychol Med* (1999) 29(4):991–5. doi: 10.1017/S0033291798007727
46. Whaley SE, Pinto A, Sigman M. Characterizing interactions between anxious mothers and their children. *J Consult Clin Psychol* (1999) 67:826–36. doi: 10.1037/0022-006X.67.6.826
47. Griffiths J, Norris E, Stallard P, Matthews S. Living with parents with obsessive-compulsive disorder: children's lives and experiences. *Psychol Psychother Theory Res Pract* (2012) 85:68–82. doi: 10.1111/j.2044-8341.2011.02016.x
48. Riordan D, Appleby L, Faragher B. Mother–infant interaction in post-partum women with schizophrenia and affective disorders. *Psychol Med* (1999) 29:991–5. doi: 10.1017/S0033291798007727
49. Lunkenheimer ES, Albrecht EC, Kemp CJ. Dyadic flexibility in early parent-child interactions: relations with maternal depressive symptoms and child negativity and behaviour problems. *Infant Child Dev* (2013) 22:250–69. doi: 10.1002/icd.1783
50. Murray L, Fiori-Cowley A, Hooper R, Cooper P. The impact of postnatal depression and associated adversity on early mother-infant interactions and later infant outcome. *Child Dev* (1996) 67:2512–26. doi: 10.1111/j.1467-8624.1996.tb01871.x
51. Behrendt HF, Konrad K, Goecke TW, Fakhrabadi R, Herpertz-Dahlmann B, Firk C. Postnatal mother-to-infant attachment in subclinically depressed mothers: dyads at risk? *Psychopathology* (2016) 49:269–76. doi: 10.1159/000447597
52. Letourneau N, Salmani M, Duffett-Leger L. Maternal depressive symptoms and parenting of children from birth to 12 years. *West J Nurs Res* (2010) 32:662–85. doi: 10.1177/0193945909359409
53. Turner SM, Beidel DC, Roberson-Nay R, Tervo K. Parenting behaviors in parents with anxiety disorders. *Behav Res Ther* (2003) 41:541–54. doi: 10.1016/S0005-7967(02)00028-1
54. Crosby Budinger M, Drazdowski TK, Ginsburg GS. Anxiety-promoting parenting behaviors: a comparison of anxious parents with and without social anxiety disorder. *Child Psychiatry Hum Dev* (2013) 44:412–8. doi: 10.1007/s10578-012-0335-9
55. Hirshfeld D, Biederman J, Brody L, Faraone S, Rosenbaum J. Associations between expressed emotion and child behavioral inhibition and psychopathology - a pilot study. *J Am Acad Child Adolesc Psychiatry* (1997) 36(2):205–13. doi: 10.1097/00004583-199702000-00011
56. Challacombe F, Salkovskis P. A preliminary investigation of the impact of maternal obsessive-compulsive disorder and panic disorder on parenting and children. *J Anxiety Disord* (2009) 23:848–57. doi: 10.1016/j.janxdis.2009.04.002
57. DiBartolo PM, Helt M. Theoretical models of affectionate versus affectionless control in anxious families: a critical examination based on observations of parent–child interactions. *Clin Child Fam Psychol Rev* (2007) 10:253–74. doi: 10.1007/s10567-007-0017-5
58. Aktar E, Bögels SM. Exposure to parents' negative emotions as a developmental pathway to the family aggregation of depression and anxiety in the first year of life. *Clin Child Fam Psychol Rev* (2017) 20:369–90. doi: 10.1007/s10567-017-0240-7
59. Aktar E, Colonnesi C, De Vente W, Majdandžić M, Bögels SM. How do parents' depression and anxiety, and infants' negative temperament relate to parent-infant face-to-face interactions? *Dev Psychopathol* (2017) 29:697–710. doi: 10.1017/S0954579416000390
60. Weinberg MK, Beeghly M, Olson KL, Tronick E. Effects of maternal depression and panic disorder on mother-infant interactive behavior in the face-to-face still-face paradigm. *Infant Ment Health J* (2008) 29:472–91. doi: 10.1002/imhj.20193
61. Ainsworth Mary D, Salter Bell SM, Stayton DF. Infant-mother attachment and social development: socialization as a product of reciprocal

responsiveness to signals. In: *The integration of a child into a social world.* p. 99–135. doi: 10.1007/978-0-387-89959-6_2
62. Easterbrooks M, Bureau J, Lyons-Ruth K. Developmental correlates and predictors of emotional availability in mother–child interaction: a longitudinal study from infancy to middle childhood. *Dev Psychopathol* (2012) 24(1):65–78. doi: 10.1017/S0954579411000666
63. Bost KK, Shin N, Mcbride BA, Brown GL, Vaughn BE, Coppola G, et al. Maternal secure base scripts, children's attachment security, and mother - child narrative styles. In: *Attachment and Human Development.* p. 241–60. doi: 10.1080/14616730600856131
64. Spieker SJ, Oxford ML, Fleming CB, Lohr MJ. Parental childhood adversity, depressive symptoms, and parenting quality: effects on toddler self-regulation in child welfare services in involved families. *Infant Ment Health J* (2018) 39:5–16. doi: 10.1002/imhj.21685
65. Grossmann K, Grossmann KE, Spangler G, Suess G, Unzner L. Maternal sensitivity and newborns' orientation responses as related to quality of attachment in Northern Germany. *Monogr Soc Res Child Dev* (1985) 50:233. doi: 10.2307/3333836
66. De Wolff MH., van Ijzendoorn M. Sensitivity and attachment: a meta-analysis on parental antecedents of infant attachment. *Child Dev*(1997) 68(4):571–91. doi: 10.1111/j.1467-8624.1997.tb04218.x
67. Cicchetti D, Barnett D. Attachment organization in maltreated preschoolers. *Dev Psychopathol* (1991) 3:397–411. doi: 10.1017/S0954579400007598
68. Fenichel E. Relationships at risk. *Infants Young Child* (2002) 15:49–56. doi: 10.1097/00001163-200210000-00007
69. Main M, Hesse E. Parents' unresolved traumatic experiences are related to infant disorganized attachment status: Is frightened and/or frightening parental behavior the linking mechanism? In: Greenberg MT, Cicchetti D, Cummings EM, (Eds.), *The John D. and Catherine T. MacArthur Foundation series on mental health and development. Attachment in the preschool years: theory, research, and intervention.* Chicago, IL, US: University of Chicago Press. (1990) pp. 161-182. doi: 10.1016/j.ncl.2015.11.007
70. Belsky J, Pasco Fearon RM. Early attachment security, subsequent maternal sensitivity, and later child development: does continuity in development depend upon continuity of caregiving? *Attach Hum Dev* (2002) 4:361–87. doi: 10.1080/14616730210167267
71. Sroufe LA. Attachment and development: a prospective, longitudinal study from birth to adulthood. *Attach Hum Dev* (2005) 7:349–67, doi: 10.1080/14616730500365928
72. Wartner UG, Grossmann K, Fremmer-Bombik E, Suess G. Attachment patterns at age six in South Germany: predictability from infancy and implications for preschool behavior. *Child Dev* (1994) 65(4):1014–27. doi: 10.1111/j.1467-8624.1994.tb00799.x
73. Campbell SB, Brownell CA, Hungerford A, Spieker SJ, Mohan R, Blessing JS. The course of maternal depressive symptoms and maternal sensitivity as predictors of attachment security at 36 months. *Dev Psychopathol* (2004) 16:231–52. doi: 10.1017/S0954579404044499
74. Carter AS, Garrity-Rokous FE, Chazan-Cohen R, Little C, Briggs-Gowan MJ. Maternal depression and comorbidity: predicting early parenting, attachment security, and toddler social-emotional problems and competencies. *J Am Acad Child Adolesc Psychiatry* (2001) 40:18–26. doi: 10.1097/00004583-200101000-00012
75. Bakermans-Kranenburg MJ, Van IJzendoorn MH, Juffer F. Less is more: meta-analyses of sensitivity and attachment interventions in early childhood. *Psychol Bull* (2003) 129:195–215. doi: 10.1037/0033-2909.129.2.195
76. Lotzin A, Lu X, Kriston L, Schiborr J, Musal T, Romer G, et al. Observational tools for measuring parent–infant interaction: a systematic review. *Clin Child Fam Psychol Rev* (2015) 18(2):99–132.
77. Bretherton I. Emotional availability: an attachment perspective. *Attach Hum Dev* (2000) 2:233–41. doi: 10.1080/14616730050085581
78. Bretherton I. Revisiting Mary Ainsworth's conceptualization and assessments of maternal sensitivity-insensitivity. *Attach Hum Dev* (2013) 15:460–84. doi: 10.1080/14616734.2013.835128
79. Mesman J, Emmen RAG. Mary Ainsworth's legacy: a systematic review of observational instruments measuring parental sensitivity. *Attach Hum Dev* (2013) 15:485–506. doi: 10.1080/14616734.2013.820900
80. Owen MT. The NICHD study of early child care mother-infant interaction scales. *Unpubl manuscript, Timberlawn Psychiatr Res Found Dallas, TX* (1992)
81. Bradley Bradley RH, Corwyn RF. Infant temperament, parenting, and externalizing behavior in first grade: a test of the differential susceptibility hypothesis. *J Child Psychol Psychiatry* (2008) 49:124–31. doi: 10.1111/j.1469-7610.2007.01829.x
82. NICHD Early Child Care Research Network. Child-care and family predictors of preschool attachment and stability from infancy. *Dev Psychol* (2001) 37:847–62. doi: 10.1037//0012-1649.37.6.847
83. Bakermans-Kranenburg MJ, Van IJzendoorn MH, Kroonenberg PM. Differences in attachment security between African-American and white children: ethnicity or socio-economic status? *Infant Behav Dev* (2004) 27:417–33. doi: 10.1016/j.infbeh.2004.02.002
84. NICHD Early Child Care Research Network. Child-care structure→ process→ outcome: direct and indirect effects of child-care quality on young children's development. *Psychol Sci* (2002) 13:199–206. doi: 10.1111/1467-9280.00438
85. Biringen Z. *The emotional availability (EA) scales and the emotional attachment and emotional availability (EA2) clinical screener: Infancy/early childhood version; middle childhood/youth version; therapist/interventionist manual; couple relationship manual.* Boulder (2008). Available at: www.emotionalavailability.com.
86. Biringen Z, Derscheid D, Vliegen N, Closson L, Easterbrooks MA. Emotional availability (EA): theoretical background, empirical research using the EA Scales, and clinical applications. *Dev Rev* (2014) 34:114–67. doi: 10.1016/j.dr.2014.01.002
87. Easterbrooks MA, Biringen Z. The emotional availability scales: methodological refinements of the construct and clinical implications related to gender and at-risk interactions. *Infant Ment Health J* (2005) 26:291–4. doi: 10.1002/imhj.20053
88. Kogan N, Carter AS. Mother-infant reengagement foilowing the still-face: the role of maternal emotional availability in infant affect regulation. *Infant Behav Dev* (1996) 19:359–70. doi: 10.1016/S0163-6383(96)90034-X
89. Biringen Z, Damon J, Grigg W, Mone J, Pipp-Siegel S, Skillern S, et al. Emotional availability: differential predictions to infant attachment and kindergarten adjustment based on observation time and context. *Infant Ment Health J* (2005) 26:295–308. doi: 10.1002/imhj.20054
90. Dolev S, Oppenheim D, Koren-Karie N, Yirmiya N. Emotional availability in mother-child interaction: the case of children with autism spectrum disorders. *Parenting* (2009) 9:183–97. doi: 10.1080/15295190902844332
91. Crittenden PM. *CARE-Index: coding manual. Unpubl manuscript.* Miami: Family Relations Institute (2003).
92. Bowlby, J. (1969). *Attachment and loss: vol. 1. Attachment.* New York: Basic Books.
93. Ross LE, McLean LM. Anxiety disorders during pregnancy and the postpartum period: a systematic review. *J Clin Psychiatry* (2006) 67:1285–98. doi: 10.4088/JCP.v67n0818
94. Agius A, Xuereb RB, Carrick-Sen D, Sultana R, Rankin J. The co-existence of depression, anxiety and post-traumatic stress symptoms in the perinatal period: a systematic review. *Midwifery* (2016) 36:70–9. doi: 10.1016/j.midw.2016.02.013
95. Network NECCR. Child care and mother-child interaction in the first 3 years of life. *Dev Psychol* (1999) 35:1399–413. doi: 10.1037//0012-1649.35.6.1399
96. McHugh ML. Interrater reliability: the kappa statistic. *Biochem Med (Zagreb)* (2012) 22(3):276–82.
97. Parsons CE, Young KS, Stein A, Kringelbach ML. Intuitive parenting: understanding the neural mechanisms of parents' adaptive responses to infants. *Curr Opin Psychol* (2017) 15:40–4. doi: 10.1016/j.copsyc.2017.02.010
98. Derogatis LR. Symptom Checklist-90-R (SCL-90-R). In: *Administration, scoring, and procedures manual.*, 3rd. Minneapolis: National Computer Systems (1994).
99. Franke GH. Brief symptom inventory von Derogatis (BSI). Göttingen: Beltz Test (2000).
100. Cox J, Chapman G, Murray D, Jones P. Validation of the Edinburgh Postnatal Depression Scale (EPDS) in non-postnatal women. *J Affect Disord* (1996) 39(3):185–9. doi: 10.1016/0165-0327(96)00008-0
101. Tietz A, Zietlow AL, Reck C. Maternal bonding in mothers with postpartum anxiety disorder: the crucial role of subclinical depressive symptoms and maternal avoidance behaviour. *Arch Womens Ment Health* (2014) 17:433–42. doi: 10.1007/s00737-014-0423-x
102. O'Hara M, Wisner K. Perinatal mental illness: definition, description and aetiology. *Elsevier Best Pract Res Clin Obstet Gynaecol* (2014) 28:3–12. doi:

10.1016/j.bpobgyn.2013.09.002
103. Reck C, Struben K, Backenstrass M, Stefenelli U, Reinig K, Fuchs T, et al. Prevalence, onset and comorbidity of postpartum anxiety and depressive disorders. *Acta Psychiatr Scand* (2008) 118:459–68. doi: 10.1111/j.1600-0447.2008.01264.x
104. Cohn JF, Campbell SB, Matias R, Hopkins J. Face-to-face interactions of postpartum depressed and nondepressed mother-infant pairs at 2 Months. *Dev Psychol* (1990) 26:15–23. doi: 10.1037/0012-1649.26.1.15
105. Ewell Foster CJ, Garber J, Durlak JA. Current and past maternal depression, maternal interaction behaviors, and children's externalizing and internalizing symptoms. *J Abnorm Child Psychol* (2008) 36:527–37. doi: 10.1007/s10802-007-9197-1
106. Caughy MO, Huang K-Y, Lima J. Patterns of conflict interaction in mother-toddler dyads: differences between depressed and non-depressed mothers. *J Child Fam Stud* (2009) 18:10–20. doi: 10.1007/s10826-008-9201-6
107. Laucht M, Esser G, Schmidt MH. Heterogene entwicklung von kindern postpartal depressiver mütter. *Z Klin Psychol Psychother* (2002) 31:127–34. doi: 10.1026//1616-3443.31.2.127
108. Laurent HK, Ablow JC. The missing link: mothers' neural response to infant cry related to infant attachment behaviors. *Infant Behav Dev* (2012) 35:761–72. doi: 10.1016/j.infbeh.2012.07.007
109. Bögels SM, Van Melick M. The relationship between child-report, parent self-report, and partner report of perceived parental rearing behaviors and anxiety in children and parents. *Pers Individ Dif* (2004) 37:1583–96. doi: 10.1016/j.paid.2004.02.014
110. Kim P, Rigo P, Leckman JF, Mayes LC, Cole PM, Feldman R, et al. A prospective longitudinal study of perceived infant outcomes at 18-24 months: neural and psychological correlates of parental thoughts and actions assessed during the first month postpartum. *Front Psychol* (2015) 6:1772. doi: 10.3389/fpsyg.2015.01772
111. Lok P, Pop-Purceleanu M, Tendolkar I. Anxiety disorders during pregnancy and the post-partum period. *Tijdschr Psychiatr* (2015) 57(6):415–23.
112. Majer M, Ising M, Künzel H, Binder EB, Holsboer F, Modell S, et al. Impaired divided attention predicts delayed response and risk to relapse in subjects with depressive disorders. *Psychol Med* (2004) 34:1453–63. doi: 10.1017/S0033291704002697
113. Lee RSC, Hermens DF, Porter MA, Redoblado-Hodge MA. A meta-analysis of cognitive deficits in first-episode major depressive disorder. *J Affect Disord* (2012) 140:113–24. doi: 10.1016/j.jad.2011.10.023
114. Madigan S, Plamondon A, Browne D, Jenkins J. Stability of observed maternal behavior across tasks, time, and siblings. *Parenting* (2016) 16:108–24. doi: 10.1080/15295192.2016.1134990
115. Murray L, Cooper P, Creswell C, Schofield E, Sack C. The effects of maternal social phobia on mother-infant interactions and infant social responsiveness. *J Child Psychol Psychiatry* (2007) 48:45–52. doi: 10.1111/j.1469-7610.2006.01657.x
116. Spangler G. Individual dispositions as precursors of differences in attachment quality: why maternal sensitivity is nevertheless important. *Attach Hum Dev* (2013) 15:657–72. doi: 10.1080/14616734.2013.842065
117. Simons RL, Beaman J, Conger RD, Chao W. Childhood experience, conceptions of parenting, and attitudes of spouse as determinants of parental behavior. *J Marriage Fam* (1993) 55:91–106. doi: 10.2307/352961
118. Belsky J, Sligo J, Jaffee SR, Woodward L, Silva PA. Intergenerational transmission of warm-sensitive-stimulating parenting: a prospective study of mothers and fathers of 3-year-olds. *Child Dev* (2005) 76:384–96. doi: 10.1111/j.1467-8624.2005.00852.x
119. Bailey H, DeOliveira C, Wolfe V, Evans E, Hartwick C. The impact of childhood maltreatment history on parenting_A comparison of maltreatment types & assessment methods. *Child Abuse Neg* (2012) 36(3):236–46. doi: 10.1016/j.chiabu.2011.11.005
120. Gaillard A, Le Strat Y, Mandelbrot L, Keïta H, Dubertret C. Predictors of postpartum depression: prospective study of 264 women followed during pregnancy and postpartum. *Psychiatry Res* (2014) 215:341–6. doi: 10.1016/j.psychres.2013.10.003
121. Kivijarvi M, Raiha H, Virtanen S, Lertola K, Piha J. Maternal sensitivity behavior and infant crying, fussing and contented behavior: the effects of mother's experienced social support. *Scand J Psychol* (2004) 45:239–46. doi: 10.1111/j.1467-9450.2004.00400.x
122. Mertesacker B, Bade U, Haverkock A, Pauli-Pott U. Predicting maternal reactivity/sensitivity: the role of infant emotionality, maternal depressiveness/anxiety, and social support. *Infant Ment Health J* (2004) 25:47–61. doi: 10.1002/imhj.10085
123. Sidor A, Köhler H, Cierpka M. Einfluss der sozioökonomischen Risikobelastung auf mütterliche Feinfühligkeit, Stressbelastung und Familienfunktionalität. *Prax Kinderpsychol Kinderpsychiatr* (2018) 67:257–3. doi: 10.13109/prkk.2018.67.3.257
124. Tamis-LeMonda CS, Briggs RD, McClowry SG, Snow DL. Maternal control and sensitivity, child gender, and maternal education in relation to children's behavioral outcomes in African American families. *J Appl Dev Psychol* (2009) 30:321–31. doi: 10.1016/j.appdev.2008.12.018

15

Prenatal Alcohol Exposure and Child Psychosocial Behavior: A Sibling Fixed-Effects Analysis

Kayoko Ichikawa[1*], *Takeo Fujiwara*[2] *and Ichiro Kawachi*[2,3]

[1] Department of Health Informatics, Kyoto University School of Public Health, Kyoto, Japan, [2] Department of Global Health Promotion, Tokyo Medical and Dental University, Tokyo, Japan, [3] Department of Social and Behavioral Sciences, Harvard T.H. Chan School of Public Health, Boston, MA, United States

Correspondence:
Kayoko Ichikawa
ichikawa.kayoko.35a@kyoto-u.ac.jp

Background: The association between low levels of alcohol consumption during pregnancy and children's health remains unclear because of the difficulty in ruling out residual genetic and environmental confounding factors. In this study, using a within-family sibling fixed effects design, we sought to examine the association between low prenatal alcohol exposures (PAE) and children's overall psychosocial behavior in a Japanese cohort.

Methods: We used maternal and sibling data from the Japanese Study of Stratification, Health, Income and Neighborhood 2012-2013. Households were recruited from the Tokyo metropolitan area through clustered random sampling. Children under 18 years old who have siblings (n = 1,600) and their mothers were selected. PAE status was retrospectively measured, and classified by binominal and continuous measurements. Outcome measures of children's psychosocial behavior were assessed with the Child Behavior Checklist T-score.

Results: Low PAE was significantly associated with the offspring's anxiety problems (β = 1.54, 95%CI = 0.26, 2.82) and internalizing problems (β = 2.73, 95%CI = 0.87, 4.60), and marginally significant with the offspring's total problem scores (β = 2.34, 95%CI = −0.24, 4.92). There was no significant difference in PAE between boys and girls when it comes to behavioral problems.

Conclusions: Low PAE was associated with children's anxiety, internalizing problems and overall problems, taking into account possible unobserved genetic and environmental confounding influences.

Keywords: alcohol-related disorders, developmental disabilities, maternal-fetal relations, pregnancy, prenatal alcohol exposure

INTRODUCTION

The U.S. Centers for Disease Control, the U.S. Surgeon General, the American College of Obstetricians and Gynecologists, and the American Academy of Pediatrics uniformly advise women not to consume alcohol during pregnancy (1–5). However, the debate on whether "moderate consumption" of alcohol can be safely practiced during pregnancy continues (6–9). For example, a large-scale study in Denmark recently reported that antenatal exposure to binge drinking was associated with internalizing and externalizing behavioral problems among boys (5). However, the study found no association with lower doses of alcohol exposure. In fact, children of expectant mothers who consumed moderate amounts of alcohol were found to have better mental health than those whose mother abstained from alcohol–a controversial result that was widely reported in the media.

Although it is widely accepted that binge drinking during pregnancy increases the risk of fetal alcohol syndrome (10, 11), whether low-to-moderate levels of alcohol consumption during pregnancy can affect children's health remains controversial (12–14). A recent meta-analysis which assessed both normal and abnormal development as continuous variables concluded that mild-to-moderate prenatal alcohol exposure (PAE) during all trimesters was not associated with child psychosocial outcomes such as cognition and mental development (12). However, it suggested that further studies were needed to rule out residual confounding factors.

There are several reasons why it is challenging to investigate the effects of PAE on children's behavioral problems. First, mothers tend to under report their drinking levels during pregnancy because of prevailing social norms (14). Second, any correlation between maternal drinking during pregnancy and child outcomes is likely to be confounded by a range of unobserved factors including family environment and shared genetic influences. Third, it is ethically infeasible to design a randomized controlled trial to investigate the association between PAE and child behavioral outcomes. As an alternative to directly manipulating the exposure of interest, some sort of quasi-experimental approach is needed, such as the within-family sibling fixed-effects design. To our knowledge, there is a limited number of studies that have used quasi-experimental design to infer causality of deferential low PAE on behavior problems among twins, siblings, or cousins (15, 16). Hence, there has been a call for the implementation of more quasi-experimental study using natural experiment (17).

Notably, studies that considered observed and unobserved confounding factors are rare (16, 18, 19). The basic idea of a sibling fixed-effects design is to leverage the within-family, between-sibling differences in exposure to maternal drinking during pregnancy (e.g., mother drank during first pregnancy, but not during subsequent pregnancies), which effectively differentiates sibling-invariants observed and unobserved confounding variables, such as genetic influences or maternal temperament/personality, or family environment (19, 20).

The findings from the few existing studies using the sibling fixed-effects approach (16, 18, 19) suggest that even low-to-moderate PAE is a risk factor for children's externalizing problems such as attention deficit hyperactivity disorder, infant difficulties and children's behavioral problems. However, the literature remains sparse, especially in the Asian context where alcohol consumption among women is low compared to Western societies (21).

Abbreviations: PAE, prenatal alcohol exposure; OLS, ordinary least squares.

In this study, we examined the association between low PAE and children's overall psychosocial behavior in a Japanese cohort using the sibling fixed-effects design.

METHODS

Participants

The J-SHINE (Japanese study of Stratification, Health, Income and Neighborhood) is an ongoing cohort study established since 2010. Details of the study have been previously described (22). Briefly, the baseline survey was carried out between 2010 and 2011, when a clustered random sample of individuals aged 25–50 years residing in four municipalities in urban or suburban settings of the Tokyo metropolitan area were invited to participate. The household survey asked about the health of all children under the age of 18 years co-residing with the subjects. A follow-up survey was conducted between 2012 and 2013. In the baseline survey, 13,920 individuals were randomly selected from the "*koseki*" registration system, a compulsory domiciliary registration system in Japan that included all residents in target area (N = 594,249). Among the individuals invited to participate, 4,385 men and women responded (31.6% response rate), including 2,184 households with children under 18 years. By wave 2, the number of households with children increased to 2,244, and of these, 1,520 households (67.7%) agreed to participate in the follow-up survey (including 2,470 children under 18 years). Written informed consent was received from all the participants in the study. We excluded children who did not have the outcome data and the prenatal mothers who drink alcohol more than 2 times per week (N = 33, 1.7% of all sample) because we focused on low-level drinkers. Therefore, the number of children in the study was 1,933. In addition, we used only sibling data for the fixed-effects models, the total number of children who had siblings and who had outcome data was 1,600 (mean age 114.1 months ± 52.5 *SD*). Among them, 1,046 had two siblings, 518 had three siblings, and 36 had four siblings. If the number of siblings was more than two in one family, we compared each sibling pair separately. For example, if the number of the children were three (A, B, C) in one household, we compared A-B, A-C, and B-C.

The J-SHINE was conducted using computer-assisted personal interviewing (CAPI), unless the participants requested a face-to-face interview. This study was carried out in accordance with the recommendations of ethical guidelines for medical and health research involving human subjects. The study protocol was approved by the ethics committee of the Graduate School of Medicine of the University of Tokyo. All subjects provided written informed consent in accordance with the Declaration of Helsinki.

MEASUREMENTS

Prenatal Alcohol Drinking

The J-SHINE study asked mothers to report their drinking behavior during each pregnancy retrospectively. Response categories included: (1) 2 times or more per week, (2) 1–4 times

TABLE 1 | Demographic characteristics of children and families for individual level.

Variables	All sample (n = 1933) n (%)	Siblings sample (n = 1600) n (%)
AREA CHARACTERISTICS		
Tokyo urban area (Adachi)	393 (20.3)	332 (20.8)
Tokyo urban area (Mitaka)	389 (20.1)	306 (19.1)
Tokyo suburban area (Kashiwa)	646 (33.4)	546 (34.1)
Tokyo suburban area (Tokorozawa)	505 (26.1)	416 (26.0)
FAMILY CHARACTERISTICS		
Mother's age (years old) (mean, SD)	37.5 (5.5)	37.2 (5.3)
Father's age (years old) (mean, SD)	39.4 (6.3)	39.2 (6.2)
MOTHER'S EDUCATION		
< = 12 years	946 (49.0)	388 (24.3)
>12 years	875 (45.3)	1186 (74.1)
unknown	112 (5.8)	26 (1.6)
FATHER'S EDUCATION		
< = 12 years	427 (22.1)	371 (23.2)
>12 years	1441 (74.6)	1181 (77.8)
unknown	30 (1.6)	48 (3.0)
Working mother	875 (45.3)	707 (44.2)
Working father	1631 (84.4)	1363 (85.2)
NUMBERS OF FAMILY		
< = 4	1351 (60.0)	1054 (65.9)
> = 5	574 (27.0)	541 (33.8)
Unknown	8 (0.4)	5 (0.3)
FAMILY INCOME		
<JPY 5 million[a]	438 (22.7)	362 (22.6)
JPY 5–7.5 million	572 (30.0)	484 (52.9)
JPY 7.5–10 million	391 (20.2)	329 (20.6)
>JPY 10 million	369 (19.1)	288 (18.0)
unknown	163 (8.4)	137 (8.6)
Domestic violence	631 (32.6)	538 (33.6)
Prenatal smoking	67 (3.5)	59 (3.7)
CHILDREN'S CHARACTERISTICS		
Number of siblings		
1	333 (17.3)	-
2	1046 (54.1)	1046 (65.4)
3	518 (26.8)	518 (32.4)
4	36 (1.9)	36 (2.3)
Sex (male)	971 (50.2)	800 (50.0)
Age (months) (mean, SD)	113.9 (53.7)	114.1 (52.5)
PRENATAL ALCOHOL CONSUMPTION		
1-4 times/month	110 (5.7)	98 (6.1)
rare	401 (20.7)	347 (21.7)
never	1083 (56.0)	886 (55.4)
unknown	339 (17.5)	269 (16.8)
CBCL *T* SCORE, *N*, MEAN (*SD*)		
4-18 Years old		
Physical problem	52.3 (4.8)	52.1 (4.7)
Social problem	53.3 (5.3)	53.0 (5.1)
Thought problem	51.0 (3.8)	51.0 (3.8)
Delinquency	52.9 (5.2)	52.9 (5.2)
2-18 YEARS OLD		
Withdrawal	53.4 (5.4)	53.2 (5.4)
Anxiety problem	52.7 (4.9)	52.6 (4.9)
Attention problem	53.0 (5.7)	52.8 (5.6)
Aggressiveness	53.4 (5.5)	53.4 (5.5)
Internalizing problem	49.6 (7.8)	49.3 (7.8)
Externalizing problem	49.6 (8.4)	49.5 (8.4)
Total problem	48.4 (9.7)	48.0 (9.7)

[a]*JPY, Japanese Yen; JPY 120 is approximately equal to US 1 dollar.*

per month, (3) rarely (but not zero), and (4) never. We excluded those who responded with "2 times or more per week" to focus on low prenatal alcohol drinking during pregnancy, and combined "1–4 times per month" and "rarely," so that PAE was binarized into "never" vs. "ever."

Outcome Variable: The CBCL4-18/2-3 (Child Behavior Check List 4-18/2-3)

The outcome variable, that is, children's psychosocial developmental problems, was assessed with the CBCL4-18 checklist which targets children aged 4 to 18 years, and the CBCL2-3 which targets children aged 2 to 3 years (23, 24). The CBCL is a scale that assesses internalizing, externalizing, and total behavior problems using 113 items, with good psychometric properties (24). A higher score denotes more problematic behavior. Ratings were completed by caregivers (mother, n = 1316, 83.7%). The T score of each CBCL score was calculated using the standardized distribution among Japanese children and mean score represents the 50th percentile, which has been shown to have good reliability and validity (23–25).

Covariates

We considered a wide range of potential correlates of PAE as control variables in adjusted models. There are two types of covariates: sibling variables that are less likely to be variant and sibling-varying variables. With respect to our sibling fixed-effects models, sibling variables that are less likely to be variant include factors that did not vary between siblings, that is, parent's age, educational level, working status, family income and domestic violence and others that are less likely to be changeable variables. In contrast, sibling-varying variables include children's age, sex, and prenatal smoking during each pregnancy.

Statistical Analysis

To estimate the relationship between maternal drinking during pregnancy and children's behavioral outcomes, we conducted ordinary least squares (OLS) regressions controlling for all observed sibling-varying and sibling-invariant variables for the full sample, as well as for the sibling sub-sample. Next, we conducted sibling fixed-effects analysis only among the siblings (i.e., singletons do not contribute to this analysis), with further adjustment of correlation of 3 or more siblings comparisons from the same family. In the fixed-effects model, the effects of PAE on children's outcomes were calculated by differentiating the unobserved, sibling-invariant shared factors, such as genetic or family environmental influences. Finally, we conducted fixed-effects models stratified by child sex (i.e., male-male, female-female, and male-female pair of siblings) as a sensitivity analysis. All analyses were performed with STATA 13.0 (StataCorp LP, College Station, TX, USA).

RESULTS

Table 1 shows the demographic characteristics of families and children comparing the full sample (n = 1,933) and the sample restricted to the siblings (n = 1,600). In the full sample, the frequencies of prenatal alcohol "1-4 times/month," "rarely," and "never" were 6.1, 21.7, and 55.4%, respectively. The vast majority of pregnant women in this Japanese cohort therefore fitted into the abstention or light drinking categories.

There was a total of 491 sibling pairs whose mother never drank during pregnancies (**Appendix 1**). Further, 37 (4.6%) mothers reported drinking during their first pregnancy but not during subsequent pregnancies. Another 31 mothers (3.9%) reported abstaining from alcohol during their first pregnancy, but consumed alcohol during subsequent pregnancies. Effects of PAE, binarized according to "ever" vs. "never," are shown in **Table 2**. In the OLS model, the effect of PAE was not significantly associated with children's psychosocial problems in both the overall sample and the sibling sample. In the unadjusted sibling fixed-effects model, prenatal drinking was significantly associated with children's delinquency (β = 1.63, 95%CI = 0.02, 3.25), anxiety problems (β = 1.50, 95%CI = 0.15, 2.85), internalizing problems (β = 2.62, 95%CI = 0.61, 4.62), and total problem scores (β = 2.39, 95%CI = 0.11, 4.66). After adjusting for sibling-varying variables, maternal drinking during pregnancy was significantly associated with offspring's anxiety problems (β = 1.54, 95%CI = 0.26, 2.82), internalizing problems (β = 2.73, 95%CI = 0.87, 4.60) and marginally significant with offspring's overall problem scores (β = 2.34, 95%CI = −0.24, 4.92). Additionally, adjusting for sibling-varying and sibling-invariant variables, such as parent's working status and maternal drinking during pregnancy, remained significantly associated with children's anxiety problems, internalizing problems and overall problem scores. In sensitivity analysis, maternal drinking during pregnancy measured with continuously (i.e., frequencies of alcohol drinking per month) was not statistically significant (**Appendix 2**).

Table 3 shows the sibling fixed-effects results of maternal drinking and children's psychosocial problems, stratified by children's sex. Drinking during pregnancy was not associated with girl's thought problems (β = −2.56, 95%CI = −7.59, 2.47) attention problems (β = −0.16, 95%CI = −2.29, 1.96), anxiety problems (β = −2.56, 95%CI = −0.80, 3.07) and aggression (β = 0.27, 95%CI = −3.17, 3.70). When it comes to the effect of drinking during pregnancy on internalizing, externalizing and total problems, there was no different between boys and girls.

TABLE 2 | OLS models and fixed-effects models of the association between PAE[a] and children's psychosocial behaviors.

	All sample, OLS, all measured variables adjusted[b]		Siblings sample, OLS, all measured variables adjusted[b]		Fixed effects model,unadjusted		Fixed effects model, adjusted[c]		Fixed effects model, adjusted[d]	
CBCL T score	**β**	**95%CI**	**β**	**95%CI**	**β**	**95%CI**	**β**	**95%CI**	**β**	**95%CI**
4-18 YEARS OLD										
Physical problem	0.29	−0.28, 0.86	0.51	−0.10, 1.11	0.94	−0.68, 2.56	1.19	−1.74, 4.11	0.90	−1.85, 3.65
Social problem	0.12	−0.53, 0.77	0.47	−0.20, 1.14	0.74	−0.95, 2.44	1.30	−0.63, 3.23	1.22	−0.76, 3.20
Thought problem	−0.35	−0.77, 0.07	−0.24	−0.67, 0.20	−0.83	−2.11, 0.44	−0.80	−3.34, 1.73	−0.86	−3.35, 1.63
Delinquency	0.48	−0.14, 1.10	0.51	−0.17, 1.19	**1.63**	**0.02, 3.25**	1.73	−0.33, 3.79	1.57	−0.50, 3.64
2–18 YEARS OLD										
Withdrawal	−0.01	−0.65, 0.62	0.19	−0.50, 0.88	−0.51	−1.95, 0.93	−0.40	−1.59, 0.79	−0.41	−1.66, 0.84
Anxiety problem	0.14	−0.43, 0.70	0.43	−0.18, 1.05	**1.50**	**0.15, 2.85**	**1.54**	**0.26, 2.82**	**1.40**	**0.09, 2.72**
Attention problem	0.27	−0.37, 0.91	0.43	−0.23, 1.10	−0.53	−2.20, 1.13	−0.44	−2.57, 1.69	−0.58	−2.78, 1.63
Aggressiveness	0.32	−0.33, 0.96	0.49	−0.21, 1.20	1.18	−0.45, 2.80	1.15	−0.70, 2.99	1.23	−0.69, 3.16
Internalizing problem	0.41	−0.49, 1.31	0.91	−0.07, 1.88	**2.62**	**0.61, 4.62**	**2.73**	**0.87, 4.60**	**2.68**	**0.73, 4.63**
Externalizing problem	0.49	−0.48, 1.45	0.72	−0.35, 1.78	1.77	−0.45, 3.99	1.50	−1.04, 4.04	1.64	−0.94, 4.22
Total problem	0.42	−0.71, 1.55	0.95	−0.30, 2.19	**2.39**	**0.11, 4.66**	2.34[e]	−0.24, 4.92	2.32	−0.34, 4.98

[a]*Measurements of alcohol drinking is binary outcomes (never = 0, more than one time = 1).*
[b]*Adjusted by children's age and sex, parent's age, education and working status, family income, prenatal smoking, domestic violence, clustered by family ID.*
[c]*Adjusted by children's age and sex and difference levels of prenatal smoking baseline prenatal drinking status among siblings, clustered by family ID.*
[d]*Adjusted by children's age and sex, parent's education level, family income, family number, domestic violence and baseline prenatal drinking status among siblings, clustered by family ID.*
[e]*Marginally significant: p = 0.08.*
Bold values means the results which is statistically significant.

TABLE 3 | Fixed-effects model stratified by sibling's sex pairs.

	Male-male pair		Female-female pair		Male-female pair	
CBCL T score	**β**	**95%CI**	**β**	**95%CI**	**β**	**95%CI**
4–18 YEARS OLD						
Physical problem	0.01	−3.88, 3.90	1.05	−4.41, 6.51	2.11	−1.95, 6.18
Social problem	1.34	−2.28, 4.97	1.16	−1.64, 3.96	1.27	−1.71, 4.24
Thought problem	1.39	−1.35, 4.12	−2.56	−7.59, 2.47	−1.43	−4.13, 1.27
Delinquency	0.76	−3.22, 4.75	0.16	−3.06, 3.39	**3.15**	**0.52, 5.77**
2–18 YEARS OLD						
Withdrawal	−0.81	−3.41, 1.79	−1.22	−2.47, 0.03	0.33	−1.28, 1.95
Anxiety problem	2.32	−0.56, 5.20	1.13	−0.80, 3.07	1.37	−0.07, 2.82
Attention problem	1.04	−1.98, 4.06	−0.16	−2.29, 1.96	−1.60	−5.49, 2.30
Aggressiveness	1.27	−2.77, 5.30	0.27	−3.17, 3.70	1.68	−0.86, 4.22
Internalizing problem	2.35	−1.76, 6.46	2.32	−1.18, 5.81	**3.34**	**1.05, 5.63**
Externalizing problem	0.86	−3.96, 5.67	−0.10	−4.37, 4.18	2.76	−1.18, 6.69
Total problem	1.24	−3.24, 5.72	0.64	−3.26, 4.54	4.03	−0.05, 8.11

Bold values means the results which is statistically significant.

DISCUSSION

We found that low PAE during pregnancy is associated with children's anxiety, internalizing and overall problems. Our findings serve as additional evidence for the deleterious impact of maternal drinking during pregnancy on children's psychosocial behavior, and are consistent with previous animal models suggesting that even a relatively small amount of alcohol during fetal development can result in an increase in synaptic connectivity specific to the basolateral amygdala and induce a subtle anxiety-like behavior in rats (26).

Previous studies have reported inconsistent results regarding which sex is more affected by exposure to alcohol *in utero* (5, 27). Sayal et al. suggested that girls whose mother drank alcohol less than once per week during pregnancy have increased risk of behavioral problems; however, these results should be interpreted with caution because of a lack of evidence on dose-response effects (27). In contrast, another study indicated that boys are more vulnerable to PAE than girls (5), because of the brain development trajectory (28, 29). Our findings suggest that PAE is particularly deleterious for certain developmental problems such as attention problems, anxiety problems and aggression in male offspring. However, when it comes to internalizing, externalizing and overall developmental problems, there is no difference between sexes. The mechanism of how PAE affects children's behavior is still unknown and we cannot eliminate social environment completely in this study.

Our study has several limitations. First, the assessment of drinking during pregnancy was retrospectively self-reported by the mothers. Furthermore, we assessed only the frequency of drinking (as opposed to the total amount of ethanol consumed) or the timing of drinking during different trimesters of pregnancy. However, there is evidence that retrospective reports of prenatal substance use can be reliable (30, 31). Nonetheless, further study on the effects of both the timing of alcohol use and the total amount consumed is warranted. Second, the assessment of child psychosocial problems was reported by the parents, which may have given rise to information bias. However, in the sibling fixed-effects model, reports on behavior problems among siblings were made by the same parent, thereby reducing the possibility of differential misclassification. It has also been found by independent researchers that assessment by mothers is often more reliable than laboratory assessment because the latter is only a snapshot of children's behaviors (32). Finally, the sibling fixed-effects models cannot completely control for unknown sibling-varying confounders such as changes in family circumstances and social situations that differed between siblings. Although this study used sibling-invariant variables as parent's age, educational level, working status, family income and domestic violence, these factors could vary between siblings and we did not measure these variables at the time when the mothers became pregnant. Nonetheless, fixed-effects models are known to provide a more credible causal identification strategy compared with traditional OLS regression models (20, 33).

In conclusion, our study provides additional evidence that even low PAE during pregnancy may adversely affect children's psychosocial behaviors, especially anxiety problems. Our findings provide further support for the current recommendation of abstinence during pregnancy, based on the notion that there is no known safe threshold of alcohol consumption during pregnancy.

AUTHOR CONTRIBUTIONS

KI analyzed the data and drafted the paper and designed the study. IK was responsible for conception and design of the study and coauthored the paper, TF was involved in the study design, supervised the data analysis, and coauthored the paper. All authors read and approved the final manuscript.

FUNDING

This research was supporteded by Seseragi Foundation and Japan Health Foundation. These funding was not involved in study design, in the collection, analysis and interpretation of data, writing of the report and in the decision to submit the article for publication.

ACKNOWLEDGMENTS

The authors thank Professor Hideki Hashimoto and his team for providing us with the data from the J-SHINE. The authors also thank Dr. Toru Tsuboya and Dr. Yoshimitsu Takahashi for their valuable advice. This research was supporteded by Seseragi foudation, Japan.

REFERENCES

1. The U.S. Centers for Disease Control. *What You Should Know About Alcohol and Pregnancy.* Available online at: http://www.cdc.gov/Features/AlcoholAndPregnancy/ (Accessed *December 7, 2017*).
2. The U.S. Surgeon General. *Advisory on Alcohol Use in Pregnancy.* Available online at: http://www.cdc.gov/ncbddd/fasd/documents/surgeongenbookmark.pdf (Accessed *December 7, 2017*).
3. The American College of Obstetricians and Gynecologists. *At-risk Drinking and Alcohol Dependence: Obstetric and Gynecologic Implications.* Available online at: http://www.acog.org/Resources-And-Publications/Committee-Opinions/Committee-on-Health-Care-for-Underserved-Women/At-Risk-Drinking-and-Alcohol-Dependence-Obstetric-and-Gynecologic-Implications (Accessed *December 7, 2017*).
4. The American Academy of Pediatrics. *Where We Stand: Alcohol During Pregnancy.* Available online at: http://www.healthychildren.org/English/ages-stages/prenatal/Pages/Where-We-Stand-Alcohol-During-Pregnacy.aspx (Accessed *December 7, 2017*).
5. Niclasen J, Andersen AMN, Teasdale TW, Strandberg-Larsen K. Prenatal exposure to alcohol, and gender differences on child mental health at age seven years. *J Epidemiol Community Health* (2014) 68:224–32. doi: 10.1136/jech-2013-202956
6. Richardson SS, Daniels CR, Gillman MW, Golden J, Kukla R, Kuzawa C, et al. Don't blame the mothers. *Nature* (2014) 512:131–2. doi: 10.1038/512131a
7. Sowell ER, Charness ME, Riley EP. Pregnancy: no safe level of alcohol. *Nature* (2014) 513:172. doi: 10.1038/513172c
8. Robinson M, Oddy WH, McLean NJ, Jacoby P, Pennell CE, de Klerk NH, et al. Low-moderate prenatal alcohol exposure and risk to child behavioural development: a prospective cohort study. *Bjog* (2010) 117:1139–50. doi: 10.1111/j.1471-0528.2010.02596.x
9. Kelly Y, Sacker A, Gray R, Kelly J, Wolke D, Quigley MA. Light drinking in pregnancy, a risk for behavioural problems and cognitive deficits at 3 years of age? *Int J Epidemiol.* (2009) 38:129–40. doi: 10.1093/ije/dyn230
10. Mattson SN, Crocker N, Nguyen TT. Fetal alcohol spectrum disorders: neuropsychological and behavioral features. *Neuropsychol Rev.* (2011) 21:81–101. doi: 10.1007/s11065-011-9167-9
11. Sokol RJ, Delaney-Black V, Nordstrom B. Fetal alcohol spectrum disorder. *JAMA* (2003) 290:2996–9. doi: 10.1001/jama.290.22.2996
12. Flak AL, Su S, Bertrand J, Denny CH, Kesmodel US, Cogswell ME. The association of mild, moderate, and binge prenatal alcohol exposure and child neuropsychological outcomes: a meta-analysis. *Alcohol Clin Exp Res.* (2014) 38:214–26. doi: 10.1111/acer.12214
13. Dixon DR, Kurtz PF, Chin MD. A systematic review of challenging behaviors in children exposed prenatally to substances of abuse. *Res Dev Disabil.* (2008) 29:483–502. doi: 10.1016/j.ridd.2007.05.006
14. Kesmodel US, Mortensen EL, Lifestyle During Pregnancy Study G. Different perspectives on the methodology of studying the potential effects of different alcohol drinking patterns in early pregnancy on the neuropsychological development of young children Reply. *Bjog* (2012) 119:1673–5 doi: 10.1111/1471-0528.12009
15. Knopik VS, Heath AC, Jacob T, Slutske WS, Bucholz KK, Madden PA, et al. Maternal alcohol use disorder and offspring ADHD: disentangling genetic and environmental effects using a children-of-twins design. *Psychol Med.* (2006) 36:1461–71. doi: 10.1017/S0033291706007884
16. D'Onofrio BM, Van Hulle CA, Waldman ID, Rodgers JL, Rathouz PJ, Lahey BB. Causal inferences regarding prenatal alcohol exposure and childhood externalizing problems. *Arch Gen Psychiatry* (2007) 64:1296–304. doi: 10.1001/archpsyc.64.11.1296
17. Gray R, Mukherjee RA, Rutter M. Alcohol consumption during pregnancy and its effects on neurodevelopment: what is known and what remains uncertain. *Addiction* (2009) 104:1270–3. doi: 10.1111/j.1360-0443.2008.02441.x
18. Knopik VS, Heath AC, Bucholz KK, Madden PAF, Waldron M. Genetic and environmental influences on externalizing behavior and alcohol problems in adolescence: a female twin study. *Pharmacol Biochem Behav.* (2009) 93:313–21. doi: 10.1016/j.pbb.2009.03.011
19. Chen J-H. Maternal alcohol use during pregnancy, birth weight and early behavioral outcomes. *Alcohol Alcohol.* (2012) 47:649–56. doi: 10.1093/alcalc/ags089
20. Duncan GJ, Magnuson KA, Ludwig J. The endogeneity problem in developmental studies. *Res Hum Dev.* (2004) 1:59–80. doi: 10.1080/15427609.2004.9683330
21. Organization WH. *Global Status Report on Alcohol and Health 2014.* (2014) Available online at: http://www.who.int/substance_abuse/publications/global_alcohol_report/en/
22. Takada M, Kondo N, Hashimoto H, Comm JSDM. Japanese study on stratification, health, income, and neighborhood: study protocol and profiles of participants. *J Epidemiol.* (2014) 24:334–44. doi: 10.2188/jea.JE20130084
23. Achenbach T, Edelbrock C, Howell C. Empirically based assessment of the behavioral/emotional problems of 2- and 3- year-old children. *J Abnorm Child Psychol.* (1987) 15:629–50.
24. Achenbach TM. *Child Behavior Checklist/4-18. CBCL/4-18.* Burlington, VT: Department of Psychiatry, University of Vermont (1991).
25. Standardization of the Japansese version of the child behavior checklist/4-18. *Psychiatr Neurol PaediatrJpn.* (2001) 41:243–52. Available online at: https://ci.nii.ac.jp/naid/10020330513#cit
26. Cullen CL, Burne THJ, Lavidis NA, Moritz KM. Low dose prenatal ethanol exposure induces anxiety-like behaviour and alters dendritic morphology in the basolateral amygdala of rat offspring. *PLoS ONE* (2013) 8:e54924. doi: 10.1371/journal.pone.0054924
27. Sayal K, Heron J, Golding J, Emond A. Prenatal alcohol exposure and gender differences in childhood mental health problems: a longitudinal population-based study. *Pediatrics* (2007) 119:E426–34. doi: 10.1542/peds.2006-1840
28. Andersen SL. Trajectories of brain development: point of vulnerability or window of opportunity? *Neurosci Biobehav Rev.* (2003) 27:3–18. doi: 10.1016/S0149-7634(03)00005-8
29. Goodlett CR, Johnson TB. Temporal windows of vulnerability within the third trimester equivalent: why "knowing when" matters. In: *Alcohol and Alcoholism: Effects on Brain and Development.* Hannigan JH, Spear LP, Spear NE, Goodlett CR, editors. Mahwah: Lawrence Erlbaum Associates Publishers (1999). p. 59–91
30. Reich W, Todd RD, Joyner CA, Neuman RJ, Heath AC. Reliability and stability of mothers' reports about their pregnancies

with twins. *Twin Res.* (2003) 6:85–8. doi: 10.1375/twin.6.2.85

31. Heath AC, Knopik VS, Madden PA, Neuman RJ, Lynskey MJ, Slutske WS, et al. Accuracy of mothers' retrospective reports of smoking during pregnancy: comparison with twin sister informant ratings. *Twin Res.* (2003) 6:297–301. doi: 10.1375/136905203322296656
32. Fox NA, Henderson HA. Does infancy matter? Predicting social behavior from infant temperament. *Infant Behav Dev.* (1999) 22:445–55.
33. Gilman SE, Loucks EB. Invited commentary: does the childhood environment influence the association between every X and every Y in adulthood? *Am J Epidemiol.* (2012) 176:684–8. doi: 10.1093/aje/kws228

APPENDIX

TABLE A1 | Distribution of prenatal alcohol consumption among siblings pair (pair =799) N (%).

Both siblings were not exposed to alcohol	491 (61.5)
Senior child exposed, junior child not exposed	37 (4.6)
Senior child not exposed, junior child exposed	31 (3.9)
Both siblings were exposed to alcohol	240 (30.0)

TABLE A2 | OLS models and fixed-effects models of the association between PAE[a] and children's psychosocial behaviors.

	All sample, OLS, all measured variables adjusted[b]		Siblings sample, OLS, all measured variables adjusted[b]		Fixed effects model,unadjusted		Fixed effects model, adjusted[c]		Fixed effects model, adjusted[d]	
CBCL T score	**β**	**95%CI**	**β**	**95%CI**	**β**	**95%CI**	**β**	**95%CI**	**β**	**95%CI**
4-18 YEARS OLD										
Physical problem	0.25	−0.26, 0.76	0.53	−0.02, 1.07	1.25	−0.09, 2.60	1.47	−0.34, 3.27	1.10	−0.47, 2.67
Social problem	0.34	−0.24, 0.92	0.54	−0.06, 1.13	0.76	−0.64, 2.16	0.94	−1.01, 2.89	0.82	−1.22, 2.86
Thought problem	−0.20	−0.58, 0.18	−0.11	−0.50, 0.28	−0.49	−1.55, 0.56	−0.37	−2.20, 1.47	−0.52	−2.41, 1.36
Delinquency	0.47	−0.09, 1.03	0.47	−0.14, 1.08	1.16	−0.18, 2.50	1.12	−0.16, 2.41	0.85	−0.49, 2.20
2–18 YEARS OLD										
Withdrawal	0.17	−0.39, 0.73	0.45	−0.16, 1.07	−0.72	−1.92, 0.49	−0.50	−1.62, 0.61	−0.62	−1.78, 0.53
Anxiety problem	0.17	−0.33, 0.67	0.47	−0.08, 1.01	0.49	−0.65, 1.62	0.57	−0.87, 2.01	0.41	−1.00, 1.82
Attention problem	0.50	−0.07, 1.06	**0.68**	**0.09, 1.27**	0.37	−1.03, 1.77	0.51	−1.36, 2.37	0.29	−1.70, 2.29
Aggressiveness	**0.69**	**0.12, 1.25**	**0.93**	**0.31, 1.54**	0.74	−0.61, 2.08	0.74	−1.02, 2.51	0.64	−1.16, 2.44
Internalizing problem	0.58	−0.22, 1.38	**1.08**	**0.21, 1.95**	1.02	−0.67, 2.71	1.35	−0.18, 2.87	1.25	−0.30, 2.80
Externalizing problem	**1.14**	**0.28, 1.99**	**1.35**	**0.41, 2.29**	1.22	−0.65, 3.08	1.39	−0.83, 3.62	1.36	−0.89, 3.60
Total problem	**1.01**	**0.01, 2.01**	**1.42**	**0.31, 2.52**	1.12	−0.79, 3.04	1.31	−0.76, 3.38	1.14	−1.01, 3.30

[a] *Measurements of alcohol drinking was frequencies of alcohol drinking per month (continuous variables).*
[b] *Adjusted by children's age and sex, parent's age, education and working status, family income, prenatal smoking, domestic violence, clustered by family ID.*
[c] *Adjusted by children's age and sex and difference levels of prenatal smoking baseline prenatal drinking status among siblings, clustered by family ID.*
[d] *Adjusted by children's age and sex, all measured variables about family and baseline prenatal drinking status among siblings, clustered by family ID.*
Bold values means the results which is statistically significant.

16

The Danish High Risk and Resilience Study —VIA 11: Study Protocol for the First Follow-Up of the VIA 7 Cohort–522 Children Born to Parents with Schizophrenia Spectrum Disorders or Bipolar Disorder and Controls being Re-Examined for the First Time at Age 11

Anne A. E. Thorup[1,2,3], Nicoline Hemager[1,2,3], Anne Søndergaard[1,3], Maja Gregersen[1,3], Åsa Kremer Prøsch[1,3], Mette F. Krantz[1,3], Julie M. Brandt[1,3], Line Carmichael[1,3], Marianne Melau[3], Ditte V. Ellersgaard[1,3], Birgitte K. Burton[1,2], Aja N. Greve[1,4], Md Jamal Uddin[1,3], Jessica Ohland[1,3], Ayna B. Nejad[2,5], Line K. Johnsen[2,5], Anna Hester Ver Loren van Themaat[2,5], Anna K. Andreassen[1,4], Lotte Vedum[1,4], Christina B. Knudsen[1,4], Henriette Stadsgaard[1,4], Jens Richardt M. Jepsen[1,2,6], Hartwig Roman Siebner[5], Leif Østergaard[7], Vibeke F. Bliksted[1,4,7], Kerstin J. Plessen[1,2,8], Ole Mors[1,4] and Merete Nordentoft[1,3]*

[1] The Lundbeck Foundation Intiative for Integrative Psychiatric Research (iPSYCH), Aarhus, Denmark, [2] Research Unit, Child and Adolescent Mental Health Center, University of Copenhagen, Copenhagen, Denmark, [3] Mental Health Center Copenhagen, Research Unit, University of Copenhagen, Copenhagen, Denmark, [4] Psychosis Research Unit, Aarhus University Hospital, Risskov, Denmark, [5] Danish Research Centre for Magnetic Resonance, Section 714, Hvidovre Hospital, University of Copenhagen, Copenhagen, Denmark, [6] Center for Neuropsychiatric Schizophrenia Research (CNSR) and Center for Clinical Intervention and Neuropsychiatric Schizophrenia Research, Mental Health Centre Glostrup, University of Copenhagen, Copenhagen, Denmark, [7] Center of Functionally Integrative Neuroscience, Aarhus University, Department of Neuroradiology, Aarhus University Hospital, Aarhus, Denmark, [8] Division of Adolescent and Child Psychiatry, Department of Psychiatry, Lausanne University Hospital, Lausanne, Switzerland

***Correspondence:**
Anne A. E. Thorup
Anne.Amalie.Elgaard.Thorup@regionh.dk

Introduction: Offspring of parents with severe mental illness have an increased risk of developing mental illnesses themselves. Familial high risk cohorts give a unique opportunity for studying the development over time, both the illness that the individual is predisposed for and any other diagnoses. These studies can also increase our knowledge of etiology of severe mental illness and provide knowledge about the underlying mechanisms before illness develops. Interventions targeting this group are often proposed due to the potential possibility of prevention, but evidence about timing and content is lacking.

Method: A large, representative cohort of 522 7-year old children born to parents with schizophrenia, bipolar disorder or controls was established based on Danish registers. A comprehensive baseline assessment including neurocognition, motor functioning, psychopathology, home environment, sociodemographic data, and genetic information was conducted from January 1, 2013 to January 31, 2016. This study is the first follow-up of the cohort, carried out when the children turn 11 years of age. By assessing the cohort at this age, we will evaluate the children twice before puberty. All instruments have been selected with a longitudinal perspective and most of them are identical to those used at inclusion into the study at age 7. A diagnostic interview, motor tests, and a large cognitive battery are conducted along with home visits and information from teachers. This time we examine the children's brains by magnetic resonance scans and electroencephalograms. Measures of physical activity and sleep are captured by a chip placed on the body, while we obtain biological assays by collecting blood samples from the children.

Discussion: Findings from the VIA 7 study revealed large variations across domains between children born to parents with schizophrenia, bipolar and controls, respectively. This study will further determine whether the children at familial risk reveal delayed developmental courses, but catch up at age 11, or whether the discrepancies between the groups have grown even larger. We will compare subgroups within each of the familial high risk groups in order to investigate aspects of resilience. Data on brain structure and physical parameters will add a neurobiological dimension to the study.

Keywords: parental schizophrenia, parental bipolar disorder, early signs of mental illness, longitudinal cohort, psychopathology, MR scanning

INTRODUCTION

For decades, familial high-risk studies have shown that individuals who are born to parents with schizophrenia and affective disorders have a higher risk of developing mental disorders and neurocognitive impairments than non-predisposed individuals (1–3). Cohort studies of children with familial risk with assessments carried out over several time points in their lives allow us to study the early processes that precede illness manifestation. Such studies increase our understanding of the etiology of these complex diseases, and they give us an excellent starting point for developing a specialized and focused preventive approach in terms of early intervention for high risk individuals.

A meta-analysis concluded that ~55% of all familial high risk (FHR) children will experience some kind of mental illness during early adult life (1), and a third will have a severe mental illness (SMI). Offspring of parents with SMI have a higher risk of developing the same disorders as their parents, but also of developing other mental disorders (4). Former FHR studies have reported neuro-integrative problems, social impairments, deficits in attention, information processing and other neurocognitive functions, poorer neuromotor functions and early symptomatology such as anxiety, sleep and mood disorders (2, 3), among offspring of parents with SMI. Moreover, in the premorbid phase the early signs of later schizophrenia (SZ) or bipolar disorder (BD) can present themselves already in childhood as e.g., anxiety, depression, or other non-psychotic disorders (5, 6). The first results from The Danish High Risk and Resilience Study—VIA 7 confirmed this by showing that already by age seven, children born to parents diagnosed with SZ and BD present much higher rates of a psychiatric diagnosis as well as cognitive deficits (only FHR SZ) across several domains, and motor problems (7–10). However, research is sparse when it comes to the question whether these abnormalities or developmental delays diminish over time, indicating that the individuals only suffer from those deficits and symptoms in a transitory manner and then catch up compared with the typically developing children, or whether the problems become even worse. A comprehensive review (11) synthesizing the data of neurocognition in individuals with FHR of schizophrenia concluded on the basis of 30 studies and nine cognitive domains that mild cognitive deficits (i.e., intermediate/between healthy controls and individuals diagnosed with schizophrenia) are reliably present in young FHR individuals, and that longitudinal studies should aim to elucidate the trajectories of cognitive changes to improve early intervention strategies. Concerning individuals at FHR of bipolar disorder there is evidence that neurocognitive deficits also play a role (12), although studies are smaller and tests are seldom repeated at different ages. It is therefore relevant to carry out careful examinations of early signs or symptoms of mental disorders among high risk children several times before puberty to learn more about these individuals and the trajectories of their emerging symptoms or difficulties.

Abbreviations: ADHD, attention deficit and hyperactivity disorder; BASYS, The Bipolar and Schizophrenia Young Offspring Study; BD, bipolar disorder; DNA analytic, deoxyribonucleic acid; FHR, familial high risk; FHR-BP, familial high risk for bipolar disorder; FHR-SZ, familial high risk for schizophrenia; FORBOW (study), Families overcoming risks and building opportunities for well-being; GWAS, genome wide association analyses; MANOVA/MANCOVA, multivariate analyses of variances/covariance; MR/MR scan, magnetic resonance scanning; PLEs, psychotic like experiences; PTSD, post-traumatic stress disorder; SIPS/SOPS, Structured Interview for Prodromal Syndromes and Scale for Prodromal Symptoms; SZ, schizophrenia.

Puberty is a period characterized by massive changes in brain structures and connectivity as well as changes in physical appearance, hormonal status and psychological and social constitution (13, 14). It is also a period with high incidence rates for mental disorders and for some, it is a period with changes of behavior, including risk taking activities and new relational patterns, for example higher degrees of independency. From a developmental perspective it is a period in life that is of high importance, but also very complex to study since both age and hormonal status as well as social and psychological aspects matter when comparing individuals in e.g., a cohort. Social mechanisms like bullying or other forms of social defeat that take place in childhood and early adolescence are frequently reported and have systematically been shown to be directly related to later emergence of mental illnesses like depression (15) and other negative life outcomes. Attributional style or coping, however, have been less investigated and may be of importance.

Brain changes in schizophrenia are present in drug naïve adult patients, and the strongest risk factors exert their influence already in the pre- or perinatal period (16, 17). Lately, the study of endophenotypes and biomarkers has advanced the field of SZ and BD as well as our understanding of the neurodevelopmental nature of both disorders (18, 19). This approach will also allow for early identification and intervention of serious mental illness (20). Despite the fact that only populations of young individuals before the mean age for the onset of the disorder are genuinely "at high risk" (19), few studies to date have examined adolescents at risk with the same means of brain mapping, and none before the onset of puberty. Taken together, the existing literature suggests the study of familial high-risk individuals as fruitful for the understanding of correlates for vulnerability and resilience (compensatory mechanisms), but findings have been inconsistent. In particular, magnetic resonance scans (MR scans) before puberty will permit the study of brain changes during early disease formation and provide important information on differences between individuals with and without familial risk.

Patients with SZ and BD have a higher risk of *somatic comorbidity* than the background population, and they have higher mortality rates due to medical diseases and untreated physical conditions (21). It is likely that early markers of physical illness can be traced already in childhood, either because of common life style factors in the family and/or because of a shared genetic vulnerability to mental disorders and physical illnesses, but evidence is limited. It is therefore relevant to examine early markers of evolving physical illness in children with FHR for mental illness and to analyze whether variations can be explained solely by differences in life style factors such as nutrition, environment, sleep, and physical activity. Also, very little is known about whether e.g., frequency of absence from school and the children's health service use differ between the groups. A Danish register study demonstrated, however, that children with FHR for SMI are more likely not to complete elementary school or to score lower grades than children without a predisposition for mental illness (22).

Family functioning is very often influenced when one of the parents (or both) are suffering from a severe mental illness, also in cases when the child does not live with the affected parent, but only with the co-parent (23). The daily routines can suddenly be disrupted by behavior or needs due to the mentally ill parents and resources, both materially, socially, culturally, and emotionally may be scarce. Dysfunctional family patterns are often seen in several dimensions of family life such as problem solving, communication, role functioning, affective responsiveness, affective involvement and behavior control in families with parental mental illness (24). These dimensions are thoroughly described by the authors behind Family Assessment Device, a self-administrated and widely used questionnaire based on social and system theoretical principles to measure family functioning [FAD (25)].

Briefly, the first *results from the VIA 7 study* showed considerable associations between parental mental illness and several domains of child functioning. Children born to parents diagnosed with schizophrenia showed markedly impaired neurocognitive functioning on the majority of applied measures; i.e., processing speed, working memory, executive functioning, visuospatial functions, sustained attention, and declarative memory (7). At the same time, we found an increased risk of displaying mental health problems or even mental disorders among both groups of children with familial high risk, but in particular among the children with familial high-risk of schizophrenia. Of children with FHR for SZ 38.7% had a life time diagnosis, while this was found in 35.6% of the children with FHR for BD, and in 15.2% of the controls. Also dimensional measures of psychopathology showed this (8). Especially anxiety, ADHD, and stress and adjustment disorders were more prevalent in both of the FHR-groups. Children with FHR for SMI also showed impairments in motor functioning (9) and in sustained attention and interference control (10). Further, children with FHR for both mental disorders were found to be at a greater risk of growing up under low socioeconomic status and reported more adverse life events than the controls based on interviews with the caregivers (unpublished data). Results further indicate an increased risk for living in a home environment with insufficient levels of stimulation and support for children predisposed for SZ and to a lesser extent also BD, and also social cognition and language development was found to be impaired in the FHR-SZ group (manuscript in preparation).

Increasing our knowledge about both the risk and the protective factors that influence these children's development is important to improve our chances for identifying the most vulnerable groups of children. More knowledge concerning the underlying psychological and neurobiological mechanism will guide future developments of early interventions with a preventive approach.

AIMS

In a cohort of children with familial high risk for schizophrenia or bipolar disorder our aims are:

1) To improve insight into early disease processes in schizophrenia and bipolar affective disorder including symptom formation, impairments or delays of maturation in different domains of cognitive functioning incl. social

cognition, paralleled by difference of brain structure and of patterns of brain activation compared to controls.
2) To investigate the development over time (i.e., from age 7 to age 11) of children with familial high risk compared to controls in the domains of neurocognition, psychopathology, social cognition, motor function and adverse life events and to identify and describe possible associations between familial high risk and factors that increase resilience in children.
3) To identify the influence of genetic and environmental exposures and their interactions.
4) To identify early amendable risk factors such as lack of stimulation and support, traumatic events during childhood, insufficient parenting, low socioeconomic status, neurocognitive and social cognitive deficits, and early, subtle signs of psychopathology.
5) To improve knowledge about physical health status among children with familial high risk for severe mental illness.

DESIGN

The Danish High Risk and Resilience Study is a representative nationwide cohort study consisting of 522 children born to parents with schizophrenia, bipolar disorder or neither of these disorders. The participating families were recruited from Danish registers and investigated thoroughly during 2013–2016 when the children were seven years old. The first assessment is referred to as the VIA 7 study, for details please see study protocol for the VIA 7 study (26).

The cohort consists of 522 individuals, now 11 years old (see **Figure 1**):

a) 202 children with at least one parent diagnosed with schizophrenia spectrum psychosis
b) 120 children with at least one parent diagnosed with bipolar disorder
c) 200 children with neither of the parents treated in mental health services for the above diagnoses.

The children of parents with SZ and controls were matched on municipality, sex and exact age of the child. The representative cohort is based on data from The Danish Civil Registration System (27) linked to the Danish Psychiatric Central Research Register (28). Saliva from the children and blood samples from the parents were used for genome wide association analyses (GWAS, PsychChip). The children and their parents were thoroughly examined with interviews, neurocognitive, social cognitive and motor tests, questionnaires, home visits, and observations. Assessments were supplemented with data from questionnaires sent to school teachers. Outcomes for the children were assessed thoroughly in the domains of neuromotor functioning, neurocognitive, social cognitive functioning, social functioning, and psychopathology. Also, parents were interviewed about their mental health, and data on their neurocognitive as well as social cognitive functioning was collected.

Compared to previous studies this cohort is unique due to the very large representative sample of children, all of the same age at the time of assessment, which allows inference about development in the repeated cross-sectional examinations and ultimately it will allow us to follow developmental pathways in the longitudinal design. By including genetic material in combination with thorough estimates of environmental factors, measures of illness severity, and level of functioning of the parents we have a unique possibility of investigating the gene-environment interplay.

The full assessment battery in the VIA 7 study lasted ~3 days (5–6 h per day), as does the VIA 11 study-battery and the vast majority of the families completed the whole battery in the VIA 7 study. Parents were offered feedback on their child's performance, all participants received a gift card, and all families were informed that a follow-up at age 11 was planned.

METHODS

In the VIA 11 study we are aiming at re-assessing all children exactly 4 years from the date when they were included in the VIA 7 study. The adult who is taking care of the child on a regular basis and who is registered with the same address as the child is invited to give information (i.e., interviews and questionnaires) about the child's actual well-being and behavior ("primary caregiver"). This is often but not always one of the biological parents. The completion of the entire test battery lasts at least three days, and when organizing the appointments

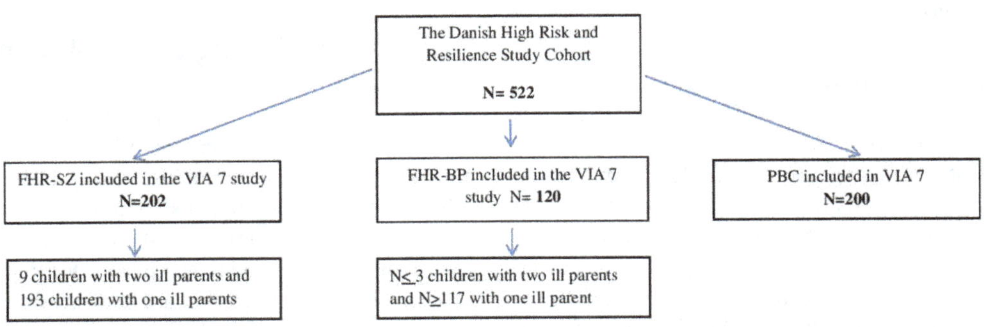

FIGURE 1 | Flowchart of the Danish High Risk and Resilience Study illustrating all children being assessed in the VIA 7 study and who are now being assessed again.

all kinds of flexible arrangements are being made to meet the families' specific needs without compromising the quality of the data collection.

All outcome measures are examined with validated instruments, specifically developed and selected for this age group, sensitive to small changes and suitable for later follow-up (**Tables 1, 2**). We will take advantage of the fact that most variables will be measured twice, making analyses of developmental predictors and associations possible between level of functioning at age seven and age 11, e.g., by multivariate analysis. Moreover, our analytic strategy will capitalize on the fact that the genetic exposures can be modeled directly with polygenic risk scores. Analyses will include measurement of the current environment to which the child is exposed. For each of the outcome domains listed below, we will analyse

1) the differences between the three groups of children at age 11,
2) the differences in associations of outcomes from age seven to age 11 in the three groups
3) the extent to which direct measures of environmental factors (e.g., home environment) and direct measures of genetic risk (e.g., polygenic risk scores for SZ and BD) are responsible for variations in outcomes and development.

The analyses will thematically be divided into groups and will be carried out by Ph.D. students and postdoc researchers. Researchers are based in two centers, one in Copenhagen (Research Unit at Mental Health Center Copenhagen, Gentofte Hospital) and one in Aarhus (Psychosis Research Unit, Aarhus University Hospital Risskov) and have close collaboration at all levels including regular face-to-face meetings and video conferences. The outcomes are organized in the domains listed in **Tables 1, 2** and described below.

DOMAINS AND INSTRUMENTS

Neuromotor Function

Fine motor speed is being assessed with Finger Tapping Test (30), while manual dexterity, ball skills and balance are assessed with Movement Assessment Battery for Children-2, Movement ABC-2 (29). Physical activity will be measured by a sensor in an easily wearable adhesive patch [SENS motion® (31)] which can directly measure sleep disturbances and level of physical activity during a 1-week observation period.

Neurocognitive Function

The comprehensive test battery includes Word Selective Reminding and Memory for Stories [TOMAL-2 (33)], Rey Complex Figure Test and Recognition Trial (34), Rapid Visual Information Processing [CANTAB (35)], Conners' CPT-II [Continuous Performance Test II (36)], Verbal Fluency 1–3 and Trail Making Test 2–4 [D-KEFS (38)], Symbol Search and Coding [WISC-IV (39)], Stockings of Cambridge, Intra-Extra Dimensional Shift, Spatial Recognition Memory, Spatial Span, and Spatial Working Memory [CANTAB (35)], Letter-Number Sequencing and Arithmetic [WISC-IV (39)], Cambridge Gambling Task [CANTAB (35)], and Reynolds Intellectual Screening Test [part of the RIAS (43)].

Social cognition is measured by Animated Triangles (41), Beeds Test (44) (tendency to jump to conclusion), Frederic's Stories (42), and the Social Cognition paradigm from the Human Connectome Project (78).

Psychopathology

General psychopathology and psychotic-like experiences (PLEs) will be examined with the diagnostic interview K-SADS-PL (45) including a specialized assessment of sub-threshold psychotic-like experiences (79). Magical Thinking Questionnaire (47) is included to ensure optimal information about tendency to magical ideation that is not covered by the K-SADS-PL-interview.

The aberrant salience-hypothesis (80) suggests that patients with schizophrenia have deviances in attributional style. Results from the VIA 7 study showed that familial high-risk children more often reported being bullied (unpublished results), which could be a sad truth, but it could also be partly explained by deviances in attributional style. We have developed and included a predefined social situation in a virtual reality scenario that will help us identify any liability to social anxiety and paranoid ideas. By using a virtual reality scenario, we will be able to investigate if a subgroup of the children is more inclined than the others to appraise an ambiguous social situation as threatening or bullying using a virtual reality scenario. We will apply a Danish children's version of the State Social Paranoia Scale (55), which asks about positive, neutral and paranoid appraisal of the virtual reality environment.

Executive functioning including affective regulation and flexibility will be assessed with the questionnaire Behavior Rating Inventory of Executive Function [BRIEF (51)] from both caregiver and teacher. Autism spectrum traits are evaluated with Social Responsiveness Scale [SRS (59)] also completed by the child's caregiver and the teacher. Dimensional measures of psychopathology will be covered with Child Behavior Checklist [CBCL (48)], ADHD rating scale [ADHD-RS (49)], and Strengths and Difficulties Questionnaire [SDQ (57); both by parent and teacher] while the ratings of the clinical impression of the child during the testing are registered with the Test Observation Form [TOF (81)].

Social Functioning and Behavior

Self-esteem will be coved by "I think I am"-questionnaire [Sådan er jeg (53)]. Social development is captured by the Vineland-2 Parental interview (58) and with the Strengths and Difficulties Questionnaire [SDQ (57)]. Data from the school will also be included via questionnaires sent to the teacher (see **Table 1** for details). Bullying is included with the questionnaire developed by Olweus for the child itself (54). Resilience is measured by a short version of Child Youth Resilience Measurement [CYRM (56)] as well as by associating the life situation and context of the child with their course of psychopathology.

TABLE 1 | Domains and instruments used for testing the children at age 11 in the Danish High Risk and Resilience Study VIA 11.

Domains	Outcomes	In VIA 7	Child	Primary caregiver	Teacher	Type of instrument
Neuromotor and physical measures	Motor development and milestones	Yes	Movement ABC (29)			Test in clinic
	Anthropometry	Yes	Height, weight, waist			Observations in clinic
	Motor speed and dexterity	Yes	Finger tapping (30)			Test in clinic (or home)
	Physical activity and sleep	No	SENS chip (31)	Anamnestic interview		Chip on tight for one week (32) Interview with primary caregiver
Neurocognition	Verbal Memory and visual memory	Yes	Word Selective Reminding and Memory for Stories from Tomal-2 (33) RCFT (Rey Complex Figure Test and Recognition Trial (34) and Spatial Recognition Memory from CANTAB (35)			Test in clinic or at home
	Attention	Yes	RVP (Rapid Visual Information Processing;3-5-7 mode) from CANTAB (35). Conners CPT (Continuous Performance Test (36)			Computer test
	Communication and pragmatic/social interaction	Yes			CCC-2 (Children's Communication Checklist-II) (37)	Questionnaire
	Speed of Processing	Yes	Verbal Fluency 1-2 and Trail making Test 2-4 from D-KEFS (38) and Symbol Search, and Coding test from WISC-IV (39)			Test in clinic or home
	Executive functions (planning and flexibility)	Yes	SOC (Stockings of Cambridge) and IED (Intra-Extra Dimensional Set Shift) from CANTAB (35) and Verbal Fluency 3 from D- KEFS (38)			Computer test
	Executive functions (visual and verbal working memory)	Yes	SSP (Spatial Span) and SWM (Spatial Working Memory) from CANTAB (35) and Letter-number Sequencing and Arithmetic from WISC-IV (39)			Computer test and test in clinic or home
	Executive functions (error monitoring)	Yes	Flanker Task (40) – before and during fMRI			Computer test
	Social cognition	Yes No	Animated Triangles (41) before and during fMRI (without the goal directed animation) Frederic's stories (42)			Computer test Practical test
	Intelligence	Yes	RIST (Reynolds Intellectual Screening Test) (43)			Test in clinic or home
	Decision making	No Yes	Beads' Test (44) Cambridge Gambling Task from CANTAB (35)			Computer test
Psychopathology	Psychiatric symptoms, incl. depression, anxiety, psychotic symptoms, thought disorders, PLEs, obsessive-compulsive symptoms, eating disorders, sleep disturbances, self harming behavior and traumatic life events	Yes Yes No Yes	Kiddie-SADS-PL interview (45) PLE assessment (46) Magical Ideation Questionnaire (47)	Kiddie-SADS-PL interview (45) Anamnestic interview CBCL (48) (Child Behavior Checklist)	TRF (48) (Teachers Rating Form)	Interview (categorical psychopathology) Questionnaires, (dimensional psychopathology)

(Continued)

TABLE 1 | Continued

Domains	Outcomes	In VIA 7	Child	Primary caregiver	Teacher	Type of instrument
Do	Attention/hyperactivity	Yes		ADHD-Rating Scale (49)	ADHD-Rating Scale (49)	Questionnaire
	Affect regulation/flexibility	Yes	CEMS (50) (Children's Emotion Management Scale)	BRIEF (Behavior Rating Inventory of Executive Function (51)	BRIEF (Behavior Rating Inventory of Executive Function (51)	Questionnaire
Do	Anxiety	Yes	STAIC (State-Trait Anxiety Inventory for Children (52)			Questionnaire
Social functioning and behavior	Self-esteem	Yes	Sådan er jeg' ['I think I am' (53)]			Questionnaire
	Bullying	No	Olweus Bully/Victim Questionnaire (54)			Questionnaire
			SSPS (State Social Paranoia Scale (55)			Questionnaire after Virtual Reality scenario
	Resilience	No	CYRM (Child and Youth Resilience Measure short version (56)			
	Social Functioning	Yes		SDQ (Strengths and Difficulties Questionnaire (57)	SDQ for teachers (Strengths and Difficulties Questionnaire (57)	Questionnaire (emotional symptoms, conduct problems, hyperactivity/ inattention)
		Yes			CCC-2 [Child Communication Checklist (37)]	
	Social development	Yes		Vineland Adaptive Behavior Scales –II (58)		Interview
	Autism spectrum traits	Yes		SRS–2 (Social Responsiveness Scale (59)	SRS-2 (Social Responsive ness Scale (59)	Questionnaire
Environment and emotional climate	Stimulation and support in actual rearing environment	Yes	HOME Inventory, Early Adolescent version (60)	HOME inventory, Early Adolescent version (60)		Interview made in the home with both child and parent
	Life events and trauma	No	CTS [Childhood Trauma Screener (61)]	Anamnestic interview focusing on age 7-11		Questionnaire and semi-structured interview
	Perceived support from social network	Yes		SPS [Social Provision Scale (62)]		Questionnaire
	Attachment style	Yes, but new test	Secure Base Script Test (63)			Test in clinic or home
	Expressed emotions/emotional family climate/familiar relations	Yes No		FMSS [Five Minute Speech Sample (64)] FAD [Family Assessment Device (25)]		Interview Questionnaire
	Stress	Yes	Hair test for cortisol			Hair sample
			Items from DLSS [Daily Life Stressor Scale (65)]			Questionnaire
	Use of social media	No		Anamnestic interview		Questionnaire

(Continued)

TABLE 1 | Continued

Domains	Outcomes	In VIA 7	Child	Primary caregiver	Teacher	Type of instrument
Physical health	Puberty status	No	Tanner stages (66, 67)			Illustrations
			Hormone level			Blood sample
	Physical health	No	HbA1c. leucocytes, CRP			Blood sample
			Exercise on bicycle,			Test (Copenhagen only)
Genetic and epigenetic analyses	Polygenic risk scores	Yes	Dry blood spots from Danish Neonatal Screening Biobank and blood samples			Day 1, hospital
	Inflammatory and infectious markers.	Yes	Dry blood spots from Danish Neonatal Scrbeening Biobank and blood samples			Day 1, hospital
Brain scan	Functional and structural MRI	No	MR Scanning and EEG			Day 2, Scan at hospital
	Electrophysiology	No	The Copenhagen Psychophysiological Test Battery (CPTB) (prepulse inhibition, P50 gating, mismatch negativity)			Day 2, before the scan at hospital

TABLE 2 | Instruments for the assessment of the parents' mental health status, actual level of functioning and parenting issues in the Danish High Risk and Resilience Study - VIA 11.

Domains	In VIA 7	Parent/actual caregiver	Co- parent	Type of test
Mental health status (previous 4 years)	Yes (lifetime)	SCAN [Schedules for Clinical Assessment in Neuropsychiatry (68)] for the person him/herself and the other parent	do	Interview
Daily Functioning	Yes	PSP [Personal and Social Performance Scale (69)]	do	Interview
Actual state of illness	Yes	SANS [Scale for the Assessment of Negative Symptoms (70)]	do	Interview
Do	Yes	SAPS [Scale for the Assessment of Positive Symptoms (71)]	do	Interview
Do	Yes	Hamilton Rating Scale for Depression (72)	do	Interview
Do	Yes	YMRS [Young Mania Rating Scale (73)]	do	Interview
Affective regulation	Yes	ALS [Affective Liability Scale (74)]	do	
Family functioning	No	Family Assessment Device, short version [FAD-12 (25)]		Questionnaire
Perceived support from social network	Yes	Social Provision Scale [SPS (62)]	do	Questionnaire
Social Response, adult	No	Social Responsiveness Scale -Adult, self-report [SRS-A (75)]	do	Questionnaire
Relation to child and relation to other parent	Yes	FMSS [Five Minute Speech Sample (64)]		Interview (recorded and transcribed)
Adverse childhood experiences	No	ACE Study Questionnaire [Adverse Childhood Experiences Questionnaire (76)]	do	Questionnaire
Attachment style	Yes	PAM questionnaire (77)	do	Questionnaire
Knowledge about mental illness and talking to children about mental illness if relevant	No	Included in anamnesis		Interview

Environment

Familial environment in the home is measured by the use of a semi-structured interview, HOME, that must take place at a home visit with the caregiver and the child being present at the same time [Home Observation for Measurement of the Environment (82)]. We chose the version called Early Adolescence (EA-HOME) which is appropriate for children from age 11. An anamnestic interview with the primary caregiver includes sociodemographic data, data on the child's health service use, adverse life events, school performance and leisure activities as well as social network. Childhood trauma is measured directly from the child through the section in the K-SADS-PL (45) about post-traumatic stress disorder (PTSD) combined with the Childhood Trauma Screener [CTS (61)]. Attachment style categorization will be based on Secure Base Script Test [SBST (63)] while level of stress will be captured by Daily Life Stressor Scale [DLS (65)] and from level of hair cortisol in a hair sample.

The parents' level of daily functioning is measured with Personal and Social Performance Scale [PSP (69)] and is used as a measure of the environment together with Five Minute Speech Sample (64), which contains data about the primary caregiver's impression of the relationship with the child.

Physical Health Status

We will describe the children's physical condition including a long range of tests relevant for risk of physical illness at age 11. This will include: VO_2max, anthropometry, Body Mass Index, white blood cells, C-reactive protein, HbA1c, and level of cortisol in hair samples. Puberty status will be determined by analyses of sex-hormones in blood tests and with the Tanner test (66, 67), which is letting the child look at drawings of different stages of puberty, and choose which stage is closest to the child's actual development.

Genetic and Epigenetic Analyses

Saliva and peripheral blood are being sampled from the children and will be analyzed with DNA-analytic results from the dried blood spot from birth and from saliva-sample results collected at age seven with the purpose of studying epigenetic changes.

Structural and Functional Magnetic Resonance Imaging (fMRI) an Electroencephalography (EEG)

We will examine the children with anatomical and functional magnetic resonance imaging (MRI) of the whole brain at 3.0 Tesla at Aarhus University, Center for Functionally Integrative Neuroscience (CFIN) and Hvidovre Hospital's, Danish Research Center for Magnetic Resonance (DRCMR). We will acquire 3D T1-weighted (MP2RAGE) and high-quality diffusion weighted imaging (DWI) data to calculate a set of measures that will allow us to detect regional changes in brain microstructure and structural brain connectivity (DWI based tractography) across groups. The measures include fractional anisotropy, apparent diffusion coefficient, and diffusion kurtosis indices. These measures will be used to compare regional changes in brain microstructure, as indexed by diffusion weighted imaging (DTI) across groups. Functional MR scans will map task related changes in brain activity and connectivity during three experimental tasks: the Eriksen Flanker paradigm, which addresses cognitive control and motivation, the Social Cognition (Animated Triangles) paradigm from the Human Connectome Project (78) which tap into theory of mind, and a Self-Reference paradigm to probe the ability to relate external events to oneself.

It is our intention to use these MR-scans carried out at age 11 as a basis for identifying developmental trajectories of brain changes during disease formation as we plan to repeat the same MR protocol later in adolescence (at age 15 or 16). The trajectory in children developing schizophrenia is expected to include reduced maturation of inhibitory pathways and excessive pruning of excitatory pathways leading to altered excitatory–inhibitory balance in the prefrontal cortex. We also anticipate structural and functional alterations of the brain's connectivity. Although some data support each of these possible neurodevelopmental mechanisms for schizophrenia, no study has previously provided possibilities for identifying measures of abnormal structural brain maturation (such as less or excessive pruning, less maturation of major limbic/cognitive fiber tracts, abnormal global brain connectivity, dysfunctional processing), and differences in integration in key circuits that will be probed with task-based fMRI and EEG in young individuals at risk for those disorders before puberty. We plan to correlate the abundant biological, clinical, and neurocognitive information already collected at age seven to future imaging data to see whether earlier data are predictive of imaging outcomes.

In a subgroup of ~50% of the participants, EEG will be performed at DRCMR to record functional task-related cortical activity during an auditory 40 Hz stimulation paradigm, a mismatch negativity paradigm, and a Flanker paradigm which is closely matched to the one used during functional MR to enable data integration. We selected these tasks based on consistent evidence for deficits in neural synchrony and event-related potentials (ERPs), evoked by using those paradigms in patients with SZ (83, 84) and, although to a lesser degree, in patients with BD (85). Reduced power of cortical activity and reduced amplitudes of event-related potentials in neural mechanisms are assumed to be related to both automatic sensory processes as to higher-order cognitive functions (86) and provide a window into some of the neurobehavioral symptoms (87). No study before has studied these neural correlates in a large sample of children at familial high risk for schizophrenia and bipolar disorder.

PROCEDURES AND PERMISSIONS

Contact and Procedures

All families have been informed by the completion of the first assessment in the VIA7 study that a follow-up was planned at age 11. To maintain contact with the participants of the cohort, Christmas cards and birthday cards have been sent to the children each year and a short survey consisting of two questionnaires [the "I think I am" (53) and the Child Behavior Check List CBCL (48)] was sent out to each family when the child turned 9 years of age; this survey is called the VIA 9 study.

As in the VIA 7 study, the first contact for the assessment is made by sending out a hard copy letter and an illustrative folder to the child's address (see **Figure 2**), followed by a phone call by the research coordinator, who invites the family to an information meeting. All parents give informed consent before data collection can start and for those who are divorced or separated and have joint custody over the child, informed consent from both parents is mandatory. We meet all families with a very friendly and flexible approach, taking into account any individual concerns or obstacles that they may have with regard to participation. The first results from the

VIA 7 study are available for those participants who ask for them.

The data collection takes place during 3–4 meetings, each lasting up to ~5 h. The caregiver and the child are assessed simultaneously by two researchers, and whenever possible the assessor testing the child is kept blinded for the familial high-risk status and for the potential diagnosis from the first assessment at age seven to avoid any subjective influences. The first two days take place in the clinic, the third day is at the MR-scan facility, while the fourth day is in the family's home in order to complete the home environment assessment. However, some children may need more time or cannot concentrate sufficiently and thus need shorter but more frequent meetings. The child receives a gift card after each day completed and at the end of the whole assessment, the parents are offered a feedback on their child's performance and results. If any specific concern is raised on the basis of the interviews and testing, the researchers will guide the parents to relevant support or even make the referral or inform the social authorities or hospital service, if necessary. All diagnoses retrieved from the diagnostic interviews K-SADS-PL (45) and the SCAN interviews (68) are discussed and confirmed or declined at weekly clinical conferences, with a child and adolescent psychiatrist (A. Thorup) being present together with the research team members.

Permissions and Data Protection

The study was approved by the local Ethical committee (Protocol number: H 16043682) and the Data Protection Agency (ID-number RHP-2017-003, I-suite no. 05333).

The majority of tests that we used in the VIA 7 study were chosen at the outset (among other reasons) because they would also be suitable at age 11 and this is a considerable advantage when aiming to study relatively small changes over time (**Tables 1, 2**).

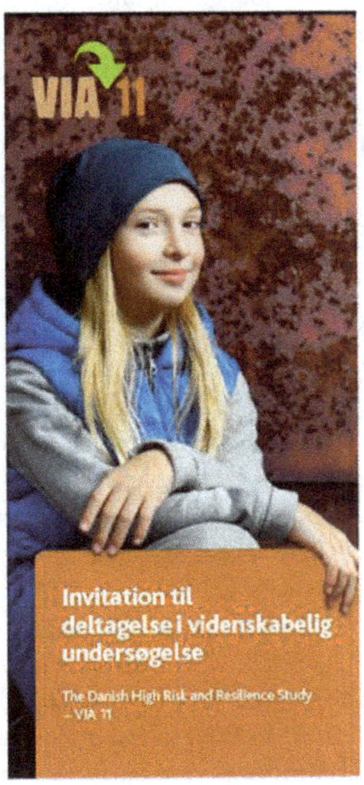

FIGURE 2 | Lay out for the invitation to all families in the VIA 11 study.

Statistical Analyses

Several descriptive and inferential statistical tools will be applied to analyse the data. For example, for descriptive analyses, frequency distribution, mean or median, and graphical representation will be applied. For inferential analysis, linear regression and/or analysis of variance or covariance (ANOVA/ANCOVA) will be the standard method for analyzing the association between exposure variables (i.e., high-risk status) and continuous outcome measures (e.g., psychopathology). If a variable does not follow a normal distribution even after possible transformations, non-parametric methods (e.g., Kruskal–Wallis test) or non-linear statistical models can be an alternative approach. Moreover, to control for the Type I error probability as well as the correlation between multiple outcome variables, multivariate analyses of variances/covariance (MANOVA/MANCOVA) will be applied. Furthermore, dichotomous/count outcome measures will be analyzed with generalized linear models (e.g., logistic or Poisson regression). To account for longitudinal effect from VIA 7 to VIA 11 data, linear mixed effect model for the continuous outcome and the generalized estimating equation for the dichotomous outcome will be applied. Based on our specific research question, we may consider clinically meaningful interaction terms (e.g., high-risk status and other covariates) in the models. Furthermore, as we are collecting genetic data for children and parents, to account for genetic background, polygenic risk scores (e.g., for Schizophrenia, education) would be considered as a covariate in the statistical models. In the case of missing data, multiple imputations will also be considered given that data are missing at random (MAR). However, in case of participating families with lower functioning there might be the chance that missing data are not at random (i.e., non-ignorable missing), but solely due to the inability or unwillingness to complete instruments, test, or questionnaires. Thus, we will apply sensitivity analyses for investigating the possible violations of the missing at random assumption. For families not participating at all, we will have the opportunity to include data from Danish registers in the sensitivity analyses. To handle the latent factors like resilience and vulnerability, we will apply structural equation modeling (SEM) or different kinds of path analyses. In addition, multiple regression will be applied for analyses of predictors and associations from age 7 to age 11 regarding changes in mental and physical symptoms.

RESULTS

Results will be presented within the context of both cross sectional and longitudinal analyses, i.e., comparing the results from the first assessment at age seven with the results found at age 11. Cross sectional results will be reported in all new areas or instruments like MR scans, Virtual Reality setting, SENS motion data, and blood sample data, while developmental trajectories will be investigated for those measures that are repeated, i.e., most of the cognitive measures, psychopathology, motor development, as well as many of the questionnaires, and the home environment evaluation (see **Tables 1, 2**).

Results concerning the actual psychopathology and the association to the mental health status at age seven will be investigated, including data on attributional style (tendency to report being excluded/bullied) and physical health. Data on social cognition will be linked to data on the developmental trajectories of Psychotic Like Experiences (PLE's; i.e., intensity, frequency, and severity) from age seven to age 11. Neurocognitive data will be analyzed to learn more about the extent to which these children's deficits or advantages measured at age seven remain stable, deteriorate or diminish over time. Brain scan data will focus on potential differences between high risk groups in terms of structural properties, neural networks, and connectivity.

DISCUSSION

This protocol describes the research strategy for the first follow-up of the unique familial high-risk cohort consisting of 522 children all the same age called The Danish High Risk and Resilience Study. This second wave is called the VIA 11 study since all children are now 11 years of age. The advantages of this cohort are especially that all children have the same age and that all families of the cohort have been recruited from national registries. Further, the comprehensive battery and the multidimensional approach will allow us to combine results from many research areas in order to add knowledge to the field of familial high risk, developmental psychopathology, brain development and risk, and resilience assessment.

The field of familial high risk studies is not new, actually the first study with this design was described and conducted by Barbara Fish (88) in New York in the early fifties, and from this study came the "pandysmaturation"-hypothesis, giving inspiration to the neurodevelopmental hypothesis of understanding the etiology of schizophrenia. In the field of schizophrenia research several familial high-risk studies have been conducted since Fish' study and recently reviewed by Hameed (89). However, we believe that the possibility of recruiting the participants from registries and not from clinics (i.e., biased toward including only those in treatment or with severe courses), with all children having the same age is a major advantage. From the perspective of neurodevelopmental psychopathology, age greatly matters when comparing results of cognitive tests, social and behavioral functioning and developmental milestones.

There are other important familial high-risk studies that are ongoing and should be mentioned here. One is the Canadian FORBOW study by Uher et al. (90) which is still recruiting both parents with schizophrenia, major depression and bipolar disorder and their offspring and testing various types of prevention and early interventions in the cohort, while also conducting annual assessments. The Spanish study led by Sanchez-Gistau (91, 92), called The Bipolar and Schizophrenia Young Offspring Study (BASYS), is a multi-center, naturalistic study which aims to evaluate psychopathology and neuropsychological and neuroimaging variables in child and adolescent offspring of patients with schizophrenia or bipolar disorder in two child and adolescent psychiatry departments in Madrid and Barcelona. The sample consists of 41 offspring of parents with schizophrenia, 90 offspring of parents with bipolar disorder and 107 controls. The age span is wide, 6–17 years and all participants are recruited via parents seeking treatment. The Dutch Bipolar Offspring Study led by Manon Hillegers in the Netherlands is a longitudinal fixed cohort study established in 1997 and followed up until early adulthood (93). It consists of 140 offspring from 86 families where one of the parents suffered from bipolar disorder. Many interesting results have been reported from this cohort, e.g., that the impact of life events especially in the early phases of the illness may be mediated by a passive reactive coping style. Further, a study led by Iacono et al. (94) has recent data on a smaller group of offspring of parents with bipolar disorder. However, all studies have much wider age ranges and smaller Ns.

Conducting a Longitudinal Study

Conducting a longitudinal study and aiming for several assessments of both parents and children over time is an ambitious and demanding project. Longitudinal studies must be well-prepared and sufficiently financially supported and the team behind the study must set a long-term plan, have a strong collaboration and develop clear and good ways of communication with regular meetings and other forms of contact. Research questions must be based on a theoretical framework and reflect current state of the art and must map onto the aims of the study. Recruitment procedures of participants and strategies for retaining participants in the study are crucial and must be planned and discussed with potential participants/pilot users. The assessor group must be properly trained, have regular meetings and good collaboration, and high levels of interrater reliability is essential. Data must be handled in accordance with rules of data protection and analyzed on the basis of a statistical, preset strategy. Finally, results must be published for both professionals and the population (95). Communication of results that reveal some aspects that could be interpreted as negative for the participants must be planned and handled with empathy.

Clinical Implications

Developmental trajectories will inform us on how the delays and abnormalities observed at age seven will evolve and influence the individual's risk of mental symptoms or reduced level of daily functioning at age 11. For example, much more knowledge is needed if we are aiming for understanding, treating or giving advice to children and their parents when children report psychotic like experiences (PLEs). Are PLEs at age seven just a normal, transient phenomenon that we as clinicians should not worry about? What is the impact if PLEs are found to correlate with an increased risk of psychopathology at age 11 and should persistent PLEs (i.e., found at both age seven and age 11) be considered as more severe early risk factor? We intend to investigate the nature of all possible PLEs mentioned by the children in the VIA 11 study in a very thorough way to be able to analyze data at a detailed level. Results from the VIA 7 study indicated that PLEs are much more common among FHR-SZ children (Ellersgaard et al, in preparation) and do correlate with poorer functioning, and this fact is important to follow very closely to help us learn more about their value as a risk marker for later mental illness, as proposed by others (96). A large cohort study reported that up to 2/3 of a population of school children aged nine to 11 would report some kind of PLEs on a self-report measurement, and for those individuals who reported the PLEs to be persistent after 2 years, a correlation with an increased risk for internal and external psychopathology later in life was found (96). However, methodological considerations are important, since other studies find much lower rates (97), for example the frequency was 5.9% based on a clinical interview in a large birth cohort of 12-year-old twins. In the VIA 11 study we initially considered using a self-report instrument, but concluded that due to the long test battery, the data collectors will have time to build a good relationship with the child and thus confidentiality will most likely be high, allowing the child to tell the interviewer if she or he has had any PLEs. Still, a well-validated rating scale for PLEs among children and adolescents with a clear and informative manual would be a considerable contribution to the field for the future. An adapted version of the SIPS/SOPS instrument (79) could be a place to start.

In a more general perspective, we hope that the results from this important cohort will shed light on the problems that these families face and struggle with every day. We appeal for authorities, institutions, and organizations, who are responsible for providing help and support to the whole population, to pay extra attention to families where severe mental disorders are involved, sometimes in two generations (see **Box 1**).

Limitations

The comprehensive and thorough test battery is also quite time consuming which may lead to some families not being able to complete all instruments, tests, and questionnaires. Although we try to motivate every family to participate again, some degree of attrition is inevitable, and that this could be expected to be more pronounced in the group of lower functioning families, but it could also be in the busy and well-functioning ones. In the VIA 7 study, however, many families were positive about their participation and for some, the feedback on their child's performance and the results that we provided, meant a lot to them. We also offer all families a feed back after completed testing in the VIA 11, and in those cases, where the situation calls for immediate help or support from authorities, we try to guide the family, or we send referrals and information to the municipalities.

Since a large group of testers are working with the same instruments, we will be ensuring very carefully that all instruments are used, and results interpreted in the same way by having monthly meetings where we discuss any issues or problems and where we score clinical examples together. Testers often work together in pairs, but in varying combinations also with colleagues from the other center.

Most tests are chosen with the follow-up perspective, allowing us to compare results from the VIA 7 study to the VIA 11 study directly. However, this was not possible in some cases and it will thus be necessary to look into the comparability of tests. This is for example the case for the measure of attachment, where the method used in the VIA 7 study was the Story Stem Assessment Profile [SSAP (98)], which is suitable for age four to nine. In the VIA 11-study we use the Secure Base Script Test [SBST (63)], which is recommended from age 9 to 14. However, both tests are based on the same theoretical basis that a narrative setting and an invitation to create a story that is inspired from everyday situations will tap into the child's inner world and working models of adult- and self-presentations. Optimally, we would conduct a validity study with e.g., 30 nine-year-old children performing both tests and then see how the attachment profiles correspond in the two tests.

Box 1 | Case Benjamin

Benjamin is a curious 11-year-old boy,who lives with his mother and his younger brother. Benjamin's mother has been diagnosed with bipolar disorder when Benjamin was four years old and she divorced Benjamin's father a few years ago. Benjamin visits his father every other weekend, sometimes more frequent, if his mother is depressed and in need of hospitalization. For most part of his life,Benjamin was told that his mother was hospitalized due to influenza, but recently Benjamin learned that it was because of her 'thoughts in her mind', that his mother sometime had to go away and letting him and his brother stay with their father and his new wife, and their baby twins.

Benjamin is usually a happy boy who likes to go to school, play football and Minecraft. However, he is also a rather anxious boy; who is not comfortable with sleeping at his friends or going too far away from home. He has also developed a sleep disorder as it takes him a very long time to fall asleep every night. At school and at home Benjamin sometimes gets very angry and has tantrums,although it is now much less frequent than when he was younger. He is doing fine in school and has one good friend. For a while,Benjamin was seriously bullied by some boys from another class. He was afraid to tell his mother about the bullying, because he wanted to protect her from getting sad. Eventually,the teacher found out and contacted Benjamin's mother. Now, the bulling has stopped but Benjamin still thinks a lot about having been bullied. Maybe that is why he sometimes have problems concentrating in school.

Benjamin participated in the VIA 7 study and the VIA 11 study and was fond of it, although the assessment at the hospital lasted three full days and was quite demanding. He talked to a psychologist in the VIA 11study about the sounds and voices that he had been hearing almost monthly for the past 8 months. The sounds and voices always seem to come when he is nervous or on his own, and although he realizes that they are not real, they make him feel uneasy. A few times he had shouted back at them. He had never talked to anybody about this before and found it as a relief to share it with a friendly person.

We decided to use two scanner facilities, one in Aarhus and one in Copenhagen to be able to cover all of Denmark apart from the similar scanner systems across sites, and to introduce the site variable in the data analyses, so that bias due the site will be detected. Finally, we will pay close attention to securing equal distribution of the scans of the cohort between the two centers in terms of HR-status of the children, so the two centers can analyze data independently.

Mean age of onset of puberty has lowered for the last decades (99), and for some children at age 11 the process of puberty has already started. We will be able to control for this difference in our analyses by using data from the blood tests and data regarding Tanner state of puberty as covariates.

Perspectives

It is highly relevant to carry out careful examinations of early signs or symptoms of mental disorders among high-risk children several times before and during puberty to measure longitudinal patterns of symptoms. Especially, it is important to determine constellations and interactions with external influences that determine the event of a more negative progression of symptoms and function vs. constellations that facilitate resilience in an individual with a similar vulnerability. The current study allows us to explore these patterns, including a wide array of measures, reaching from phenotyping, to measures of brain structure and function.

The children at age 11 are facing puberty, which is a period characterized by massive changes in brain structures and connectivity as well as changes in physical appearance, hormonal status and psychological, and social constitution (13). Paradoxically, even though self-regulatory control develops at a fast pace during puberty, it is also a period with changes of behavior, including risk taking activities and new relational patterns, for example higher degrees of independency, and a period with high incidence rates for mental disorders. From a developmental perspective puberty is a period in life that is highly formative but also complex to study because both age, hormonal status and social and psychological aspects matter when comparing individuals in e.g., a cohort. This is why cohorts that focus on a narrow age range may be helpful in determining differences of development and behavior inter-individually, or systematically across specific groups. Social mechanisms, such as bullying or other forms of social defeat that may take place in childhood and adolescence, are frequently reported and are related to later emergence of mental illnesses like depression and psychosis (15) and other negative life outcomes.

It will be of immense value if a better understanding of the early phases of the development of mental disorders, neurodevelopmental changes including brain development and the needs of these children will permit early interventions with potential prevention or preemption of psychosis. Increased knowledge about the impact of the thoroughly described and closely investigated environmental risk factor like home environment, parenting style and relation, parental functioning and mental health, social network, socioeconomic status, and adverse life events will create the basis for developing specific supportive and preventive interventions. These children have for decades been known to be at an increased risk of mental illness. The more we know about the early development of their potential course of illness and resilience factors, the better we can provide early and specific help.

AUTHOR CONTRIBUTIONS

AET wrote the manuscript together with MN. All co-authors NH, AS, MG, ÅP, MK, JB, LC, MM, DE, BB, AG, MU, JO, AN, LJ, ALT, AA, LV, CK, HS, JJ, OM read the manuscript, commented etc. MU was responsible for the statistics section. KP, HRS, LØ, and VB were responsible for all content regarding the MR scans.

FUNDING

This study was supported by the Lundbeck Foundation Initiative for Integrative Psychiatric Research (iPSYCH), the Mental Health Services of the Capital Region of Denmark, the Research Fund in Capital Region of Denmark, The Independent Research Fund Denmark and The Innovation Foundation. The sponsors had no role in the design and conduct of the study; collection, management, analysis and interpretation of the data, preparation, review or approval of the manuscript for publication.

ACKNOWLEDGMENTS

We would like to acknowledge the following persons for their highly valued contribution to the development of the project: Physiotherapist Camilla Tjott, Child and Adolescent Mental Health Center, Capital Region of Denmark, for being responsible for learning and accreditation of Movement ABC for all assessors.

Psychologist, Ass. Prof. Elia Psouni, University of Lund, Sweden for being responsible for learning and accreditation of Secure Base Script Test and for collaboration. Research assistant, nurse Heidi Jensen, Mental Health Center Copenhagen for helping us with the Data Protection Declaration. Collaborators at Khora Virtual Reality, Copenhagen, Anders B. R. Pedersen and Peter Fisher for helping us develop the VR-environment. Specialist in data technology, Kasper Lykkegaard CEO in SENS-Innovation, Copenhagen, for collaboration about the SENS chip. PhD, MSc Troels Thorsteinsson for implementing the bicycle-test in Copenhagen. Ass. prof. Torben E. Lund, University of Aarhus for assistance with the MR scans in Aarhus. Psychologist Lars Clemmensen for implementation of the Revised Frederick's stories. Data manager, MSc Mette Rubæk, Child and Adolescent Mental Health Center, Copenhagen for setting up the database. Creative director Jørgen Høj for creating the logo and the lay out for all visual material. Psychologist Martin Wilms and Sinnika Birkehøj Roed, Mental Health Center Copenhagen, for data collection and data interpretation in the VIA 11 group. All students helping with the management of the project.

REFERENCES

1. Rasic D, Hajek T, Alda M, Uher R. Risk of mental illness in offspring of parents with schizophrenia, bipolar disorder, and major depressive disorder: a meta-analysis of family high-risk studies. *Schizophr Bull.* (2013) 40:28–38. doi: 10.1093/schbul/sbt114
2. Niemi LT, Suvisaari JM, Tuulio-Henriksson A, Lonnqvist JK. Childhood developmental abnormalities in schizophrenia: evidence from high-risk studies. *Schizophr Res.* (2003) 60:239–58. doi: 10.1016/S0920-9964(02)00234-7
3. Birmaher B, Axelson D, Monk K, Kalas C, Goldstein B, Hickey MB, et al. Lifetime psychiatric disorders in school-aged offspring of parents with bipolar disorder: the Pittsburgh Bipolar Offspring study. *Arch Gen Psychiatry* (2009) 66:287–96. doi: 10.1001/archgenpsychiatry.2008.546
4. Thorup AAE, Laursen TM, Munk-Olsen T, Ranning A, Mortensen PB, Plessen KJ, et al. Incidence of child and adolescent mental disorders in children aged 0-17 with familial high risk for severe mental illness - a Danish register study. *Schizophr Res.* (2017) S0920-9964(17)30686-2. doi: 10.1016/j.schres.2017.11.009
5. Duffy A, Horrocks J, Doucette S, Keown-Stoneman C, McCloskey S, Grof P. Childhood anxiety: an early predictor of mood disorders in offspring of bipolar parents. *J Affect Disord.* (2013) 150:363–9. doi: 10.1016/j.jad.2013.04.021
6. Pine DS, Fox NA. Childhood antecedents and risk for adult mental disorders. *Annu Rev Psychol.* (2015) 66:459–85. doi: 10.1146/annurev-psych-010814-015038
7. Hemager N, Plessen KJ, Thorup A, Christiani C, Ellersgaard D, Spang KS, et al. Assessment of neurocognitive functions in 7-year-old children at familial high risk for schizophrenia or bipolar disorder: the Danish high risk and resilience study VIA 7. *JAMA Psychiatry* (2018) 75:844–52. doi: 10.1001/jamapsychiatry.2018.1415
8. Ellersgaard D, Jessica Plessen K, Richardt Jepsen J, Soeborg Spang K, Hemager N, Klee Burton B, et al. Psychopathology in 7-year-old children with familial high risk of developing schizophrenia spectrum psychosis or bipolar disorder - the Danish high risk and resilience study - VIA 7, a population-based cohort study. *World Psychiatry* (2018) 17:210–9. doi: 10.1002/wps.20527
9. Burton BK, Thorup AAE, Jepsen JR, Poulsen G, Ellersgaard D, Spang KS, et al. Impairments of motor function among children with a familial risk of schizophrenia or bipolar disorder at 7 years old in Denmark: an observational cohort study. *Lancet Psychiatry* (2017) 4:400–8. doi: 10.1016/S2215-0366(17)30103-7
10. Burton BK, Vangkilde S, Petersen A, Skovgaard LT, Jepsen JR, Hemager N, et al. Sustained attention and interference control among 7-year-old children with a familial high risk of schizophrenia or bipolar disorder-a nationwide observational cohort study. *Biol Psychiatry Cogn Neurosci Neuroimag.* (2018) 3:704–12. doi: 10.1016/j.bpsc.2018.04.012
11. Agnew-Blais J, Seidman LJ. Neurocognition in youth and young adults under age 30 at familial risk for schizophrenia: a quantitative and qualitative review. *Cogn Neuropsychiatry* (2013) 18:44–82. doi: 10.1080/13546805.2012.676309
12. Bora E, Ozerdem A. A meta-analysis of neurocognition in youth with familial high risk for bipolar disorder. *Eur Psychiatry* (2017) 44:17–23. doi: 10.1016/j.eurpsy.2017.02.483
13. Berenbaum SA, Beltz AM, Corley R. The importance of puberty for adolescent development: conceptualization and measurement. *Adv Child Dev Behav.* (2015) 48:53–92. doi: 10.1016/bs.acdb.2014.11.002
14. Blakemore SJ. The social brain in adolescence. *Nat Rev Neurosci.* (2008) 9:267–77. doi: 10.1038/nrn2353
15. Moore SE, Norman RE, Suetani S, Thomas HJ, Sly PD, Scott JG. Consequences of bullying victimization in childhood and adolescence: a systematic review and meta-analysis. *World J Psychiatry* (2017) 7:60–76. doi: 10.5498/wjp.v7.i1.60
16. Howes OD, Murray RM. Schizophrenia: an integrated sociodevelopmental-cognitive model. *Lancet* (2014) 383:1677–87. doi: 10.1016/S0140-6736(13)62036-X
17. Cannon M, Jones PB, Murray RM. Obstetric complications and schizophrenia: historical and meta-analytic review. *Am J Psychiatry* (2002) 159:1080–92. doi: 10.1176/appi.ajp.159.7.1080
18. Insel TR. Rethinking schizophrenia. *Nature* (2010) 468:187–93. doi: 10.1038/nature09552
19. Cooper D, Barker V, Radua J, Fusar-Poli P, Lawrie SM. Multimodal voxel-based meta-analysis of structural and functional magnetic resonance imaging studies in those at elevated genetic risk of developing schizophrenia. *Psychiatry Res.* (2014) 221:69–77. doi: 10.1016/j.pscychresns.2013.07.008
20. Shoemaker EZ, Tully LM, Niendam TA, Peterson BS. The next big thing in child and adolescent psychiatry: interventions to prevent and intervene early in psychiatric illnesses. *Psychiatr Clin North Am.* (2015) 38:475–94. doi: 10.1016/j.psc.2015.05.010
21. Nordentoft M, Wahlbeck K, Hallgren J, Westman J, Osby U, Alinaghizadeh H, et al. Excess mortality, causes of death and life expectancy in 270,770 patients with recent onset of mental disorders in Denmark, Finland and Sweden. *PLoS ONE* (2013) 8:e55176. doi: 10.1371/journal.pone.0055176
22. Ranning A, Laursen T, Agerbo E, Thorup A, Hjorthoj C, Jepsen JRM, et al. School performance from primary education in the adolescent offspring of parents with schizophrenia and bipolar disorder- a national, register-based study. *Psychol Med.* (2017) 48:1–8. doi: 10.1017/S0033291717003518
23. Saunders JC. Families living with severe mental illness: a literature review. *Issues Ment Health Nurs.* (2003) 24:175–98.
24. Friedmann MS, McDermut WH, Solomon DA, Ryan CE, Keitner GI, Miller IW. Family functioning and mental illness: a comparison of psychiatric and nonclinical families. *Fam Process.* (1997) 36:357–67. doi: 10.1111/j.1545-5300.1997.00357.x
25. Epstein N, Baldwin L, Bishop D. The McMaster family assessment device. (1983) 1983.
26. Thorup AA, Jepsen JR, Ellersgaard DV, Burton BK, Christiani CJ, Hemager N, et al. The Danish High Risk and Resilience Study - VIA 7 - a cohort study of 520 7-year-old children born of parents diagnosed with either schizophrenia, bipolar disorder or neither of these two mental disorders. *BMC Psychiatry* (2015) 15:233. doi: 10.1186/s12888-015-0616-5
27. Pedersen CB, Gøtzsche H, Møller JØ, Mortensen PB. *The Danish Civil Registration System - A Cohort of 8 Million People.* (2006) (Accessed 11/1/2006).
28. Mors O, Perto GP, Mortensen PB. The Danish Psychiatric Central Research Register. *Scand J Public Health* (2011) 39(Suppl. 7):54–7. doi: 10.1177/1403494810395825
29. Henderson S, Sugden D, Barnett A. *The Movement Assessment Battery for Children, 2nd Edn.* London: The Psychological Corporation. (2007).
30. Letz R, Baker EL. *Finger Tapping Test.* Winchester, MA: Neurobehavioral Systems (1988).
31. Bartholdy C, Gudbergsen H, Bliddal H, Kjaergaard M, Lykkegaard KL, Henriksen M. Reliability and construct validity of the sens motion(R) activity measurement system as a tool to detect sedentary behaviour in patients with knee osteoarthritis. *Arthritis* (2018) 2018:6596278. doi: 10.1155/2018/6596278
32. Pulver AE, Liang KY, Brown CH, Wolyniec P, McGrath J, Adler L, et al. Risk factors in schizophrenia: Season of birth, gender, and familial risk. *Br J Psychiatry* (1992) 160:65–71. doi: 10.1192/bjp.160.1.65
33. Reynolds CR, Voress JK. *Tomal 2 Test of Memory and Learning, 2nd Ed.* (2007)
34. Meyers JE, Meyers KR. *Rey Complex Figure Test and Recognition Trial.* Odessa, FL: Psychological Assessment Resources. (1995).
35. Sahakian BJ, Owen AM. Computerized assessment in neuropsychiatry using CANTAB: discussion paper. *J R Soc Med.* (1992) 85:399–402.
36. Conners CK. *Conners CPT: Conners' Continuous Performance Test Computer Program: User's Manual.* Toronto, ON: Multi-Health Systems (1995).
37. Bishop DV. Development of the Children's Communication Checklist (CCC): a method for assessing qualitative aspects of communicative impairment in children. *J Child Psychol. Psychiatry.* (1998) 39:879–91.
38. Delis DC, Kaplan E, Kramer JH. *D-KEFS.* San Antonio, TX: The Psychological Corporation (2001).
39. Wechsler D. *WISC-IV The Wechsler Intelligence Scale for Children—4th ed.* San Antonio, TX: The psychological Corporation (2003).
40. Eriksen BA, Eriksen CW. Effects of noise letters upon the identifaction of a target letter in a nonsearch task. Percept Psychophys. (1974) 16:143–9.
41. Klein AM, Zwickel J, Prinz W, Frith U. Animated triangles: an eye tracking investigation. *Quart J Exp Psychol.* (2009) 6:1189–97. doi: 10.1080/17470210802384214

42. Clemmensen L, van OJ, Skovgaard AM, Vaever M, Blijd-Hoogewys EM, Bartels-Velthuis AA, et al. Hyper-theory-of-mind in children with Psychotic Experiences. *PLoS ONE* (2014) 9:e113082. doi: 10.1371/journal.pone.0113082
43. Reynold C, Kamphaus RW. *Reynold's Intellectual Assessment Scale (RIAS)*. Lutz, FL: Psychological Assessment Resources Inc. (2003).
44. Hassanali N, Ruffell T, Browning S, Bracegirdle K, Ames C, Corrigall R, et al. Cognitive bias and unusual experiences in childhood. *Eur Child Adolesc Psychiatry* (2015) 24:949–57. doi: 10.1007/s00787-014-0644-6
45. Kaufman J, Birmaher B, Brent D, Rao U, Flynn C, Moreci P, et al. Schedule for Affective Disorders and Schizophrenia for School-Age Children-Present and Lifetime Version (K-SADS-PL): initial reliability and validity data. *J Am Acad Child Adolesc Psychiatry* (1997) 36:980–8. doi: 10.1097/00004583-199707000-00021
46. Lencz T, Smith CW, Auther A, Correll CU, Cornblatt B. Nonspecific and attenuated negative symptoms in patients at clinical high-risk for schizophrenia. *Schizophr Res.* (2004) 68:37–48. doi: 10.1016/S0920-9964(03)00214-7
47. Bolton D DP, Madronal-Luque, Baron-Cohen S. *Magical Thinking in Childhood and Adolescence: Development and Relation to Obsessive Compulsion*. London, UK: British Journal of Developmental Psychology (2002). p. 479–94.
48. Achenbach TM, Edelbrock, C. *CBCL, Manual for Child Behavior Checklist and Revised Child Behavior Profile*. University of Vermont, Burlington (1983).
49. Szomlaiski N, Dyrborg J, Rasmussen H, Schumann T, Koch SV, Bilenberg N. Validity and clinical feasibility of the ADHD rating scale (ADHD-RS) A Danish Nationwide Multicenter Study. *Acta Paediatr.* (2009) 98:397–402. doi: 10.1111/j.1651-2227.2008.01025.x
50. Zeman J, Shipman, K., Penza-Clyve, S. Development and initial validation of the Children's Sadness Management. *J Nonverbal Behav.* (2001) 25:540–7. doi: 10.1023/A:1010623226626
51. Gioia GA, Isquith PK, Guy SC, Kenworthy L. Behavior rating inventory of executive function. *Child Neuropsychol.* (2000) 6:235–8. doi: 10.1076/chin.6.3.235.3152
52. Spielberger C, Edwards CD, Lushene J, Montouri J, Platzek D. *The State-Trait Anxiety Inventory for Children (STAIC)*. Palo Alto, CA: Consulting Psychologists Press. (1973).
53. Suonpää E, Kresanov K, Ouvinen-Birgerstam P, Piha J. Self-concept of Finnish children on the second grade of normal elementary school. *Acta Paedopsychiatr.* (1989) 52(Spielberger):157–64.
54. Solberg MEOD. *Prevalence Estimation of School Bullying With the Olweus Bully/Victim Questionnaire*. Bergen: Aggressive Behavior (2003). p. 238–68.
55. Freeman D, Pugh K, Green C, Valmaggia L, Dunn G, Garety P. A measure of state persecutory ideation for experimental studies. *J Nerv Ment Dis.* (2007) 195:781–4. doi: 10.1097/NMD.0b013e318145a0a9
56. Liebenberg L, Ungar M, LeBlanc JC. The CYRM-12: a brief measure of resilience. *Can J Public Health* (2013) 104:e131-e5.
57. Obel C, Dalsgaard S, Stax HP, Bilenberg N. [Strengths and Difficulties Questionnaire (SDQ-Dan). A new instrument for psychopathologic screening of children aged 4-16 years]. *Ugeskr Laeger* (2003) 165:462–5.
58. Sparrow SS, Balla DAC, *D.V. Vineland*. Circle Pines, MN: American Guidance Service (1984).
59. Constantino JN, Gruber CP. *SRS*. Los Angeles, CA: Western Psychological Services (2005).
60. Caldwell BM, Bradley RH. Home *Observation for Measurement of the Environment: Administration Manual*. Tempe, AZ: Family & Human Dynamics Research Institute, Arizona State University (2003).
61. Grabe HJ, Schulz A, Schmidt CO, Appel K, Driessen M, Wingenfeld K, et al. [A brief instrument for the assessment of childhood abuse and neglect: the childhood trauma screener (CTS)]. *Psychiatr Prax.* (2012) 39:109–15. doi: 10.1055/s-0031-1298984
62. Cutrona CE, Russell, D. *SPS: Social Provisions-Scale*. Report No.: 1. (1987).
63. Psouni E, Apetroaia A. Measuring scripted attachment-related knowledge in middle childhood: the Secure Base Script Test. *Attach Hum Dev.* (2014) 16:22–41. doi: 10.1080/14616734.2013.804329
64. Daley D, Sonuga-Barke EJ, Thompson M. Assessing expressed emotion in mothers of preschool AD/HD children: psychometric properties of a modified speech sample. *Br J Clin Psychol.* (2003) 42(Pt. 1):53–67. doi: 10.1348/014466503762842011
65. Kearney CA, Drabman RS, Beasley JF. The trials of childhood: the development, reliability, and validity of the daily life stressors scale. *J Child Family Stud.* (1993) 2:371–88. doi: 10.1007/BF01321232
66. Marshall WA, Tanner JM. Variations in pattern of pubertal changes in girls. *Arch Dis Child.* (1969) 44:291–303.
67. Marshall WA, Tanner JM. Variations in the pattern of pubertal changes in boys. *Arch Dis Child.* (1970) 45:13–23.
68. Wing JK, Babor T, Brugha T, Burke J, Cooper JE, Giel R, et al. SCAN. schedules for clinical assessment in neuropsychiatry. *Arch Gen Psychiatry* (1990) 47:589–93. doi: 10.1001/archpsyc.1990.01810180089012
69. Morosini PL, Magliano L, Brambilla L, Ugolini S, Pioli R. Development, reliability and acceptability of a new version of the DSM-IV Social and Occupational Functioning Assessment Scale (SOFAS) to assess routine social functioning. *Acta Psychiatr Scand.* (2000) 101:323–9.
70. Andreasen NC. *Schedule for Assessment of Negative Symptoms*. (1983)
71. Andreasen NC. *Schedule for Assessment of Positive Symptoms*. (1984).
72. Hamilton M. Development of a rating scale for primary depressive illness. *Br J Soc Clin Psychol.* (1967) 6:278–96. doi: 10.1111/j.2044-8260.1967.tb00530.x
73. Young RC, Biggs JT, Ziegler VE, Meyer DA. A rating scale for mania: reliability, validity and sensitivity. *Br J Psychiatry.* (1978) 133:429–35. doi: 10.1192/bjp.133.5.429
74. Oliver MNI, Simons JS. The affective lability scales: development of a short-form measure. *Pers Individ Diff.* (2004) 37:1279–88. doi: 10.1016/j.paid.2003.12.013
75. Constantino JN, Todd RD. Intergenerational transmission of subthreshold autistic traits in the general population. *Biol Psychiatry* (2005) 57:655–60. doi: 10.1016/j.biopsych.2004.12.014
76. Felitti VJ, Anda RF, Nordenberg D, Williamson DF, Spitz AM, Edwards V, et al. Relationship of childhood abuse and household dysfunction to many of the leading causes of death in adults. The Adverse Childhood Experiences (ACE) Study. *Am J Prev Med.* (1998) 14:245–58. doi: 10.1016/S0749-3797(98)00017-8
77. Berry K, Wearden A, Barrowclough C. Adult attachment styles and psychosis: an investigation of associations between general attachment styles and attachment relationships with specific others. *Soc Psychiatry Psychiatr Epidemiol.* (2007) 42:972–6. doi: 10.1007/s00127-007-0261-5
78. Barch DM, Burgess GC, Harms MP, Petersen SE, Schlaggar BL, Corbetta M, et al. Function in the human connectome: task-fMRI and individual differences in behavior. *Neuroimage* (2013) 80:169–89. doi: 10.1016/j.neuroimage.2013.05.033
79. Miller TJ, McGlashan TH, Rosen JL, Cadenhead K, Cannon T, Ventura J, et al. Prodromal assessment with the structured interview for prodromal syndromes and the scale of prodromal symptoms: predictive validity, interrater reliability, and training to reliability. *Schizophr Bull.* (2003) 29:703–15. doi: 10.1093/oxfordjournals.schbul.a007040
80. Kapur S. Psychosis as a state of aberrant salience: a framework linking biology, phenomenology, and pharmacology in schizophrenia. *Am J Psychiatry* (2003) 160:13–23. doi: 10.1176/appi.ajp.160.1.13
81. McConaughy SH AT. *Manual for the Test Observation Form (TOF) for Ages 2-18*. Burlington, VT: University of Vermont, Research Center for Children, Youth, & Families (2004).
82. Bradley RH, Caldwell BM. Home observation for measurement of the environment: a revision of the preschool scale. *Am J Ment Defic.* (1979) 84:235–44.
83. Thune H, Recasens M, Uhlhaas PJ. The 40-Hz auditory steady-state response in patients with schizophrenia: a meta-analysis. *JAMA Psychiatry* (2016) 73:1145–53. doi: 10.1001/jamapsychiatry.2016.2619
84. Umbricht D, Krljes S. Mismatch negativity in schizophrenia: a meta-analysis. *Schizophr Res.* (2005) 76:1–23. doi: 10.1016/j.schres.2004.12.002
85. O'Donnell BF, Vohs JL, Hetrick WP, Carroll CA, Shekhar A. Auditory event-related potential abnormalities in bipolar disorder and schizophrenia. *Int J Psychophysiol.* (2004) 53:45–55. doi: 10.1016/j.ijpsycho.2004.02.001
86. Naatanen R, Sussman ES, Salisbury D, Shafer VL. Mismatch negativity (MMN) as an index of cognitive dysfunction. *Brain Topogr.* (2014) 27:451–66. doi: 10.1007/s10548-014-0374-6
87. O'Donnell BF, Vohs JL, Krishnan GP, Rass O, Hetrick WP, Morzorati SL. The auditory steady-state response (ASSR): a translational biomarker for schizophrenia. *Suppl Clin Neurophysiol.* (2013) 62:101–12. doi: 10.1016/B978-0-7020-5307-8.00006-5

88. Jablensky A, McNeil TF, Morgan VA. Barbara fish and a short history of the neurodevelopmental hypothesis of schizophrenia. *Schizophr Bull.* (2017) 43:1158–63. doi: 10.1093/schbul/sbx094
89. Hameed MA, Lewis AJ. Offspring of parents with schizophrenia: a systematic review of developmental features across childhood. *Harv Rev Psychiatry* (2016) 24:104–17.doi: 10.1097/HRP.0000000000000076
90. Uher R, Cumby J, MacKenzie LE, Morash-Conway J, Glover JM, Aylott A, et al. A familial risk enriched cohort as a platform for testing early interventions to prevent severe mental illness. *BMC Psychiatry* (2014) 14:344. doi: 10.1186/s12888-014-0344-2
91. de la Serna E, Sugranyes G, Sanchez-Gistau V, Rodriguez-Toscano E, Baeza I, Vila M, et al. Neuropsychological characteristics of child and adolescent offspring of patients with schizophrenia or bipolar disorder. *Schizophr Res.* (2017) 183:110–5. doi: 10.1016/j.pnpbp.2015.08.014
92. Sanchez-Gistau V, Romero S, Moreno D, de la Serna E, Baeza I, Sugranyes G, et al. Psychiatric disorders in child and adolescent offspring of patients with schizophrenia and bipolar disorder: a controlled study. *Schizophr Res.* (2015) 168:197–203. doi: 10.1016/j.schres.2015.08.034
93. Mesman E, Nolen WA, Reichart CG, Wals M, Hillegers MH. The Dutch bipolar offspring study: 12-year follow-up. *Am J Psychiatry* (2013) 170:542–9. doi: 10.1176/appi.ajp.2012.12030401
94. Iacono V, Beaulieu L, Hodgins S, Ellenbogen MA. Parenting practices in middle childhood mediate the relation between growing up with a parent having bipolar disorder and offspring psychopathology from childhood into early adulthood. *Dev Psychopathol.* (2017) 30:1–15. doi: 10.1017/S095457941700116X
95. Language, Reading Research C, Farquharson K, Murphy KA. Ten steps to conducting a large, multi-site, longitudinal investigation of language and reading in young children. *Front Psychol.* (2016) 7:419. doi: 10.3389/fpsyg.2016.00419
96. Downs JM, Cullen AE, Barragan M, Laurens KR. Persisting psychotic-like experiences are associated with both externalising and internalising psychopathology in a longitudinal general population child cohort. *Schizophr Res.* (2013) 144:99–104. doi: 10.1016/j.schres.2012.12.009
97. Polanczyk G, Moffitt TE, Arseneault L, Cannon M, Ambler A, Keefe RS, et al. Etiological and clinical features of childhood psychotic symptoms: results from a birth cohort. *Arch Gen Psychiatry* (2010) 67:328–38. doi: 10.1001/archgenpsychiatry.2010.14
98. Hodges J, Hillman, S. Story Stem Assessment Profile (SSAP). (2007). (Unpublished data).
99. Abreu AP, Kaiser UB. Pubertal development and regulation. *Lancet Diabetes Endocrinol.* (2016) 4:254–64. doi: 10.1016/S2213-8587(15)00418-0

17

Prenatal Depression and its Associated Risk Factors Among Pregnant Women in Bangalore: A Hospital Based Prevalence Study

B. Sheeba[1], Anita Nath[2], Chandra S. Metgud[3], Murali Krishna[4], Shubhashree Venkatesh[1], J. Vindhya[1] and Gudlavalleti Venkata Satyanarayana Murthy[5]*

[1] Research Assistant, Indian Institute of Public Health Hyderabad, Public Health of Foundation of India, Bangalore, India, [2] Wellcome Trust DBT India Alliance, Intermediate Fellow in Clinical and Public Health, Indian Institute of Public Health Hyderabad, Public Health Foundation of India, Hyderabad, India, [3] Professor, Department of Community Medicine, Pt. Jawahar Lal Nehru Memorial Medical College, Belgavi, India, [4] Consultant, FRAME, Mysore, India, [5] Indian Institute of Public Health Hyderabad, Public Health Foundation of India, Hyderabad, India

***Correspondence:**
Sheeba B
sheeba.b@iiphh.org

Background: Depression is the commonest psychological problem that affects a woman during her perinatal period worldwide. The risk of prenatal depression increases as the pregnancy progresses and clinically significant depressive symptoms are common in the mid and late trimester. There is a paucity of research on depression during the prenatal period in India. Given this background, the present study aimed to assess the prevalence of prenatal depression and its associated risk factors among pregnant women in Bangalore, Southern India.

Methods: The study was nested within an on-going cohort study. The study participants included 280 pregnant women who were attending the antenatal clinic at Jaya Nagar General Hospital (Sanjay Gandhi Hospital) in Bangalore. The data was collected by using a structured questionnaire which included. Edinburgh Postnatal Depression Scale (EPDS) to screen for prenatal depression.

Results: The proportion of respondents who screened positive for prenatal depression was 35.7%. Presence of domestic violence was found to impose a five times higher and highly significant risk of developing prenatal depression among the respondents. Pregnancy related anxiety and a recent history of catastrophic events were also found to be a positive predictors of prenatal depression.

Conclusion: The high prevalence of prenatal depression in the present study is suggestive of its significance as a public health problem. Health care plans therefore can include screening and diagnosis of prenatal depression in the antenatal care along with other health care facilities provided.

Keywords: prenatal depression, pregnant women, domestic violence, marital discord, social support, pregnancy related anxiety, Banglaore

INTRODUCTION

The relationship between a pregnant woman and her developing fetus is possibly the most earnest and overwhelming but perplexing of all human relationships. Pregnancy entails physiological, hormonal and psychological changes which could increase the probability of mental and emotional changes resulting in depression, anxiety or psychological distress in the pregnant mother (1).

Maternal and Child Health Programmes in developing countries are commonly focused upon improving the nutritional status and less importance is given toward a woman's emotional and mental health during and after pregnancy (2, 3). Poor mental health of the woman during pregnancy could have profound consequences for the mother and her child in terms of adverse pregnancy outcomes and offspring development (4–7). Most of the existing data, research, and practice policies with regard to perinatal mental disorders center on the postnatal period and there is less research related depression during pregnancy (8, 9).

Depression is the most common psychological problem that affects a woman worldwide during the perinatal period (3, 10). About 15 % of women are known to be depressed at some point during their lifetime and more predominantly during pregnancy and after childbirth (11). The risk of prenatal depression increases significantly as the pregnancy progresses and clinically significant depressive symptoms are common in the mid and late trimester (12). The prevalence rates of prenatal depression differ between high, middle and low—income countries. Studies from various countries around the world show a prevalence rate ranging from as low as 4% to as high as 81% (13–16). The prevalence rate is reported to be lower in high income countries like Australia 7% (17), Hong Kong 4.4% (18), Finland 7.7% (19), and higher in many of the low-income countries like Pakistan 64.6% (20), Bangladesh 18% (13), Nigeria 24.5% (14), and Ethiopia 24.94% (15). The prevalence of depression in India is varies from 9.18% in one study to 36.7 % reported in another study (21, 22).

Even though prenatal depression is an important public health problem, most studies related to maternal depression are focused on post-natal depression and its outcomes; hence there is paucity of research on depression during the prenatal period, especially from India (8). The importance of screening for depression during pregnancy is that prenatal depression, if not treated and diagnosed early, may continue as postnatal depression (23–25) later on and could also result in an adverse influence on birth outcomes and offspring development. Given this background, the present study aimed to assess the prevalence of prenatal depression and its associated risk factors among pregnant women in Bangalore, Southern India.

MATERIALS AND METHODS

Study Setting and Participants

The study sample included of pregnant women who were attending the antenatal clinic at Jaya Nagar General Hospital (also known as Sanjay Gandhi Hospital), which is a public sector hospital in Bangalore. The study was nested within an ongoing cohort study, the study protocol of which was published earlier (26). The eligibility criteria included women above or equal to 18 years of age, with confirmed pregnancy of <6 months (<24 weeks) and having no obstetric or medical complication in the present pregnancy. The study analyzed the data of 280 pregnant women who had enrolled and completed the baseline visit for the study between August 2017 and April 2018.

Data Collection

Data was obtained from the pregnant women by means of an interview, after obtaining written informed consent. A participant information sheet that explained the purpose and nature of the study was issued to those who were willing to participate in the study. The respondents were ensured about privacy and confidentiality of data. The interview process employed the use of a structured questionnaire installed in an Android tablet App. The App included questions about socio-demographic data, obstetric history, medical history and measures for depression, social support, marital discord, domestic violence, and pregnancy related anxiety described below. Data related history of any mental illness and recent catastrophic event was also recorded. Calibrated instruments were used to measure height and weight and calculate the Body Mass Index (BMI). Data on hemoglobin estimation was obtained from hospital records. Depression, being the outcome variable was measured using Edinburg Postnatal Depression Scale (EPDS).

Study Measures

Depression

EPDS is a widely used 10-item self-reporting instrument, specifically designed for assessing both prenatal as well as postnatal depression. It has a sensitivity of 86%, specificity of 78% and positive predictive value of 73% (27). EPDS has been validated for detecting depression in both antepartum and postpartum mothers in many countries. This scale consists of 10 short questions with a choice of four answers that closely reflects about how she was feeling over the past 7 days. Scores are recorded as 0, 1, 2, and 3 according symptom severity. Certain question items (i.e., 3, 2, 1, and 0) are scored in a reverse manner. Respondents who score 13 and above are likely to be suffering from depression and should seek medical attention.

Social Support

The Multidimensional Scale of Perceived Social Support Scale (MSPSS) used to measure social support includes 12 questions, and is validated for use in the South Asian population (28, 29). These questions directly address the adequacy of social support and have a 7-point rating scale ranging from "very strongly disagree" to "very strongly agree." The scale assesses the perceptions of social support adequacy from three specific sources: family, friends, and "significant other." A score of <2 is considered as low support, a score of 3–5 as moderate support while score of more than five indicates high support.

Marital Discord

The Revised Dyadic Adjustment Scale (30, 31) measures seven dimensions of relationship among partners within three categories: decision making, values and affection. It consists of 14 items in which the respondents can rate their relationship on a 6-point scale. Scores range from 0 to 69; higher the score greater, is the relationship and *vice versa*. The cut- off score was taken as 48.

Spouse Physical and Sexual Violence

Spouse physical and sexual violence was measured using the Modified Conflict Tactics Scale (32). It is effective and useful in measuring domestic violence in diverse cultural settings. The scale has 9 questions wherein the respondents affirm whether domestic violence was present or absent.

Socio Economic Scale

The socio-economic class of the respondents was measured by the Modified Kuppuswamy Socio Economic Scale (33). The scale uses education, occupation of the head of the family and monthly family income to calculate socio-economic status. The scores awarded to education and occupation of the head of the family remains unchanged. Revised Consumer Price Index–IW (industrial workers) is used to calculate the monthly income range. The socio-economic status is classified as upper class, upper middle class, lower middle class, upper lower class and lower class.

Pregnancy Related Anxiety

The 10-item Pregnancy Related Anxiety Questionnaire (PRAQ) was used to screen for pregnancy anxiety (34). It appears to have good psychometric and predictive validity for child-birth and childhood outcomes. Each item is scored on a 4-point scale with cut-off scores of 28 and 24 for nulliparous and multiparous women and the internal consistency (Cronbach's alpha) of PRAQ was seen to be 0.79. A score of more than 28 was considered as anxious.

Statistical Analysis

Data were retrieved from the data server. This was followed by data cleaning and analysis using SPSS version 22. Descriptive statistics such as percentage, means and standard deviation were used to summarize the socio demographic data. An EPDS score of 13 and above pointed toward the likelihood of presence of depression. The independent variables were categorized to analyze the association between each independent and outcome variable using a bivariate analysis to calculate the Crude Odd's Ratio with 95% Confidence Interval. Those variables that were associated at a P-value of < 0.2 in the bivariate analysis were entered into a multivariate logistic regression model to calculate the Adjusted Odd's Ratio and to eliminate the effects of confounding. Variables with a P-value of <0.05 in the multivariate analysis were considered to be significant.

Ethical Considerations

The study was approved by the Ethical Committee of Indian Institute of Public Health Bangalore campus (IIPHHB/TRCIEC/118/2017). Written informed consent was obtained from the pregnant mothers and they were assured of confidentiality and privacy of records.

RESULTS

Socio Demographic Characteristics of the Respondents

Table 1 shows the frequency distribution of socio demographic characteristics of the respondents. Of the 280 pregnant mothers, majority (72.9%) of them belonged to the age group of more than 20 years, the mean age of the respondents being 23.02 ± 3.40 years. Over two-thirds among them (72.1%) were Muslim and 40.4% had completed High school. While 92.1% were housewives, the spouses of over half of the respondents (51.8%) were semi- skilled workers. According to the Kuppuswamy Socio economic status scale, more than half of the respondents (57.5%) belonged to Upper Lower class. Nearly seventy percent of the

TABLE 1 | Socio demographic characteristics of the study participants (N =280).

Socio demographic characteristics	Frequency (n = 280)	Percentage (%)
AGE GROUP (IN YEARS)		
≤20	76	27.1
>20	204	72.9
RELIGION		
Hinduism	73	26.1
Christianity	05	1.8
Islam	202	72.1
EDUCATIONAL QUALIFICATION OF THE RESPONDENTS		
Illiterate	07	2.5
Primary school	08	2.9
Middle school	77	27.5
High school	113	40.4
PUC or diploma	52	18.6
Graduate	23	8.2
EDUCATIONAL QUALIFICATION OF THE HUSBANDS		
Illiterate	36	12.9
Primary school	20	7.1
Middle school	71	25.4
High school	95	33.9
PUC or diploma	36	12.9
Graduate and post-graduate	22	7.8
OCCUPATION OF THE RESPONDENTS		
Unskilled worker	11	3.9
Semi-skilled worker	10	3.6
Clerical or farmer	01	0.4
Housewife	258	92.1
OCCUPATION OF THE HUSBANDS		
Unemployed	01	0.4
Unskilled worker	96	34.3
Semi-skilled worker	145	51.8
Skilled worker	35	12.5
Clerical or farmer	01	0.4
Semi professional	02	0.7
SOCIO ECONOMIC STATUS		
Upper middle class	36	12.9
Lower middle class	83	29.6
Upper Lower class	161	57.5

pregnant mothers had no blood relationship with their husbands, where as a notable 13.2% said that their husbands were a first cousin from their mother's side.

Prevalence and Magnitude of Prenatal Depression Among the Pregnant Women

Of the 280 pregnant mothers, the proportion of those who screened positive for prenatal depression was 35.7% (100) suggesting a high probability of clinical depression (**Figure 1**). The mean EPDS score among the respondents was 10.61± 7.48.

Association of Prenatal Depression With Socio-Demographic Characteristics

The association of socio-demographic factors like age group, educational qualification, occupation, and socio-economic status of the respondents with depression was non-significant on bivariate analysis (p-value >0.05). This is seen from **Table 2**.

Association of Prenatal Depression With Obstetric History (Table 3)

On bivariate analysis, the number of pregnancies (gravida) and unplanned pregnancy showed an association with depression at a P-value of < 0.2. However, there was no significant association observed from multivariate logistic regression analysis.

Association Between Social Support, Marital Discord, Domestic Violence, Prenatal Anxiety, Consanguinity, and Catastrophic Events With Prenatal Depression (Table 4)

Association with low social support and presence of marital discord was significant on bivariate analysis but not in multivariate logistic regression. Presence of domestic violence was found to impose a five times higher and highly significant risk of developing prenatal depression among the respondents (COR = 5.438; 95% CI: 1.6–17.5, AOR = 5.916; 95% CI: 1.7–20.5). Pregnancy related anxiety was also found to be a positive predictor of prenatal depression (COR = 1.731; 95%

TABLE 2 | Association of socio demographic characteristics with depression among the pregnant women (N = 280).

Socio demographic Characteristics	Depressed mothers (>13) (n = 100)	Non-depressed mothers (<13) (n = 180)	Bivariate analysis-crude odd's ratio (95% CI)	P-value
AGE GROUP (IN YEARS)				
≤20	29 (29%)	47 (26.1%)	1.156 (0.670–1.994)	0.603
>20	71 (71%)	133 (73.9%)	1	
EDUCATIONAL QUALIFICATION OF THE RESPONDENTS				
<High school	77 (77.0%)	126 (70.0%)	0.710 (0.403–1.250)	0.236
≥High school	23 (23.0%)	54 (30.0%)	1	
EDUCATIONAL QUALIFICATION OF THE HUSBANDS				
<High school	49 (49%)	78 (43.3%)	1.256 (0.769–2.052)	0.362
≥High school	51 (51%)	102 (56.7%)	1	
OCCUPATION OF THE RESPONDENTS				
Working	08 (8.0%)	15 (8.3%)	1.045 (0.427–2.559)	0.922
Housewife	92 (92.0%)	165 (91.7%)	1	
OCCUPATION OF THE HUSBANDS				
Skilled worker	12 (12%)	26 (14.4%)	1	
Semi/unskilled worker	88 (88%)	154 (85.6%)	1.238 (0.595–2.575)	0.568
SOCIO ECONOMIC STATUS				
Upper middle class	12 (12.0%)	24 (13.3%)	1	
Lower middle class	26 (26.0%)	57 (31.7%)	0.912 (0.396–2.100)	0.829
Upper lower class	62 (62.0%)	99 (55.0%)	1.253 (0.584–2.686)	0.563

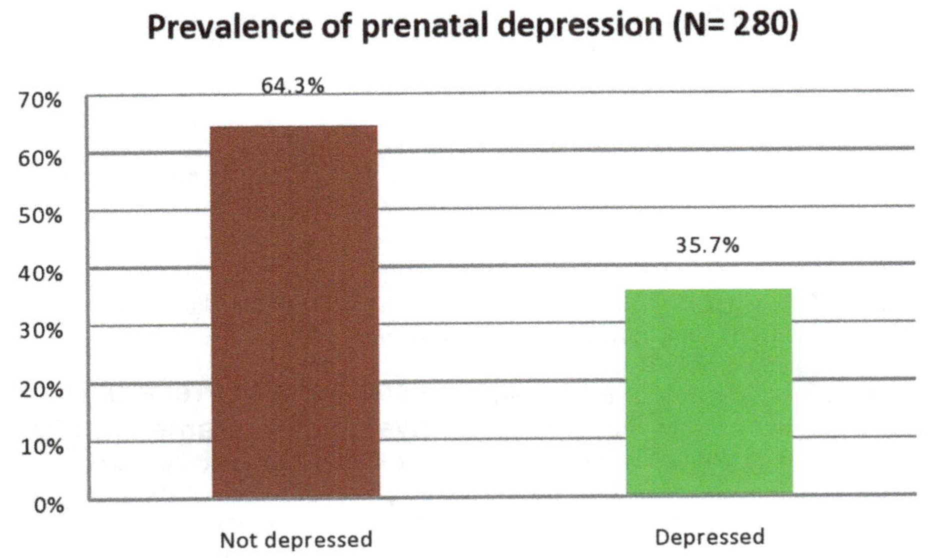

FIGURE 1 | Prevalence of prenatal depression among the pregnant women (N = 280).

TABLE 3 | Association of depression with obstetric history of the pregnant women (*N* = 280).

Obstetric history	Depressed mothers (>13) (*n* = 100)	Non-depressed mothers (<13) (*n* = 180)	Bivariate analysis crude OR (95% CI)	*P*-value	Multivariate analysis adjusted OR (95% CI)	*P*-value
GRAVIDITY						
Primigravida	37 (37.0%)	81 (45.0%)	1		1	
Multigravida	63 (63.0%)	99 (55.0%)	1.393 (0.844–2.299)	0.195	1.386 (0.793–2.424)	0.252
PARITY						
Primipara	43 (43.0%)	86 (47.8%)	1			
Multipara	57 (57.0%)	94 (52.2%)	1.213 (0.741–1.984)	0.442		
HISTORY OF ABORTION						
Yes	25 (25.0%)	37 (20.6%)	0.776 (0.435–1.385)	0.391		
No	75 (75.0%)	143 (79.4%)	1			
PREGNANCY UNPLANNED						
Yes	52 (52.0%)	74 (41.1%)	1.552 (0.949–2.538)		1.604 (0.925–2.782)	
No	48 (48.0%)	106 (58.9%)	1	0.080	1	0.092

TABLE 4 | Association of maternal depression with social support, marital discord, and domestic violence among the pregnant mothers (*N* = 280).

Maternal characteristics	Depressed mothers (>13) (*n* = 100)	Non-depressed mothers (<13) (*n* = 180)	Bivariate analysis crude OR (95% CI)	*P*-value	Multivariate analysis adjusted OR (95% CI)	*P*-value
SOCIAL SUPPORT						
High support (1–2.9)	44 (44.0%)	94 (52.2%)	1		1	
Moderate support (3–5)	24 (24.0%)	54 (30.0%)	0.949 (0.521–1.729)	0.865	0.839 (0.436–1.616)	0.600
Low support (5.1–7)	32 (32.0%)	32 (17.8%)	2.136 (1.164–3.919)	0.014	1.785 (0.915–3.481)	0.089
MARITAL DISCORD						
No	32 (32.0%)	79 (43.9%)	1		1	
Yes	68 (68.0%)	101 (56.1%)	1.662 (0.995–2.776)	0.052	1.517 (0.862–2.671)	0.149
SPOUSE PHYSICAL AND SEXUAL VIOLENCE						
Yes	11 (11.0%)	04 (2.2%)	5.438 (1.684–17.564)	0.005	5.916 (1.703–20.558)	0.005*
No	89 (89.0%)	176 (97.8%)	1		1	
PREGNANCY RELATED ANXIETY						
Absent	47 (47.0%)	109 (60.6%)	1		1	
Present	53 (53.0%)	71 (39.4%)	1.731 (1.057–2.836)	0.029	2.016 (1.134–3.587)	0.017*
CONSANGUINITY						
No	77 (77.0%)	121 (67.2%)	1			
Yes	23 (23.0%)	59 (32.8%)	0.613 (0.350–1.073)	0.086	0.728 (0.397–1.334)	0.304
CATASTROPHIC EVENTS						
No	64 (31.4%)	140 (68.6%)	1		1	
Yes	36 (47.4%)	40 (68.6%)	1.969 (1.149–3.374)	0.014	2.148 (1.203–3.837)	0.010*

**Positively significant according to multivariable analysis.*

CI: 1.05–2.8, AOR = 2.016; 95% CI: 1.13–3.5). The blood relationship with the husband did not show any significant association with prenatal depression on bivariate analysis and multivariable analysis. Presence of catastrophic events over the past 1 year imposed a two times higher and significant risk of developing prenatal depression among the respondents (COR = 1.969; 95% CI: 1.14–3.37, AOR = 2.148; 95% CI: 1.20–3.83, *p*-value = 0.010). History of mental illness was not included in the analysis because only one respondent had history of this kind and was undergoing treatment with medications.

Association of Prenatal Depression With Physiologic Parameters (Table 5)

Table 5 shows the association between physiologic parameters with prenatal depression. Presence of anemia (COR = 1.621; 95% CI: 0.9–2.7, AOR = 1.586; 95% CI: 0.91–2.75) showed some strong association with prenatal depression although this was

TABLE 5 | Association of prenatal depression with physiological parameters ($N = 280$).

Physiological parameters	Depressed mothers (>13) ($n = 100$)	Non-depressed mothers (<13) ($n = 180$)	Bivariate analysis crude OR (95% CI)	*P*-value	Multivariate analysis adjusted OR (95% CI)	*P*-value
BODY MASS INDEX						
Normal	56 (56.0%)	96 (53.3%)	1			
Underweight	12 (12.0%)	21 (11.7%)	0.980 (0.448–2.141)	0.959		
Obese	32 (32.0%)	63 (35.0%)	0.871 (0.508–1.491)	0.614		
ANEMIA						
Present	41 (41.0%)	54 (30.0%)	1.621 (0.973–2.701)	0.063	1.586 (0.912–2.756)	0.102
Absent	59 (59.0%)	126 (70.0%)	1		1	

not statistically significant. No association found between BMI and depression.

DISCUSSION

In this study we have measured the prevalence of prenatal depression among pregnant women and its association with certain risk factors such as socio-demographic characteristics, obstetric history, social support, marital discord, spouse physical and sexual violence, and physiologic measurements which included body mass index and hemoglobin level.

The mean age of respondents was 23.02 ± 3.40 years, which reflects upon the Indian cultural tradition of early marriage and parenthood. The prevalence of depression during pregnancy was 37.8% which is suggestive of a high probability of depression (using an EPDS cutoff score ≥13) among the respondents. The prevalence of prenatal depression makes it a significant public health issue in the study region. EPDS has been validated for use in India and Karnataka (26). Our study used a cut off score of more than or equal to 13 to identify women with depression; this yields a sensitivity of 100% and specificity of 84.9% in Indian settings (27). Another study from Karnataka showed an almost similar prevalence of 36.8% (21) whereas George et al., Ajinkya et al., and Bavle et al. observed much lower prevalence rates of 16.3% in coastal south India (35), 9.18% in Navi Mumbai (22), and 12.3% in Bangalore (36), respectively. This difference could be attributed to diversity in the socio-economic status, socio-cultural and psychosocial factors such as social support which might vary across different regions in the country. Moreover, this study was conducted in a public sector hospital setting, which in itself could pose as a risk factor and predictor for prenatal depression (28) due to inadequate quality of care in such settings.

In our study, majority of the study participants belonged to the low income group. Although we could not document a significant association with socio-economic status, the risk of depression during, and after pregnancy is higher among the socially disadvantaged group (10, 37, 38). It is hypothesized that low income increases the likelihood of poor living conditions, financial struggle and influences interpersonal relationships which could lead to psychosocial stress. Over a third of the study participants were high school graduates though over 90% were not working; however there was no association of education and occupation with depression. Bavle et al. (36) in their study among pregnant women in Bangalore observed that being educated but not employed outside the house could predispose to depression during pregnancy. Study findings from other low income settings point toward a significant association of a woman's occupation with depression: women who were housewives or employed in the private sector or as a laborer or merchant business were prone to get depressed during pregnancy (39, 40). Other socio-demographic factors such as age, husband's education, and occupation did not predict the occurrence of depression in the present study even though some studies have identified young age as a risk factor (41, 42). In Asian settings, having an unemployed or uneducated husband increases the probability of depression (43, 44).

Among the obstetric history variables, unplanned pregnancy increased the odds of depression on bivariate analysis. However, no significant association was observed on multivariate logistic regression analysis. Other studies show that the chance of getting depressed is higher in case of an unplanned pregnancy (15, 37, 45). Similarly multigravidity appeared to be risk factor for depression on bivariate analysis but not on logistic regression analysis although some studies do report a significant relationship (36, 46).

In this study, among the psychosocial factors, presence of spouse physical and sexual violence and pregnancy related anxiety were significant risk factors for prenatal depression in the multivariable analysis. Earlier research has also reported a strong relationship between domestic violence and the risk of depression in pregnancy in high as well as middle to low—income settings (47, 48). Moderate and low social support were significantly related on bivariate but not on multivariate analysis. The linkage between poor social support and prenatal depression has been well-documented (49, 50). Low social support may increase mental stress by inducing feelings of insecurity, predispose toward substance abuse (51), and promote interpersonal conflict (52). The findings from the present study are concurrent with the study results reported by Nongrum et al. India (53), George et al. in Southern India (35), Silva et al. in Brazil (42), and Bernard et al. in Jamaica (54). Depression and anxiety show frequent co-existence and anxiety may emerge as a strong predictor for depression (24, 37). Mohamad et al. (55) and Edward et al. (56) also demonstrated that anxiety strongly increased the risk of suffering from depression during pregnancy. Even a history of mental illness can pose as a risk factor for depression (57, 58); however in our study only one respondent appeared to have such a history. Marital discord appeared predict presence of depression on bivariate but not on multivariate analysis; other studies report that this is e a well-established risk factor due to its influence on social support (59, 60). Likewise consanguinity seemed to be associated with depression only on bivariate testing. Consanguineous marriages are fairly prevalent in South India and clinical observations have reported a high prevalence of depression in such communities (61) which could be genetically driven (62). A major catastrophic event in the past 1 year was an important risk factor which was significantly associated with prenatal depression in this study; this is consistent with the study results reported by Leigh et al. (63) and Shakeel et al. (58). Another study reported that negative life events may lead to persistent higher levels of depressive symptoms since positive life events can decrease the severity of depression over time (64).

Among the physiologic measurements, anemia was significantly associated with depression on bivariate although not so on multivariate analysis. This is in agreement with the study findings reported by Lukose et al. (65); however Yilmaz et al. depicted the existence of such an association between depressive symptoms and anemia in the third trimester of pregnancy (66). Body mass index was not linked with the risk of prenatal depression in the present study. Research done in other countries reportedly point toward an interconnection between obesity and depression (67, 68). The causal pathway could include inflammation (62), hormonal imbalance (69), or sleep disturbance (70).

STUDY STRENGTHS AND LIMITATIONS

This study focuses on prenatal depression which has received less attention than postnatal depression. All the instruments/scales used to measure the study variables had good psychometric properties. Our study had few a limitations. Antenatal care at such hospitals is mostly availed by pregnant women from the lower and middle—income groups in a community. Hence the findings from this study cannot be extrapolated to pregnant women belonging to the high income group as there could be variations in the psychosocial factors and standard of living. As a part of the cohort study protocol, we excluded women with high risk pregnancies and those with a history of intake of steroidal medication over the past 1 year; this could limit the generalizability of the study findings. Adverse obstetric complications during pregnancy can modulate the mental health of a woman during pregnancy. In the south-east Asian context, conflict with in-laws is also a significant risk factor, although this item was not recorded in the present study but will be included in future data collection. We used the EPDS scale which is a self -reporting screening measure for identifying women at risk for depression. Even though EPDS has a high sensitivity and specificity and can be easily administered by a trained health worker, it is important to confirm the presence of depression by using a structured clinical interview to confirm diagnosis.

CONCLUSION

The present study showed a high prevalence of prenatal depression which is suggestive of its public health importance in the study region. Spouse physical and sexual violence, pregnancy related anxiety and a history of catastrophic events were important predictors of prenatal depression. Obstetric practice should include screening and diagnosis of prenatal depression as a part of routine antenatal care in low and middle—income countries.

ETHICS STATEMENT

This study was carried out in accordance with the recommendations of the Ethical Committee of Indian Institute of Public Health Bangalore campus (IIPHHB/TRCIEC/118/2017) with written informed consent from all subjects. All subjects gave written informed consent in accordance with the Declaration of Helsinki. The protocol was approved by the Ethical committee of Indian Institute of Public Health Bangalore campus.

AUTHOR CONTRIBUTIONS

AN and MK: conceptualization. BS, SV, and JV: formal analysis. AN and GM: funding acquisition. CM: methodology. AN and SB: writing-original draft preparation.

FUNDING

This project is funded by Welcome Trust DBT India Alliance (Clinical and Public Health Research Fellowship), grant number IA/CPHI/16/1/502634.

ACKNOWLEDGMENTS

We would like to extend our sincere thanks to the staffs of Jaya Nagar General Hospital for supporting us during data collection.

REFERENCES

1. DiPietro JA. Psychological and psychophysiological considerations regarding the maternal-fetal relationship. *Infant Child Dev.* (2010) 19:27–38. doi: 10.1002/icd.651
2. Rahman A, Patel V, Maselko J, Kirkwood B. The neglected 'm' in MCH programmes-why mental health of mothers is important for child nutrition. *Trop Med Int Health.* (2008) 13:579–83. doi: 10.1111/j.1365-3156.2008.02036.x
3. Bowen A, Muhajarine N. Antenatal depression. *Can. Nurse.* (2006) 102:26–30.
4. Grote NK, Bridge JA, Gavin AR, Melville JL, Iyengar S, Katon WJ. A meta-analysis of depression during pregnancy and the risk of preterm birth, low birth weight, and intrauterine growth restriction. *Arch Gen Psychiatry.* (2010) 67:1012–24. doi: 10.1001/archgenpsychiatry.2010.111

5. Accortt E, Cheadle A, Dunkel SC. Prenatal depression and adverse birth outcomes: an updated systematic review. *Matern Child Health J.* (2014) 19 1306–37. doi: 10.1007/s10995-014-1637-2
6. Van den Bergh B, Mulder E, Mennes M, Glover V. Antenatal maternal anxiety and stress and the neurobehavioural development of the fetus and child: links and possible mechanisms. A review. *Neurosci Biobehav Rev.* (2005) 29:237–58. doi: 10.1016/j.neubiorev.2004.10.007
7. Plant DT, Pawlby S, Sharp D, Zunszain PA, Pariante CM. Prenatal maternal depression is associated with offspring inflammation at 25 years: a prospective longitudinal cohort study. *Transl Psychiatry.* (2016) 6:e936. doi: 10.1038/tp.2015.155
8. Satyanarayana VA, Lukose A, Srinivasan K. Maternal mental health in pregnancy and child behavior. *Indian J Psychiatry.* (2011) 53:351–61. doi: 10.4103/0019-5545.91911
9. Howard L, Molyneaux E, Dennis C, Rochat T, Stein A, Milgrom J. Non-psychotic mental disorders in the perinatal period. *Lancet.* (2014) 384:1775–88. doi: 10.1016/S0140-6736(14)61276-9
10. Fatoye FO, Adeyemi AB, Oladimeji B. Emotional distress and its correlates among Nigerian women in late pregnancy. *J Obstet Gynecol.* (2004) 24:504–9. doi: 10.1080/01443610410001722518
11. Rochat T, Tomlinson M, Newell M, Stein A. Depression among pregnant women testing for HIV in rural South Africa: implications for VCT. In:*9th International AIDS Impact Conference.* Botswana (2009).
12. Manikkam I, Burns JK. Antenatal depression and its risk factors: an urban prevalence study in KwaZulu-Natal. *South Afr Med J.* (2012) 102:940–4. doi: 10.7196/samj.6009
13. Nasreen H, Kabir Z, Forsell Y, Edhborg M. Prevalence and associated factors of depressive and anxiety symptoms during pregnancy: a population based study in rural Bangladesh. *BMC Womens Health.* (2011) 111:22. doi: 10.1186/1472-6874-11-22.
14. Thompson O, Ajayi I. Prevalence of antenatal depression and associated risk factors among pregnant women attending clinics in Abeokuta North Local Government Area, Nigeria. *Depres Res Treat.* (2016) 2016:4518979. doi: 10.1155/2016/4518979
15. Biratu A, Haile D. Prevalence of antenatal depression and associated factors among pregnant women in Addis Ababa, Ethiopia: a cross-sectional study. *Reprod Health.* (2015) 12:99. doi: 10.1186/s12978-015-0092-x
16. Jafri SAM, Ali M, Ali R, Shaikh S, Abid M, Aamir IS. Prevalence of depression among Pregnant Women attending Antenatal Clinics in Pakistan. *Acta Psychopathol.* (2017) 3:54. doi: 10.4172/2469-6676.100126
17. Eastwood J, Ogbo F, Hendry A, Noble J, Page A. The impact of antenatal depression on perinatal outcomes in Australian women. *PLoS ONE.* (2017) 12:e0169907. doi: 10.1371/journal.pone.0169907
18. Lee DT, Chan SS, Sahota DS, Yip AS, Tsui M, Chung TK. A prevalence study of antenatal depression among Chinese women. *J Affect Disord.* (2004) 82:93–9. doi: 10.1016/j.jad.2003.10.003
19. Pajulo M, Savonlahti E, Sourander A, Helenius H, Piha J. Antenatal depression, substance dependency and social support. *J Affect Disord.* (2001) 65:9–17. doi: 10.1016/S0165-0327(00)00265-2
20. Humayun A, Haider I, Imran N, Iqbal H, Humayun N. Antenatal depression and its predictors in Lahore, Pakistan. *East Mediterran Heath J.* (2013) 19:327–32. doi: 10.26719/2013.19.4.327
21. Pai Keshava K, Shruthi SH, Hulegar AA, Sandeep KR. Prevalence of antenatal depression and gender preference: A cross sectional study among Mangalore population, Karnataka, India. *J Pharm Biomed Sci.* (2013) 29:1011–4.
22. Ajinkya S, Jadhav PR, Srivastava NN. Depression during pregnancy: prevalence and obstetric risk factors among pregnant women attending a tertiary care hospital in Navi Mumbai. *Ind Psychiatry J.* (2013) 22:37–40. doi: 10.4103/0972-6748.123615
23. Heron J, O'Connor TG, Evans J, Golding J, Glover V, ALSPAC Study Team. The course of anxiety and depression through pregnancy and the pospartum in a community sample. *J Affect Disord.* (2004) 80:65–73. doi: 10.1016/j.jad.2003.08.004
24. Verreault N, Da Costa D, Marchand A, Ireand K, Drista M, Khalife S. Rates and risk factors associated with depressive sympotms during pregnancy and with postpartum onset. *J Psychosom Obset Gynaecol.* (2014) 35:84–91. doi: 10.3109/0167482X.2014.947953
25. Tachibana Y, Koizumi T, Takehara K, Kakee N, Tsujii H, Mori R, et al. Antenatal risk factors of postpartum depression at 20 weeks of gestation in Japanese sample: psychosocial perspectives from a Cohort study in Tokyo. *PLoS ONE.* (2015) 10:e0142410. doi: 10.1371/journal.pone.0142410
26. Nath A, Murthy G, Babu G, Di Renzo G. Effect of prenatal exposure to maternal cortisol and psychological distress on infant development in Bengaluru, southern India: a prospective cohort study. *BMC Psychiatry.* (2017) 17:255. doi: 10.1186/s12888-017-1424-x
27. Cox JL, Holden JM, Sagovsky R. Detection of postnatal depression: development of the 10-item Edinburgh Postnatal Depression Scale. *Br J Psychiatry.* (1987) 150:782–6.
28. Zimet GD, Dahlem NW, Zimet SG, Farley GK. The multidimensional scale of perceived social support. *J Pers Assess.* (1988) 52:30–41.
29. Ng CG, AmerSiddiq AN, Aida SA, Zainal NZ, Koh OH. Validation of the Malay version of the Multidimensional Scale of Perceived Social Support (MSPSS-M) among a group of medical students in Faculty of Medicine, University Malaya. *Asian J Psychiatr.* (2010) 3:3–6. doi: 10.1016/j.ajp.2009.12.001
30. Busby DM, Christensen C, Crane DR, Larson JH. A revision of the dyadic adjustment scale for use with distressed and non-distressed couples: construct hierarchy and multidimensional scales. *J Marital Family Ther.* (1995) 21:289–308.
31. Crane DR, Middleton KC, Bean RA. Establishing criterion scores for the Kansas marital satisfaction scale and the revised dyadic adjustment scale. *Am J Family Ther.* (2000) 28:53–60. doi: 10.1080/019261800261815
32. Straus M, Gelles R. *Physical Violence in 8145 American Families: Risk Factors and Adaptations to Violence. Family Relations.* New Bmnswick, NJ: Transaction Publishing. (1990), 49–73.
33. Shaikh Z, Pathak R. Revised Kuppuswamy and B G Prasad socio-economic scales for 2016. *Int J Community Med Public Health.* (2017) 4:997–9. doi: 10.18203/2394-6040.ijcmph20171313
34. Huizink A, Delforterie M, Scheinin N, Tolvanen M, Karlsson L, Karlsson H. Adaption of pregnancy anxiety questionnaire–revised for all pregnant women regardless of parity: PRAQ-R2. *Arch Womens Mental Health.* (2015) 19:125–32. doi: 10.1007/s00737-015-0531-2
35. George C, Lalitha A, Antony A, Jacob K. Antenatal depression in costal South India: Prevalence and risk factors in the community. *Int J Soc Psychiatry.* (2015) 62:141–7. doi: 10.1177/0020764015607919
36. Bavle AD, Chandahalli AS, Phatak AS, Rangaiah N, Kuthandahalli SM, Nagendra PN. Antenatal depression in a tertiary care Hospital. *Indian J Psychol Med.* (2016) 38:31–5. doi: 10.4103%2F0253-7176.175101
37. Adewuya AO, Ola BA, Aloba OO, Dada AO, Fasoto OO. Prevalence and correlates of depression in late pregnancy among Nigerian women. *Depress Anxiety.* (2007) 24:15–21. doi: 10.1002/da.20221
38. Black MM, Baqu AH, Zaman K, McNary SW, Le K, El Arifeen S, et al. Depressive symptoms among rural Bangladeshi mothers: implications for infant development. *J Child Psychol Psychiatry.* (2007) 48:764–72. doi: 10.1111/j.1469-7610.2007.01752.x
39. Ayele T, Azale T, Alemu K, Abdissa Z, Mulat H, Fekadu A. Prevalence and associated factors of antenatal depression among women attending antenatal care service at gondar university hospital, northwest Ethiopia. *PLoS ONE.* (2016) 11:e0155125. doi: 10.1371/journal.pone.0155125
40. Gemta W. Prevalence and factors associated with antenatal depression among women following antenatal care at Shashemane health facilities, South Ethiopia. *Ann Glob Health.* (2015) 81:90. doi: 10.1016/j.aogh.2015.02.709
41. Lancaster CA, Gold KJ, Flynn HA, Yoo H, Marcus SM, Davis MM. Risk factors for depressive symptoms during pregnancy: a systematic review. *Am J Obstetr Gynecol.* (2010) 202:5–14. doi: 10.1016/j.ajog.2009.09.007
42. Silva MMJ, Leite EPRC, Nogueira DA, Clapis MJ. Depression in pregnancy. Prevalence and associated factors. Invest. *Educ. Enferm.* (2016) 34:342–50. doi: 10.17533/udea.iee.v34n2a14
43. Rahman A, Creed F. Outcome of prenatal depression and risk factors associated with persistence in the first postnatal year: prospective study from Rawalpindi, Pakistan. *J Affect Disord.* (2007) 100:115–21. doi: 10.1016%2Fj.jad.2006.10.004t
44. Andajani-Sutjahjo S, Manderson L, Astbury J. Complex emotions, complex problems: understanding the experiences of perinatal depression among

new mothers in urban Indonesia. *Cult Med Psychiatr.* (2007) 31:101–22. doi: 10.1007/s11013-006-9040-0

45. Martha A, Mesfin T, Tadese A, Dessalegn B. Prevalence and predictors of antenatal depressive symptoms among women attending Adama Hospital Antenatal Clinic, Adama, Ethiopia. *Int J Nurs Midwifery.* (2017) 9:58–64. doi: 10.5897/IJNM2016.0239
46. DiPietro JA, Costigan KA, Sipsma HL. Continuity in self-report measures of maternal anxiety, stress, and depressive symptoms from pregnancy through two years postpartum. *J Psychosom Obstet Gynaecol.* (2008) 29:115–24. doi: 10.1080/01674820701701546
47. Gazmararian JA, Lazorick S, Spitz AM, Ballard TJ, Saltzman LE, Marks JS. Prevalence of violence against pregnant women. *JAMA.* (1996) 275:1915–20.
48. Gazmararian JA, Petersen R, Spitz AM, Goodwin MM, Saltzman LE, Marks JS. Violence and reproductive health: current knowledge and future research directions. *Matern Child Health.* (2000) 4:79–84. doi: 10.1023/A:1009514119423
49. Westdahl C, Milan S, Magriples U, Kershaw TS, Rising SS, Ickovics JR. Social support and social conflict as predictors of prenatal depression. *Obstetr Gynecol.* (2007) 110:134–40. doi: 10.1097%2F01.AOG.0000265352.61822.1b
50. Ren J, Jiang X, Yao J, Li X, Liu X, Pang M. Depression, social support, and coping styles among pregnant women after the Lushan Earthquake in Ya'an, China. *PLoS ONE.* (2015) 10:e0135809. doi: 10.1371/journal.pone.0135809
51. Ahluwalia IB, Mack KA, Mokdad A. Mental and physical distress and high-risk behaviors among reproductive-age women. *Obstet Gynecol.* (2004) 104:477–83. doi: 10.1097/01.AOG.0000137920.58741.26
52. Grimstad H, Schei B, Backe B, Jacobsen G. Interpersonal conflict and physical abuse in relation to pregnancy and infant birth weight. *J Womens Health Gend Based Med.* (1999) 8:847–53. doi: 10.1089/152460999319165
53. Nongrum R, Thomas E, Lionel J, Jacob KS. Domestic violence as a risk factor for maternal depression and neonatal outcomes: a hospital-based cohort study. *Indian J Psychol Med.* (2014) 36:179–81. doi: 10.4103%2F0253-7176.130989
54. Bernard O, Gibson R, McCaw-Binns A, Reece J, Coore-Desai C, Shakespeare-Pellington S, et al. Antenatal depressive symptoms in Jamaica associated with limited perceived partner and other social support: a cross-sectional study. *PLoS ONE.* (2018) 13:e0194338. doi: 10.1371/journal.pone.0194338
55. Mohamad Yusuff AS, Tang L, Binns CW, Lee AH. Prevalence of antenatal depressive symptoms among women in Sabah, Malaysia. *J Matern Fetal Neonatal Med.* (2015) 29:1170–4. doi: 10.3109/14767058.2015.1039506
56. Edwards B, Galletly C, Semmler-Booth T, Dekker G. Antenatal psychosocial risk factors and depression among women living in socioeconomically disadvantaged suburbs in Adelaide, South Australia. *Aust N Z J Psychiatr.* (2008) 42:45–50. doi: 10.1080/00048670701732673t
57. Faisal-Cury A, Menezes P, Araya R, Zugaib M. Common mental disorders during pregnancy: prevalence and associated factors among low-income women in Sao Paulo, Brazil: depression and anxiety during pregnancy. *Arch Womens Ment Health.* (2009) 12:335–43. doi: 10.1007/s00737-009-0081-6
58. Shakeel N, Eberhard-Gran M, Sletner L, Slinning K, Martinsen EW, Holme I, et al. A prospective cohort study of depression in pregnancy, prevalence and risk factors in a multi-ethnic population. *BMC Pregnancy Childbirth.* (2015) 15:5. doi: 10.1186/s12884-014-0420-0t
59. Lau Y, Keung DW. Correlates of depressive symptomatology during the second trimester of pregnancy among Hong Kong Chinese. *Soc Sci Med.* (2007) 64:1802–11. doi: 10.1016/j.socscimed.2007.01.001
60. Crawford DW, Houts RM, Huston TL, George LJ. Compatibility, leisure, satisfaction in marital relationship. *J Marriage Family.* (2002) 64:433–49. doi: 10.1111/j.1741-3737.2002.00433.x
61. Rao TSS. The Genetics of affective disorder-a pedigree study. *Indian J Psychiatry.* (1993) 35:127–30.
62. Rao TSS, Prabhakar AK, Jagannatha Rao KS, Sambamurthy K, Asha MR, Ram D, et al. Relationship between consanguinity and depression in a south Indian population. *Indian J Psychiatry.* (2009) 51:50–2. doi: 10.4103%2F0019-5545.44906
63. Leigh B, Milgrom J. Risk factors for antenatal depression, postnatal depression and parenting stress. *BMC Psychiatr.* (2008) 8:24. doi: 10.1186%2F1471-244X-8-24
64. Zayas LH, Jankowski KRB, McKee MD. Prenatal and postpartum depression among low-income Dominican and Puerto Rican women. *Hisp J Behav Sci.* (2003) 25:370–85. doi: 10.1177%2F0739986303256914
65. Lukose A, Ramthal A, Thomas T, Bosch R, Kurpad AV, Duggan C, et al. Nutritional factors associated with antenatal depressive symptoms in the early stage of pregnancy among urban South Indian women. *Matern Child Health J.* (2014) 18:161–70. doi: 10.1007/s10995-013-1249-2
66. Yilmaz E, Yilmaz Z, Çakmak B, Gültekin IB, Çekmez Y, Mahmutoglu S, et al. Relationship between anemia and depressive mood in the last trimester of pregnancy. *J Matern Fetal Neonatal Med.* (2017) 30:977–82. doi: 10.1080/14767058.2016.1194389
67. Schuette SA, Kominiarek MA, Wisner KL, Massey SH. Pre-pregnancy body mass index and third-trimester depressive symptoms in a healthy privately insured sample. *AJP Rep.* (2018) 8:e13–7. doi: 10.1055/s-0038-1625974
68. Castanon N, Lasselin J, Capuron L. Neuropsychiatric comorbidity in obesity: role of inflammatory processes. *Front Endocrinol.* (2014) 5:74. doi: 10.3389/fendo.2014.00074
69. Joseph JJ, Golden SH. Cortisol dysregulation: the bidirectional link between stress, depression, and type 2 diabetes mellitus. *Ann N Y Acad Sci.* (2017) 1391:20–34. doi: 10.1111/nyas.13217
70. Broussard JL, Van Cauter E. Disturbances of sleep and circadian rhythms: novel risk factors for obesity. *Curr Opin Endocrinol Diabetes Obes.* (2016) 23:353–9. doi: 10.1097/MED.0000000000000276

Key Informants Specify Core Elements of Peer Supports for Parents with Serious Mental Illness

Joanne Nicholson and Anne Valentine*

Institute for Behavioral Health and Lurie Institute for Disability Policy, The Heller School for Social Policy and Management, Brandeis University, Waltham, MA, United States

***Correspondence:**
Joanne Nicholson
jnicholson@brandeis.edu

Background: Researchers have documented the lack of evidence-based interventions for parents with serious mental illness (SMI). Given the prevalence of parenthood among individuals with SMI, the value placed on parenthood, and their diverse vulnerabilities, a robust, theoretically sound and empirically tested model of peer supports would likely provide a valuable complement to psychiatric services. In this paper, we lay the groundwork for a model of peer supports using a program theory development process and guided by stages of evidence-informed innovation outlined by the National Implementation Research Network.

Methods: This study employed a developmental design in the initial stage of a larger study of the development, implementation, and testing of peer supports to address three questions: (1) What needs of parents with SMI are particularly well-suited to peer supports? (2) What do peers have to offer parents? and (3) What is unique about peer supports for parents? A purposeful sampling strategy was used to recruit key informants ($n = 22$) familiar with peer supports, family-focused care and the experiences of families living with parental mental illness. Individual interviews were conducted face-to-face or on the telephone and a full-day group interview was conducted using a workshop format. Interview data were analyzed qualitatively to identify themes reflecting potential core program elements.

Results: Consistent themes drawn from data comprise four core program elements: engage, explore, plan, and access and advocate. These core activities are likely founded on practice principles that include a focus on families and their strengths, cultural sensitivity, and acknowledgment of the trauma experienced by many parents. The findings raised a number of challenges in contemplating peer supports for parents with SMI, including the need for ongoing support for peers.

Discussion: In developing this model, aspects of organizational context must be considered along with specification of the characteristics of parents with SMI suited to this approach and the attributes of peers providing support. A fully-articulated model must include parallel theories of change for the workforce, as well as for participating parents, to support well-being in the context of peer relationships and the success of parents with SMI in family life.

Keywords: parents with serious mental illness, peer supports, family-focused care, psychiatric services, program theory, evidence-based practice

INTRODUCTION

Numerous researchers have documented the lack of targeted evidence-based interventions for parents with serious mental illnesses (e.g., schizophrenia, bipolar disorder, major depressive disorder) (1, 2). Effective psychiatric treatment is recommended, of course, dependent on a person's history, diagnosis, preferences and response. However, inattention to issues of importance to individuals with serious mental illnesses (SMI) who are parents, and the probable impact of unaddressed issues on a person's participation and progress in treatment, suggest the potential benefit of attending to a parent's circumstances and priorities, particularly if they are contributing to stress. Given the prevalence of parenthood among individuals with SMI (3, 4); the value placed on parenthood by these individuals (5, 6); and their diverse vulnerabilities (e.g., limited resources and supports) (7), a robust, theoretically sound, empirically tested model of peer supports for parents with SMI would likely provide a valuable complement to traditional psychiatric treatments. In this paper, we lay the groundwork for a model of peer supports for parents using a program theory development process (8) and guided by stages of evidence-informed innovation outlined by the National Implementation Research Network (NIRN) (9).

Peer-delivered service models have increased markedly over the past two decades and are now an integral component of the behavioral health care system in the USA (10, 11). Peer support is based on the idea that individuals with lived experience of mental health and/or substance use disorders who have made progress in recovery may be uniquely positioned to offer support, validation, and hope to others (12, 13). Within the field, peer support specialists are persons who identify as having mental health conditions who receive formal, skills-based training to deliver services in the behavioral health care system (14). Peer support specialists occupy a variety of roles in behavioral health care that vary by setting, credentialing requirements, and service model (6, 15). In the USA, states are authorized to bill Medicaid, the public insurer, for peer support services to assist individuals in recovery from mental illness and substance use disorders.

A growing body of literature supports the benefits of peer-delivered services in behavioral health care (16). Much of this literature suggests positive outcomes as demonstrated by increasing consumer engagement and retention in care, linking individuals to community-based support services, fostering hope, addressing social isolation, increasing activation and self-care, and reducing inpatient utilization of services (11, 13, 16–21). However, recent meta-analyses of peer-delivered services, particularly for individuals with SMI, provide a more tentative assessment of the empirical evidence and raise questions about the methodological rigor of published studies (18, 22, 23). Adequate categorization and clarity surrounding the role, objectives and performance of peers is often lacking (24–26). Theory-based program models of peer support with well-defined change mechanisms are needed (22, 25, 27), as is increased attention to implementation processes and barriers that might affect participation and anticipated outcomes (22, 25).

The task of specifying the core program elements and underlying processes of a model of peer supports for parents with SMI, along with clear specification of the role of parent peer specialists, is informed by review of the literature regarding peer supports in mental health in general (13, 20, 28, 29). Authors describe and link peer support processes to conceptual underpinnings. Chief among these, by definition, is the importance of lived experience with mental illness and within the system of services (13, 20, 29). The peer specialist's use of positive self-disclosure and the perception of commonalities shared with and by the patient or client contribute to relationship engagement and foster hope for change (13, 20, 29). The peer relationship is enhanced by the emotional engagement that develops in this work through trust, acceptance, understanding and empathy (13, 20, 29). Peer specialists have the ability to role model progress in recovery and coping. They may be more likely than clinical practitioners to take a strengths-based approach, rather than focusing on psychopathology, and facilitate access to social and practical support, both informal and formal (13, 20). The peer specialist role has been described as having benefit to the peer specialist as well as to the patient or client, via the assumption of the helper role (13, 29).

However, the possible emotional closeness between peer specialist and patient or client, in combination with the fact that the peer specialist role definition often lies somewhere between that of traditional mental health clinician and patient or client, may contribute to difficulties (29). The peer specialist may be vulnerable to over involvement, unsustainable boundaries and burnout (29), suggesting the need for ongoing training and support. The organizational or agency context (e.g., hospital in-patient setting, community mental health agency or health center) in which peer support is offered must be considered as well (29). Authors recommend that the process of creating peer positions should include the active involvement of non-peer staff, organizational leaders and people in recovery, especially those who may serve as champions in the effort (20).

This paper reports on the initial, preparatory and foundational stage of a multi-stage study to develop, implement and assess the effectiveness of peer supports for parents with SMI. It reports on work done together with diverse stakeholders in laying the groundwork for model development of peer supports targeting parents with SMI. The initial tasks include developing program theory linked with core elements and processes, and identifying essential qualities and characteristics of parent peer specialists. Research questions include: (1) What needs of parents with SMI are particularly well-suited to peer supports? (2) What do peers have to offer parents? and (3) What is unique about peer supports for parents (i.e., what distinguishes them from peer supports in general)? Findings from this initial exploration will inform the next stages of the project: first, further elaboration of the peer supports model for parents with SMI and, second, the installation, implementation and testing of the resultant innovative, empirically informed model.

METHODS

Design

The study reported here employed a developmental design as the initial stage of the larger study of the development, installation, implementation and testing of parent peer supports. A developmental design has the purpose of helping develop an innovation, intervention or program (30). Feedback loops inform ongoing program, staff and organizational development. This approach is particularly relevant in situations in which programs or models are being adapted to new conditions, contexts or target populations (30), that is, the exploration and installation stages outlined in the NIRN framework for the implementation of evidence-based programs and other innovation (9). The larger study methods combine three iterative approaches to program theory building (8): (a) a review of the academic and gray literature (deductive approach); (b) interviews with key informants (articulating stakeholder mental models); and (c) Implementation Team meetings as the potential program model is considered for installation at the community-based agency (inductive approach). In this paper, we report findings from interviews with key informants. The extensive literature review, reported above only briefly, focused on the experiences and needs of parents with SMI and the development, implementation and testing of peer supports in general. Implementation Team meetings are underway as we prepare to install peer supports for parents with SMI in the community agency context.

Key Informant Interviews: Articulating Stakeholder Mental Models

Mental models for programs reflect the ways in which stakeholders describe what a program would look like, how it would work, and how success would be determined, particularly as stakeholders consider the characteristics, needs and experiences of the target population (8). The selection of key informants is informed by the notion that engaging stakeholders provides access to expertise, facilitates the development of a shared understanding of the potential program and promotes empowerment, communication and uptake of the final result (8). Diverse perspectives are included to develop a more comprehensive program theory.

Sample Recruitment

A purposeful sampling strategy was used to recruit initial key informants familiar with peer supports, family-focused care and the specific needs and challenges of families living with parental mental illnesses. A preliminary list of potential study participants was constructed by the investigators, chosen to reflect diverse, relevant perspectives including state agency policymakers and funders, provider agency managers and staff, experienced peer specialists, parents with SMI, program developers and researchers. Additional informants were added to the sample as they were identified by study participants. Potential participants were sent a recruitment email informing them of the study and inviting their participation in an interview to discuss peer supports for parents with SMI, including relevant factors to consider in developing the proposed model and ideas about how to implement, sustain and assess the effectiveness of the model. All invitees agreed to participate ($n = 22$). The investigators were included as participants given the co-production nature of the project and their partnership role in facilitating key informant engagement and contributing to the design of the ultimate parent peer supports model (8, 30).

Interview Procedures

Interviews were conducted by one of the investigators, experienced clinical researchers, either face-to-face or on the telephone, at the convenience of the participants, between March 2016 and July 2017. A study overview including the interview items was emailed to participants prior to the scheduled session. The individual interviews lasted 1–2 h. One full-day group interview was conducted using a workshop format with expert stakeholders to draw out rich perspectives on key elements of program theory in an iterative, face-to-face manner (8). At the beginning of each session, informed consent was obtained and participants completed a brief background survey (e.g., age, gender, race/ethnicity, education, training/discipline, organizational affiliation, and years in their current role). For those individuals interviewed by telephone, informed consent forms were emailed in advance, signed and returned by the participant. Study procedures were reviewed and approved by the state agency research review committee and the institutional review boards of the investigators' universities.

The investigators employed a semi-structured interview protocol informed by a series of open-ended questions as suggested in the NIRN Exploration Stage of innovation development (9). The questions were used to orient conversation. By way of introducing the topic of peer supports for parents, the interview began by asking participants for their perspectives on the needs of parents with SMI. Follow-up questions elicited information on current programs and practices, potential resources for the proposed parent peer supports, anticipated implementation and sustainability challenges, and additional stakeholders to contact. The interview concluded with an open-ended question asking whether the participant had anything else to add. The investigators began reviewing data as they became available, so that earlier interviews informed later interviews as knowledge was obtained. Verbatim notes were taken during all interviews, reviewed and transcribed by the study investigators using standard word processing software, and de-identified to maintain the participants' privacy. In addition, for the workshop session, extensive notes were made on easel sheets along with verbatim notes to facilitate group discussion. These were transcribed as well.

Analysis

A framework approach to the interviews was employed, given that a starting set of issues to investigate was identified prior to data collection. These included recommended considerations in the NIRN exploration stage of innovation related to implementation context, such as the identification of essential resources, potential barriers, and lessons learned from prior initiatives (9). Open-ended interview questions were developed to provide for unstructured responses to these implementation topics as well as to allow for rich responses from study participants regarding the specific needs and experiences of parents with SMI (31, 32). While the overall framework of the interviews as focusing on developing and implementing peer supports was identified in advance, themes related to essential elements and considerations for the development and implementation of peer supports for parents with SMI emerged from the data, in a grounded theory type of approach, as thematic coding progressed (33). The investigators worked independently initially, recording notes of themes that emerged from the data, as well as informed by the research objectives. They reviewed and updated themes based on the frequency of themes within a response and the emphasis granted certain themes by participants. Together, investigators revisited and updated themes and came to consensus regarding the codes and the language used to define them. Coding was facilitated through the use of Dedoose software (34). The investigators generated memos regarding impressions and emerging themes and relationships, and reviewed findings as they supported, diverged from or augmented prior knowledge.

Trustworthiness of the qualitative analysis process and findings was established in multiple ways (35). Transcripts were reviewed and coded independently, impressions compared, and differences reconciled to achieve complete agreement in all cases. Trustworthiness was further established through member checking (33). Preliminary findings were reviewed by independent stakeholders on the study's Implementation Team and actively working in the field.

RESULTS

Participants

Massachusetts, the seventh smallest state in the US, is located in the Northeast region of the country. The state population is estimated at 6.93 million. The state's capital, Boston, is the most populous city; more than 80% of Massachusetts residents live within the greater Boston metropolitan area. Prevalence estimates suggest that more than a half a million adults in Massachusetts experience SMI; unmet need for care is high. While Massachusetts is lauded as among the best states in the nation regarding access to behavioral health care, many individuals with SMI and substance use disorders struggle to find services.

Twenty-two informants participated in the study. The majority of informants were female (77%), over 45 years of age (77%), and Caucasian (86%), reflecting the characteristics of the Massachusetts human services workforce. Most had a four-year university degree or more in education (81%). The education of the remaining participants ranged from some high school to some college, with two completing a high-school equivalency diploma or trade school. Just over one-third of the participants (36%) were in their current positions for a dozen years or more; two were unemployed outside the home. Just over half (59%) described themselves as being in practitioner roles (e.g., social work, rehabilitation counseling, clinical psychology); 23% were in policy and program administration positions; and 18% were in other roles (e.g., mental health advocate; parent at home). Informants represented community mental health and state human service agencies, and included community leaders from varied practice settings and academic researchers, as well as advocates and parents with SMI. Their familiarity with peer supports and as service providers and recipients was extensive. Their experiences varied from working as peer support specialists and educators, to directing and supervising peer and recovery services to receiving peer services as patients or clients. Several informants were funders and administrators of peer services. A significant number identified as individuals with lived experience of mental illness or as having family members with lived experience. All were parents. The notion of peer support work in the US implies that those who direct or supervise these programs are often peers themselves, with lived experience of mental illness and as service recipients. It would be incorrect to assume that only those parents unemployed outside the home had ever received services. Participants were asked to designate their primary role as they identified it at the time of the study, but were encouraged to draw from their range of experiences.

Research Question #1: What Needs of Parents With SMI Are Well-Suited to Peer Supports?

The gaps in supports and resources for parents with SMI were frequently noted by key informant participants. In addition, parents with SMI may have questions or concerns that are specific to their situations or circumstances. Needs that are common among all parents may be exacerbated in situations in which parents live with mental illnesses.

Gaps in Supports and Resources

Many participants touched on the lack of personal or professional support that parents with SMI experience, the pronounced sense of not knowing with whom to talk, and the implications of this isolation. As one key informant noted, "Often parents say they have no one who they rely on." Participants observed that because so many parents with SMI do not have a "non-threatening person with whom they can confide" they may compartmentalize their needs and fear disclosure about salient information including the "use of psychiatric medication" and "childcare challenges." Participants suggested that among parents with SMI, fear of the child welfare system and child protective services is a significant source of stress that may exacerbate parental isolation. Such parents might avoid seeking services lest disclosure of their psychiatric diagnoses or challenges in childrearing result in their children being taken from them. As one participant suggested, "the child welfare system exists to protect children, but there has to be a way for parents who are struggling to reach out—without the fear of having their children removed [from their care]." Participants also pointed out that parental isolation and the lack of support give rise to doubts and fears about a common concern of parents with serious mental illness, that is, if and when to disclose their illness to their children and others.

Concerns Specific to Parents With SMI

Peers, given their own experiences, may be best suited to discussing a number of issues that specifically relate to family life and serious mental illness. Participants strongly endorsed the use of peer supports for parents who may be "contemplating having another child" as peers may have experience with balancing the demands of parenting multiple children and managing serious mental illness. Peers may have insight into complex or stressful family relationships, for example, and suggestions for parents who have complicated relationships with their own parents, yet must "rely on [them] for child support."

Many participants noted the crucial support that a peer may provide in helping parents reframe their experiences, to "deconstruct stigma" as they make negative assumptions about the relationship between their own illness and their children's behavior, and to "normalize the day-to-day challenges of parenting" that exist independent of a psychiatric diagnosis. Parents may blame themselves and their illnesses as contributing to behavior in children that actually may be developmentally appropriate (e.g., temper tantrums in toddlers). According to one informant, "It's common to ascribe any difficulties in parenting to depression, but there are normal experiences and challenges of parenting that exist apart from major depression." Further, parents with serious mental illness may need extra support in "the pragmatic steps necessary to get through the day," for example, figuring out "how to get their kids to the bus on time in morning" or "how to get them enrolled in a good afterschool program." In helping parents with serious mental illness navigate these day-to-day challenges, peers may suggest alternative strategies that help to change parents' perspectives from that of feeling overwhelmed by demands and "failing" to one of coping and succeeding in managing everyday family life.

Parents may benefit from peer supports for situations unique to them. As participants pointed out, parents who do not have custody of their children may have supervised visitation as required by child protective services or may hope for reunification with their children. Peers may have experience with child welfare and advice for navigating the system successfully. They may be preferred, willing and able to supervise parents' visits with their children. A key informant described, "This is complicated, but it's worth taking on. How can a parent interact with a child, particularly if they have limited contact?" Another informant suggested, "Parents may need support for grieving the loss of parenthood—for those who opt not to have children" and for those who have lost custody or contact. Parents with SMI may need help repairing and renewing bonds with children. For older parents, peers may be helpful in assisting them to reconnect with their adult children.

Generic Parenting Issues Magnified

Participants also remarked on the needs of parents with SMI that are generic to all parents. Concerns about housing, healthcare, and education were frequently cited. However, many suggested that even the very basic needs of vulnerable individuals take on a different quality and urgency for parents with SMI who are primary caretakers of minor children. As one informant noted, "Do I have enough money to pay my electric bill this month?" may mean something very different for individuals who are parents than for those individuals responsible only for themselves. For parents with SMI caring for children, failing to provide for the essentials of daily living may exacerbate their doubts about their parenting abilities, mentioned above, and draw the attention and concern of others.

Research Question #2: What Do Peers Have to Offer Parents?

Peers may be sensitive to the importance of empowerment and the contribution of successful planning and problem-solving to feelings of self-efficacy and recovery. They may be well-suited to helping parents access and advocate for supports and resources for themselves and their families.

Plan

Peers can draw from their own experiences to help parents solve problems, envision change and make concrete plans to achieve their goals. "Peers workers facilitate peer-driven goal planning." Because of their unique perspective as peers, they may be better able to partner with the parent to "go to a school meeting; go to a doctor's appointment; go to get a prom dress…help plan a [parent-child] visit, plan birthday parties; talk about court and steps to get children back." They may have tested strategies, not only for managing day-to-day life but, specifically, household, money and time management. According to an informant, the peer can focus on "whatever it takes for families to be successful." Peers may see "that there is more than one way forward" and appreciate that recovery is not a straightforward path; there will likely be set-backs and relapses along the way. Peers may be more inclined than non-peers to recognize that "It's about helping the client with self-determination, autonomy and self-advocacy" and that by succeeding in planning and problem-solving, parents begin to see and believe that change is possible and that they are capable of making it happen.

Access and Advocate

One informant indicated, "The role of peer support is to provide information and support as needed." Parents may not know how to access resources, that is, "how to get adequate support" from friends or family or how to "navigate communication" across a network of professional providers. Peer specialists who are parents may be better acquainted with community resources useful to other parents and especially to those living with mental illness. Peer specialists may facilitate "referral to grassroots, community-based programs; in-home recovery services; and community-based supports" and may also be helpful in "talking with family members at the request of the client [parent]" to help the parent build natural supports. Advocacy is a key element of the process of accessing and building supports and resources. An informant pointed out, "A significant element of advocacy is integrated into the peer-based model of care. The [parent peer specialist] must understand this context, and the role of advocacy and networking with other providers serving families."

Research Question #3: What Is Unique About Peer Supports for Parents?

Informants suggested that peers could offer a unique and specialized approach to supporting parents with SMI in terms of their posture or approach to engaging with parents as well as the specific skills and expertise they employ to explore parents' strengths, resources and supports, and elicit motivation to make desired changes. Specific challenges were suggested that reflect both the benefits as well as the vulnerabilities inherent in the peer-parent relationship.

Engage

Participants indicated that peers may readily be able to engage with parents with SMI with greater authenticity than can traditional mental health clinicians. As one pointed out, peers create "relationships that feel normal, not clinical." They can "get real with parents in a way traditional mental health workers can't." The assumption is that peer relationships are based on the concept of mutuality, which "tends to make people more open." Mutuality is sparked by the perception of similarities and sharing of lived experiences. Peer specialists are trained in the use of self-disclosure to enhance relationship-building. A parent who has lost contact with children, for example, may feel better supported by someone who can talk openly about feelings attached to similar experiences and provide examples of ways in which they coped. Informants recommended a life span approach to parenting, that is, providing peer supports to parents at all stages of family life.

Participants suggested the importance of cultural sensitivity. In addition to cultural variations in the framing of mental illness and treatment, for example, the ways in which parents talk about mental illness with their children or their approach to child behavior management may differ from culture to culture. The notions of authenticity, mutuality and cultural sensitivity led to discussion of the match and fit between parents and peers. Participants emphasized the importance of choice. As one informant who is a parent with SMI pointed out, "some pairs fit better than others....Either side should be able to decline the match or ask for a re-match.... [You] need to consider the parent's needs and the peer specialist's needs in making the match." According to another informant, "Not everyone wants peer support. For some, it's not the right time." The question of whether peer supports for parents must be provided by persons who are parents emerged and, if so, what aspects of parenting should be considered as criteria for the match (e.g., age of children, custodial or non-custodial status, etc.). And in weighing the criteria for fit, the felt connection between peer and parent may matter more than particular aspects of lived experience.

The notion of choice was echoed by participants who emphasized the importance of peers taking a non-judgmental approach, given that parents with SMI so often feel judged. The value of a non-judgmental approach plays out in working together with parents to explore their families' strengths and vulnerabilities, plan for themselves and their children, and deal with the consequences of their actions. According to one informant, "People have to be given choices, including potentially risky or harmful choices," suggesting that parents may make choices that peers consider ill-advised. Another suggested, "Peer workers endorse the dignity of risk." Parents with SMI are often viewed negatively, with little regard paid to their efforts or capacity to care for their children. A peer specialist may take a more "normalizing" approach focusing less on "clinical appraisal" to make "more room for exploration of feelings that are stigmatized in clinical settings." Allowing thoughts and feelings to be expressed without fear of censure may reduce the level of blame or shame parents feel about their choices.

Explore

Peers may be especially helpful in assisting parents to identify strengths and reframe their capacity to make change in their lives. In the words of an informant, "You may be combatting a family's story or narrative. Parent peer specialists may be able to support the client around this better than others...can change the story and uplift the children." By helping parents to "figure out the life they want to live...in contrast to the treatment world, which she describes as 'so clinical,'" the parent peer specialist instills hope for change. A parent informant described a particular peer specialist as bringing "creativity, fun and positivity to her work" that allowed the parent to explore and envision a more positive future. This helps parents "to become unstuck," to participate in planning and to muster the energy and resources to achieve goals.

Peers may provide examples of success to parents with SMI, according to key informants. Peer specialists are often selected into their positions by virtue of the progress they have made in their own treatment and recovery. Parent peer specialists may offer examples and role model successful efforts to cope with the demands of parenting and illness management or negotiate more positive relationships with children and family members. They may draw from their own life experiences, not only to build relationships through perceived mutuality, but to provide examples of ways in which they themselves have coped or made changes that might work for the parent.

Lived Experience of Family Life May Convey Challenges

Peer specialist training may involve exposure to practice skills and approaches that are generally relevant to parents with SMI (e.g., shared decision-making, problem-solving, skills-building). The work of peers is further informed by their own family values and lived experience of family life, as well as their experiences with mental illnesses. Consequently, in drawing from and disclosing their family experiences, peers may become vulnerable in ways that differ from or are experienced more keenly than when providing more generic supports. Peer specialists may understand that "boundaries between peer and client are more permeable [than those between a traditional clinician and client]" and "boundaries and use of self-disclosure are [therefore] emphasized in...training." The focus on family life in working with parents has the positive potential to provide rich opportunities for sharing, but carries the risk of reminding the peer of family experiences or memories, possibly traumatic, that were painful or unpleasant. Adding family experiences to the shared lived experience of mental illness and recovery not only multiplies the opportunities for mutuality, but increases the pool of potentially painful or unresolved issues for the peer as well as for the parent.

The peer specialist may also be inclined to extend themselves for parents in ways they might not for patients or clients who are not parents, particularly because the well-being of children may be involved. As one informant pointed out, "Peers, for example, shouldn't be driving people to appointments, unless it's in the service of their work...talking to the client, introducing them to a support group." And, "Peers are not taxi drivers or junior counselors." Another informant suggested, "Peers cannot be held responsible for client behaviors, nor should they be asked to do favors for clients, including holding money or assisting with medications." These issues could become particularly salient and potentially confusing to the parent peer specialist when children are involved in the home, for example, when a parent is unable to drive a child to a doctor's appointment or has no food in the kitchen. However, as another informant concluded, "Sometimes people need to be taken care of; that's what staff do. Sometimes people need someone to be with them; that's what peers do."

DISCUSSION

Parents With SMI May be Helped by Peer Supports

Diverse informants, including parents themselves, agree that parents with SMI are often isolated, dealing with gaps in available supports and resources. They may be challenged by situations or circumstances related to parenting while managing mental illness, including very practical, day-to-day challenges of raising children, relationships with children across the life span, and issues other parents face but that are exacerbated by the challenges of navigating treatment and recovery. Peers offer special knowledge, drawn from personal feelings and their own experiences, that may serve as a resource to parents. What is unique about peer supports for parents is the potential for relationship building and the capacity for open discussion based on the sharing of the lived experience of managing mental illness, family relationships and parenthood, and the authenticity and mutuality all this inspires. Parent peer specialists potentially offer examples of success, serve as role models, reframe deficits and set-backs, normalize parenting experiences, and disclose information about themselves with purpose and intent. The lived experience that peers share also may include expertise in navigating the health care and social service systems as a parent with SMI. For example, they may be aware of community resources or problem-solving strategies that have worked for them.

Potential Challenges

The findings raise a number of challenges in contemplating peer supports for parents with SMI. Some are broadly relevant to peer support and others are particular to the role of parent peers (e.g., boundaries within the parent-peer relationship, the judicial use of self-disclosure, the potential for raising the peer specialist's own concern for painful family issues, and the peer's values associated with families, parenting and children). To some extent, these challenges exist across the range of peer supports (i.e., substance abuse recovery coaches, peer supports in elder care), but because young children may be involved—either living in the home or not—a more cautious approach may be warranted.

Working with parents, especially parents of young children, underscores the need for explicit, ongoing training and perhaps a willingness to re-examine norms or standards of practice, particularly given the assumptions, values and range of feelings that often surround parenting and family life. For example, the idea of a peer's role in honoring parent choice was noted by several informants, the underlying notion being that peer specialists are there to honor and support the autonomy of their peers. In reality, this aspect of peer support is not terribly distinct from the approach of traditional mental health clinicians, in the sense that clinicians may not weigh-in directly and/or advise patients or clients specifically about everyday decision-making. However, honoring patient or client choice is essential to peer support, in part, because in supporting autonomy, peers support clients' wellness, as opposed to their illness, and their potential for growth and recovery (21). This may be the mechanism behind a peer's authentic use of self. It is certainly one of the most salient and important aspects of peer support. For parents whose lives may be heavily intertwined with people telling them what to do (e.g., partners, extended family members, child protective service workers), the dignity of choice, of having a support person who does not mandate or require a particular response seems nothing short of essential.

However, there may be instances when the question is not really about the autonomy or wellness of the parent but, rather, the implications of the parent's behavior or actions for a young child. This may present new challenges for peer support specialists; indeed, supporting a parent's autonomy to make less than ideal decisions may convey far-reaching implications. With respect to peer supports for parents, this suggests two related ideas. First, peer specialists working with parents in the home may experience more moments of dissonance or distress than they might otherwise in working with adults with no children or in settings outside the home. The peer specialist working in the home may have greater exposure to the consequences of a parent's decision-making (e.g., an empty refrigerator). Peer support specialists may benefit from targeted training, coaching and support from supervisors and peers, and from knowledge about specific supports and resources for the parents and families with whom they work, to deal with this increased exposure. The very opportunity for enhanced relationship-building conveyed by shared lived experience also may result in peers being aware of issues about which more traditional office-based clinicians have no knowledge.

Second, peer supports may not be right for everyone—the parent or the peer. Even well-trained peer specialists may not feel comfortable "intruding" in the parent's family life. Peer support specialists may be asked to interact with family members, school personnel and other professionals. This may be distinct from work undertaken by other peer support specialists. It may not be lived experienced of parenting, *per se*, that makes the work successful but, rather, the ability to tolerate ambivalence and utilize personal disclosure in a way the fosters a sense of possibility, regardless of family circumstance. This suggests that peers who work with parents may not necessarily have to be parents themselves. Similar issues have been raised in discussions of "peerness," the fit and match of peer specialists and patients or clients (28, 36). Even individuals who are not parents themselves have lived experience of being parented and family life.

Study Limitations

This was an exploratory study with a developmental design. While the number of participants was relatively small, they drew from considerable breadth and depth of experience—as professionals and as parents. The needs and experiences of parents with SMI identified by informants were consistent with those identified in previous research and in other countries. In subsequent stages of the study we propose to specify fully, implement and test a model of peer supports for parents with SMI that will be in many ways determined by the context in which it sits. Peer support models have developed in the USA to fit not only the regional or local service system context and need, but to fit the fiscal structure of the American health care system and reimbursement for services. Therefore, the study findings generally reflect parent/family and system characteristics and conditions known to Massachusetts, though the participants included a number of national experts from other locations. While a peer support model for parents with SMI may well have international application, given the similarities in the needs and experiences of parents across countries, aspects of the implementation context must be considered if the model is to be adapted and replicated in other sites.

CONCLUSIONS AND IMPLICATIONS FOR FUTURE PRACTICE AND RESEARCH

Moving forward to inform a model of peer supports for parents, consistent themes drawn from data obtained to address the original research questions can be grouped into four core program elements: engage, explore, plan, and access and advocate. These core elements or categories of activity are likely founded on practice principles that include a focus on families and their strengths, cultural sensitivity, and acknowledgment of the trauma experienced by many parents living with mental illness, at home (e.g., when they lose custody of children) and in the system of services (e.g., if they are approached by others through the lens of negative attitudes and expectations). Further translation of core elements and practice principles into peer support activities, and the implementation and testing of the peer supports model for parents with SMI remain the focus of next steps in the multi-stage study. We anticipate that parent peer specialists will require additional training and coaching to supplement content covered in the state's mandatory training of peer support workers. The training and coaching materials will be targeted and relevant to the population of parents served. The content of these materials will be determined in consultation with key informants and other engaged stakeholders.

As noted in the introduction, a number of questions have emerged about the efficacy and impact of peer supports in behavioral health services. However, in thinking about peer supports for parents, the question isn't about whether peer support makes a difference, but under what circumstances and with whom (21). This question needs to be asked not only of the potential parent patient or client, but of the potential peer support specialist as well. Not everyone has an affinity for this work. This is a simple statement, yet one that needs to be explicitly addressed. Clearly, those who choose to provide peer supports to parents must be supported themselves (24), if their goals and the goals of the parents with whom they work are to be met.

Aspects of the organizational context must be considered along with specification of the characteristics of parents suited to this approach and the attributes of peer specialists providing support. The job description of peers working with parents with SMI must be well-specified, with adequate training, coaching and supports spelled-out and provided, to ensure that peer specialists are activating core program elements and processes, without putting their own well-being at risk. The role of peer specialists vis a vis the roles of others in the service provision setting must be clearly articulated, with organizational players prepared for and supported to promote productive collaboration and respect for the contributions of each. It is fair to assume that, amongst clinicians, there are individuals with experiences of mental illness and family life, though they may not disclose nor explicitly draw from their lived experience as do peer specialists. All staff members may require organizational leadership and support in taking a family-focused approach. A fully-articulated model of peer supports for parents with SMI, therefore, must include parallel theories of change for the workforce as well as for participating parents, to support well-being in the context of peer relationships and the success of parents in family life.

ETHICS STATEMENT

This study was carried out in accordance with the recommendations of the Dartmouth College Committee for the Protection of Human Subjects (CPHS#00030199) and the Massachusetts Department of Mental Health Institutional Review Board (Protocol#2017-04) and approved by these committees. Written informed consent was obtained from all participants.

AUTHOR CONTRIBUTIONS

JN: designed the study; JN and AV: collected the data, performed analyses, interpreted results, prepared sections of the manuscript, and contributed to manuscript revision, read, and approved the submitted version.

FUNDING

This work is funded by the National Institute on Disability, Independent Living, and Rehabilitation Research (grant #90DPGE0001-01-01) and the Massachusetts Department of Mental Health. This statements presented in this publication are solely the responsibility of the authors and do not necessarily represent the views of the funders.

ACKNOWLEDGMENTS

The authors would like to acknowledge the contributions of the Parent Peer Support Project Implementation Team, Robert Walker, Kathleen Biebel, Kelly English, and Cornelia Kammerer in reviewing findings and drafts of the manuscript.

REFERENCES

1. Nicholson J, Friesen BJ. Developing the evidence base for families living with parental psychiatric disabilities: crossing the bridge while we're building It. *Psychiatr Rehabil J.* (2014) 37:157–61. doi: 10.1037/prj0000092
2. Reupert A, Price-Robertson R, Maybery D. Parenting as a focus of recovery: a systematic review of current practice. *Psychiatric Rehabil J.* (2017) 40:361–70. doi: 10.1037/prj0000240
3. Maybery D, Nicholson J, Reupert A. Parental mental illness: estimating prevalence to inform policy and practice. In Reupert A, Maybery D, Nicholson J, Gopfert M, Seeman MV, editors. *Parental Psychiatric Disorder: Distressed Parents and their Families 3rd edn.* (2015) Cambridge: Cambridge University Press, p. 20–28.
4. Nicholson J, Biebel K, Williams V, Katz-Leavy J. Prevalence of parenthood in adults with mental illness: Implications for state and federal policy, programs, and providers. In Manderscheid RW, Henderson MJ, ediotrs. *Mental Health, United States, 2002, DHHS Pub No. (SMA) 3938* Rockville, MD: Substance Abuse and Mental Health Services Administration, Center for Mental Health Services, (2004). p. 120–137.
5. Reupert A, Maybery D, Nicholson J, Gopfert M, Seeman MV. *Parental Psychiatric Disorder: Distressed Parents and Their Families 3rd edn.* Cambridge, U.K.: Cambridge University Press (2015).
6. Weston SM, Martin ED, Shippen ME, Kraska MF, Curtis RS. Parents with serious mental illness served by peer support specialists. *Int J Psychosoc Rehabil.* (2017) 21:79–89.
7. Luciano AP, Nicholson J, Meara ER. The economic status of parents with serious mental illness in the U.S. *Psychiatric Rehabil J.* (2014) 37:242–50. doi: 10.1037/prj0000087
8. Funnell SC, Rogers PJ. *Purposeful Program Theory.* San Francisco, CA: John Wiley & Sons, Inc (2011).
9. Blasé K, van Dyke M, Fixsen D. *Stages of Implementation Analysis: Where Are We?* Chapel Hill, NC: National Implementation Research Network (NIRN) (2013).
10. Myrick K, Vecchio P. Peer support services in the behavioral healthcare workforce: state of the field. *Psychiatric Rehabil J.* (2016) 39:197–203. doi: 10.1037/prj0000188
11. Rogers ES, Swarbrick M. Peer-delivered services: current trends and innovations. *Psychiatric Rehabil J.* (2016) 39:193–6. doi: 10.1037/prj0000223
12. Mead S, Hilton D, Curtis L. Peer support: a theoretical perspective. *Psychiatric Rehabil J.* (2001) 25:134–41. doi: 10.1037/h0095032
13. Solomon P. Peer support/peer provided services underlying processes, benefits, and critical ingredients. *Psychiatric Rehabil J.* (2004) 27:392–401. doi: 10.2975/27.2004.392.401
14. USDHHS. *Core Competencies for Peer Workers in Behavioral Health Services.* Rockville, MD: USDHHS SAMHSA (2015).
15. Swarbrick M, Schmidt L, Gill K. *People in Recovery as Providers of Psychiatric Rehabilitation Servivces: Building on the Wisdom of Experience.* McLean, VA: U. S. Psychiatric Rehabilitation Association (2010).
16. Rogers ES, Farkas M, Anthony W, Kash M, Maru M, Brucker D. *Systematic Review of Peer Delivered Services Literature 1989-2009* Boston, MA: Center for Psychiatric Rehabilitation, Boston University (2009).
17. Bologna MJ, Pulice RT. Evaluation of a peer-run hospital diversion program: a descriptive study. *Am J Psychiatric Rehabil.* (2011) 14:272–86. doi: 10.1080/15487768.2011.622147
18. Chinman M, George P, Dougherty RH, Daniels AS, Ghose SS, Swift A, et al. Peer support services for individuals with serious mental illnesses: assessing the evidence. *Psychiatric Services.* (2014) 65:429–41. doi: 10.1176/appi.ps.201300244
19. Cook JA, Copeland MA, Corey L, Buffington E, Jonikas JA, Curtis LC, et al. Developing the evidence base for peer-led services: Changes among participants following Wellness Recovery Action Planning (WRAP) education in two statewide initiatives. *Psychiatric Rehabil J.* (2010) 34:113–20. doi: 10. 2975/34.2.2010.113.120
20. Davidson L, Bellamy C, Guy K, Miller R. Peer support among persons with severe mental illnesses: a review of evidence and experience. *World Psychiatry.* (2012) 11:123–8. doi: 10.1016/j.wpsyc.2012.05.009
21. Repper J, Carter T. A review of the literature on peer support in mental health services. *J Mental Health.* (2011) 20:392–411. doi: 10.3109/09638237.2011.583947
22. Lloyd-Evans B, Mayo-Wilson E, Harrison B, Istead H, Brown E, Pilling S, et al. A systematic review and meta-analysis of randomised controlled trials of peer support for people with severe mental illness. *BMC Psychiatry.* (2014) 14:1–12. doi: 10.1186/1471-244X-14-39
23. Pitt V, Lowe D, Hill S, Prictor M, Hetrick SE, Ryan R, et al. Consumer-providers of care for adult clients of statutory mental health services. *Cochr Data Base System Rev.* (2004) 2:CD004807. doi: 10.1002/14651858. CD004807
24. Cronise R. Collaborative learning: a next step in the training of peer support providers. *Psychiatric Rehabil J.* (2016) 39:292–4. doi: 10.1037/prj 0000218
25. Davidson L. Peer support: coming of age and/or miles to go before we sleep? An introduction. *J Behav Health Services Res.* (2015) 42:96–9. doi: 10.1007/s11414-013-9379-2
26. Jacobson N, Trojanowsk L, Dewa CS. What do peer support workers do? A job description. *BMC Health Serv Res.* (2012) 12:205. doi: 10.1186/1472-6963-12-205
27. Simoni JM, Franks JC, Lehavot K, Yard SS. Peer interventions to promote health: conceptual considerations. *Am J Orthopsychiatry.* (2011) 81:351–9. doi: 10.1111/j.1939-0025.2011.01103.x
28. Muralidharan A, Lucksted A, Peeples AD, Goldbert RW. Defining "peerness" in peer-delivered health and wellness interventions for serious mental illness. *Psychiatric Rehabil J.* (2017) 40:116. doi: 10.1037/prj00 00249
29. Watson E. The mechanisms underpinning peer support: a literature review. *J Mental Health Early Onli.* (2017) 1–12.doi: 10.1080/09638237.2017. 1417559
30. Patton MQ. *Developmental Evaluation: Applying Complexity Concepts to Enhance Innovation And Use.* New York, NY: The Guilford Press (2011).
31. Edwards M, Wood F, Davies M, Edwards A. The development of health literacy in patients with a long-term health condition: the health literacy pathway model. *BMC Public Health.* (2012) 12:130. doi: 10.1186/1471-2458-12-130
32. Ritchie J, Spenser L. Qualitative data analysis for applied policy research. In Bryman A, Burgess RG, editors. *Analysing Qualitative Data.* Oxford, UK: Routledge (1994). p. 173–194.
33. Lincoln YS, Guba EG. *Naturalistic Inquiry.* Newbury Park, CA: Sage Publications, Inc (1985).
34. Leiber E, Weisner T. *Dedoose.* Los Angeles, CA: SocioCultural Research Consultants, LLC (2011).
35. Elo S, Kääriäinen M, Kanste O, Polkki T, Utriainen K, Kyngas H. Qualitative Content Analysis: a Focus on Trustworthiness. *SAGE Open.* (2014) 4:1–10. doi: 10.1177/2158244014522633
36. Nicholson J, Valentine A. Defining "Peerness": developing peer supports for parents with mental illnesses. *Psychiatric Rehabil J.* (2018) 41:157–9. doi: 10.1037/prj0000301

19

Identity in Personal Recovery for Mothers with a Mental Illness

Rochelle Helena Hine[1*]*, Darryl John Maybery*[2] *and Melinda Jane Goodyear*[2]

[1] *Mental Health Services, South West Healthcare, Warrnambool, VIC, Australia,*

[2] *Department of Rural Health, Monash University, Moe, VIC, Australia*

Correspondence:
Rochelle Helena Hine
rocki8@clearmail.com.au

Developing a "positive identity" is considered a core component of personal recovery, and mothering offers meaning in life and a valued identity. Few studies have highlighted the factors influencing identity within a personal recovery paradigm for mothers with mental illness. This study explores how mothers describe their identity in relation to recovery, including the factors that influence identity. Using constructivist grounded theory methodology, in-depth interviews were conducted with 17 women who were mothers and experienced mental illness. Women defined their self-concept broadly, accentuating motherhood, but also including vocational, community and social roles. Analysis revealed six categories: defining self, becoming a mother, being a "good" mum, feeling different, doing it my way and speaking out. Valuing identity in parenting was found to be linked to recovery. Services may facilitate personal recovery by supporting mothers to enhance a self-concept associated with mothering, as well as other diverse attributes and roles.

Keywords: gender, identity, mental illness, motherhood, personal recovery

INTRODUCTION

Personal recovery is a unique journey for those experiencing a mental illness, however common underlying characteristics and processes are now becoming better understood (1). Distinct from clinical recovery, which emphasizes a remission of psychiatric symptoms, personal recovery is grounded in the subjectivity of people who have live experience of mental illness (2). Personal recovery is concerned with holistic life functioning and social participation and agency, regardless of the presence of ongoing symptoms (3). Recovery experiences are unique and individual, and also differ for men and women due to the influence of gender (4).

Identity, and particularly the development of a positive sense of self that is less illness dominated and more strength based, is one of the key processes of the CHIME personal recovery framework developed by Leamy et al. (1). Resulting from a systematic review of personal recovery literature, the CHIME framework highlights Connectedness, Hope, Identity, Meaning and Empowerment as core categories that transform in a recovery journey. The significance of redefining and reclaiming a valued identity may comprise "determining the direction of one's life, grieving for lost opportunities, and yearning for belonging and acceptance" (5).

The ways in which mothers with mental illness describe their identity and the influences upon it within the process of personal recovery, has remained peripheral within recovery discourse. The aim of this study is to explore the ways in which mothers with mental illness describe their identity, and the factors that support or hinder development of a positive identity. Critical research aims to reveal and question social inequalities that are embedded within stereotypes (6). This current study adopts a gendered lens to examine the identity experiences of mothers with mental illness, and to investigate multiple identity possibilities including and beyond motherhood.

Identity Theory

Identity is broadly defined as one's self concept and is constructed through self-awareness of what and who one is "like" and "not like" (7). Identity is constructed within one's social and cultural context (8) and is therefore related to the construct of connectedness. Identity is a highly contested concept within feminist theory. An overarching theme is that gender based identity is predominantly oppressive. Butler (9) has problematized the concept of gender identity as the reproduction of the subordination of women, and explored the ways in which it is reproduced through linguistics. She also questions whether identity is a stable and continuous entity, and if it is static, the social regulatory structures that produce this outcome:

> 'To what extent is 'identity' a normative ideal rather than a descriptive feature of experience? And how do the regulatory practices that govern gender also govern culturally intelligible notions of identity? In other words, the 'coherence' and 'continuity' of 'the person' are not logical or analytic features of personhood, but rather socially instituted and maintained norms of intelligibility' (p.23).

Côté, defines identity as multifaceted and states that "manifestations of identity exist at three levels of analysis; the subjectivity of the individual, behavior patterns specific to the person and the individual's membership in societal groups" [(10), p. 8]. Within psychology, these differentiations have more broadly been separated into two categories: personal and social identity.

Personal identity relates to the internal characteristics including attributes and values that one recognizes as inherent to one's self concept. Social identity meanwhile, reflects how individuals view themselves as affiliating with and belonging to particular societal groups. Vocational, family, community, political, or gender-based categorizations are realms in which social identity may exist.

A fundamental debate in identity theory is whether the self is essentially a stable and enduring entity, or whether it is constantly changing and evolving (7). According to self-schema theory, the core identity constructs of an individual are thought to remain stable over time, although there may be some change in the more peripheral aspects of one's identity (11). Rosenfield (12) used schemas relating to self-salience, to explain disparities in mental health outcomes across gender, race and class, where a social determinants framework was ineffective in accounting for results that were inconsistent with structural inequality. Self-salience is associated with the relative importance individuals place on self, vs. the collective (13, 14). Rosenfield (12) cites the gendered socialization processes that contribute to the social construction of femininity and masculinity, and recognizes how these differ in relation to race and culture (15). Historical and enduring social conditioning underlies the gendered internal self-salience tendencies that predispose white women to experiencing more internalizing problems (e.g., depression) and white men to have a greater prevalence of externalizing problems (e.g., aggression) (12).

In contrast, self-categorization theory is based on the assumption that individuals' identity can and does change and evolve in response to the social and environmental context in which people live, and in response to external and internal processes associated with major life events. Ontorato and Turner (7) compared the two theories and found evidence to support self-categorization theory, with two studies demonstrating "the dynamic nature of self" (p. 276) that is context dependent. Self-categorization is a useful theory to inform exploration of the influences on identity development occurring through recovery from mental illness. Underlying assumptions imply that recovery emerges through social and psychological processes of personal change and development (1). The depth and breadth of self-reflection and change embedded in many of the subjective narratives of those with lived experience in mental illness and recovery, suggest that recovery entails a transformation at a deep psychological level, not merely some pruning or enhancement on the margins. Thus, self-categorization theory relates to this study.

Although gender identity can be a source of solidarity amongst women, it is more frequently problematized within feminist debate as a site for the reproduction of existing power differentials and maintenance of patriarchy. Within feminist theory:

> "…the reproduction of normative identities cannot be understood simply as a question of positioning within language but as a lived social relation that necessarily involves the negotiation of conflict and tension" [(16), p. 185].

For women who are mothers with mental illness, those conflicts and tensions may be the precipitant as well as the result of the psychiatric diagnosis and subsequent treatment and recovery. One method of developing deeper understanding of lived social relations is through amplification of the voices of those women who are marginalized in dominant discourse. This study aims to contribute to that endeavor.

Mental Illness and Identity

Mental illness has been characterized as a loss of self (5), as psychiatric symptoms may conceal or distort an individual's skills, knowledge, values and attributes. Social identity can also be disrupted as the illness often manifests in ways that prevent people from continuing in social roles that they had previously occupied and enjoyed (17). Individuals have spoken of enduring confusion, grief and regret as they seek to reconstruct a sense of self and reconcile the differences in their identities before, during and after the mental illness experience (18).

Researchers have explored the relationship between psychiatric symptoms and disruptions or incongruence in self-concept (19, 20) including models of conceptualizing and mitigating the impact of complex trauma on ones' identity and healing (21). Wisdom et al. (5) found loss of self to be the most prominent focus of narratives, with the illness "often described as taking away… their previously held identity" (p. 491).

Feminist writers have observed that historically, society's response to mental illness in women has resulted in sanctions for deviance and non-conformity to the prevailing cultural expectations [e.g., (23)]. A focus on social "integration" and adaptation of the individual, rather than advocacy for social change to create more equal and accessible social environments that foster diversity and inclusion, are evident in critiques of the recovery paradigm (4, 22).

Mothering With a Mental Illness

Mothering with mental illness is increasingly common (24, 25). Studies conducted with mothers with mental illness have emphasized the importance of a mothering identity to women in providing meaning and purpose (26), love and connection (26), and fulfillment (27).

Researchers have highlighted that parenting stress can compromise mental health (28–30), and discovered that mothering confidence and competence can be undermined by the scrutiny and prejudice imposed by over-zealous service providers (26, 31) and family members (32), who are often operating within a risk aversion framework.

Shor and Moreh-Kremer (33) emphasized the strengths for women with mental illness in being able to claim a normative maternal identity, thereby reducing their vulnerability to stigma and alienation. Within that study mothering identity was compared to mental illness identity, without consideration of other potential sources of identity in women's lives. While there may be individual benefits to conforming to gendered norms, if this is through developing a public persona that is incongruent with one's internal value system, and acceptance of oppressed social status, there will also be psychological costs (23).

AIM

The aim of this study was to explore how a cohort of Australian women who were mothers with mental illness described their identity, and how this related to personal recovery from mental illness. The research furthermore aimed to explore the factors and processes that mothers with mental illness describe as influencing their identity.

METHOD

Constructivist grounded theory (CGT) methods were employed to gather and analyse rich descriptive qualitative data (34). Grounded in feminist understandings of gender inequality that can result in and exacerbate the effects of mental illness, the research aimed to amplify the voices of women from a marginalized population group (35). Congruent with feminist approaches to research, CGT challenges the objectivity claims of positivist methods, instead advocating for transparency in acknowledgment of the values, perspectives, experiences and biases of the researcher which all influence the research decisions, processes, and outcomes (34). CGT emerged in the 1990's [e.g., (36, 37)] in response to the epistemological assumption that if "social reality is multiple, processual, and constructed, then we must take the researcher's position, privilege, perspective and interactions into account as an inherent part of the research reality" [(34), p. 13]. While traditional grounded theory methods emphasize that researchers arrive at their own data fresh, without prejudice or influence from previous studies (38) this sequencing is not required for undertaking constructivist grounded theory as the background research and theoretical context investigated, contributes to the unique subjectivity of the researcher. As all experiences in the social world influence the perspectives, language, assumptions and biases a researcher brings to each project (34), it would be exceedingly ineffectual to refrain from reviewing literature as just one of infinite potential influences. Hence in this study, literature on identity and gender were explored prior to the data collection with participants, with a more focused search ensuing after the categories were formulated.

Procedures

Following ethics approval from two health service and one university Human Research and Ethics Committees, mental health clinicians from a regional clinical mental health service supported recruitment processes by promoting the study amongst eligible women on their caseloads. Steps were taken to ensure no harm or distress was caused, and that women felt comfortable to end or pause the interview at any time. All interviews were conducted by a researcher who was also an experienced social worker employed as a senior mental health clinician and informed consent was obtained in writing. Local services guides were developed and distributed to participants in the event that the interviews triggered psychological response requiring follow up.

Nine women were recruited via clinical mental health services, and the remaining 8 from the general community via social and print media (promoted on Twitter and in local newspaper articles). Interviews were conducted by one researcher (RH), and consistent with CTG procedures, four of these 17 women were interviewed on more than one occasion as part of theoretical sampling. These participants were invited to participate in a second interview due to specific characteristics they possessed, that meant they were able to provide data that could increase understanding of phenomena relating to emerging codes. A total of 21 interviews were conducted, the mean duration being 42 min. The participants were at different stages of recovery. None of the women were in an acute crisis or experiencing active symptoms at the time of the data collection, although one woman had been hospitalized within the last month, and 6 were engaged with a clinical mental health service at the time of the interview. Three women were supported by a community mental health service and the remaining eight reported not receiving any specific mental health service at that time.

Interviews were conducted in person within a confidential space at various community health venues that were accessible to participants. Interviews were audio recorded and transcribed verbatim. The interview schedule was open ended and flexible, containing questions pertaining to women's experiences of personal and social identity. The interview schedule is available as a **Supplementary Material**. To set the context, women were asked about their mental illness and recovery journeys. Women were then asked broad questions regarding how they describe themselves, their social roles, personal characteristics, if and how the way they see themselves has changed over time, about their mothering and parenting, how they envisage others see them, and what or who influences how they view themselves in various settings (e.g., work, mothering/family, community). The total recruitment and interview time frame was from July 2015 to February 2016.

Data Analysis

Data analysis occurred concurrently with data collection, coding and reflection beginning immediately after transcription of the first interview and continuing after each interview. Analysis consisted of initial coding following close reading of all data on multiple occasions. Memo writing, purposive sampling, focused coding, mind-mapping were subsequently undertaken to enable development of categories (34), hence the categories emerged directly from the data. Regular dynamic discussion amongst the three member research team stimulated analysis and questions relating to the emerging categories. This led to second interviews with some participants to provide additional details to define the properties of emerging categories, as consistent with purposive sampling.

Participants

Participant characteristics are summarized in **Table 1**. A total of 21 interviews were conducted with 17 women who were all mothers with a psychiatric diagnosis. The women were a heterogeneous group and varied in relation to their living arrangements, socio-economic status and cultural background. Ages ranged from 23 to 53 year, with an average age of 36.29.

RESULTS

The study resulted in identification of six categories surrounding the concept of identity. The categories name psychological or social processes that were predominant within the data collectively. "Defining self" explores how women describe their self-concept and highlights the important elements of personal and social identity. As mothering was a core component of participants' identity, the categories "becoming a Mother" and "being a 'good Mum'" illuminate the relationship between women's mothering role, their mental illness and their recovery journey. The relationship between an illness identity and a mothering identity is explored in these sections. The category "feeling different" focuses on the women's experience of lacking a social identity and the implications of this on their personal identity. The final two categories reflect women's recovery progress, and highlight the importance of developing a positive identity, for attaining other personal recovery outcomes such as empowerment and meaning in life.

Defining Self

In describing their sense of self, all of the participants sought to contextualize their current temporal personal identity within their life histories, and inter-relational experiences, beginning in childhood. Ten women shared accounts of trauma from interpersonal violence occurring within childhood and/or adult relationships, and it is not known whether the remaining women may have also experienced violence but not disclosed. Through articulating key formative events, the women sought to construct identity narratives that provided meaning to explain their current circumstances, including their mental illness diagnosis.

Personal and social identities were described by participants as changing and evolving, while also containing stable components that persisted over time as illustrated by the assertion "I've always been this way" (P7). Participants described their identity in relation to their personal attributes, social roles and key relationships. Not all women were able to eloquently describe themselves, however there were exceptions:

> "(I'm) a woman, a mother you know, I'm a feminist, I'm an atheist, I'm left wing, very left wing in a lot of ways. I'm very politically minded, I'm very also socially conscious I guess. I do a lot of social activism. I'm bisexual so I've done a lot of campaigning for marriage equality and stuff like that. I'm very creative... I do a lot of crafty stuff. I love having kids because it gives you an excuse to colour in... I do a lot of puzzles, I watch probably way too much television and movies, I'm a huge film buff. I love politics as well" (P11).

Moral characteristics such as honesty, independence, generosity and creativity were viewed positively in the ways in which women viewed themselves, and they validated this through reflecting on how others might see them "I think people would describe me as nice and caring" (P13). Recognition of their own resilience was also evident ($n = 9$) in comments such as "...sometimes I look back on what I've coped with and I think, wow" (P5).

For other women, there was recognition that attributes that had been characterized as strengths prior to the mental illness experience could also become barriers to the help seeking that may be required to address mental health challenges:

> "I would describe myself as very independent. Probably too independent... I like individual sports like running and tennis. I've never really played team sports. I like to achieve, like at work I became fairly obsessed with achieving at work. But that was another thing after having the baby. It was very different..." (P2).

The social roles that the women identified embodying were relational, vocational, and community orientated. They included mother, sister, daughter, partner, friend, worker, health professional, student, mental illness advocate or educator, committee member and volunteer. Relationships with others in these spheres contributed to how they viewed themselves, and their personal identity could be particularly susceptible to messages they received from significant others regarding their performance within those roles.

Four women referred to their religious affiliation as being important in defining their moral and ethical framework. Although three women spoke of attending church related activities, they did not view themselves as sharing many characteristics with other members of their church except for their religious beliefs, therefore this was salient for personal rather than social identity.

Cultural identity was discussed by five women, two of whom were of Aboriginal descent (P7 and P8). Cultural disconnection was apparent with one of the women who indicated she knew

TABLE 1 | Participant characteristics.

Age; cultural background	No. of children and age	Housing type and lives with	Self-reported diagnosis and did diagnosis occur prior to motherhood?	Income source	Current mental health service engagement
38; Irish and French	3:10 years, 8 years, 6 years	Private rental Lives alone	Bipolar, OCD, BPD Yes	Government payment	None
35; Australian	2:2 years, 10 months, pregnant at time of interview	Own home on farm Lives with husband and children	Anxiety and depression No	Farm income	None
44; Australian	2:13 years, 11 years	Own home Lives with husband and children	Anxiety and depression No	Husband's full time wage	None
39; English and Australian	1:15 years	Own home Lives with partner and child	PND, anxiety and depression No	Own full time wages	None
39; Finnish and Italian, adoptive family Australian	1:14 years	Private rental Lives with child	BPD and bipolar disorder. No	Government payment and part time wages	Community MHS
40; Australian	1:2 years	Public housing Lives with child	Drug induced psychosis Yes	Government payment	Clinical MHS
29, Aboriginal	8:15 11 10 8 4 3 plus 2 younger in foster care	Public housing Lives with eldest 4 children	Anxiety and depression, paranoia, bi-polar disorder No	Government payment	Clinical MHS
31; Aboriginal	6:14 years, 12 years, 9 years, 4 years 2 years, 8 months	Transitional housing Lives with youngest 3 children	Anxiety, PTSD No	Government payment	Clinical MHS
43; Australian	1:15 years	Own home Lives with husband and child	Bipolar Disorder Yes	Government payment	Community MHS
26; Australian	1:6 months	Private rental Lives with partner and child	Bipolar Disorder Yes	Partner's full time wage	Clinical MHS
34; Australian	3:9 years, 8 years, 5 years	Private rental Lives with children	PTSD and depression, PND No	Government payment	None
53; Australian	3:17 years, 16 years, 13 years	House on the family owned farm Lives with husband and children	PND and depression No	Farm income, and wages from 3 part time jobs	None
28; Australian	2:5 years, 2 years	House on the family owned farm Lives with husband, children and boarder	Depression Yes	Part time wages and farm income	None
44; Australian and English	1:9 years	Private rental Lives with mother and child	Depression and anxiety No	Government payment	Community MHS
23; Australian	1:10 months	Own home Lives with partner, step child and son	Depression and anxiety Yes	Full time wages and partners' wages	Clinical MHS
45; Australian and German	2:14 years, 12 years	Own home Lives with husband and children	Anxiety, OCD and depression Yes	Part time wages and husband's full time wage	None
26; Caucasian	1:14 months	Parents' home Living with parents and child	Depression, Anxiety and PND No	Husband's full time wage	Clinical MHS

BPD, Borderline personality disorder; MHS, Mental Health Service; OCD, Obsessive compulsive disorder; PND, Postnatal depression; PTSD, Post traumatic stress disorder.

little of her heritage as her Aboriginal father had died when she was young. Another Aboriginal woman had experienced significant trauma during childhood and in adult life and had lacked opportunities to develop cultural knowledge or connection, stating "I want to know my culture, but I don't want to *do* my culture" (P8).

Participants articulating devalued personal identities were more likely to be in roles or relationships where they derived little pleasure or fulfillment:

> "I have issues with my work and because my boss is bully... when they cut my hours I took it really personally and I couldn't go to work the next day–I just cried" (P16).

Some women had difficulty describing themselves, identifying their strengths and imagining themselves in the future: "at the moment I can't see past tomorrow... I'd really like to enjoy things in my life a little bit more" (P15).

Identity across different domains could manifest in either positive, socially valued ways, or as negative and socially devalued. For example, a mothering identity could be positive if one perceived oneself to be a "good" mother, and felt a sense of belonging to a mothers' group. Alternatively, a mothering identity could be experienced as negative if one considered herself to be deficient and incompetent, thereby judging herself as a "bad" mother. Similarly, if a woman held a position of esteem within the community as a committee member in a sporting club, this would foster positive personal and social identity across other domains, whereas a lack of community recognition or a sense of social distance could contribute to a devalued identity reinforcing isolation and social exclusion.

Becoming a Mother

> "When I gave birth, I felt connected to something bigger and stronger than myself. I'm not religious, but I'm spiritual. So I felt connected to the bigger scheme of things like connected to other women and the feminine force of the universe" (P11).

Becoming a mother was a particularly significant component of women's self-concept. It could transform a woman's personal and social identity, fostering a deep sense of connection and meaning. However, it could also negatively impact a woman's view of herself if she struggled to feel competent in the role. Diversity was apparent in the responses the women had to embodying a mothering role and identity. For some it was an identity they immediately embraced and had always expected. The majority of participants ($n = 12$) had always had aspirations of parenting, and one woman with her partner had been planning the pregnancy for some time, including changing psychiatric medication and exploring fertility options. Having a baby brought a sense of empowerment and fulfillment for 8 of the participants. For one woman it was an opportunity to exercise her own autonomy and make choices that would not necessarily be endorsed by her own mother;

> "I breastfed until 21 months and I loved it. And my mum said 'don't you think it's time you gave it up?' at six months. And I'm like, hey, I felt something was right" (P5).

However, the experience did not always live up to expectations, especially in the early days and weeks.

> "I hid it from the maternal and child health nurse that I wasn't coping and then on the Friday I'd had enough and so I rang (family services worker) and said 'I need your help'" (P10).

For four women, all of whom had relished the idea of motherhood since childhood, childbirth was accompanied by debilitating postpartum depression when they had thought they were emotionally prepared. This left them with guilt and regret for the aspects of early parenting that they missed.

Experiencing breastfeeding difficulties was a source of significant stress and eroded self-confidence for four women. One woman delayed disclosing her decision to bottle feed to her new parent's group, fearing social rejection:

> "It took me probably two weeks to tell them that I wasn't breastfeeding, because I was just so anxious about it because everyone else was breastfeeding and I was like, oh they're going to want to kick me out of the group, yeah they won't want to talk to me ever again. But once I told them they were really supportive" (P17).

Having responsibility for a child prompted two women to re-assess their social behavior and temper their anger. They explained how accepting the responsibility associated with caring for an infant had led them to cease drug use, necessitating the severing of social relationships that would undermine this new healthy lifestyle choice. This assisted in them feeling greater competence in managing emotions, which led to a more positive identity.

Becoming a mother could have positive or negative implications for the women's personal identity. This was partially influenced by the availability of supportive relationships and assistance to adjust to the early parenting phase. How women perceived themselves to be performing in the mothering role profoundly shaped their identity, as did the quality of their relationships with family members and health professionals and the ways in which their inherent value was reflected through interactions within these relationships.

Another factor was whether the women's mental illnesses emerged before or after they became a mother. While 6 women had been given a psychiatric diagnosis prior to becoming a mother, an additional 7 participants expressed the belief that the mental health issues that eventually led to the subsequent diagnosis (after motherhood) had existed for many years, in some cases from childhood or adolescence. In these situations women described the mental illness label as providing an explanation for psychological, cognitive and behavioral events, along with the opportunity for enhanced social identity through developing peer relationships.

Being a "Good Mum"

A "Good Mum" was defined as accepting responsibility for one's children, prioritizing her children's needs over her own, being present and responsive and "making it fun" (P7); using humor and actively engaging in play. Attending to children's emotional needs and being available was a part of this: "I want to be the person that my kids will come and talk to me when something's going on, you know. Instead of hiding that away" (P7). All of the women interviewed expressed a desire to be identified by others as a "good mother." Furthermore, they wanted to embrace this label for themselves, although for three participants reconciling their thoughts and emotions regarding the mothering role with an ideal self-as-mother, was problematic. One woman rationalized that she wasn't a good mother because

> "...most of the time I feel like I'm just getting through... it's the extras that play with the mind and question how well you are doing. Am I stimulating them enough? Am I doing the right things for learning at this age?" (P2).

Characteristics of being a "good" mother ranged from meeting children's basic needs for nutrition, sleep and intellectual stimulation to being physically and emotionally available to children; "a good mother is showing love to their child, their little one, talking to them, validating their feelings... understanding his point of view" (P5). It involved persisting through hard days. Persisting entailed getting up in the mornings despite exhaustion or symptoms of depression, putting "a smile on a lot in front of them and for them" (P7) and for two mothers, remaining in undesirable employment to provide financial stability. In speaking about striving to be a good mother, two participants referred overtly to the sexism embedded in their own interpersonal relationships that saw them taking primary responsibility for child rearing while their husbands enjoyed more leisure time.

Eight women expressed sadness and regret regarding their own upbringing. Attributing their subsequent mental illness to the cumulative impact of trauma, abuse, neglect and disadvantage, participants felt that if they had been raised in a family with a responsive adult figure attentive to their needs, their lives may have taken a different path. This fuelled a desire to be present and considerate and sensitive to their children's traits, strengths and needs, even within challenging socio-economic circumstances.

> "Making sure I do a good job and (my child) gets a good education and just the little things, speaking to him nicely. I've never ever yelled at him, I don't believe in that and I don't like people who smack their children" (P6).

Despite best intentions, there were times when women's stress levels were high and their mental health was compromised. They became aware of how difficult this high expectation of parenting was in such times. For five women, serious physical health conditions such as pneumonia also took a toll. At this time children.

> "...learnt to become very independent and it was hard to parent them at that time. I didn't have the energy to discipline them and I noticed a lot of things went out the window—just their manners and the way they behaved and stuff—like I just couldn't be a good parent" (P16).

Breaking the pattern of cycles of intergenerational poverty, trauma and substance use were important to women in demonstrating their parenting attributes. They hoped for easier life circumstances for their children and hoped to guide them toward healthy choices:

> "It's being able to see beyond their pain and just walk with them and be their friend and guide them and show them this is what Mum and Dad have been through and this is why we don't want you to go down this path" (P1).

Viewing oneself as a good mother therefore had a positive impact on personal identity, while feeling incompetent or guilty had the opposite effect. Women used different measures to assess their parenting capabilities however an increased capacity for self-reflection and self-compassion was associated with greater progress toward recovery.

Feeling "Different"

A sense of disconnection and alienation from peers and family members pervaded development of a valued and intact self-concept for a number of women and they related experiences stemming from childhood to illustrate this. For some this was characterized by additional sensitivity, "I was a very clingy needy child" (P16) or having different needs and abilities to siblings "when we were younger I would clean (my sister's) room or do stuff for her just so I could spend time with her. Because we're very different" (P10). These examples suggest an unmet need for nurturing and connection in childhood. Resulting from this was a fragmented sense of self that was dominated by rejection.

For others it was about possessing a unique skill set or perspective on life, "the way my mind works I've never known anything different...and because of that I got treated different" (P7). Being able to deflect childhood labels of deviance and learning to embrace their own uniqueness fostered a sense of wellbeing, but was difficult to achieve outside the context of a supportive relationship. Women who felt validated by supportive intimate partners were better able to reflect of their childhood experiences of exclusion and externalize the cause of this experience.

Doing It My Way

This category was associated with increased confidence in one's experience and competence in mothering and signified a recovery milestone. Over time, women's self-awareness grew, and they became more insightful as to their own strengths, values and needs. This informed the resources and strategies they accessed to support their mental health and wellbeing. They gradually became proficient at seeking the support they required, whether that involved psychiatric medication, talking therapy, social connection, creating art, returning to study or if it was a viable economic option, taking respite from employment.

A key recovery milestone was reached when women grew in confidence and self-belief, enabling them to recognize and confront people in their lives that they saw as exerting disproportionate influence. In relation to parenting choices and styles, four women spoke of rejecting the preferred methods of others and asserting themselves. A sense of empowerment emerged when they were able to exert control over their baby's wellbeing. For one woman, ensuring that her own mother was not verbally or physically violent toward her in her infant son's presence was of paramount importance, and she asserted herself around her expectations through threatening to withdraw access to her son.

Another participant reflected on receiving what she defined as a "one size fits all" (P5) approach to parenting and attributes much of her mental anguish to the circumstances of her adoption. Being able to successfully breast feed her baby for 18 months was an empowering experience for this mother, and perhaps the most powerful example of her defying her adoptive mother with great success for the health and wellbeing of herself and her son.

Living on her in-law's rural property, another woman (P2) explained how she withdrew from her husband's parents as a strategy to maintain her independence and to reduce the feelings of inadequacy her mother-in-law instilled. In declining offers of child care from the children's grandmother, this woman sacrificed the potential for respite from her two young children, in the interests of sustaining her need for independence and autonomy.

Self-expression through choosing unusual clothing was how another participant asserted her own style. Creativity was employed to physical represent her mood, and she shared how her curious outfits at times draw smiles from community members, which then made her feel "that little bit happier." On one occasion she related dressing in a pink ball gown with a purple top hat to go to the supermarket:

> "I just got up feeling... I'm in a mood today, what can I wear? And I will spend hours because I need to find (the right outfit) and I won't wear something that won't match my personality, if I don't I think that matches my personality for today I won't wear it" (P7).

Speaking Out

The category of speaking out included disclosing, becoming a mental health advocate/educator, addressing stigma and challenging stereotypes. Although in speaking out, mental illness became dominant in women's personal identity, it was viewed positively and enabled social identity through peer networks to flourish. Enduring the ups and downs of mental illness was seen as a valuable asset that enabled women to take on an educator role, to connect with others through shared experience and to be knowledgeable in ways that others were not.

> "My mental health journey has meant that I've got experience in that to be able to connect with people on that level and that's what I want to be able to do" (P13).

Sometimes the desire to engage in community education stemmed from experiences of discrimination that woman believed arose from ignorance.

> "I was angry with the way society treated us. And just cast us aside like we were nothing... you can't necessarily see the pain that we carry with us. Its soldiers. And that's what I call it. We're all soldiers. We're all in this together..." (P1).

When women began speaking out, they embraced their illness as a core component of self. The illness symptoms, treatments, and ramifications were integrated into their lives and were a part of how they viewed themselves and presented themselves to others:

> "...doing the mental illness education was a really big part of my recovery so to go back and give out to the community, our point of view of how we feel, that's recovery too" (P1).

Participants expressed being selective in how and to whom they disclosed. Generally there was a correlation between the relative perceived safety of the participant's social environment and the extent of their disclosing. Women who felt supported and who had a multi-faceted, secure and positive social identity within their community were more likely to fully disclose. Past involvement with child protection was a deterrent that led women to conceal or minimize the impact of their mental illness.

DISCUSSION

The majority of women who participated in this study described multifaceted identities that represented their mothering and familial roles, their employment or vocational occupations, community relationships, hobbies and interests, religious and cultural status as well as the ways in which they defined their political or social values and attitudes. These descriptions encompass broader dimensions of identity than have previously been reported in studies with this cohort (39). Each of these could be considered positive and socially valued, or negative and socially devalued, with implications for social and personal identity, depending on the perceived competence and autonomy in the role. For instance, self-identifying as either a "good" or "bad" mother. Mothering was found to be a particularly powerful influence on women's self-concept, and participants identified the characteristics of being a "good Mum" as self-sacrifice, being present and enjoying the role. These concepts are congruent with the prevailing Western ideals of mothering that are grounded in traditional gendered roles that are oppressive to women (40). The findings emphasized the importance of identity to recovery, consistent with the CHIME framework (1).

Also significant, were women's expectations of the future. Impending opportunities and obstacles were related to women's ideas about their own competence, social status, agency and aspirations. The findings also highlight that identity is inseparable from social connection with participants described the ways in which their sense of self was heavily shaped by interactions with others (41). **Figure 1** represents conceptually the ways in which the women described the factors influencing

WHO AM I RIGHT NOW?

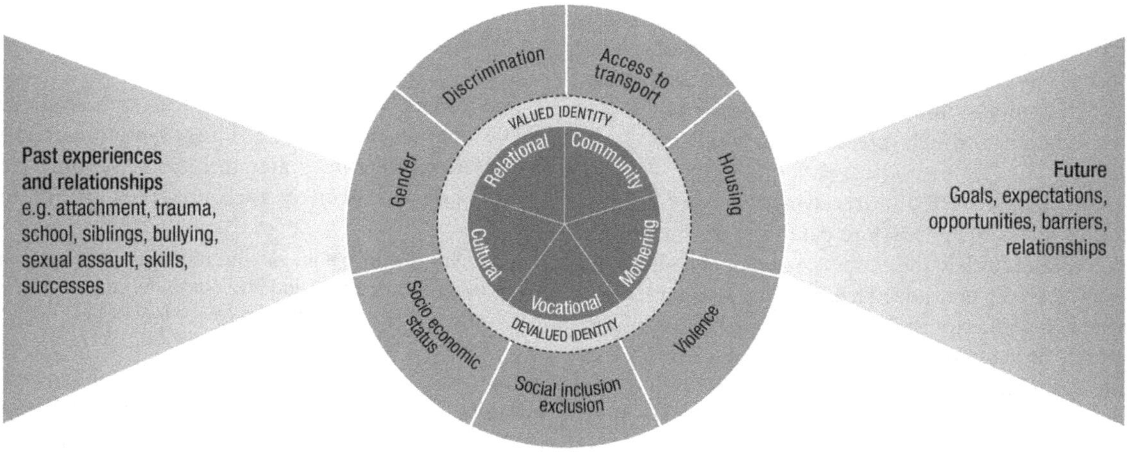

FIGURE 1 | Influences on personal and social identity for mothers with mental illness.

their personal identity. This figure was developed from the theoretical concepts that emerged from the data. Women described their identity being dependent on how they conceived their self-concept across a range of social domains. Each of these domains could be viewed as socially valued and positive or devalued and negative. Women spoke of being influenced not only by events and relationships from their past, but also their beliefs and aspirations regarding the future, thereby hope was a critical ingredient for a positive identity.

The categories of "doing it my way" and "speaking out" were indicators of significant integration of the illness experience into a woman's personal and social identity. Although the illness identity was at the forefront in "speaking out," it was constructed positively, intrinsically linked to meaning in life and empowerment, which are other recovery processes identified by Leamy et al. (1). Women emphasized recovery outcomes attained through being supported to identify their strengths, validate and normalize their challenges and self-reflect on the development of their identity across their life span. Often, however, prejudiced attitudes of others, especially associated with their mothering capacity, undermined women's self-concept.

Mothering Identity

Consistent with previous parenting studies [e.g., (26)], participants spoke of disconnection from other mothers. This was associated with socio-economics, parenting styles and difficulty infiltrating closed (well-established) social groups. Feeling disconnected, socially isolated and "different" is a common experience for mothers with mental illness [e.g., (42)] and is considered a barrier to both sustaining a positive social identity and to recovery (43) and wellbeing more generally (41).

Identifying as a "good" mother was symbolic of women's reflective capacity and internalization of social and cultural expectations as they related to the morality of parenting and the quality of relationships to children. Narratives reflected how women compared their mothering experiences to archetypes represented in their social environment. This finding echoed Venkataraman and Ackerson's (44) study on sources of parenting norms in popular culture, the media and parenting literature. Importantly, the signals women perceived from service providers, portrayed a deep understanding of how society assesses "good" mothering, and an intense desire to be viewed as competent. This facet of personal identity was susceptible to women's own internalized self-criticisms, in addition to the censorious messages conveyed by health professions or family members.

Having a psychiatric diagnosis was a core component of identity for some women, however this was not always experienced negatively, as disclosure could also bring meaning, purpose and connection, when used to educate, support or advocate around mental illness. For other women, having experienced mental health difficulties was just one relatively insignificant facet of a rich and varied life history. In this study a distinction between positive and negative identity was apparent, however this was not necessarily associated with the extent to which women embraced the illness as part of their personal identity.

Identity, Mental Illness and Trauma

The data also parallels Agnew and colleagues' study that "highlighted the complex and intertwined nature of traumatic experience, personality organization, and self/identity" [(19), p. 8]. Crucially important in defining a self-concept within the current study, were women's experiences from the past, including trauma resulting from physical, psychological or sexual abuse, the quality of early life attachments, transience in housing and schooling, relationships with siblings and parents, experiences at school and access to physical and economic resources. These factors, along with the ways in which women conceptualize them have also been previously highlighted (32, 42, 45, 46). In this study, these factors shaped the identity journey and the way the women saw themselves in the present.

For some women, having a diagnosis provided meaning and understanding that made sense of their symptomatic experiences. Additionally, this enabled them to connect with a peer network of others who shared similar thoughts, feelings and behavior and this offered validation. Mental health education and activism constituted a positive interpretation of lived experience that could simultaneously maintain the mental illness part of identity at the forefront.

Identity and Change

Identity is assumed to be fluid and dynamic within self-categorization theory (7), and while the participant interviews in this study are a snapshot in time, identity was described by participants as flexible, changing and evolving. This was evident in women's descriptions of themselves over time, and the ways in which they connected with others including disconnecting from unhealthy relationships and becoming more discerning or alternatively, learning to trust. However, there was also reference to consistent and enduring components of identity associated with preferences and strategies for managing stress and mental health difficulties. Crossley (47) adopted a narrative approach in investigating the disruptive impact of trauma, identifying the capacity for trauma to unseat previously coherent conceptualizations associated with self. Crossley (47) found that assumptions regarding one's usual patterns of thoughts, behavior and emotions are undermined along with one's temporal awareness that ordinarily provides meaning and context. This is congruent with women's descriptions of managing distress, in the early period of the illness. For the participants in Crossley's study, narratives become prominent in creating meaning, when customary psychological processes fail under the vast strain of traumatic occurrence.

Not only was it observed that events from women's past shaped their current identity, but their perceptions of their future lives including hopes, plans and aspirations were also influential in defining how they perceived themselves in the present. Identity development appeared to be a non-linear process that was highly permeable to social influence.

Recommendations for Research, Policy and Practice

The findings demonstrate mothering identity to be important for mental illness treatment and recovery. Women primarily related as mothers in articulating their self-concept and strove to be recognized as proficient in this role, highlighting their skills, strengths and underpinning parenting values as critical components of their identity. Therapeutic interventions need to explore mothering relationship to self and others, as "therapeutic understanding that takes into account the deficiencies within diagnostic criteria and acknowledges the diverse nature of self and identity of an individual may improve the therapeutic relationship" (19). Within such interventions, women need to feel safe and secure to explore their identity "journey" including the interactions and events that have led to their current self-concept.

A strong therapeutic alliance is critical to cultivating a safe space within which women can begin to address the issues that underpin their healing and recovery (48). Women spoke of the importance of this particularly in the early parenting phase, while adjusting to a new mothering role, and not yet feeling confident in their parenting knowledge and skills. The women who participated in this study indicated that validation of normalcy of parenting challenges can be useful at this time, as well as a more conversational approach that moves beyond the assessment checklists, to the development of an authentic relationship that offered individualized support, rather than reinforcing a sense of being "monitored" and judged.

Elevating the significance of identity and self may reveal areas of intervention that can support more flexible, nuanced and realistic expectations surrounding women's multiple roles and activities. Identity work, integrating past experiences that may challenge individual's assumptions regarding their identity (43) and reflecting on emotional and behavioral responses, is acknowledged as a core component of the recovery process (1, 48).

Beyond this, the current research suggests that investigation of identity and self in the context of social and environmental conditions must incorporate critical reflection on the dominant norms that may be oppressive and result in devalued status within various identity domains. Challenging and contextualizing these dominant assumptions may be particularly significant for marginalized population groups (e.g., Indigenous, people identifying as GLBTI), who are demonstrated to be at increased risk of developing mental health difficulties (49).

Discussions at this deeper conceptual level may be perceived as challenging to establish in the midst of psychological distress, and practitioner judgment in ascertaining readiness for such discussions is essential. However, avoiding these topics can pathologise individual responses to issues that are associated with layers of structural inequality. Future research should also focus upon overcoming workforce barriers within mental health and family services to engaging in identity work with women who have a mental illness.

Mental health policy needs to recognize and reflect the importance of identity work as a crucial part of practice. A disproportionate focus on medication and risk management within clinical mental health continues to stifle recovery oriented practice that encompasses a holistic view of people including consideration of their diverse and multi-faceted roles and relationships.

CONCLUSION

The importance of developing and sustaining an identity that is multifaceted and socially valued has been under-acknowledged within mental health services, despite positive identity development being repeatedly identified as a key characteristic of the recovery process. Fostering a positive self-concept, particularly associated with one's parenting role, can assist in facilitating personal recovery in mental illness.

For women who are mothers with mental illness, gendered norms around the mothering role can result in the imposition of unrealistic expectations of women's functioning, particularly if they are living in impoverished social and economic circumstances. Identity work needs to incorporate consideration of the personal level including past experiences, relationships, thoughts, emotions and behavior, as well as the broader environmental context.

ETHICS STATEMENT

This study was carried out in accordance with the recommendations of the Australian National Statement on Ethical Conduct in Human Research. The protocol was approved by South West Healthcare Multi-disciplinary HREC, Monash University HREC and Ballarat Health Services and St John of God Hospital HREC. All subjects gave written informed consent in accordance with the Declaration of Helsinki.

AUTHOR CONTRIBUTIONS

RH, DM, and MG developed the research design and methodology together. RH undertook the literature review and the data collection and led data analysis. DM and MG contributed to data analysis and all researchers were involved in initial coding and conceptual analysis as well as developing the findings. RH wrote the manuscript with editing/contributions from DM and MG.

REFERENCES

1. Leamy M, Bird V, Le Boutillier C, Williams J, Slade M. Conceptual framework for personal recovery in mental health: systematic review and narrative synthesis. *Br J Psychiatry.* (2011) 199:445–52. doi: 10.1192/bjp.bp.110.083733
2. Jacobson N. *In Recovery: The Making of Mental Health Policy.* 1st ed. Nashville, TN: Vanderbilt University Press (2004).
3. Slade M. The contribution of mental health services to recovery. *J Mental Health.* (2009) 18:367–71. doi: 10.3109/09638230903191256
4. Morrow M, Jamer B, Weisser J. *The Recovery Dialogues: a Critical Exploration of Social Inequities in Mental Health Recovery.* Vancouver: Centre for the Study of Gender, Social Inequities and Mental Health (CGSM). (2011). Available online at: https://www.researchgate.net/publication/264877917_The_Recovery_Dialogues_A_Critical_Exploration_of_Social_Inequities_in_Mental_Health_Recovery
5. Wisdom JP, Bruce K, Saedi GA, Weis T, Green CA. 'Stealing me from myself': identity and recovery in personal accounts of mental illness. *Aust N Z J Psychiatry.* (2008) 42:489–95. doi: 10.1080/00048670802050579
6. Wilkinson R. Socioeconomic determinants of health: health inequalities: relative or absolute material standards? *Br Med J.* (1997) 314–591. doi: 10.1136/bmj.314.7080.591
7. Ontorato RS, Turner JC. Fluidity in the self-concept: the shift from personal to social identity. *Eur J Soc Psychol.* (2004) 34:257–78. doi: 10.1002/ejsp.195
8. Weinreich P, Saunderson W. *Analysing Identity: Cross-cultural, Societal and Clinical Contexts.* East Sussex: Routledge (2003).
9. Butler J. *Gender Trouble.* New York, NY: Routledge (1990).
10. Côté J. Identity studies: how close are we to developing a social science of identity? - An appraisal of the field. *Identity.* (2006) 6:3–25. doi: 10.1207/s1532706xid0601_2
11. Markus H, Crane M, Bernstein S, Siladi M. Self-schemas and gender. *J Personal Soc Psychol.* (1982) 42:38–50.
12. Rosenfield S. Triple jeopardy? Mental health at the intersection of gender, race and class. *Soc Sci Med.* (2012) 74:1791–801. doi: 10.1016/j.socscimed.2011.11.010
13. Gibson P. Gender and Self-Salience. In: Cockerham W, Dingwall R, Quah S, editors. *The Wiley Blackwell Encyclopedia of Health, Illness, Behavior, and Society.* (2014). doi: 10.1002/9781118410868.wbehibs184
14. Rosenfield S, Lennon M, Raskin White H. The self and mental health: self-salience and the emergence of internalizing and externalizing problems. *J Health Soc Behav.* (2005) 46:323–34. doi: 10.1177/002214650504600402
15. Hill Collins P. *Black Feminist Thought: Knowledge, Consciousness and the Politics of Empowerment.* Boston, MA: Unwin Hyman (1990).
16. McNay L. Agency and experience: gender as a lived experience. In: Adkins L, Skeggs B, editors. *Feminism after Bourdieu.* Oxford: Blackwell Publishing (2004). p. 173–90.
17. Charmaz K. The body, identity and self: adapting to impairment. *Soc Q.* (1995) 36:657–80. doi: 10.1111/j.1533-8525.1995.tb00459.x
18. Heron J, Gilbert N, Dolman C, Shah S, Beare I, Dearden S, et al. Information and support needs during recovery from postpartum psychosis. *Arch Women. Ment Health.* (2012) 15:155–65. doi: 10.1007/s00737-012-0267-1
19. Agnew G, Shannon C, Ryan T, Storey L, McDonnell C. Self and identity in women with symptoms of borderline personality: a qualitative study. *Int J Qual Stud Health Well-being.* (2016) 11:30490. doi: 10.3402/qhw.v11.30490
20. Oyserman D, Elmore K, Smith G. Self, self-concept, and identity. In: Leary MR, Tangney JP,editors. *Handbook of Self and Identity.* New York, NY: Guildford Press (2012). p. 69–104.
21. Herman JL. *Trauma and Recovery: The Aftermath of Violence - From Domestic Abuse to Political Terror.* New York: Basic Books (1992).
22. Onken S, Craig C, Ridgway P, Ralph R, Cook J. An analysis of the definitions and elements of recovery: a review of the literature. *Psychiatr Rehabil J.* (2007) 31:9–22. doi: 10.2975/31.1.2007.9.22
23. Ussher JM. *Women's Madness: Misogyny or Mental Illness?* Amherst, MA: University of Massachusetts Press. (1991).
24. Maybery DJ, Reupert AE, Patrick K, Goodyear M, Crase L. Prevalence of parental mental illness in Australian families. *Psychiatr Bull.* (2009) 33:22–6. doi: 10.1192/pb.bp.107.018861
25. Vigod SN, Seeman MV, Ray JG, Anderson GM, Dennis CL, Grigoriadis S, et al., Temporal trends in general and age-specific fertility rates among women with schizophrenia (1996-2009): a population-based study in Ontario, Canada. *Schizophr Res.* (2012) 139:169–75. doi: 10.1016/j.schres.2012.05.010
26. Montgomery P, Tompkins C, Forchuk C, French S. Keeping close: mothering with serious mental illness. *J Adv Nursing.* (2006) 54:20–8. doi: 10.1111/j.1365-2648.2006.03785.x
27. Blegen NE, Hummelvoll JK, Severinsson E. Experiences of motherhood when suffering from mental illness: a hermeneutic study. *Int J Mental Health Nursing.* (2012) 21:419–27. doi: 10.1111/j.1447-0349.2012.00813.x
28. Ackerson BJ. Coping with the dual demands of severe mental illness and parenting: the parents' perspective. *Fam Soc.* (2003) 84:109–18. doi: 10.1606/1044-3894.69
29. Mowbray CT, Bybee D, Hollingsworth L, Goodkind S, Oyserman D. Living arrangements and social support: effects on the well-being of mothers with mental illness. *Soc Work Res.* (2005) 29:41–55. doi: 10.1093/swr/29.1.41
30. Reupert A, Maybery D, Kowalenko N. Children whose parents have a mental illness: prevalence, need and treatment. *MJA Open.* (2012) 1:7–9. doi: 10.5694/mjao11.11200

31. Seeman M. Intervention to prevent child custody loss in mothers with schizophrenia. *Schizophr Res Treat.* (2012) 2012:796763. doi: 10.1155/2012/796763
32. Perera DN, Short L, Fernbacher S. "Its not that straightforward": when family support is challenging for Mothers living with mental illness. *Psychiatr Rehabil J.* (2014) 37:170–5. doi: 10.1037/prj0000074
33. Shor R, Moreh-Kremer M. Identity development of mothers with mental illness: contribution and challenge of motherhood. *Soc Work Ment Health.* (2016) 14:215–26. doi: 10.1080/15332985.2015.1017135
34. Charmaz K. *Constructing Grounded Theory.* 2nd ed. London: Sage (2014).
35. Hesse-Biber S. Feminist research: exploring, interrogating, and transforming the interconnections of epistemology, methodology and method. In: Hess-Biber, editor. *Handbook of Feminist Research.* 2nd ed. Thousand Oaks, CA: Sage Publications (2015). p. 2–27.
36. Bryant A. Re-grounding grounded theory. *J Inform Technol Theor Appl.* (2002) 4:25–42. Available online at: https://aisel.aisnet.org/jitta/vol4/iss1/7
37. Clark A. Situational analyses: grounded theory after the postmodern turn. *Symbol Interact.* (2003) 26:553–76. doi: 10.1525/si.2003.26.4.553
38. Glaser B. *Basics of Grounded Theory Analysis.* Mill Valley, CA: Sociology Press (1992).
39. Hine R, Maybery D, Goodyear M. Identity in recovery for mothers with a mental illness: a literature review. *Psychiat Rehabil J.* (2016). 41:16–28. doi: 10.1037/prj0000215
40. Hays S. *The Cultural Contradictions of Motherhood.* New Haven, CT: Yale University Press (1996).
41. Townsend KC, McWirther BT. Connectedness: a review of the literature with implications for counseling, assessment and research. *J Counsel Dev.* (2005) 83:191–201. doi: 10.1002/j.1556-6678.2005.tb00596.x
42. Carpenter-Song EA, Holcombe BD,Torrey J, Hipolito M, Peterson LD. Recovery in a family context: experiences of mothers with serious mental illness. *Psychiatr Rehabil J.* (2014) 37:162–9. doi: 10.1037/prj0000041
43. Tan R, Gould RV, Combes H, Lehmann S. Distress, trauma, and recovery: adjustment to first episode psychosis. *Psychol Psychother.* (2014) 87:80–95. doi: 10.1111/j.2044-8341.2012.02073.x
44. Venkataraman M, Ackerson BJ. Parenting among mothers with bipolar disorder: strengths, challenges, and service needs. *J Fam Soc Work.* (2008) 11:389–408. doi: 10.1080/10522150802441825
45. Mowbray CT, Oyserman D, Bybee D, MacFarlane P, Rueda-Riedle A. Life circumstances of mothers with serious mental illnesses. *Psychiatr Rehabil J.* (2001) 25:114–23. doi: 10.1037/h0095034
46. Morrow M. *Violence and Trauma in the Lives of Women With Serious Mental Illness.* Vancouver, Canada: British Columbia Centre for Excellence in Women's Health. (2002). Available online at: http://bccewh.bc.ca/wp-content/uploads/2012/05/2002_Violence-and-Trauma-in-the-Lives-of-Women-with-Mental-Illness.pdf
47. Crossley M. Narrative psychology, trauma and the study of self/identity. *Theor Psychol.* (2000) 10:527–46. doi: 10.1177/0959354300104005
48. Shepherd A, Sanders C, Doyle M, Shaw J. Personal recovery in personality disorder: systematic review and meta-synthesis of qualitative methods studies. *Int J Soc Psychiatry.* (2016) 62:41–50. doi: 10.1177/0020764015589133
49. Marmot M. Social determinants of health inequalities. *Lancet.* (2005) 365:1099–104. doi: 10.1016/S0140-6736(05)74234-3

20

Overcoming Clinician and Parent Ambivalence: General Practitioners' Support of Children of Parents with Physical or Mental Illness and/or Substance Abuse

Marit Hafting[1], Frøydis Gullbrå[2], Norman Anderssen[2,3], Guri Rørtveit[2,4], Tone Smith-Sivertsen[2] and Karin van Doesum[5,6,7]*

[1] Regional Center for Child and Youth Mental Health and Child Welfare, Uni Research Health, Bergen, Norway, [2] Research Unit for General Practice, Uni Research Health, Bergen, Norway, [3] Department of Psychosocial Science, University of Bergen, Bergen, Norway, [4] Research Group for General Practice, Department of Global Public Health and Primary Care, University of Bergen, Bergen, Norway, [5] Clinical Psychology, Radboud University Nijmegen, Nijmegen, Netherlands, [6] Impluz, Prevention Team Mental Health, Deventer, Netherlands, [7] Regional Center of Child and Youth Mental Health and Child Welfare, Artic University of Tromsø, Tromsø, Norway

***Correspondence:**
Marit Hafting
marit.hafting@uni.no

Children who are next of kin to parents with physical or mental illness and/or substance abuse need access to mental health support and several cost-effective interventions are available. Because most parents in the target group often consult general practitioners (GPs), GPs may have a crucial role in identifying burdened children and ensuring their follow-up. However, this important topic has received little attention in clinical discussions and research. In response to the knowledge gap, we conducted the research project Burdened Children as Next of Kin and the General Practitioner. Four sub-studies have been completed and published: a sub-study with qualitative analysis of focus group interviews with GPs (paper 1), a qualitative analysis of focus group interviews with adolescents as next of kin (paper 2), and a qualitative analysis of individual interviews with parents with illness and/or substance abuse (paper 3). The results from these sub-studies were incorporated in a survey sent to members of a nationwide GP organization (paper 4). The aim of the present sub-study was to gain further knowledge about conditions for the encounters between GPs and parents with impairments to be supportive for the children as next of kin. The material of the present sub-study derived from the project's four previous sub-studies and comprised a secondary analysis of the four prior sub-studies. We conducted an overarching thematic analysis of these sub-studies' results sections. We searched for statements from the GPs, the adolescents, and the parents on their experiences and evaluations of the needs of the children and their families, and the possible ways of accommodating these needs in general practice. The analysis shows that both GPs and parents were ambivalent about addressing the topic of the patients' children during consultations. This was the case although the GPs were in a good position to identify these vulnerable children, and the parents were worried about their children's situations. Possible strategies for GPs to overcome this ambivalence can be to (1) strengthen their competence in the topic, (2) gradually build trusting relationships with parents, and (3) gradually gain contextual knowledge about the families' situations. GPs can do this by performing ordinary GP tasks and acknowledging the parents' efforts to give their children good daily lives.

Keywords: children as next of kin, parents with impairments, general practitioners, health prevention, health promotion, qualitative research

INTRODUCTION

Approximately 20–30% of children 0–18 years at some point in time experience a parent with physical or mental illness and/or substance abuse (1–4). While the prevalence of children living with parents with illness and/or substance abuse varies, as the definitions of these parental problems are often not the same, the negative effects that this situation can have on the children are clear. These children are at risk of poor psychosocial outcomes and health problems (5–7). In addition, the children describe difficulties in their daily lives, health problems, school problems, loneliness, and instability in the family situation (8–13).

During the last few decades, children's legal rights have been strengthened (14). In Norway, a law was enacted in 2010 concerning care for children as next of kin to parents with severe physical illness, mental illness, and substance abuse. Health personnel who have parents in treatment are obligated to inform their children (with their parents' informed consent) about their parents' situations and ensure follow-up if necessary (15). The same year, Sweden enacted an identical law (16).

Families affected by illness and substance abuse face many challenges that can be exacerbated by stigmatization, parental prognosis, exposure to violence and trauma, and the impairment's impact on the family economy. Children as next of kin to parents with the abovementioned problems experience varying risk and protective factors, and the impairments have different impacts on their lives and developments. Despite these differences, the children have in common, at least in periods, that their parents often struggle to fulfill their parental tasks and give their children the developmental support that they need (17, 18). They are children at risk but are often described as "invisible" in public life and to support services, and thus are difficult to reach for health promoting and prevention (17, 19). Identifying these children and giving the family necessary support is an important preventive task. Evidence-based interventions are available (7, 20–22), including home visits, individual and group sessions for parents, support groups for children, and family intervention programs. However, there is a need for more high-quality studies on the effectiveness of these programs and how they adapt to different children and family situations (23, 24).

A study from the United Kingdom (UK) reported that 23% of children between 9 and 17 years of age with mothers with depression met the criteria for a DSM IV diagnosis. However, only 33% of the children with a diagnosis had been identified and were in treatment (25). The mothers were mainly recruited from general practices. The authors called this a situation of missed opportunities because the professionals in contact with the mothers could have identified these children and offered them appropriate follow-up. It was our belief that general practitioners (GPs) might be in a good position to change this situation. Most patients with parental responsibilities who suffer from mental illness, severe somatic illness, and/or substance abuse will repeatedly consult a GP, often the same GP, several times over the years (26). Although this topic has been raised in clinical discussions and research (27–29), there is still a knowledge gap concerning how the GPs could support patients' children as next of kin. Therefore, we conducted the research project Burdened Children as Next of Kin and the General Practitioner. The results of four sub-studies have been published (10, 30–32).

In these four studies, we found that the GPs were in a good position to identify the children, but they experienced substantial obstacles to ensure them follow-up care. Parents and adolescents, however, wanted the GPs to address their family situations in the encounters. This had to be enacted within a trusting relationship where parents and adolescents felt that their struggles to manage their challenges were recognized.

This article presents the results from the fifth sub-study of the project. This is a thematic analysis of the four sub-studies' result sections. The aim is to gain further knowledge about how GPs can take on a child-focus and support children as next of kin when their parents with illnesses and/or substance abuse seek the GP for their own health problems.

Context and Setting

In Norway, where this project took place, general practice provides an open access for people with all types of health-related problems, and the GPs are often the patients' first medical contact within the healthcare system. GPs cooperate with others in the primary healthcare setting, giving the patients coordinated care. They also act as gatekeepers and coordinate entrance into secondary care by referrals. A patient list system is operational, and almost all citizens are enlisted with a personal GP, which facilitates continuity of the doctor-patient relationship. The children are usually enlisted with their mothers' GP. GPs primarily work at their office in which they receive patients for consultations.

Theoretical Assumptions

The prevailing consultation model among Norwegian GPs is the patient-centered consultation model (33) which encourages the GPs to explore and understand the patient's expectations, background, and feelings. Then, in dialogue with the patient, the GPs combine these insights with the examination-results and his or her medical knowledge. According to this model, the GPs must explore the context, including family matters and the children's situations. However, if the patients for some reason do not want the GPs to address the children's situations, the subject might be omitted even though the GPs ethically and legally have obligations toward the children.

Patient trust is often a precondition for the patient to allow for and engage in difficult conversations about vulnerable themes with a medical professional (34, 35). In a study from Skirbekk et al. on patient-GP consultations (36), trust is conceptualized as the patient's implicit willingness to accept the physician's judgment in matters of concern to the patient. Several studies on general practice concluded that an attitude of recognition from the GP can encourage the patient to share his or her story (37, 38). Here, an attitude of recognition is described as relational, mutual, and based on respect for the person as a subject, as an authority of one's own experiences. This attitude may make it easier for the GP and the patient to tolerate their different viewpoints during the encounter. The concepts of patient-centeredness, patient trust, and patient recognition provide theoretical support for our analysis (39).

As this project's sub-studies were completed, the researchers discussed the implications of the results. GPs mostly meet their patients in a doctor's office. These consultations between the GPs and the parents are the central arena that can allow the GPs to learn about the children's situations and, in collaboration with the parents, ensure follow-up care of the children. Our research suggests that while the GP may be a crucial figure in helping the children of parents with impairments, there are many missed opportunities in practice (31). Therefore, this secondary analysis of our results might deepen the understanding of the possibilities and limitations of these consultations.

MATERIALS AND METHODS

There are four sub-studies in our project considered in the present analysis (10, 30–32) (**Table 1**): a qualitative analysis of focus group interviews with GPs (paper 1), a qualitative analysis of focus group interviews with youth as next of kin (paper 2), a qualitative analysis of individual interviews with parents with illnesses and substance abuse (paper 3), and a survey sent to members of a nationwide GP organization that incorporated the results of the previous sub-studies (paper 4). The current sub-study comprised a secondary analysis of the four prior sub-studies. The results sections of these four sub-studies provide the data analyzed in the present study. The empirical material of this study allows us to combine the perspectives of GPs, youths and parents on how to support burdened children. To reach a deeper understanding of this topic, a thematic analysis (40) is appropriate as it allows for a systematic treatment of the material. This method involves searching the dataset to find repeated patterns of meaning. The analysis is structured and consists of different steps, as described below. During the analysis the researcher continuously compared the codes and themes they developed with the text as a whole to ensure that the results were grounded in the original data set.

After defining the aim, two of the authors (MH) and (FG) read the four articles several times to *familiarize* themselves with the material seen as a whole and recorded their preliminary ideas. Then we searched the results sections specifically for elements that described the informants' experiences and evaluations of the needs of the children and their families, and the possible ways of accommodating these needs in general practice. We marked these elements with *codes*. We found that the text dealt with 37 different codes relevant to our aim. We gathered the textual elements with the corresponding codes. We then determined how the codes from the different sub-studies were interconnected by comparing and integrating them, and then developed preliminary subthemes and overarching themes. Each *subtheme* should cohere together meaningfully, and there should be clear distinctions between them. This process ended with 11 subthemes. We grouped the subthemes under three *overarching themes* that organize the results section of this analysis. The 11 subthemes are used as subheadings (**Figure 1**). To assure the quality of this analytic process, a third author (KvD) compared the four sub-studies with the list of codes and development of subthemes. At this stage, we searched the text for citations that would best illustrate the subthemes. During this analysis, we evaluated the developed codes, subthemes, and overarching themes against the four sub-studies to ensure that they were based on the empirical material.

RESULTS

The adolescents described a lack of knowledge about their parents' situations and that they wanted to be offered follow-up on their often-stressful life situations. During the analysis, we found that their needs were acknowledged by the GPs and the parents, but both groups expressed ambivalent feelings about addressing the children's situations in the consultations.

The major overarching themes and sub-themes derived from analysis are (1) The parents had mixed feelings about receiving support on parenting (sub-themes "Parents acknowledged their children's need for information and to talk about their experiences," "Parents lacked knowledge about support services for their children," and "Parents gave double messages"), (2) GPs often missed their opportunities to support parents and children ("GPs faced obstacles in the general practice framework," "GPs feared jeopardizing the doctor-patient relationship," and "GPs lacked knowledge about talking to the children"), and (3) How can the GP lay the ground for reduced ambivalence of talking about the children? (sub-themes "Recognizing the parents' struggle for an ordinary family life," "Taking the initiative," "Awareness of the therapeutic alliance," "Gaining contextual knowledge and building multidisciplinary networks," and "Building competence").

Overarching Theme 1: The Parents had Mixed Feelings About Receiving Support on Parenting

Parents Acknowledged Their Children's Need for Information and to Talk About Their Experiences

During the focus group interviews, the adolescents indicated that they had incomplete knowledge about their parents' conditions and expected outcomes. This caused worries and uncertainty and made their daily lives unpredictable. They described a

TABLE 1 | Overview of the four articles in the project Burdened Children as Next of Kin and the General Practitioner.

	Aim	Design/data collection	Participants	Parental problems	Analysis
Paper 1	Explore GPs thoughts and experiences with handling the special needs of children as next of kin in general practice	Qualitative interview study/4 focus group interviews	27 GPs, 9 women, 38–65 years of age, 6–33 years in GP		Thematic analysis (40)
Paper 2	Explore significant experiences of adolescents as next of kin that the GP should identify and recognize	Qualitative interview study/4 focus group interviews	15 adolescents, 12 women, 16–25 years of age	5 physical illness 5 substance abuse 5 mental illness	Systematic text condensation (41)
Paper 3	Identify important factors for the GP to bear in mind during encounters with ill and substance-abusing parents to enable the GP to provide appropriate support to the children	Qualitative interview study/Individual semi-structured interviews	12 parents with a total of 28 children, 9 women	4 physical illness 2 substance abuse 8 mental illness	Systematic text condensation (41)
Paper 4	Investigate the experiences of GPs concerning their involvement with their ill patients' children and their evaluation of the opportunity to help these children	Web-based survey with some open questions	499 GPs 244 men		Numeric data analyzed by cross tables, t-tests, chi-square testing and multiple regression. Text material from the open questions analyzed by thematic analysis (40)

daily struggle to balance their own needs for an ordinary adolescence—participating in social activities and focusing on school performances—with the boundaries and burdens caused by their parents' problems. For these adolescents, it was important to have someone to talk to about their family situation and who acknowledged their challenges. This individual could be the healthy parent, a teacher, a friend, a family member, a support group, and someone from the health care system, including the GP. A girl with a mother with mental illness, now living in a foster home, said the following (paper 2):

> It is so nice to talk to some adults who can tell you that this is NOT how you should live. You should not wash the dishes after a huge dinner that you didn't eat. That is not how life should be for a kid. You should be out playing, because it is sunny outside. That kind of information is incredibly important.

The majority of parents recognized their children's lack of information and emotional burdens. However, giving such information to the children was perceived as difficult. Often, due to the parents' own medical condition, they did not sense their children's worries. For example, consider the statement from one mother with severe chronic back pain (paper 3):

> ......because all kids get worried when the mother stays in bed all day, and when they peep into the bedroom, she is laying there crying with pain. Of course, my kids got worried. They were terrified. They thought that I would die. They did not see the difference whether I laid there not being able to move because of back pain, or if I had cancer. For them, there was no difference. I did not manage to sense these worries.

Some parents expressed that their children avoided talking about their parents' problems at home. Often, choosing the best time to inform the children of their problem was difficult. Moreover, the parents were unsure what information was relevant to share. Many parents wanted concrete and individualized advice on how to talk to their children about their situations. For this purpose, they said that a helper close by would be the best person to seek counseling from. Some parents wanted their children to be offered help from professionals.

Parents Lacked Knowledge About Support Services for Their Children

The adolescents described constraints in their lives caused by their parents' impairment. It was important for them to relax and take part in social activities such as going out with friends and joining sports activities. They needed "time-outs." One 16-year-old girl living alone with a father with schizophrenia echoed this sentiment (paper 2):

> I just wanted to have time out with them, my friends, where nobody knew about my dad. I found that relaxing. I didn't want to be pitied for living with him, I just wanted to be seen as an ordinary girl.

In addition, parents missed having relieving activities for themselves and their children, help for daily household concerns, and financial support. They often did not have the energy, social network, or competence to search for support services. Parents wanted their GP to ask questions about their family's needs and to help them to find relevant support. A mother with bipolar disorder who lived alone with two children said the following (paper 3):

> It is important that the GPs have knowledge about where they can recommend us to get help when it comes to the children. Once the doctor knows that we have children, there should be

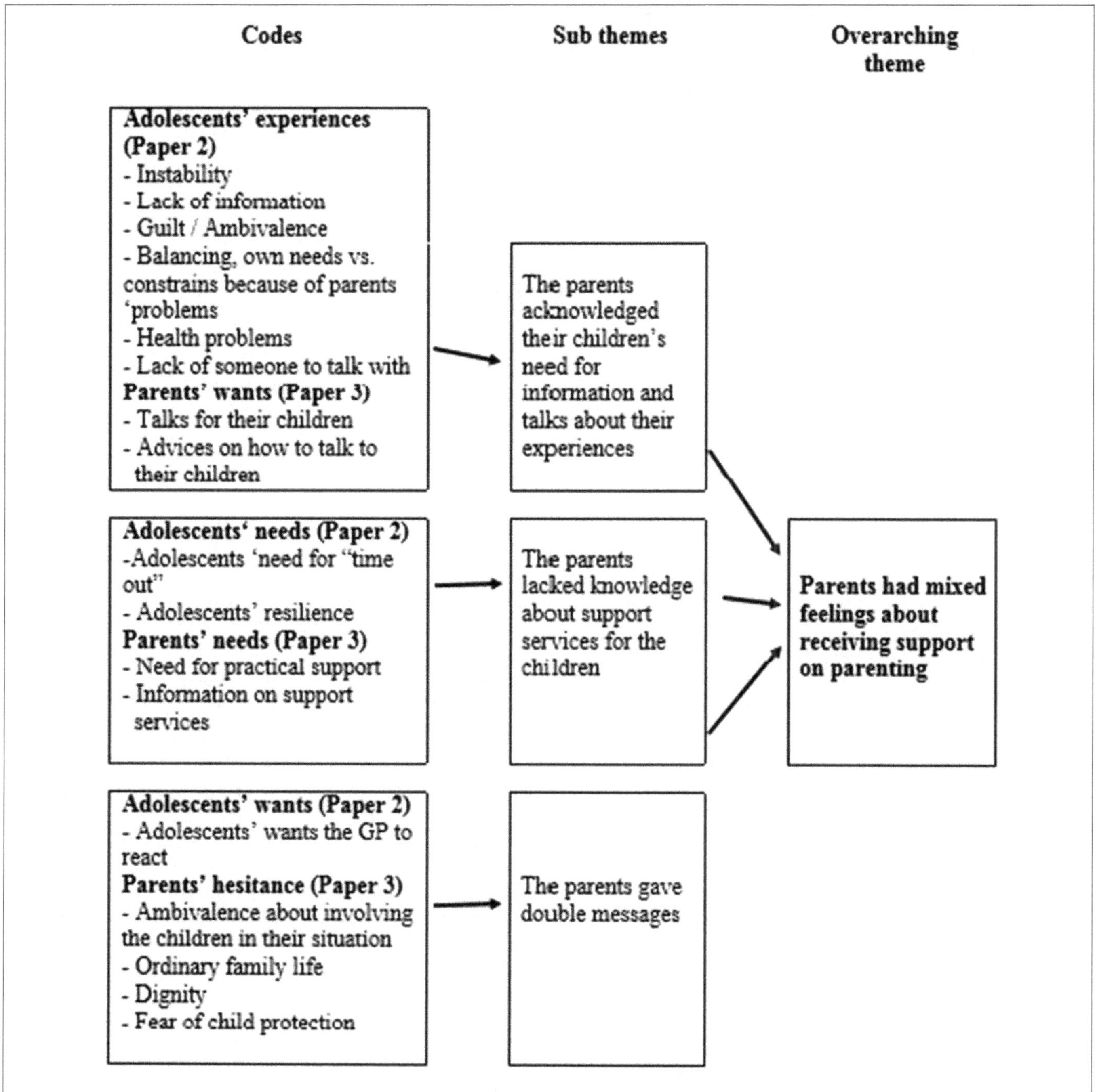

FIGURE 1 | Analysis process from codes over sub-themes to overarching themes. Result section "Patients had mixed feelings about receiving support on parenting" as an example.

> an alarm ringing telling them: "Okay, now these kids need to be protected." The doctor should tell the parents: "I have some advice for you, and some helpers you can contact, and here are the phone numbers," .... a brochure to hand out or stuff—I think that can be very helpful.

Parents Gave Double Messages

The youths often wished for more information and to have talks about their life experiences. In particular, they wanted to know more about their parents' conditions, how to understand their sometimes-deviant behaviors, their disease progressions and help to understand their own life situation and the rationale for their struggles. They wanted someone to talk to about their experiences. The parents acknowledged their children's needs to be informed and supported. In addition, they realized that advice on parenting could be beneficial. Despite this, they revealed ambivalent stances on the topic and gave what could be termed a double message; they both wanted and did not want their children's situation to be a topic in the consultations. Some openly stated that they were afraid of being considered bad parents. Likewise, some feared their children would be taken from them if they revealed the problems at home. Some GPs in the survey noticed this resistance and attributed it to the parents' fear of losing custody. The adolescents, however, wanted the GPs to intervene. For instance, one girl blamed the GP for not contacting the child protection services after a consultation she had attended with her mother who was heavily drunk. Related to this, many parents wanted to preserve their dignity and social acceptance. They described their struggle to keep up the appearance of an ordinary family life. Last, the parents were unsure about how much information should be provided to the children, as knowing too much about their parents' problems could cause their children unnecessary concerns. A single mother with a personality disorder living with an 8-year-old son maintained, as did many parents, that keeping up the impression of a normal family was in a child's best interest (paper 3):

> I have simply avoided talking about it. I have been afraid about making our situation abnormal, that he might think we are living differently. That he would be ashamed. For this is what is normal for him.

Overarching Theme 2: GPs Often Missed Their Opportunities to Support Parents and Children

GPs Faced Obstacles in the General Practice Framework

Some GPs knew their patients' children from local communities and from collaboration with the health visitors in the geographic area. Others pointed out that they only had a "peephole" into their patients' everyday lives, and the patients regulated the GPs' knowledge of their families. As one GP said: "It is easy to hide from a GP." Due to the continuity of care, this "peephole" sometimes gradually broadened through knowledge gained over time during ordinary GP tasks.

In particular, the GPs emphasized three factors within the GP framework that hampered their opportunities to address the children's situations during consultations: busy practices with heavy workloads, short consultations, and the registry system where family members could be enrolled with different GPs. Most of the respondents in the survey (paper 4) answered that they felt responsible for their patients' children when they were enrolled on their own list. However, only half of the GPs felt the same responsibility when the child was enrolled with another GP. The following glimpse from an interview between the interviewer (FG) and a GP illustrates this point (paper 1):

> FG: "Does the general practitioner already have so many tasks that this becomes difficult to handle during the workday?"
>
> GP: "I think that's a good point, especially in a situation where the rest of the family is not on your list. Then you think there are other people involved who will take care of them. The rest of the family can be people you don't know and whom you have never seen."

However, these children might have GPs who do not know about their parent's problems. If a child's GP does not routinely ask about his or her parents' condition, this GP may not recognize if the child is at risk. This is often the situation for children of ill or substance-abusing fathers because at birth Norwegian children are automatically enrolled with the same GP as their mother.

GPs Feared Jeopardizing the Doctor-Patient Relationship

Relational constraints—such as focusing on the parents during the consultations and thus, forgetting to address the children—caused problems for the GPs. In addition, the GPs were also concerned about the possibility of hurting or losing their vulnerable patients if they brought up the children's situations. Some GPs said that they avoided the topic because they did not want to add guilt and place burdens on parents who were already struggling. One female GP expressed this notion (paper 1):

> It is difficult, because then it's as though I am also saying that her problem is her children's problem. Then I am putting the blame on her, and here she has come to get help for herself. I am just placing one more burden on her shoulders, I should think.

Similarly, some GPs avoided the topic because they thought they could offend their patients. These GPs viewed that ending a long-term doctor-patient relationship would be a disadvantage for the patient and the family.

GPs Lacked Knowledge About Talking to the Children

The GPs often engaged in discussions about parenting, giving advice to both ill and healthy parents. A female GP told a relevant story about a family with an 8-year-old boy (paper 1):

> The mother had asked me for advice on how to inform her son about the father's drug problem. (....) Then, the father died in an overdose. Afterwards I gave advice on how to tell this son about death and why it happened. Naturally, I also visited their home a few times after he died and talked with the little 8-year-old boy. That was not easy!

The GPs who addressed the children's situations were confident in informing and advising their parents. However, GPs felt more uncomfortable about talking directly to the children.

Overarching Theme 3: How Can the GP Lay the Ground for Reduced Ambivalence of Talking About the Children?

The parents gave a double message on whether to thematize the children's situations in the encounters with the GPs. The GPs said that they often avoided the topic of their patients' children out of fear of placing more burdens on their struggling patients or of losing the therapeutic alliances. However, the data-set contained thoughts and experiences from both the parents and the GPs on how to overcome this mutual ambivalence who might hamper identification of and support to the children.

Recognizing the Parents' Struggle for an Ordinary Family Life

Many parents tried to make ordinary daily lives for their children. Overall, they wanted their impairment to have as little negative impact as possible. Parenthood gave them social belonging and self-respect. Crucially, it sent a message to them and those around them that they managed parenting despite their problems. One mother with substance abuse framed it this way (paper 3):

> For the last 6 months, a woman from child protection has been coming to my home twice a week to take urine tests. In addition, she does an inspection in our home. I wanted it that way. I wanted these people to come home to me, to let them see that we manage just as well as our neighbors.

For these parents, admitting that they needed support threatened their self-image of being a competent parent who managed daily life in an ordinary family. Therefore, before they could admit their shortcomings and collaborate with the GP, many parents needed recognition for their efforts and love of their children.

Taking the Initiative

Despite their expressed ambivalent feelings, parents interviewed in Paper 3 wanted their GPs to address their children's situations. However, the parents did not want to put forward the topic themselves. Rather, they had to be prompted by the GP. The adolescents expressed the same sentiment: They wanted the GP to ask about their family and situation at home during ordinary consultations. The adolescents' expectations of the GP could be negatively formed by their parents' previous medical experiences such as delayed cancer diagnosis or psychiatric diagnoses. The GP might misunderstand this hesitant attitude or ambivalence from parents and children as avoidance or that the topic was not relevant.

Awareness of the Therapeutic Alliance

Sometimes, the GPs worried that their rapport with patients would be affected negatively if they addressed the children's situations (see above "GPs feared jeopardizing the alliance"). The parents, however, told stories of how they had previously tolerated direct speech from a trusted helper, someone whose alternative viewpoints and corrections they could accept. The parents often had a trusting relationship with one professional, a person who had provided continuity of care and demonstrated strong personal involvement. One father who had recently lost his wife to cancer expressed this view (paper 3):

> Support from the GP, a cancer nurse, or health visitor is really important. To have helpers genuinely interested in helping you and not just doing a job because it is their duty to do so. You tell more to a person you know and trust than to a person you see only once. These helpers have been there during the illness. It started with the GP, the GP has been there all the time, and it is there you go if new troubles come up.

Gaining Contextual Knowledge and Building Multidisciplinary Networks

It was important for the parents to have helpers who knew their situation well, including the social and family settings. In addition, the parents appreciated when the GP had adequate knowledge about support services and participated in multidisciplinary meetings. In these meetings, the GP could contribute with valuable information. For the parents, it was important that the different helpers collaborated, as stated by a single mother of two children (paper 3):

> My GP is very active participating in collaborative meetings. Then she gets more information about my situation—more than if she just sees me at her office. In those meetings, we talk about almost everything. It is of great importance that the GP participate. Otherwise, she would have had no insight. I am not that often at the GP's office.

Some GPs emphasized that collaborating with health visitors in preventive child health networks provided them with knowledge about local societies and the families' daily lives. House calls could also give important information and generally made it easier to become aware of the children's situation. Most importantly, however, continuity of care gave the GP gradual insights into the families and their social situations. Some GPs did not participate in multidisciplinary meetings, but those who did experienced that they could also support the parents this way.

Building Competence

In the survey (paper 4), the participant GPs were asked about what would help them to ensure the support of these vulnerable families. In particular, younger GPs and GPs who were not specialists in general practice reported "more competence about children as next of kin." Some of the GPs wanted more training in talking to children about sensitive matters. Notably, many of them did not know about the 2010 law (15) that requires them to, given the parents' informed consent, ensure that children receive information and follow-up. The GPs called for, among other things, net-based courses, booklets, and overviews of the services for families in primary care and social services.

DISCUSSION

The parents and the GPs who participated in the four sub-studies generally accepted that the parents' health problems might have a negative impact on their children's current and future wellbeing, health, and psychosocial adaptation. Despite this, both groups were ambivalent about addressing the children's situations during encounters in doctors' offices, and the topic was often omitted. This analysis suggests recommendations for how GPs can overcome these barriers: namely (1) recognize the parents' good intentions, (2) ask directly about their children, (3) learn more about children as next of kin, (4) learn more about how to talk to children, (5) build a trusting alliance with the parents and rely on it, and (6) participate in multidisciplinary networks concerning these families. Some of these elements are previously described from general practice and specialist health services (10, 29, 30, 42). Our research, however, points out opportunities to incorporate these elements into a clinical context in general practice.

Many authors recommend using a family-focused approach in general practice to reach children in need (26, 29). Based on a qualitative study of GPs in Denmark, Holge-Hazelton and Tulinius (19) defined "cases with a child in need" in general practice as "a case that directly or indirectly involves problems with a specific child, an as-yet unborn child, or one or both parents of a family, currently or potentially threatening the wellbeing of the family and the child." They found that in general practice, most cases with a child in need are found during indirect consultations; indirect in the sense that the child is not present, or the primary cause of the consultation itself may not be the child. This is in accordance with the aim of our study: to indirectly support children as next of kin during consultations with their parents. However, the results from the present analyses suggest that a family focus is a necessary, but not sufficient prerequisite. In addition, the GP usually has to prompt parents to bring up the children's situations and overcome the ambivalent feelings both in themselves and the parents.

Our results showed that the GPs were often unsure whether the parent tolerated their inquiry into family matters. Their concern was that some parents might think this topic was not a GP's business, be offended, leave the office and—in the worst case—leave their patient registry. Broholm-Jorgensen et al. (43) recently published a study on GPs' strategies for retaining patients during preventive health checks. Opportunistic health checks during consultations for other topics might be provocative for patients. The researchers found that respect was a core element for the GP to succeed in a professional urge to promote better health practices in smokers, overweight persons, etc. They identified two complementary fields of respect: the GP's respect for the patient's autonomy and the patient's respect for the GP's professional authority. If the GP balanced the emphasis on his or her authority with their respect for the patient's autonomy, there was an increased chance that the patient would come back for another consultation. During such consultations, there would ideally be an exchange of mutual respect. Because GPs have ethical and legal obligations to address children of parents with illnesses and substance abuse during consultations with these parents, it is crucial—given the result from the aforementioned study—that GPs treat the topic of children with respect. Trust and recognition might be useful concepts to apply here as well.

The parents wanted information and advice from a trusted helper from whom they could accept direct speech and alternative viewpoints. This lead into the question of how the GP can evaluate the strength and quality of the patient's trust. Skirbekk et al. (36), having studied GPs' consultations, concluded that doctor-patient trust is mostly indirectly, and rarely openly, addressed by doctor and patient. The patient gives the doctor a "mandate of trust" in which the patient sets the conditions for what is an accepted topic during the consultation. This mandate can be limited or broad, and it may change during the consultation. The GP might negotiate the mandate of trust by taking the initiative to talk openly about the patient–doctor relationship. To what extent does the patient trust the GP? What are his or her doubts and mistrust if the topic of the children's situation is addressed? An open talk might disclose that the patient already indirectly has given the GP an open mandate, or that the patient does not have enough trust in the doctor to reveal problems at home that might affect the children. Then these concerns might become a topic in the consultation.

As the study of Broholm-Jorgensen et al. demonstrated (43), recognition may be a crucial aspect of the exchange of mutual respect. When asked about daily family lives, most parents in the present study first emphasized how well they managed their ordinary routines. Later, some revealed difficulties, such as worries about their children and needing support for themselves and their children. As described in the section "Theoretical assumptions," an attitude of recognition allows for the acceptance of another person's experiences and opinions. This attitude has been shown to be beneficial to a doctor–patient relationship in which the patient may gradually accept the doctor's viewpoints. For example, after the parent has told the GP about the efforts that he or she puts into maintaining as ordinary a life as possible for the children and the GP has verbally recognized this efforts, the parent may respond and give the GP trust in return and respect the GPs authority and advice about the children's need for support. However, the GP is responsible for laying the groundwork for this process to develop.

If the GPs manage to overcome the mutual ambivalence to address the family situation during consultations, this might benefit not only the children but also the parents with impairments. In a Dutch interview study of parents with mental health and substance abuse disorders (44), the parents stated that parenthood and the demands of parenting gave meaning and structure to their lives, and thereby provided them with strength. Therefore, if the GPs come in a position to support and coach parents by taking the parents' experiences and goals as a starting point, this will be of help for both children and parents. In the parental interviews (Paper 3), we learned how important their identity as responsible parents was, but also their need for emotional and practical support.

The GPs wanted to build more competence in the topic of children as next of kin, and stated that this could raise their awareness and ensure adequate support for the children. However, the topic is inconsistently referred to in the medical education curriculum and continuing education for specialists in general practice. Therefore, medical schools, governmental health authorities, and the Norwegian Medical Association must take measures to prevent transgenerational transference of psychosocial problems. For example, child-focused and family-focused content should be strengthened in the training of medical students as well as in the continuing education for GPs, including ways to overcome barriers in raising potentially confrontational issues about children's welfare during consultations.

Strengths and Limitations

To our knowledge, the research project Burdened Children as Next of Kin and the General Practitioner is one of very few focusing on the care of these children in general practice. Because GPs are central to the primary health care of the parents in the target groups and their children, our project may act as a basis for clinical work and further research. It is a strength of the project that it combines experiences from all three relevant informant groups: children, parents, and GPs.

The empirical material for this analysis was a text composed of the result sections of the four published articles and not the original raw data from the four projects. This may constitute a limitation regarding richness. However, the aim of the present secondary analysis was to gain further knowledge about the consultation situation, where the main experiences of the actors were juxtaposed and abstracted into salient themes. This bird's eye view of the situation was possible only by looking at the main experiences after they had been identified in the previous sub-studies. That said, there were some limitations in the data collection methods used in the sub-studies. First, the parents were recruited through their GPs, and because of this it is possible that they had more positive experiences with their doctor than informants on average. We have little information from those who could reveal shortcomings in GPs' services, did not have a rapport with their GP, or had their health services covered by specialist services. Second, the material contains no direct information from "invisible" children because the adolescents were recruited from support groups. Some of them, however, told stories in retrospect about their daily lives before they were identified and helped. Third, the results section of paper 4 refers to 499 respondents to a survey sent to ~6,000 GPs. We can assume that the results then are based on answers from GPs who were more interested in the topic that the average GP (45).

Finally, some interviewer and interpreter biases may have occurred because the interviewers were GPs (FG) and child and adolescent psychiatrists (MH). How the participants presented themselves and their experiences might have been influenced by this fact (46). The GPs may have avoided telling stories about encounters where they felt that they failed and the adolescents and the parents generally avoided sharing bad experiences from encounters with GPs.

Overall, the material possibly contains less information about bad experiences of encounters with GPs where the children's life situations were addressed. We assume that there are more aspects concerning these encounters than our analysis has brought forward. Nevertheless, the suggestions we have provided for GPs to overcome mutual ambivalences during these encounters are valid and can be transferred to general practices in Norway and most likely to comparable GP and health care systems.

Implications and Advice for the GP (Memory box)

- Assume that parents are striving for and want the best for their children. Acknowledge parents' efforts to maintain ordinary daily lives for their children.
- Keep in mind that most of these parents want their children's situations to be addressed, but the parents must be prompted by a GP that they trust.
- Conduct critical evaluation of the doctor–patient relationships with parents. Undertake necessary efforts to obtain a working mandate of trust that ensures openness about the children's situations.
- Expand personal knowledge and skills on the topic, including the local psychosocial networks of families with problems, relevant support resources, and everyday challenges children as next of kin are facing.
- Give priority to and actively participate into collaborations with the other helpers for a specific family.
- Establish contact with support services. Provide children and parents with a list of possible support services for families with children as next of kin.

FURTHER RESEARCH

It is important to continue the work to develop evidence-based guidelines for GPs during encounters with parents with illnesses and/or substance abuse to ensure their children adequate information about their parent's impairments and follow-up if necessary. The following specific recommendations for research are:

1) A web-based survey with a representative sample of Norwegian GPs. The aim of the survey would be to assess (1) the distribution of views and attitudes and current practices related to what most Norwegian GPs consider to be good service to burdened children and their families in general practice, (2) how the expectations of the children and their parents (Paper 2 and 3) can be met, and (3) GPs evaluation of how the preliminary guidelines from the present sub-study can be applied in their practices.
2) A multicenter randomized controlled trial with GPs in Scandinavia. The intervention could be education on the topic of children as next of kin and clinical training in applying the preliminary guidelines from the present sub-study. The outcome measure would be if children of the GPs' patients are identified and offered follow-up. Are there differences between the intervention group and the control group? We plan to include centers in Sweden and Denmark to achieve a sample that is large enough to give statistically significant results. The context for general practice in Scandinavia is fairly equal.

ETHICAL APPROVAL

This study was carried out in accordance with recommendations of the Western Norway Regional Authority and theResearch Council of Norway. The empirical material in the present article stem from our previous four articles in the project. Two of the articles (10, 30) received approval from Regional Committee for Medical and Health Research Ethics, Western Norway (2012/2336-3). According to the Regional Committee for Medical and Health Research Ethics, the Act does not apply to the sub-studies published in the two other articles (31, 32) and the present article. All subjects gave a written informed consent in accordance with the Declaration of Helsinki.

AUTHOR CONTRIBUTIONS

MH headed the research group Children as Next of Kin and the General Practitioner and had formal responsibility in all stages of the present research process. FG and MH coded the material in the present article. FG and KvD followed the research process closely and commented during the work process. MH, FG, NA, TS-S, and GR worked together on the foundation of the project and had substantial contributions to the four published articles (10, 30–32). NA, TS-S, and GR commented on the last versions of the present article, and all the authors approved it.

FUNDING

The study was funded by the Western Regional Health Authority (911743) and the Research Council of Norway (213050/H10).

ACKNOWLEDGMENTS

We want to thank the adolescents, parents, and GPs for sharing their experiences with us in the focus groups, the individual interviews, and the survey.

REFERENCES

1. Manning V, Best DW, Faulkner N, Titherington E. New estimates of the number of children living with substance misusing parents: results from UK national household surveys. *BMC Public Health* (2009) 9:377. doi: 10.1186/1471-2458-9-377
2. Reupert AE, D JM, Kowalenko NM. Children whose parents have a mental illness: prevalence, need and treatment. *Med J Aust.* (2013) 199(3 Suppl.):7–9. doi: 10.5694/mja.11.11200
3. Barkmann C, Romer G, Watson M, Schulte-Markwort M. Parental physical illness as a risk for psychosocial maladjustment in children and adolescents: epidemiological findings from a national survey in Germany. *Psychosomatics* (2007) 48:476–81. doi: 10.1176/appi.psy.48.6.476
4. Gullbra F. (2017) *Children as Next of Kin and the General Practitioner. A Qualitative Study About the General Practitioner's Opportunity to Help*. Thesis, University of Bergen, Bergen.
5. Rutter M, Quinton D. Parental psychiatric disorder: effects on children. *Psychol Med.* (1984) 14:853–80.
6. Felitti VJ, Anda RF, Nordenberg D, Williamson DF, Spitz AM, Edwards V, et al. Relationship of childhood abuse and household dysfunction to many of the leading causes of death in adults. The Adverse Childhood Experiences (ACE) Study. *Am J Prev Med.* (1998) 14:245–58.
7. Ellis SJ, Wakefield CE, Antill G, Burns M, Patterson P. Supporting children facing a parent's cancer diagnosis: a systematic review of children's psychosocial needs and existing interventions. *Eur J Cancer Care* (2017) 26:e12432. doi: 10.1111/ecc.12432
8. Balsa AI, French MT. The impact of parental drinking on children's use of health care. *Subst Use Misuse* (2012) 47:450–60. doi: 10.3109/10826084.2011.648044
9. Bjorgvinsdottir K, Halldorsdottir S. Silent, invisible and unacknowledged: experiences of young caregivers of single parents diagnosed with multiple sclerosis. *Scand J Caring Sci.* (2014) 28:38–48. doi: 10.1111/scs.12030
10. Gullbra F, Smith-Sivertsen T, Graungaard AH, Rortveit G, Hafting M. How can the general practitioner support adolescent children of ill or substance-abusing parents? A qualitative study among adolescents. *Scand J Prim Health* (2016) 34:360–7. doi: 10.1080/02813432.2016.1253819
11. Rossow I, Felix L, Keating P, McCambridge J. Parental drinking and adverse outcomes in children: a scoping review of cohort studies. *Drug Alcohol Rev.* (2016) 35:397–405. doi: 10.1111/dar.12319
12. Trondsen MV. Living with a mentally ill parent: exploring adolescents' experiences and perspectives. *Qual Health Res.* (2012) 22:174–88. doi: 10.1177/1049732311420736
13. Werner A, Malterud K. Children of parents with alcohol problems performing normality: A qualitative interview study about unmet needs for professional support. *Int J Qual Stud Health Wellbeing* (2016) 11:30673. doi: 10.3402/qhw.v11.30673
14. UN. *Convention on the Rights of the Child* (1989). Available online at *https://treaties.un.org/Pages/ViewDetails.aspx?src=IND&mtdsg_no=IV-11&chapter$=$4&lang$=$en*
15. Norwegian Directorate of Health. *Barn som Pårørende (Children as Next of kin): Rundskriv til lov av 2.* Oslo (2010). Available online at: *https://helsedirektoratet.no/publikasjoner/barn-som-parorende*
16. The Swedish National Board of Health and Welfare. *Children as next of kin - legislation and organization in Sweden* (2010). Available online at *https://www.anhoriga.se/Global/BSA/Dokument/Rapporter_kunskaps%C3%B6versikter/infoblad%20barn%20som%20anh%C3%B6riga%20- %20lagar-eng.pdf*
17. Charles G, Stainton T, Marshall S. Young carers in Canada: an invisible population. *Relat Child Youth Pract.* (2008) 21:5–12.
18. Moore CW, Rauch PK, Baer L, Pirl WF, Muriel AC. Parenting changes in adults with cancer. *Cancer* (2015) 121:3551–7. doi: 10.1002/cncr.29525
19. Holge-Hazelton B, Tulinius C. Beyond the specific child. What is 'a child's case' in general practice? *Br J Gen Pract.* (2010) 60:e4–9. doi: 10.3399/bjgp10X482059
20. Calhoun S, Conner E, Miller M, Messina N. Improving the outcomes of children affected by parental substance abuse: a review of randomized controlled trials. *Subst Abuse Rehabil.* (2015) 6:15–24. doi: 10.2147/SAR.S46439
21. Siegenthaler E, Munder T, Egger M. Effect of preventive interventions in mentally ill parents on the mental health of the offspring: systematic review and meta-analysis. *J Am Acad Child Adolesc Psychiatry* (2012) 51:8–17.e8. doi: 10.1016/j.jaac.2011.10.018
22. van Doesum K, Hosman CMH. Prevention of emotional problems and psychiatric risks in children of parents with a mental illness in the Netherlands: II. Interventions. *Austr J Adv Ment Health* (2009) 8:264–76. doi: 10.5172/jamh.8.3.264
23. Thanhauser M, Lemmer G, de Girolamo G, Christiansen H. Do preventive interventions for children of mentally ill parents work? Results of a systematic review and meta-analysis. *Curr Opin Psychiatry* (2017) 30:283–99. doi: 10.1097/YCO.0000000000000342
24. Reupert A, Cuff, R Drost, L, Foster, K van Doesum, K.T.M., van Santvoort. F. Intervention programs for children whose parents have a mental illness: a review. *MJA Open* (2012) 1(Suppl. 1):10–22. doi: 10.5694/mjao11.11145
25. Potter R, Mars B, Eyre O, Legge S, Ford T, Sellers R, et al. Missed opportunities: mental disorder in children of parents with depression. *Br J Gen Pract.* (2012) 62:e487–93. doi: 10.3399/bjgp12X652355
26. Baulderstone MJ, Morgan BS, Fudge EA. Supporting families of parents with mental illness in general practice. *Med J Aust.* (2013) 199(3 Suppl.):S11–3. doi: 10.5694/mja11.11146
27. Hartley K, Phelan M. The needs of children of depressed mothers in primary care. *Fam Pract.* (2003) 20:390–2. doi: 10.1093/fampra/cmg409
28. Reupert A, Maybery D, Morgan B. The family-focused practice of primary care clinicians: a case of missed opportunities. *J Ment Health* (2015) 24:357–62. doi: 10.3109/09638237.2014.998803
29. Reupert A WC, Maybery D. How family orientated are primary care physicians? *J Clin Fam Stud.* (2016). 26:329–35. doi: 10.10077/s10826-016-0558-7
30. Gullbra F, Smith-Sivertsen T, Rortveit G, Anderssen N, Hafting M. Ill and substance-abusing parents: how can the general practitioner help their children? A qualitative study. *BMC Fam Pract.* (2016) 17:154. doi: 10.1186/s128875-016-0553-5
31. Gullbra F, Smith-Sivertsen T, Rortveit G, Anderssen N, Hafting M. To give the invisible child priority: children as next of kin in general practice. *Scand J Prim*

Health Care (2014) 32:17–23. doi: 10.3109/02813432.2014.874133

32. Hafting M, Anderssen, N Gullbra, F Rortveit, G Smtih-Sivertsen, T. Fastlegen i møte med barn som pårørende (The general practitioner meeting children as next of kin). *Tidsskrift Velferdsforsk.* (2018). 12:208–26. doi: 10.18261/issn.2464-3076-2018-03-02
33. Levenstein JH, McCracken EC, McWhinney IR, Stewart MA, Brown JB. The patient-centred clinical method. 1. A model for the doctor-patient interaction in family medicine. *Fam Pract* (1986) 3:24–30.
34. Fugelli P. [Trust]. *Tidsskr Nor Laegeforen* (2001) 121:3621–4.
35. Skirbekk H. (2008) *The Patient's Trust. Theoretical Analyses of Trust and a Qualitative Study in General Practice Consultations.* Thesis, University of Oslo, Oslo.
36. Skirbekk H, Middelthon AL, Hjortdahl P, Finset A. Mandates of trust in the doctor-patient relationship. *Qual Health Res.* (2011) 21:1182–90. doi: 10.1177/1049732311405685
37. Steihaug S, Gulbrandsen P, Werner A. Recognition can leave room for disagreement in the doctor-patient consultation. *Patient Educ Counsel.* (2012) 86:316–21. doi: 10.1016/j.pec.2011.06.011
38. Lind AB, Risoer MB, Nielsen K, Delmar C, Christensen MB, Lomborg K. Longing for existential recognition: a qualitative study of everyday concerns for people with somatoform disorders. *J Psychosom Res.* (2014) 76:99–104. doi: 10.1016/j.jpsychores.2013.11.005
39. Malterud K. Theory and interpretation in qualitative studies from general practice: why and how? *Scand J Public Health* (2016) 44:120–9. doi: 10.1177/1403494815621181
40. Braun V, Clarke, V. Using thematic analysis in psychology. *Qual Res Psychol.* (2006) 3:77–101. doi: 10.1191/147808887066pq063oa
41. Malterud K. Systematic text condensation: a strategy for qualitative analysis. *Scand J Public Health* (2012) 40:795–805. doi: 10.1177/14034948124 65030
42. Lauritzen C, Reedtz C, Van Doesum K, Martinussen M. Factors that may facilitate or hinder a family-focus in the treatment of parents with a mental illness. *J Child Fam Stud.* (2015) 24:864–71. doi: 10.1007/s10826-01 3-9895-y
43. Broholm-Jorgensen M, Guassora AD, Reventlow S, Dalton SO, Tjornhoj-Thomsen T. Balancing trust and power: a qualitative study of GPs perceptions and strategies for retaining patients in preventive health checks. *Scand J Prim Health Care* (2017) 35:89–97. doi: 10.1080/02813432.2017.12 88811
44. Van der Ende PC, van Busschbach JT, Nicholson J, Korevaar EL, van Weeghel J. Strategies for parenting by mothers and fathers with a mental illness. *J Psychiatr Ment Health Nurs.* (2016) 23:86–97. doi: 10.1111/jpm. 12283
45. Cunningham CT, Quan H, Hemmelgarn B, Noseworthy T, Beck CA, Dixon E, et al. Exploring physician specialist response rates to web-based surveys. *BMC Med Res Methodol.* (2015) 15:32. doi: 10.1186/s12874-015-0016-z
46. Coar L, Sim J. Interviewing one's peers: methodological issues in a study of health professionals. *Scand J Prim Health Care* (2006) 24:251–6. doi: 10.1080/02813430601008479

Permissions

All chapters in this book were first published by Frontiers; hereby published with permission under the Creative Commons Attribution License or equivalent. Every chapter published in this book has been scrutinized by our experts. Their significance has been extensively debated. The topics covered herein carry significant findings which will fuel the growth of the discipline. They may even be implemented as practical applications or may be referred to as a beginning point for another development.

The contributors of this book come from diverse backgrounds, making this book a truly international effort. This book will bring forth new frontiers with its revolutionizing research information and detailed analysis of the nascent developments around the world.

We would like to thank all the contributing authors for lending their expertise to make the book truly unique. They have played a crucial role in the development of this book. Without their invaluable contributions this book wouldn't have been possible. They have made vital efforts to compile up to date information on the varied aspects of this subject to make this book a valuable addition to the collection of many professionals and students.

This book was conceptualized with the vision of imparting up-to-date information and advanced data in this field. To ensure the same, a matchless editorial board was set up. Every individual on the board went through rigorous rounds of assessment to prove their worth. After which they invested a large part of their time researching and compiling the most relevant data for our readers.

The editorial board has been involved in producing this book since its inception. They have spent rigorous hours researching and exploring the diverse topics which have resulted in the successful publishing of this book. They have passed on their knowledge of decades through this book. To expedite this challenging task, the publisher supported the team at every step. A small team of assistant editors was also appointed to further simplify the editing procedure and attain best results for the readers.

Apart from the editorial board, the designing team has also invested a significant amount of their time in understanding the subject and creating the most relevant covers. They scrutinized every image to scout for the most suitable representation of the subject and create an appropriate cover for the book.

The publishing team has been an ardent support to the editorial, designing and production team. Their endless efforts to recruit the best for this project, has resulted in the accomplishment of this book. They are a veteran in the field of academics and their pool of knowledge is as vast as their experience in printing. Their expertise and guidance has proved useful at every step. Their uncompromising quality standards have made this book an exceptional effort. Their encouragement from time to time has been an inspiration for everyone.

The publisher and the editorial board hope that this book will prove to be a valuable piece of knowledge for researchers, students, practitioners and scholars across the globe.

List of Contributors

Marieke R. Potijk, Louisa M. Drost, Petra J. Havinga, Catharina A. Hartman and Robert A. Schoevers
University Center for Psychiatry, University Medical Center Groningen, Groningen, Netherlands

Joanne Riebschleger and Daniel L. Cavanaugh
School of Social Work MSU, Michigan State University, East Lansing, MI, United States

Shane Costello and Christine Grové
Faculty of Education - Monash, Monash University, Melbourne, VIC, Australia

Luca Steardo Jr., Vito Caivano, Gaia Sampogna, Arcangelo Di Cerbo, Giovanna Fico, Francesca Zinno, Valeria Del Vecchio, Vincenzo Giallonardo, Mario Luciano and Andrea Fiorillo
Department of Psychiatry, University of Campania Luigi Vanvitelli, Naples, Italy

Marco Torella
Department of Gynecology, University of Campania Luigi Vanvitelli, Naples, Italy

Sami Räsänen
Department of Psychiatry, Oulu University Hospital, Oulu, Finland

Mika Niemelä
Center for Life Course Health, Research, University of Oulu, Oulu, Finland
Department of Psychiatry, Oulu University Hospital, Oulu, Finland
Research Unit of Clinical Neurosciences, Department of Psychiatry, University of Oulu, Oulu, Finland

Helinä Hakko
Department of Psychiatry, Oulu University Hospital, Oulu, Finland
Research Unit of Clinical Neurosciences, Department of Psychiatry, University of Oulu, Oulu, Finland

Hannu Kallunki and Birkitta Ala-Aho
Joint Municipal Authority of Wellbeing in Raahe District, Raahe, Finland

Jaana Jokinen
Faculty of Social Sciences, University of Lapland, Rovaniemi, Finland

Tiina Ristikari
Adolescents and Families Unit, National Institute for Health and Welfare Children, Oulu, Finland

Tytti Solantaus
Finnish Association for Mental Health, Helsinki, Finland
Mental Health Unit, National Institute for Health and Welfare, Helsinki, Finland

Hanna Christiansen
Department of Clinical Child and Adolescent Psychology, Philipps University Marburg, Marburg, Germany

Annette Bauer
Personal Social Services Research Unit (PSSRU), London School of Economics and Political Science, London, United Kingdom

Batool Fatima
Human Development Programme, Aga Khan University, Karachi, Pakistan

Melinda Goodyear
School of Rural Health, Monash University, Melbourne, VIC, Australia

Ingunn Olea Lund
The Norwegian Institute of Public Health, Oslo, Norway

Ingrid Zechmeister-Koss
Ludwig Boltzmann Institute for Health Technology Assessment, Vienna, Austria

Jean Lillian Paul
Mental Health Research Program, The Village, Ludwig Boltzmann Gesellschaft, Innsbruck, Austria
Division of Psychiatry I, Department of Psychiatry, Psychotherapy and Psychosomatics, Medical University Innsbruck, Innsbruck, Austria

Adekeye Kolade and Holly Hope
Faculty of Biology, Medicine and Health, Centre for Women's Mental Health, Manchester Academic Health Science Centre, The University of Manchester, Manchester, United Kingdom

Penny Bee
Division of Nursing, Faculty of Biology, Medicine and Health, Manchester Academic Health Science Centre, School of Health Sciences, The University of Manchester, Manchester, United Kingdom

Judith Gellatly
Faculty of Biology, Medicine and Health, Centre for Women's Mental Health, Manchester Academic Health Science Centre, The University of Manchester, Manchester, United Kingdom
Division of Nursing, Faculty of Biology, Medicine and Health, Manchester Academic Health Science Centre, School of Health Sciences, The University of Manchester, Manchester, United Kingdom

Diane Hunter
NSPCC, London, United Kingdom

Lina Gega
Department of Health Sciences, Hull York Medical School, University of York, York, United Kingdom

Craig Callender
St. Nicholas Hospital, Northumberland Tyne and Wear NHS Foundation Trust, Newcastle upon Tyne, United Kingdom

Kathryn M. Abel
Faculty of Biology, Medicine and Health, Centre for Women's Mental Health, Manchester Academic Health Science Centre, The University of Manchester, Manchester, United Kingdom
Greater Manchester Mental Health NHS Foundation Trust, Manchester, United Kingdom

Charlotte Reedtz and Camilla Lauritzen
Regional Centre for Child and Adolescent Mental Health and Child Wellfare, Faculty of Health Sciences, UiT The Arctic University of Norway, Tromsø, Norway

Karin van Doesum
Clinical Psychology, Radboud University Nijmegen, Nijmegen, Netherlands
Impluz, Prevention Team Mental Health, Deventer, Netherlands
Regional Center of Child and Youth Mental Health and Child Welfare, Artic University of Tromsø, Tromsø, Norway

Giulia Signorini and Giovanni de Girolamo
Unit of Epidemiological and Evaluation Psychiatry, IRCCS Istituto Centro San Giovanni di Dio Fatebenefratelli, Brescia, Italy

Therese van Amelsvoort
Department of Psychiatry and Psychology, Maastricht University, Maastricht, Netherlands

Floor van Santvoort
Pluryn/Hoenderloogroep, Research & Development, Nijmegen, Nederlands

Allan H. Young
Department of Psychological Medicine, Institute of Psychiatry, Psychology and Neuroscience, King's College London and South London and Maudsley NHS Foundation Trust, London, United Kingdom

Philippe Conus
Service de Psychiatrie Générale, Dép. de Psychiatrie, Centre Hospitalier Universitaire Vaudois (CHUV), Lausanne, Switzerland

Richard Musil
Bipolar Disorders and Borderline Personality Disorders Unit, Clinic for Psychiatry and Psychotherapy, LMU Klinikum der Universität München, München, Germany

Thomas Schulze
Institute for Psychiatric Phenomics and Genomics (IPPG), Klinikum der Universität München, München, Germany

Michael Berk
IMPACT Strategic Research Centre, School of Medicine, Barwon Health, Deakin University, Melbourne, VIC, Australia
Orygen Youth Health Research Centre and the Centre of Youth Mental Health, The Florey Institute for Neuroscience and Mental Health and the Department of Psychiatry, University of Melbourne, Melbourne, VIC, Australia

Argyris Stringaris
Mood and Development Laboratory, Emotion and Development Branch, National Institute of Mental Health, National Institutes of Health, Bethesda, MD, United States

Geneviève Piché
Psychoeducation and Psychology Department, Université du Québec en Outaouais, Gatineau, QC, Canada

Torleif Ruud
Mental Health Services, Akershus University Hospital, Lørenskog, Norway
Institute of Clinical Medicine, University of Oslo, Oslo, Norway

Darryl Maybery
School of Rural Health, Monash University, Moe, VIC, Australia

Andrea Reupert
Faculty of Education, Monash University, Clayton, VIC, Australia

Bente Weimand
Mental Health Services, Akershus University Hospital, Lørenskog, Norway
Faculty of Health Sciences, OsloMet—Oslo Metropolitan University, Oslo, Norway

Kim Foster
School of Nursing, Midwifery and Paramedicine, Australian Catholic University, Sydney, NSW, Australia
NorthWestern Mental Health, Parkville, VIC, Australia

Anne Grant
School of Nursing and Midwifery, Queens University Belfast, Belfast, United Kingdom

Bjørg Eva Skogøy
Nordland Hospital Trust, Bodø, Norway Faculty of Health Sciences, UiT The Arctic University of Norway, Tromsø, Norway

Solveig O. Ose
Health Services Research, SINTEF, Trondheim, Norway

Corinna Reck
Department of Clinical Child and Adolescent Psychology, Faculty of Psychology, Ludwig-Maximilians-University München, Munich, Germany

Anna-Lena Zietlow
Center for Psychosocial Medicine, Institute of Medical Psychology, Heidelberg University Hospital, Heidelberg, Germany

Kathleen Otto
Department of Social Psychology, Business and Methods, Faculty of Psychology, Philipps University Marburg, Marburg, Germany

Ricarda Steinmayr and Linda Wirthwein
Department of Educational Psychology, Faculty of Education, Psychology and Sociology, Institute of Psychology, Technical University Dortmund, Dortmund, Germany

Sarah Weigelt
Department of Vision, Visual Impairment & Blindness, Faculty of Rehabilitation Science, Technical University Dortmund, Dortmund, Germany

Rudolf Stark
Department of Psychotherapy and Systems Neuroscience, Faculty of Psychology and Sports Science, Justus-Liebig-University Gießen, Gießen, Germany

Claudia Buntrock
Department of Clinical Psychology and Psychotherapy, Institute of Psychology, Friedrich-Alexander-University Erlangen-Nürnberg, Erlangen, Germany

Johannes Krisam, Christina Klose and Meinhard Kieser
Department of Medical Biometry, Institute of Medical Biometry and Informatics, Heidelberg University, Heidelberg, Germany

Christina Schwenck
Department of Special Needs Educational and Clinical Child and Adolescent Psychology, Faculty of Psychology and Sports Science, Justus-Liebig-University Gießen, Gießen, Germany

David D. Ebert
Department of Psychology, Chair for Clinical Psychology and Psychotherapy, Friedrich-Alexander University Erlangen-Nuremberg, Erlangen, Germany
Department of Clinical, Neuro- & Developmental Psychology, Vrije Universiteit Amsterdam, Amsterdam, Netherlands

Markus Stracke, Kristin Gilbert
Department of Clinical Child and Adolescent Psychology, Philipps University Marburg, Marburg, Germany

Meinhard Kieser, Christina Klose and Johannes Krisam
Institute of Medical Biometry and Informatics, University of Heidelberg, Heidelberg, Germany

Louise Arseneault, Eloise Crush and Helen L. Fisher
King's College London, Social, Genetic & Developmental Psychiatry Centre, Institute of Psychiatry, Psychology & Neuroscience, London, United Kingdom

Simon Riches
King's College London, Social, Genetic & Developmental Psychiatry Centre, Institute of Psychiatry, Psychology & Neuroscience, London, United Kingdom
South London & Maudsley NHS Foundation Trust, London, United Kingdom

Raha Bagher-Niakan and Manar Alsultan
King's College London, Department of Psychosis Studies, Institute of Psychiatry, Psychology & Neuroscience, London, United Kingdom

Ylva V. Stover, Janita L. Freili and Kamilla Rognmo
Institute of Psychology, Faculty of Health Sciences, UiT The Arctic University of Norway, Tromsø, Norway

Christine Heinisch, Sandra Gabler, Judith Fößel and Gottfried Spangler
Developmental and Educational Psychology, Institute of Psychology, Friedrich Alexander University Erlangen-Nürnberg, Erlangen, Germany

Mirijam-Griseldis Galeris
Developmental and Educational Psychology, Institute of Psychology, Friedrich-Alexander University Erlangen-Nürnberg, Erlangen, Germany
Department of Paediatric Psychiatry, Psychotherapy and Psychosomatics, Universitätsklinikum Leipzig, Leipzig, Germany

Susanne Simen
Klinik für Psychiatrie und Psychotherapie, Universitätsklinik der Paracelsus Medizinischen Privatuniversität, Klinikum Nürnberg Süd, Nürnberg, Germany

Juliane Junge-Hoffmeister
Klinik für Psychotherapie und Psychosomatik des Universitätsklinikums Carl Gustav Carus der Technischen Universität Dresden, Dresden, Germany

Kayoko Ichikawa
Department of Health Informatics, Kyoto University School of Public Health, Kyoto, Japan

Takeo Fujiwara
Department of Global Health Promotion, Tokyo Medical and Dental University, Tokyo, Japan

Ichiro Kawachi
Department of Global Health Promotion, Tokyo Medical and Dental University, Tokyo, Japan
Department of Social and Behavioral Sciences, Harvard T.H. Chan School of Public Health, Boston, MA, United States

Anne A. E. Thorup and Nicoline Hemager
The Lundbeck Foundation Intiative for Integrative Psychiatric Research (iPSYCH), Aarhus, Denmark
Research Unit, Child and Adolescent Mental Health Center, University of Copenhagen, Copenhagen, Denmark
Mental Health Center Copenhagen, Research Unit, University of Copenhagen, Copenhagen, Denmark

Birgitte K. Burton
The Lundbeck Foundation Intiative for Integrative Psychiatric Research (iPSYCH), Aarhus, Denmark
Research Unit, Child and Adolescent Mental Health Center, University of Copenhagen, Copenhagen, Denmark

Marianne Melau
Mental Health Center Copenhagen, Research Unit, University of Copenhagen, Copenhagen, Denmark

Anne Søndergaard, Maja Gregersen, Åsa Kremer Prøsch, Mette F. Krantz, Julie M. Brandt, Line Carmichael, Ditte V. Ellersgaard, Md Jamal Uddin, Jessica Ohland and Merete Nordentoft
The Lundbeck Foundation Intiative for Integrative Psychiatric Research (iPSYCH), Aarhus, Denmark
Mental Health Center Copenhagen, Research Unit, University of Copenhagen, Copenhagen, Denmark

Aja N. Greve, Anna K. Andreassen, Lotte Vedum, Christina B. Knudsen, Henriette Stadsgaard and Ole Mors
The Lundbeck Foundation Intiative for Integrative Psychiatric Research (iPSYCH), Aarhus, Denmark
Psychosis Research Unit, Aarhus University Hospital, Risskov, Denmark

Hartwig Roman Siebner
Danish Research Centre for Magnetic Resonance, Section 714, Hvidovre Hospital, University of Copenhagen, Copenhagen, Denmark

Ayna B. Nejad, Line K. Johnsen and Anna Hester Ver Loren van Themaat
Research Unit, Child and Adolescent Mental Health Center, University of Copenhagen, Copenhagen, Denmark
Danish Research Centre for Magnetic Resonance, Section 714, Hvidovre Hospital, University of Copenhagen, Copenhagen, Denmark

Jens Richardt M. Jepsen
The Lundbeck Foundation Intiative for Integrative Psychiatric Research (iPSYCH), Aarhus, Denmark
Research Unit, Child and Adolescent Mental Health Center, University of Copenhagen, Copenhagen, Denmark
Center for Neuropsychiatric Schizophrenia Research (CNSR) and Center for Clinical Intervention and Neuropsychiatric Schizophrenia Research, Mental Health Centre Glostrup, University of Copenhagen, Copenhagen, Denmark

Leif Østergaard
Center of Functionally Integrative Neuroscience, Aarhus University, Department of Neuroradiology, Aarhus University Hospital, Aarhus, Denmark

B. Sheeba, Shubhashree Venkatesh and J. Vindhya
Research Assistant, Indian Institute of Public Health Hyderabad, Public Health of Foundation of India, Bangalore, India

Anita Nath
Wellcome Trust DBT India Alliance, Intermediate Fellow in Clinical and Public Health, Indian Institute of Public Health Hyderabad, Public Health Foundation of India, Hyderabad, India

Chandra S. Metgud
Professor, Department of Community Medicine, Pt. Jawahar Lal Nehru Memorial Medical College, Belgavi, India

Murali Krishna and Gudlavalleti Venkata Satyanarayana Murthy
Consultant, FRAME, Mysore, India
Indian Institute of Public Health Hyderabad, Public Health Foundation of India, Hyderabad, India

Joanne Nicholson and Anne Valentine
Institute for Behavioral Health and Lurie Institute for Disability Policy, The Heller School for Social Policy and Management, Brandeis University, Waltham, MA, United States

Rochelle Helena Hine
Mental Health Services, South West Healthcare, Warrnambool, VIC, Australia

Darryl John Maybery and Melinda Jane Goodyear
Department of Rural Health, Monash University, Moe, VIC, Australia

Marit Hafting
Regional Center for Child and Youth Mental Health and Child Welfare, Uni Research Health, Bergen, Norway

Frøydis Gullbrå and Tone Smith-Sivertsen
Research Unit for General Practice, Uni Research Health, Bergen, Norway

Norman Anderssen
Research Unit for General Practice, Uni Research Health, Bergen, Norway
Department of Psychosocial Science, University of Bergen, Bergen, Norway

Guri Rørtveit
Research Unit for General Practice, Uni Research Health, Bergen, Norway
Research Group for General Practice, Department of Global Public Health and Primary Care, University of Bergen, Bergen, Norway

Index

A

Affective Responsiveness, 24

Antenatal Care, 182, 188-189

Anxiety Disorders, 1-2, 4-8, 19, 28-29, 47, 73-74, 76-78, 81-82, 85-87, 91, 130, 145, 152, 154-157

Assessment Form, 131-132

B

Baseline Assessment, 64, 166

Behavioral Problems, 18, 28, 50, 61-62, 79, 130, 158-159, 162

Best Treatment Option, 20-21, 24

Binary Logistic Regression, 115, 132, 139

C

Changed Clinical Practice, 232, 242

Child Protection Agencies, 71, 74, 79, 82-83

Child Protection Services, 31-34, 72-73, 79, 83, 138, 142, 217

Child Wellbeing, 1, 3, 6-8, 62, 66-67

Clinical Global Impression, 20, 24-25

Cluster Randomization, 63-64

Collective Impact, 31-32, 34

Constructivist Grounded Theory, 200, 202

Coping Strategies, 10, 15, 20, 22, 26-27, 29, 56, 118, 130

Cultural Sensitivity, 191, 196, 198

D

Defining Self, 200, 203

Depressive Disorder, 28-30, 59, 96, 119, 132, 136, 141, 157, 179

Diagnosis Severity, 134-136

Diagnostic Interview Schedule, 113

Diverse Vulnerabilities, 191-192

Domestic Violence, 160-162, 165, 182-187, 190

E

Electronic Patient Journals, 61, 129, 131, 140-141

F

Family Adversity, 31-32, 141

Family Assessment Form, 131-132

Family Burden, 20, 29

Family Composition, 132, 134

Family Coping Questionnaire, 20, 24-25

Family-focused Approach, 1-2, 4-7, 9, 83, 198, 219

Family-focused Care, 5-7, 191, 193

G

Global Assessment Of Functioning, 20, 24

H

Hierarchical Logistic Regression, 132, 135

I

Infographic Film, 5

M

Marital Status, 25-26, 73-76, 78, 80-81, 131-132

Maternal Psychosis, 111-113, 115-116

Mental Health Literacy, 10-15, 17-19, 21, 37, 41, 49, 51-52, 57, 61, 66, 130

Mental Health Professionals, 14, 23, 26-27, 141

Mental Health Service, 40, 46, 71-73, 77, 79, 83, 202, 204

Mental Health Workers, 65, 140, 196

Mental Illness, 1-2, 4-19, 21, 36-40, 42, 45-47, 49-52, 54, 58-61, 66, 68-73, 76-79, 81-89, 94-95, 97-100, 102, 107-109, 119, 121-134, 136, 138-144, 147, 166-169, 173, 178-179, 181, 183, 186, 188, 191-192, 194-203, 205-213, 215, 221

Mentally Ill Fathers, 133, 135, 138-139

Mentally Ill Mothers, 9, 133, 135, 139, 144-147, 149, 151, 153

Minor Children, 2, 10, 19, 61, 63, 68, 71-74, 77, 79, 82, 129, 131, 138, 195

Mobile Teams, 73

Motherhood, 83, 144, 200, 204-205, 210-211

Mothering Identity, 202-203, 205, 208-209

Multivariate Logistic Regression, 111, 115, 185

O

Offspring Development, 183

P

Parent Peer Specialists, 192, 196-197

Parent's Treatment, 130, 132, 134-136

Parental Mental Disorder, 19, 50, 63, 66, 231

Parental Mental Illness, 11-12, 18-19, 47, 49-51, 58-60, 68, 70-72, 79, 83-84, 86, 89, 94-95, 98, 109, 127, 131, 141, 143, 168, 191, 199, 210

Parenting, 1-11, 18, 38, 40, 50, 53, 59-62, 66, 68-70, 72, 77, 83-85, 87-89, 92-93, 95-102, 104, 107, 109-110, 114, 118-119, 130, 136, 138-139, 141-142, 144-147, 151-152, 154-157, 169, 173, 178, 181, 190, 194-197, 221

Parenting Phase, 205

Pattern Of Care Schedule, 20, 23, 25
Peer Supports, 191-199
Perinatal Depression, 20-22, 25, 27-29, 189
Personal Identity, 201, 203, 205-208
Personal Recovery, 200, 202-203, 210-211
Pharmacotherapy, 63, 109, 240
Physiologic Measurements, 187-188
Positive Attitudes, 107
Postnatal Depression, 20, 22, 24-25, 28-29, 149, 151, 182-183, 188-190, 204
Postpartum Depression, 20, 28-30, 38, 144, 146, 148, 151-152, 154-155, 157, 189-190, 205
Prevalence Of Outpatients, 72-74, 76-77, 79, 81
Preventive Interventions, 1-2, 19, 34, 38, 47, 59, 62-63, 69, 73, 84, 88-89, 94, 98-99, 109-110, 112, 120, 126, 129, 178, 221
Psychiatric Disorders, 83, 112, 119-121, 131, 136, 140, 143-144, 146-148, 151-153, 155, 179, 181
Psychoactive Substance, 134-135, 137
Psychoeducation, 1-8, 10, 12, 19, 21-22, 27, 29-30, 61, 100, 147
Psychoeducation Meetings, 4, 6-8
Psychological Counseling, 21, 23-24
Psychological Problems, 97-98, 137
Psychometric Properties, 10, 12, 15, 17, 66, 103, 160, 180
Psychotic Disorders, 27, 73, 112, 119, 167
Psychotic Phenomena, 111-113, 115-118

S

Serious Mental Illnesses, 192, 211
Sexual Violence, 184, 186-188
Social Networking Sites, 121-123, 125-127
Social Support, 11-13, 21, 28, 37, 41, 44-45, 59, 62-63, 66, 72-73, 77, 79, 85, 91-92, 102, 111-112, 114-118, 120, 130, 144, 147, 154, 157, 182-183, 185-190, 210
Socioeconomic Status, 21, 27, 112-113, 116-117, 125, 128, 154, 168-169, 178
Strengths-based Approach, 18, 127, 192
Substance Abuse Disorder, 11, 121, 126
Supportive Relationship, 206

T

Targeted Training, 5, 197
Treatment Sessions, 5, 104

W

Women's Personal Identity, 205, 207

Y

Youth At Risk, 17, 121
Youth Education And Support, 10, 13-15

www.ingramcontent.com/pod-product-compliance
Lightning Source LLC
LaVergne TN
LVHW082206200926
848484LV00008B/2217
* 9 7 9 8 8 8 7 4 0 2 6 1 1 *